Total Ankle Replacement

Beat Hintermann • Roxa Ruiz

Total Ankle Replacement

A Practical Guide to Surgical Management

Springer

Beat Hintermann
Center of Excellence for Foot and Ankle
Kantonsspital Baselland
Liestal, Switzerland

Roxa Ruiz
Center of Excellence for Foot and Ankle
Kantonsspital Baselland
Liestal, Switzerland

ISBN 978-3-031-56809-1 ISBN 978-3-031-56810-7 (eBook)
https://doi.org/10.1007/978-3-031-56810-7

This Springer imprint is published by the registered company Springer Nature Switzerland AG
The registered company address is: Gewerbestrasse 11, 6330 Cham, Switzerland

To Esteban, Mathias, Sabrina, and Valeria

Foreword

For a quarter of a century, I have watched a remarkable group of talented surgeons assembled in the picturesque enclave of Liestal, Switzerland, educate orthopaedic surgeons worldwide about the use of total ankle replacement to treat painful end-stage ankle arthritis. This undertaking began at a time when the very idea of ankle replacement was dismissed by most surgeons. The odyssey embarked upon by these authors has paved the way for other surgeons globally to restore mobility and function by replacing arthritic ankles.

Now, their highly influential body of work—and the deep thinking underpinning it—has been distilled into this exceptionally educational and exquisitely illustrated book. As readers will see from opening sections integrating the subtleties of anatomy with the mechanics of load transfer to the last sections showing the future challenges facing our field, the level of thoughtfulness and understanding of total ankle replacement is unparalleled.

In the present day, total ankle replacement surgery is recognized as being able to transform the lives of many patients suffering from debilitating ankle pain and dysfunction. It is a procedure that demands a nuanced understanding of lower limb anatomy and biomechanics, meticulous surgical execution, appraisal of the benefits and potential pitfalls of technological innovation, and compassionate patient care. This book, fastidiously curated by true experts in the field, captures this essence brilliantly.

What distinguishes this book is its comprehensive and detailed approach to the subject. The authors have skilfully demystified a complex topic, rendering it accessible to a broad readership without compromising on the depth of information. Everyone—from novice foot and ankle practitioners to seasoned practitioners—will improve their skills with this book. Chapters delve deep into the intricacies of patient selection, surgical planning, implant options, considerations for secondary surgeries, and rehabilitation strategies. The inclusion of numerous real-life case studies including detailed illustrations, standard and advanced imaging, surgical photographs, and step-by-step decision-making guides further enhances and elevates the educational value of this book.

Congratulations to the authors for distilling years of experience into this illuminating volume. May it serve as a compass for orthopaedic surgeons navigating the ever-expanding landscape of total ankle replacement, ultimately contributing to the enhanced well-being of those in our care.

Charles Saltzman
University of Utah
Salt Lake City, UT, USA

Preface

With the discouraging results from first-generation prostheses, Hamblen's answer in his editorial "Can the ankle be replaced?" (J Bone Joint Surg Br 1985, 67:689–690) was a clear no. This statement was followed by our teachers in orthopedics when we started our orthopedic career over a quarter of a century ago. The main focus of treatment of end-stage ankle osteoarthritis was how to get the ankle reliably fused, but not on patient-related outcomes. Inspired by our patients seeking solutions other than a fusion to preserve the ankle range of motion, allowing them to continue a much healthier and more active lifestyle, we were attracted by the renewed interest in total ankle arthroplasty in the 1990s. It was then our privilege to be a part of the evolution of total ankle arthroplasty.

This book is thus written as a monograph, characterized by its uniform approach through all 18 main chapters. It not only intends to be an update on the morphological and mechanical changes of the osteoarthritic ankle and the associated pathologies but also provides an up-to-date overview of the available treatment techniques in the form of an operative manual based on the lifelong experience of both authors.

It is based on lifelong meticulous documentation of cases, which is an additional workload for every surgeon but mandatory to recognize, understand, and get insight into many underlying processes that may affect patient outcomes. To be able to assess the outcome many years after surgical treatment and to be able to compare the outcome with the initial situation has the unique potential to analyze the effectiveness of selected treatment critically and, additionally, to understand failures.

We are grateful to several people for the opportunity to complete this book, starting with the staff members, co-workers, and residents who have accompanied us over the years. We especially thank and acknowledge the scientific team for building up the database. And finally, we thank all our patients; they are the ones who continuously inspire us to develop and evaluate new techniques to make things better.

Teaching and sharing the experience with others may be one of our highest privileges as surgeons. The effort invested in preparing this book has been immense; however, the learning process has been the most rewarding experience. Working together as a team on holidays, weekends, and nights was a privilege. If *Total Ankle Replacement* offers useful information to our colleagues and provides a new platform of knowledge from which others can advance and evolve further treatment of the osteoarthritic ankle and its associated pathologies, we will have reached our goal.

Liestal, Switzerland — Beat Hintermann
Liestal, Switzerland — Roxa Ruiz

Contents

About the Authors

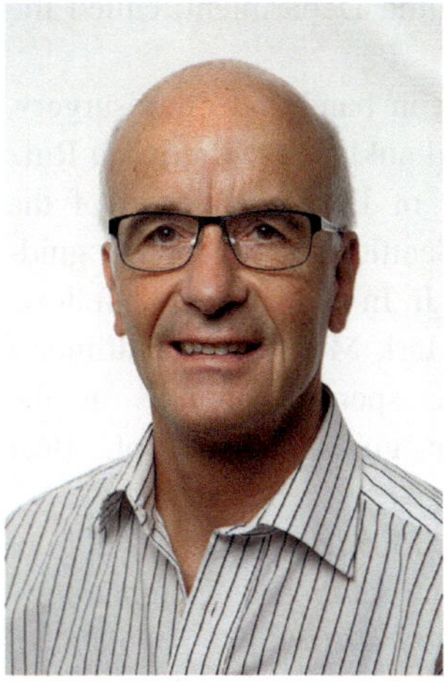

Beat Hintermann born in 1956, was trained in Orthopedic Surgery and Traumatology at the Hospitals of Neuchâtel, St. Gallen, Davos, and then at the Orthopedic Department of the University of Basel. After finishing his residency program, he completed a research fellowship in Biomechanics at the University of Calgary/Canada (Benno Nigg, 1991–1992) and two clinical traveling fellowships to Asia and the USA/United Kingdom, respectively. As an Associate Professor at the University of Basel, he was in charge of the Orthopaedic Trauma Unit at the University Hospital of Basel from 1994 to 2006. From 2006 to 2019, he has been the Chair of the Orthopaedic Department at the teaching hospital in Liestal. For over 25 years, his main orthopedic interest has been in the ankle and hindfoot. In 2019, he founded, together with Dr. Roxa Ruiz, the Center of Excellence for Foot and Ankle in Liestal, which he has chaired since. During his tenure, new and innovative techniques and procedures have been introduced, such as total ankle replacement, correcting osteotomies, arthrodeses of the hindfoot complex, ankle arthroscopy, and stabilizing procedures.

Besides having published over 250 peer-reviewed articles in Orthopedic Surgery, particularly related to ankle osteoarthritis, total ankle replacement, foot and ankle trauma, ankle arthroscopy, and ankle instability, he is the author of six medical textbooks related to reconstructive surgery of the ankle and hindfoot complex. He has received several awards for his clinical and biomechanical research.

Beat Hintermann was the main conceptor of the H3 ankle (Hintermann Series, former Hintegra), which is, after 24 years of clinical use, the best-documented three-component prosthesis on the market. The US FDA approved it by June 4, 2019. Together with Dr. Roxa Ruiz, he also developed the H2 ankle, which the US FDA approved. Currently, he is developing new concepts for revision arthroplasty of the ankle.

Over the last decade, he has put tremendous efforts into teaching orthopedic surgeons and those to-be around the world and at his clinic, which was honored by several national Foot and Ankle societies and institutions. In 2017, he was appointed as a Visiting Professor at the Ruijin University of Shanghai, China. He is regularly a faculty member of international Foot and Ankle meetings and organizer of Practical Instructional courses in Switzerland and abroad.

Beat Hintermann is married, has two children, and lives in Liestal, Switzerland. Besides running, skiing, and mountaineering, he enjoys traveling, gardening and photography.

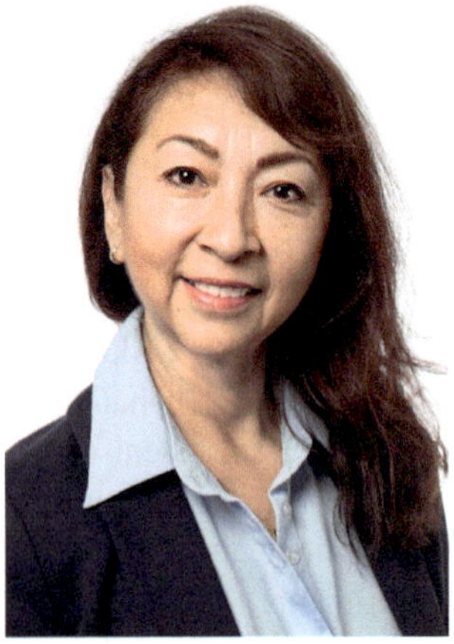

Roxa Ruiz born in 1965, finished medical school in 1992 in Lima (Peru). After that, she underwent an educational program in orthopedic trauma in Peru that also included services in the emergency departments of medical units in Lima. In 1998, she entered the Central Military Hospital of Lima as a senior resident. From 2001 onwards, she was working as a senior attending and afterwards also as the head of one of the two units of the Orthopedic Trauma Department, called the "War Service."

After having received training in hand and microsurgery, her main interest was the foot and ankle. In 2003, Roxa Ruiz did a fellowship at the Institute of Foot and Ankle of the Harborview Medical Center in Seattle/USA under the guidance of Prof. Sigvard Ted Hansen Jr. In 2008, she did a fellowship under the guidance of Dr. Mark Myerson in Baltimore/USA. Thereafter, in 2011, she spent 3 months at the Kantonsspital Liestal under the guidance of Prof. Beat Hintermann.

As a pioneer in her country, she founded the chapter of Foot and Ankle in the Peruvian Orthopaedic and Traumatology Society, for which she also served as the first presidentad. Besides other innovative techniques, she introduced total ankle replacement surgery in the country. In 2014, she got honored by being incorporated as a guest Professor in the Post Grade Unit of the Mayor University of San Marcos in Lima, Peru. Additionally, she served as an International AO Faculty in many courses, including some in Davos. Since 2016, after having been working first as a foot and ankle surgeon at the Orthopedic Clinic, she took over the position of a Medical Director of the Center of Excellence for Foot and Ankle at the Kantonsspital Baselland in Liestal, Switzerland.

Roxa Ruiz is the author of over 25 peer-reviewed articles in Orthopedic Surgery, particularly related to ankle osteoarthritis, total ankle replacement, foot and ankle trauma, and ankle instability. In 2021, she shared her vast experience in reconstructive surgery in the textbook *Foot and Ankle Instability* that she co-authored with Beat Hintermann.

Over the last years, she put tremendous efforts into teaching activities around the entire world, and she is regularly a faculty member at International Foot and Ankle meetings. She is the author of numerous scientific papers, book chapters, and co-conceptor of the H2 ankle prosthesis (Hintermann Series). Currently, she chairs the project of an innovative new concept for revision arthroplasty of the talus.

Roxa Ruiz is married, has two children and lives in Liestal, Switzerland. Besides skiing, swimming and hiking, she enjoys cooking and gardening.

Part I

General Considerations

Introduction

1

Osteoarthritis of the ankle continues to be a significant problem for patients, and its prevalence, at least post-traumatic osteoarthritis, appears to be increasing. It causes joint deformity, disability, and loss of income, affects patients' quality of life, and affects a higher percentage and younger age group than patients affected by hip or knee arthritis. Active lifestyles and the growing health consciousness of society with solid expectations have challenged foot and ankle surgeons to develop methods of treatment that improve affected ankle joint functioning.

In an era of joint replacement surgery, ankle procedures still need to achieve what has been accomplished with other joints. To some extent, an example that typifies the "ankle replacement experience" to date is that of British orthopedic surgeon John Charnley, who, frustrated by the failure of his compression arthrodesis, turned to hip arthroplasty and successfully pioneered procedures in that specialty. Decades after Charnley's failed efforts, ankle arthrodesis is still a commonly used procedure for the painful arthritic ankle. Although unilateral ankle arthrodesis may result in acceptable function (provided that the subtalar and midtarsal joints are normal and provide a compensatory mechanism), the disadvantages are significant in the long term. Besides a not negligible non-union rate, subsequent reoperations, appearance and progression of subtalar and midtarsal arthrosis, incorrect alignment of the foot to the leg, and gait disorder are the main limitations of ankle fusions.

The introduction of total ankle arthroplasty aimed to obtain a painless joint while maintaining its motor function, improving gait, and preserving function in adjacent joints. With continuous progress and improvement, ankle replacement surgery is receiving more and more recognition. The improvement is functional and is mainly perceived as beneficial to the patient from health perspectives' general, physical, psychological, emotional, and social quality. Though the range of motion achieved after the replacement surgery is not that of the original joint, the patients are generally delighted to have some motion left that allows them a more normal life. Every smile and gratitude from patients coming back all the years for control make our effort to improve treatment worthwhile. Reflecting that we could be in the place of one of them once in the future, we are convinced that making the same decision for the opportunity to preserve some movement would be the right choice. Let us take responsibility for counseling and treating our patients in the best way to meet their expectations and give them back as much normality as possible. As proven with the progress in the last years, total ankle arthroplasty has become a reliable and valuable option for treating the end-stage osteoarthritic ankle.

However, achieving effectiveness with total ankle replacement surgery requires a thorough understanding of the biomechanics and function of the ankle and the undergoing changes with the osteoarthritic process. It is mandatory to develop adequate surgical techniques and prosthetic implants that preserve the individual's original anatomy as much as possible, maintaining the bone stock and stabilizing structures. There is also a need for solutions should the treatment fail, and revision surgery may become necessary.

More complications than the hip and the knee still plague the ankle replacement surgery. The main reason may be the more complex structure of the ankle, which is composed of three bones, of which small areas are supposed to receive the component and to resist the forces created between the body and the ground. Moreover, most osteoarthritic ankles are associated with deformities and instability, making ankle replacement surgery a part of foot and ankle reconstruction. We all who deal with total ankle arthroplasty are faced with complications. Only a surgeon who does not perform surgeries has no complications. The goal is thus not to present an exhaustive list of solutions or rigid thinking but to provide a thoughtful overview and suggestions for itemizing the problems inherent in total ankle arthroplasty and management of associated problems while minimizing potential complications and pitfalls in this complex surgery.

Altogether, the procedure of total ankle arthroplasty can result in a substantial number of secondary procedures that may be named "revisions," "reoperations," or "additional procedures." The question to debate remains whether the

B. Hintermann, R. Ruiz, *Total Ankle Replacement*, https://doi.org/10.1007/978-3-031-56810-7_1

removal or exchange of one or more of the metallic components or exchange of the polyethylene meniscus in case of wear or fracture is a revision and thus should be considered a complication. We remember the farmer in whom we did a bilateral total ankle arthroplasty for hemochromatosis-caused osteoarthritis 17 years ago, at the age of 52 years. He came from far away because he was recommended for bilateral fusion surgery and was counseled to sell his farm first. The replacement surgery enabled him to keep his farm. He was worried about calling us for fear of bothering us after he felt an acute popping and pain in one of his replaced ankles caused by a polyethylene fracture. When presenting in the consultation, he first said with tears in his eyes, "Thank you, thank you for keeping me alive." After replacing the polyethylene insert, he could return to his farm and pursue his work 6 weeks later, happy that we could solve the problem and happiest that he could still assist his son on the family farm and enjoy the farmer's life. This case will appear as a complication in our statistics. However, is a worn-out, fractured polyethylene insert that can be exchanged after 17 years a complication?

We have had the privilege of treating more than 2200 patients with total ankle arthroplasty in the last 25 years. Not only did we go through a learning curve, but we also took advantage of improved techniques and designs and learned from our failures. We are thus aware that no surgeon considering starting or has just started with total ankle arthroplasty can accomplish the need for a successful ankle replacement in a more complex condition. However, is it fair to deny a patient this option because we have yet to embark on a learning curve? What hurts us more than to feel the sadness of a dissatisfied patient with a fused ankle because the surgeon could not perform a total ankle arthroplasty, thus having done a fusion?

Finally, the best treatment results from thoroughly understanding the pathology, knowing the patient's expectations, and being aware of the availability of various surgical and nonsurgical techniques. Knowing their possibilities and limitations is mandatory for success when considering surgical treatment. The main focus of this book is thus to give step-by-step instructions in the form of an operational manual based on the authors' life-long experience.

2 Anatomic and Biomechanical Characteristics of the Ankle Joint

The ankle joint forms a functional unit with the subtalar joint that is fundamental for plantigrade bipedal ambulation. The intact ankle efficiently translates the compressive, shear, rotatory, and ground reaction forces encountered when weight-bearing and during the different phases of the gait cycle. A large articular contact area provides inherent stability under static load, and the ligaments and tendons provide dynamic stability through balanced muscular forces. The effectiveness of the ankle can be inferred from its relative resistance to primary degenerative joint disease. Cartilage and ligament injury or changes in alignment caused by trauma or inflammatory disease may result in articular degeneration.

In recent decades, total ankle arthroplasty has become a viable alternative to fusion in treating end-stage degenerative diseases. To achieve successful results, however, proponents of total ankle arthroplasty must consider the biomechanical properties of this unique and complex joint. This chapter will elucidate the anatomic and biomechanical characteristics of the ankle joint from the perspective of total ankle arthroplasty.

2.1 Anatomic Considerations

The ankle joint is a highly congruent and dynamic joint consisting of three bones, collateral and syndesmotic ligaments, and surrounding tendons and muscles (Fig. 2.1). The talar body is held within a mortise formed by the distal tibia and fibula and is bound by strong ligaments. It articulates superiorly with the tibial plafond, on the medial side with the medial malleolus, and on the lateral side with the lateral malleolus. The facets of the medial and lateral malleoli are parallel to the corresponding facets of the talus [1].

Congruency of the corresponding malleolar and talar facets is provided throughout the entire range of motion [1]. Both the medial tibiotalar and talofibular contact areas

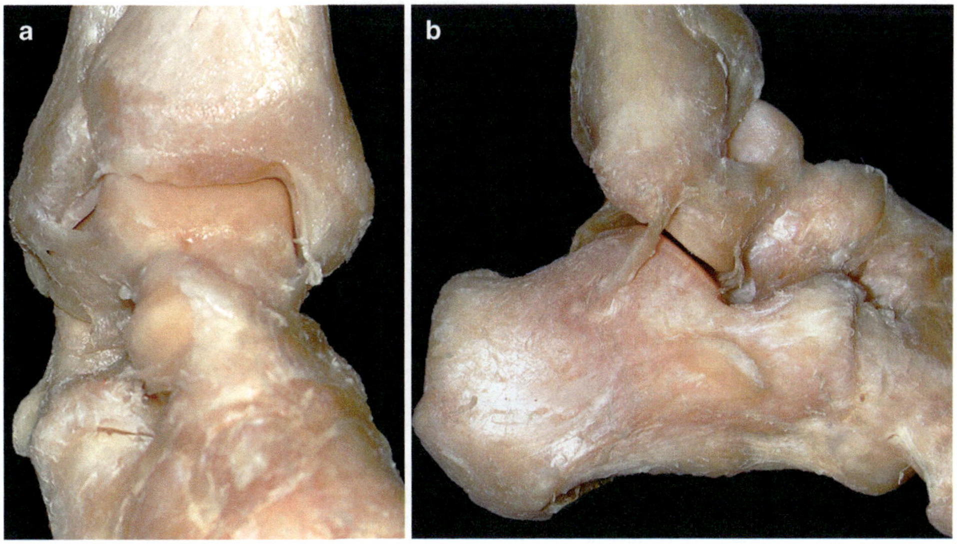

Fig. 2.1 Anatomy of the talocrural joint. The ankle is highly congruent with close joint contacts. Each ligament has a well-defined isometric position to the joint, and some ligaments cross neighboring joints. (**a**) Anterior view, (**b**) lateral view

B. Hintermann, R. Ruiz, *Total Ankle Replacement*, https://doi.org/10.1007/978-3-031-56810-7_2

increase significantly with weight-bearing and are at their maximum at 50% of stance [2].

2.1.1 Bony Configuration

The bony configuration varies markedly between the tibia, talus, and fibula.

2.1.1.1 Tibia

The distal tibial plafond and the medial malleolus form the articulating surface of the mortise. The ankle's most superior aspect articulates with the talus dome. In various studies, the anatomic morphology of the distal tibia in healthy joints was analyzed and will briefly be discussed here [1–5].

The distal tibial plafond has a concave shape with an average medial angle of 22° ± 4° (mean ± standard deviation) and shows a slight varus (Fig. 2.2) [1]. The angle measured in the coronal plane on the lateral side between the midline of the tibia and the surface of the plafond of the ankle (lateral distal tibial angle, LDTA) was found to be 96.7° ± 3.2°, ranging from 80° to 92° (Fig. 2.3) [3]. When taking the surgical axis of the tibia, determined by the tibial tuberosity and the middle of the tibial plafond, the LDTA was found to be 87.6° ± 3.1°, ranging from 80° to 96° [4]. Women showed approximately a 2.2° smaller tibiotalar angle than men. With increasing age, the LDTA diminished from 87.6° to 98.5° [5]. The same authors observed that the LDTA measured differs significantly when measurements were done on mortise ankle images (87.9° ± 2.2°) compared to whole lower leg images (85.4° ± 2.6°); thus, they suggested that lower leg images should be used to assess the LDTA [5]. From a sagittal view, the posterior edge of the distal tibial plafond was slightly lower than the anterior edge, resulting in a mean anterior distal tibial angle (ADTA) of 83° ± 3.6° ranging from 76° to 97° [6]. In the same radiological study, tibial coverage was 88.1° ± 6.7°. A decreased tibial coverage was found to be a risk factor for chronic ankle instability [7].

Interestingly, Hvid et al. [8] observed that tibial bone was considerably weaker than talar bone (40% on average). Furthermore, they found that the bone strength distribution in the distal tibia was not homogenous, with the lowest values measured in the anterolateral areas (Fig. 2.4). When comparing the bone strength measured using an osteopenetrometer of five successive 2 mm levels starting with the subchondral bone, they found a significant decrease of bone strength from the first to the second level at the tibia (Fig. 2.5). In contrast, bone strength increased at first and then decreased significantly for the talus [8]. For total ankle arthroplasty, these findings are fundamental. Hvid et al. [8] concluded that resection of >4 mm distal tibial bone might result in too weak bone to support the loads imposed by current prosthetic designs. Kofoed confirmed this in his study, showing that only 1–1.5 cm of the distal tibia is the solid subchondral bone [9].

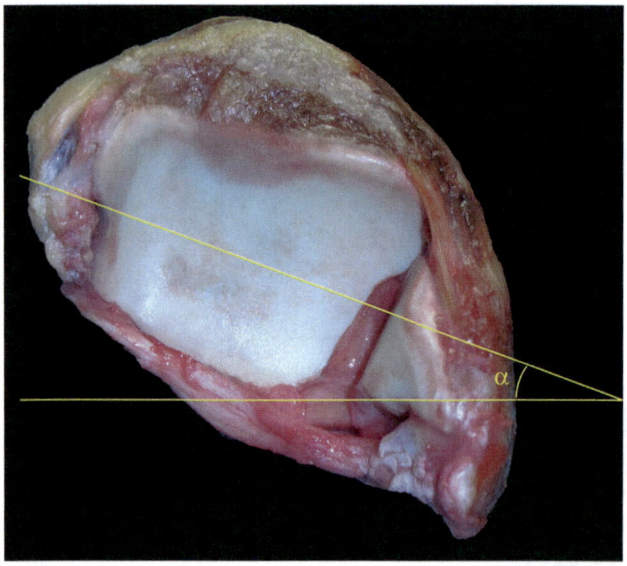

Fig. 2.2 The ankle mortise. The ankle mortise consists of two bones connected by the syndesmotic ligaments. *AITFL* anterior tibiofibular ligament; *PITFL* posterior tibiofibular ligament; *TFIL* tibiofibular interosseous ligament (see Fig. 2.10). The tibial plafond is concave and externally rotated about the coronal plane (α = medial angle)

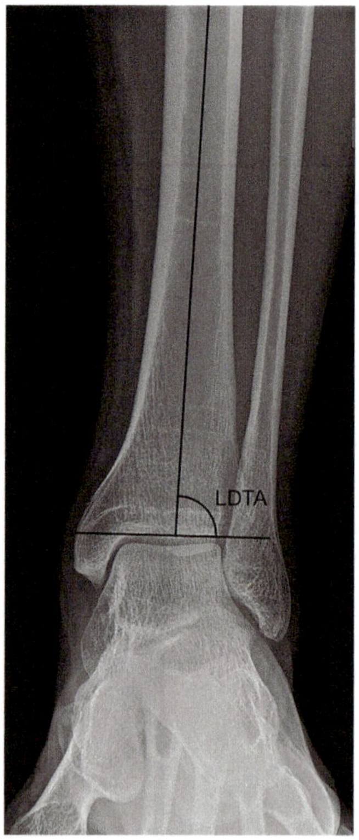

Fig. 2.3 Lateral distal tibial angle. The lateral distal tibial angle (LDTA) is the angle measured in the coronal plane on the lateral side between the midline of the tibia and the surface of the plafond of the ankle

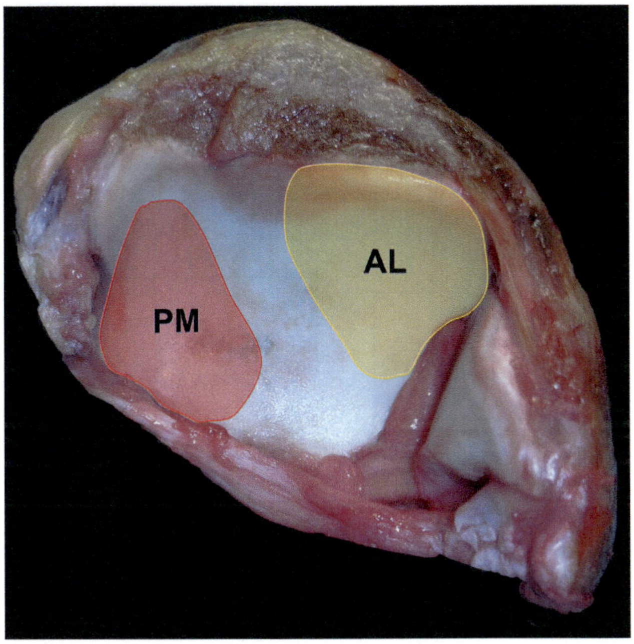

Fig. 2.4 Compressive resistance of tibial plafond. The maximal bone strength of the distal tibia is posteromedially (PM), and the minimal bone strength anterolaterally (AL)

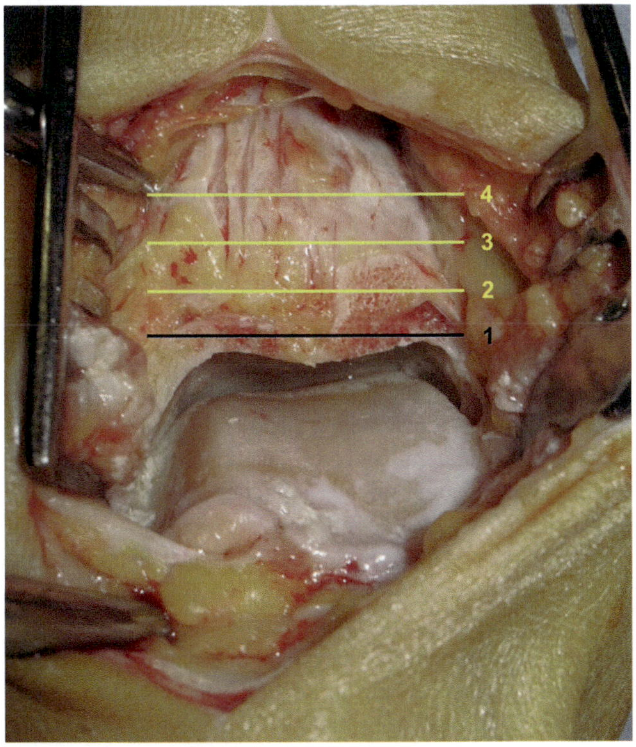

Fig. 2.5 Tibial compressive resistance. The compressive resistance of the bone greatly decreases as the cut chosen for bony resection occurs higher on the distal tibia (see text)

2.1.1.2 Fibula

The fibula terminates at the lateral malleolus in a pyramid-like shape with three surfaces: lateral, medial, and posterior. The lateral surface is convex and subcutaneous. On the medial side, the fibula is in contact with the incisura fibularis of the tibia, and over the posterior surface lie the peroneus brevis and longus tendons. The distal tibiofibular articulation is flexible with limited articulation. Moving the foot from plantarflexion into dorsiflexion is associated with axial rotation and mediolateral translation of the fibula relative to the tibia [10–13]. Axial rotation of the fibula is higher at the distal than at the proximal end [10]. Congruency of the distal tibiofibular articulation has high biomechanical importance. Minor changes in the fibular position, such as two or more millimeters of shortening, lateral shift, or five or more degrees of external rotation of the fibula, may cause a significant increase in the pressure in the tibiotalar joint [14].

2.1.1.3 Talus

The talus forms the convex side of the ankle joint. It articulates with the tibia superiorly and medially and with the fibula laterally. When looked at from the top to down, the talus has a conically shaped surface with a smaller medial radius and a medially directed apex (Fig. 2.6) [1]. The difference between the medial and lateral length of the trochlea was found to be 2.1 ± 1.1 mm, with a range of 0–6 mm [13]. In the sagittal plane, the talar trochlea has a wedge shape that articulates with the tibial plafond. The average width of the talar trochlea is 29.9 ± 2.6 mm anterior, 27.9 ± 3.0 mm in the middle, and 25.2 ± 3.7 mm posterior, generally wider in males than in females [15]. The average posterior width of the talus is less than the anterior width by 2.4 ± 1.3 mm, with a range of 0–6 mm [1]. When using a line between the tip of the medial malleolus and the fibula as the empirical axis of the ankle joint, the vertical plane of the lateral talar facet lays close to being perpendicular, with an angle of 89.2 ± 2.8° (range 80–95°). The medial talar facet's vertical axis is oblique to the ankle joint's axis with an angle of 83.9 ± 5.2° (range 70–93°) [1].

Body weight, height, and age do not affect ankle morphology in the adult population [16]. However, it has been shown that foot morphology differs between different ethnic groups [17, 18]. For instance, Chinese adults were found to have thicker and narrower trochlea tali in general and a narrower posterior talar width. In contrast, the cross-sectional area of the tibial mortise was closer to a square in Caucasian adults [15, 18].

The internal architecture of the talus is unique and reflects its biomechanical properties. Compact bone in the talus was found to be nonuniform, with thicker regions over the poste-

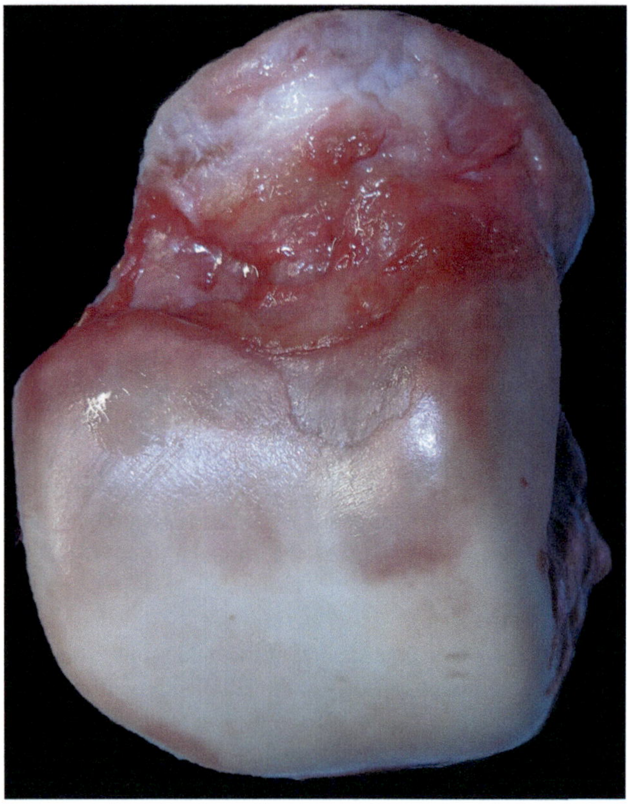

Fig. 2.6 Cranial view of the talus. The talus is covered to approximately 60% by cartilage. The tibiotalar joint forms a trochlea, which is anteriorly wider than posteriorly, and the medial radius is smaller than the lateral (see text)

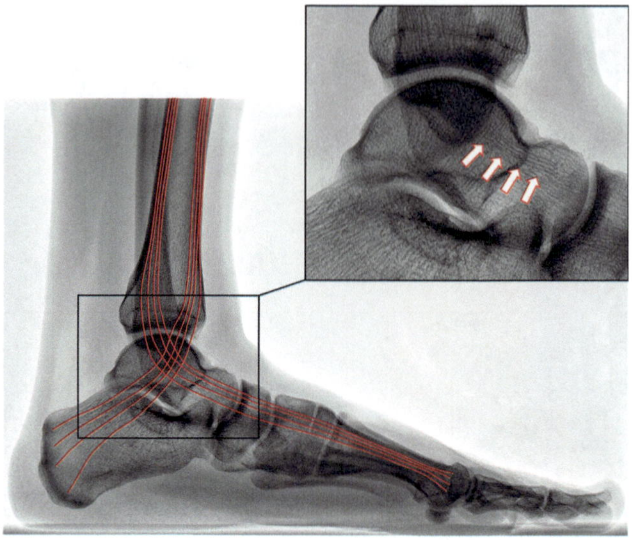

Fig. 2.7 Bony force trajectories. The main trabecular lines through the foot and ankle (main force trajectories) run close to the upper cortical shell of the talar neck (arrows). Removing part of the cortical shell of the talar neck places abnormally increased stress on the remaining less resistant cancellous bone

rior calcaneal facet, medial malleolar facet, and lateral malleolar facet [19]. Thinner regions of compact bone exist over the trochlear surface and head of the talus. The trabeculae of the talus can be divided into two sets (Fig. 2.7). The first set can be found deep to the medial part of the trochlear surface and on the anterior third of the lateral trochlear surface. Trabeculae of this set run anteriorly toward the head and neck of the talus. The second set originates from the posterior two-thirds of the trochlear surface and descends onto the posterior calcaneal facet. The neck of the talus includes sagittal plates extending from the body to the head. This internal architecture reflects the distribution and transmission of forces through the talus during gait [19, 20]. It is important to remember that the internal trabecular alignment may change due to cartilage degeneration for total ankle arthroplasty [21]. Age-related changes differed in the talar body, neck, and head [22]. The most significant loss of bone volume with age was seen in the talar body. In contrast, it was only moderate in the talar neck, primarily expressed in reduced trabecular thickness. Bone structure changes were independent of gender.

The blood supply is limited to vessels in the tarsal tunnel, deltoid ligament, and sinus tarsi [23–25]. This lack of direct blood delivery may make the talus susceptible to avascular necrosis, mainly if the blood supply is lessened due to trauma and surgery.

2.1.2 Ligamentous Configuration

The ankle joint complex and its surrounding ligaments represent a complex mechanical structure with mechanical properties highly dependent on the integrity of the ligaments [26, 27].

2.1.2.1 Lateral Ankle Ligaments

The anterior talofibular, calcaneofibular, and posterior talofibular ligaments constitute the lateral collateral ligaments of the ankle. Each lateral collateral ligament has its role in stabilizing the ankle and subtalar joint, depending on the foot's position (Fig. 2.8). In dorsiflexion, the posterior talofibular ligament is maximally stressed, and the calcaneofibular ligament is taut. In contrast, the anterior talofibular ligament is loose. In plantarflexion, however, the anterior talofibular ligament is taut, and the calcaneofibular and posterior talofibular ligaments become loose [28–30]. Slight variations exist due to the different divergence patterns between the anterior talofibular and calcaneofibular ligaments [27].

Sequential sectioning of the lateral ligaments has demonstrated the function of these ligaments in different positions and under various loading conditions. Johnson and Markolf [31] studied laxity after sectioning the anterior talofibular ligament and found that most changes occur in plantarflex-

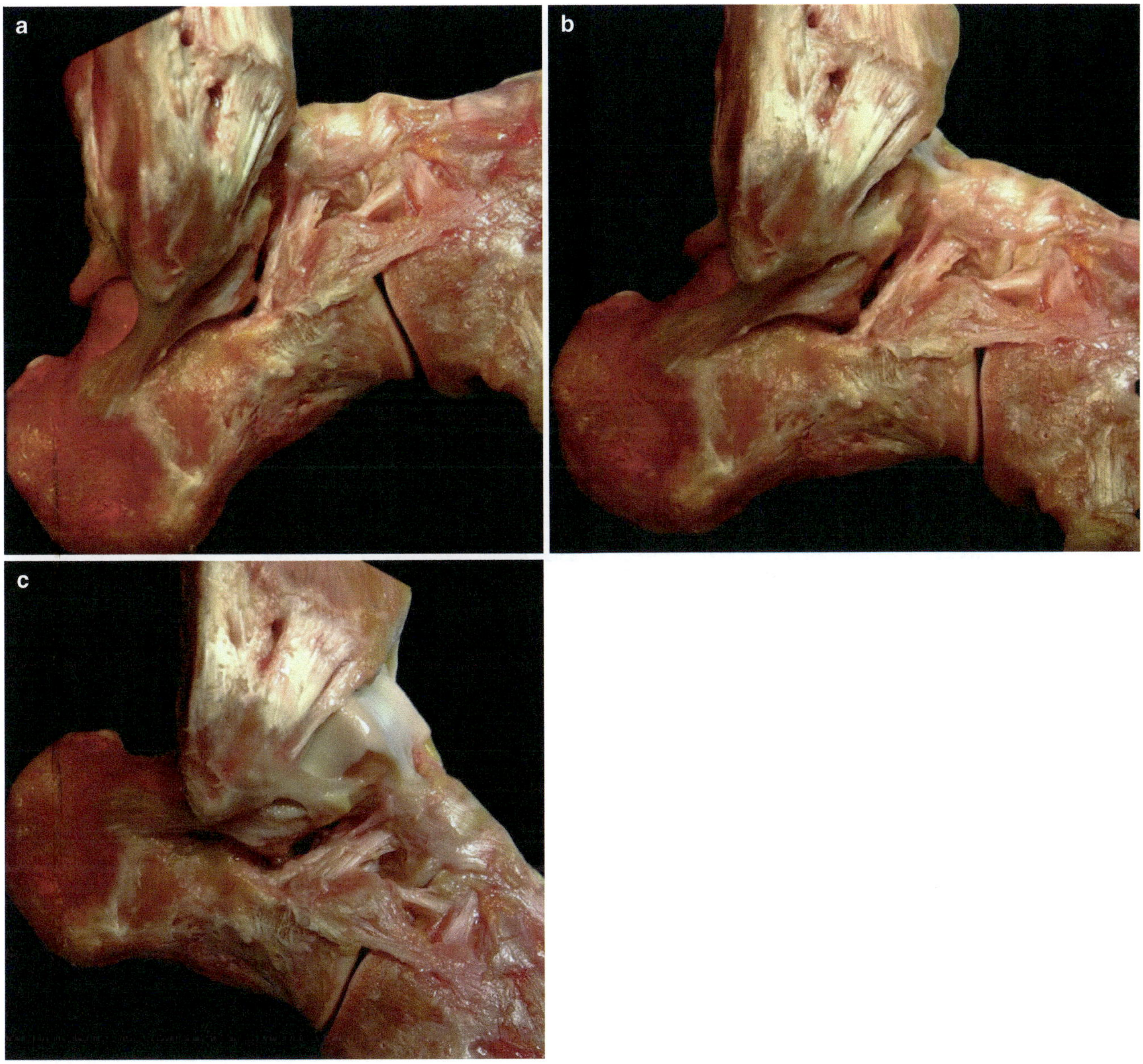

Fig. 2.8 The lateral ankle ligaments. Position and tension of lateral ankle ligaments at (**a**) dorsiflexion, (**b**) neutral position, and (**c**) plantarflexion of the foot

ion. They found a smaller change in laxity in dorsiflexion, suggesting that the anterior talofibular ligament limits talar tilt throughout the full range of motion, however, having the greatest influence on plantarflexion. Rasmussen and Tovborg-Jensen [32] further confirmed these findings, stating that talar tilt is limited in plantarflexion and neutral position by the anterior talofibular ligament and in dorsiflexion by the calcaneofibular ligament plus the posterior talofibular ligament. Hollis et al. [33], in a similar in vitro study, found that the inversion motion of the ankle increased when both the calcaneofibular and the anterior talofibular ligament were sectioned.

2.1.2.2 Medial Ankle Ligaments

Wide variations have been noted in the anatomic description of the medial ankle ligament complex (Fig. 2.9). However, it is widely accepted that the medial ankle ligaments, also known as the deltoid-spring ligament complex, prevent valgus tilting and external rotation of the talus and is composed of a superficial and deep layer. The tibiocalcaneal, tibiospring, and tibionavicular ligaments comprise the superficial portion of the deltoid complex and span over the medial malleolus to insert broadly onto the sustentaculum tali (calcaneus), navicular, talar neck, and spring ligament [27, 34–38]. The deep anterior tibiotalar, superficial posterior tibiotalar,

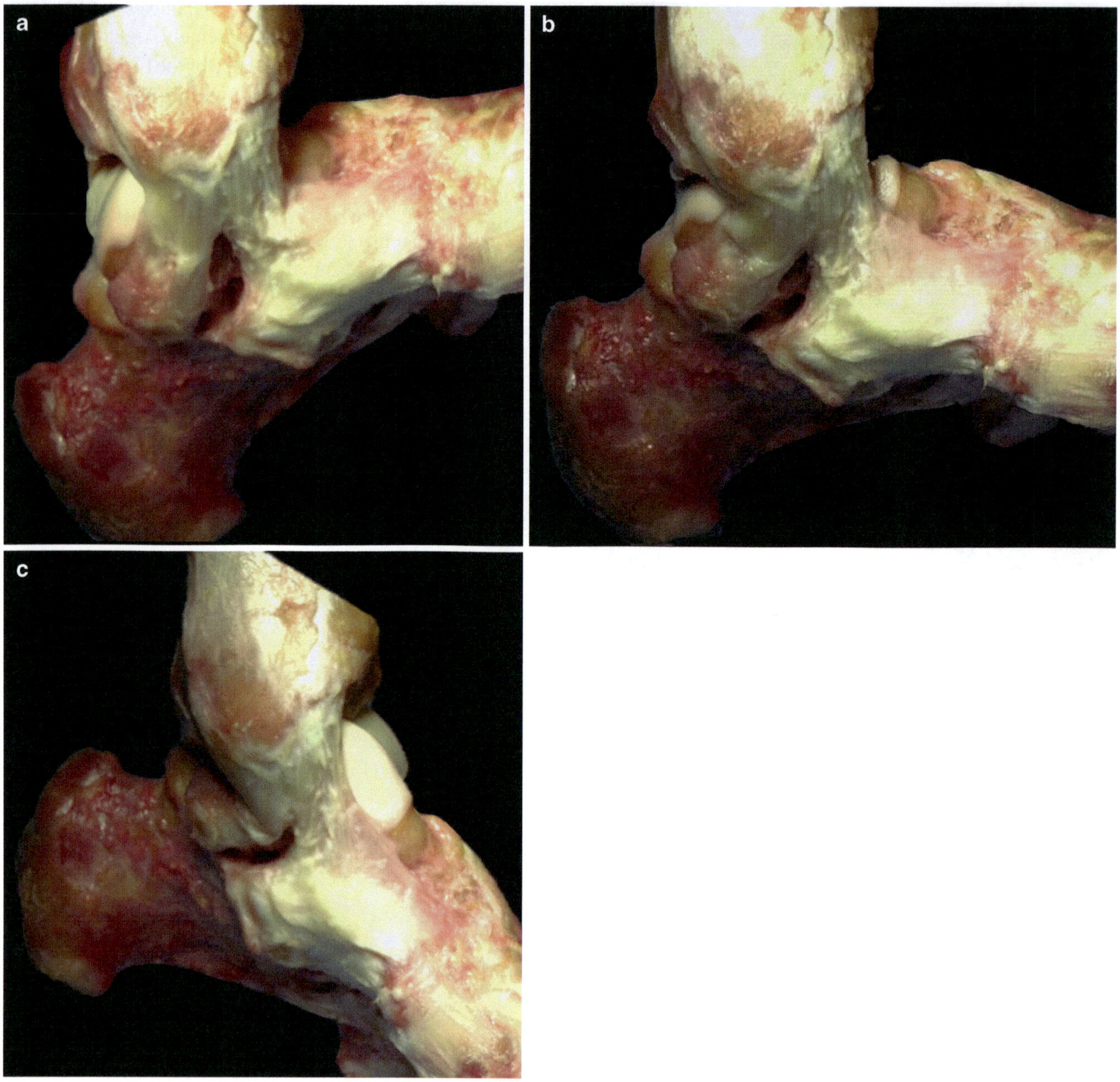

Fig. 2.9 The medial ankle ligaments. Position and tension of medial ankle ligaments at (**a**) dorsiflexion, (**b**) neutral position, and (**c**) plantarflexion of the foot

and deep posterior tibiotalar ligaments constitute the deep portion of the deltoid complex.

Close [39] found the deltoid ligament to be a strong restraint limiting talar abduction. With all lateral structures removed, he found that the intact deltoid ligament allowed only 2 mm of separation between the talus and medial malleolus. With the release of the deep deltoid ligament, the talus could be separated from the medial malleolus by 3.7 mm. The strongest superficial ligament of the deltoid complex, the tibiocalcaneal ligament, specifically limits talar abduction, whereas the deep portions additionally resist external rotation [32, 40, 41].

2.1.2.3 Syndesmotic Ligaments

Four ligaments form the syndesmotic ligament complex: anterior inferior tibiofibular ligament, posterior inferior tibiofibular ligament, tibiofibular interosseous ligament, and transverse tibiofibular ligament (Fig. 2.10). These ligaments work together with the bony restraints to maintain the integrity of the distal tibia and the fibula by resisting the axial, rotational, and translational forces [27, 42, 43]. Furthermore, although the deltoid ligament is not formally included in the syndesmotic complex, it plays a vital role in mortise stability [27, 43, 44].

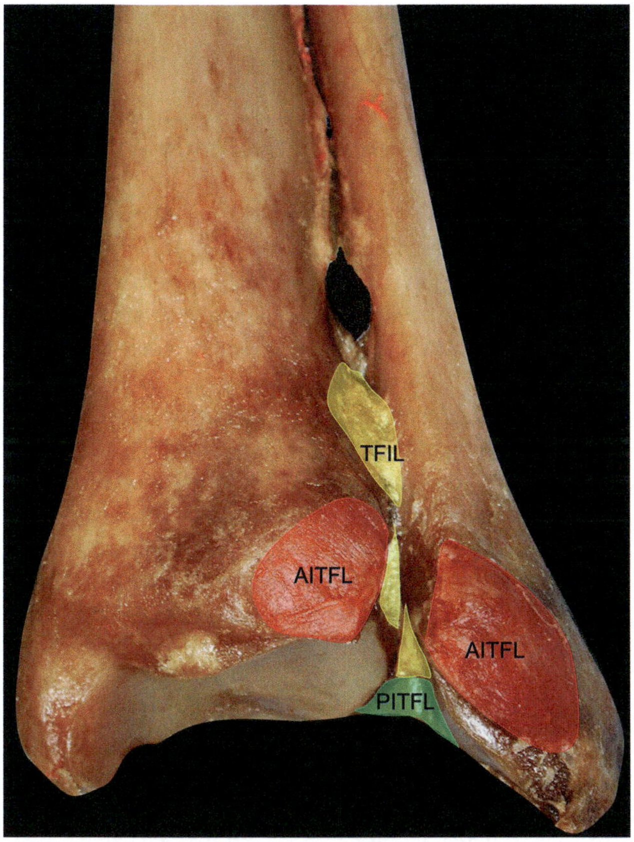

Fig. 2.10 Syndesmotic ligaments. Anterior view of the syndesmotic ligaments that are composed of the anterior inferior tibiofibular ligament (AITFL, dissected), posterior inferior tibiofibular ligament (PITFL), and tibiofibular interosseous ligament (TFIL, partially dissected). The anterior and posterior tibiofibular ligaments are at risk if the tibial resection is high. The tibiofibular interosseous ligament is the distal part of the interosseous membrane

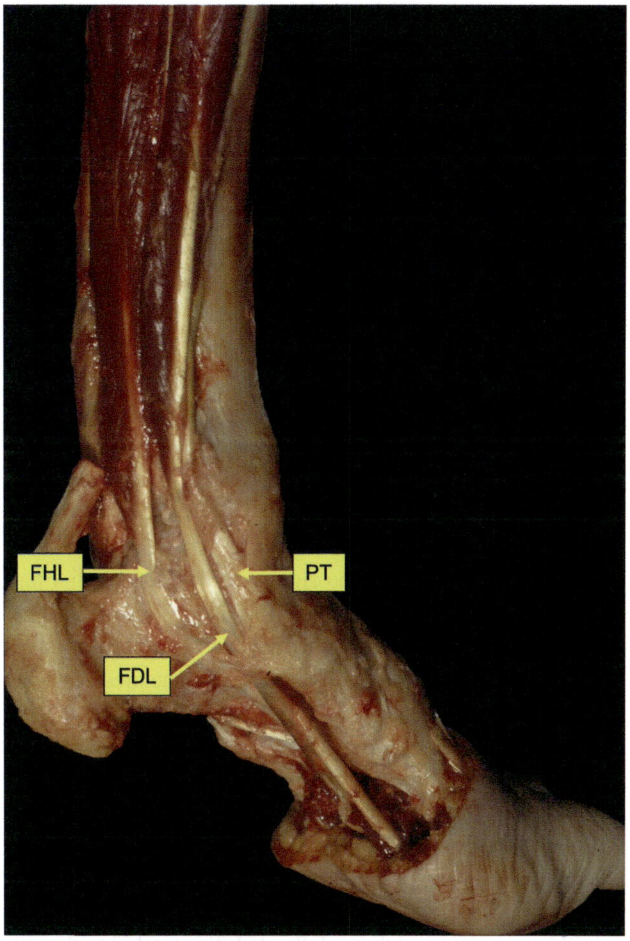

Fig. 2.11 Deep flexor tendons. The deep flexor tendons run posteromedially close to the ankle joint. The flexor hallucis longus (FHL) tendon runs in the first layer behind the posterior capsule of the ankle; thus, it is prone to be involved in scarring of the posterior capsule in posttraumatic ankle osteoarthritis or getting injured when the tibial cut is performed during total ankle arthroplasty (FDL, flexor digotorum longus; PT, posterior tibial)

2.1.3 Tendons

Both extrinsic muscles and osteoarticular and ligamentous structures influence the active and passive motion of the foot during gait. The tendons of the extrinsic muscles of the foot move a certain distance to the underlying bone during both concentric and eccentric muscle work; the amount of tendon movement depends on the moment arm of the tendon about the instantaneous joint rotation axis [45].

2.1.3.1 Peroneal Tendons

The peroneus brevis inserts on the fifth metatarsal, while the peroneus longus inserts on the first metatarsal. Compared to the peroneus brevis, the peroneus longus has a greater impact on the foot due to its lateral tether and the fact that it traverses the plantar aspect of the foot before attaching to the base of the first metatarsal.

The estimates of peroneus brevis and peroneus longus tendon moment arms indicate that they are approximately equal [45, 46]. Muscle architecture studies [47, 48] suggest that the peroneus longus has twice the strength of the peroneus brevis with equal tendon strengths, suggesting the two muscles may well function at the same force levels. The larger muscle belly of the peroneus longus may be associated with requirements for greater excursion or velocity of shortening rather than strength.

2.1.3.2 Flexor Hallucis Longus Tendon

The flexor hallucis longus tendon runs beneath the sustentaculum tali distally to insert on the distal phalanx of the great toe. The muscle belly and the tendon are in the first layer behind the posterior capsular of the ankle joint (Fig. 2.11). Thus, this muscle-tendon unit is prone to damage after an injury involving the ankle joint's posterior structures, resulting in it not functioning normally. In the case of a progressive collapsing flatfoot deformity, the flexor hallucis longus is used to stabilize the calcaneus against eversion, typically resulting in a flexion contracture of the great toe [27, 49].

2.1.3.3 Posterior Tibial Tendon

The tibialis posterior tendon runs along the posterior facet of the medial malleolus to insert with some variations on the medial arch [50, 51]. It elevates the medial arch and inverts, adducts, and plantarflexes the foot [45, 52]. During the stance phase of gait, the tibialis posterior is the primary dynamic stabilizer of the foot. As a vital contributor to the midtarsal joint locking mechanism, the posterior tibial tendon inverts the hindfoot, creating a rigid midfoot and allowing the gastrocnemius-soleus complex to transmit plantarflexion forces to the metatarsal heads [45]. With its minimal excursion and specific muscular architecture, the posterior tibial muscle is prone to scar, which results in a contracture with subsequent progressive, irreducible supination deformity; or, in progressive collapsing flatfoot deformity, its tendon may undergo degeneration and rupture.

2.1.3.4 Anterior Tibial Tendon

The tibialis anterior muscle originates from the medial part of the anterior compartment, from the upper two-thirds of the lateral surface of the tibia and the adjacent part of the interosseous membrane, and typically inserts into the medial cuneiform and first metatarsal bone [53, 54]. It runs beneath the extensor retinaculum, typically dissected when exposing the ankle joint through an anterior approach.

2.1.3.5 Achilles Tendon

During locomotion, propulsion is based on the ability to transmit forces to the forefoot. The pull of the triceps surae complex is transferred through the Achilles tendon to the calcaneus and subsequently to the metatarsal heads. During the gait cycle, the moment arm of the ground reaction force increases [55] when moving from under the heel to the midfoot and, at last, to the metatarsal heads at takeoff. Therefore, the integrity of the Achilles tendon is crucial for normal gait, especially during foot push-off.

2.2 Axis of Rotation of the Ankle

The obliquity of the ankle joint axis can vary between individuals in the coronal plane, even though the articular surfaces of the ankle joint appear to lie in a plane perpendicular to the long axis of the leg. To understand this, one must realize that the trochlea is a frustum of a cone rather than a cylinder [1]. In 1952, Barnett and Napier measured the trochlear surfaces of 152 human tali and reported that the medial and lateral curvatures of the talus were different. This indicated that the ankles' rotation axis changed its position during the arc of motion [13]. Hicks, 1 year later, defined these different axes as the "dorsiflexion axis" and "plantarflexion axis," stating that movement cannot occur about these two axes simultaneously [56]. Since then, several investigators have demonstrated that the axis of rotation of the ankle is not fixed and changes continuously throughout the range of motion [57–61].

Lundberg et al. [57] used roentgen stereo photogrammetry to analyze the axis of rotation in eight healthy volunteers. Measurements taken at 10° increments between 30° plantarflexion and 30° dorsiflexion showed that the rotation axis changed continuously, and large interindividual differences also existed. Probably the most significant finding was that plantarflexion and dorsiflexion, pronation and supination, as well as medial and lateral rotation axes for each subject when drawn in the exact figure coincided or ran very close to one central point in the trochlea of the talus, irrespective of their inclination (Fig. 2.12) [57].

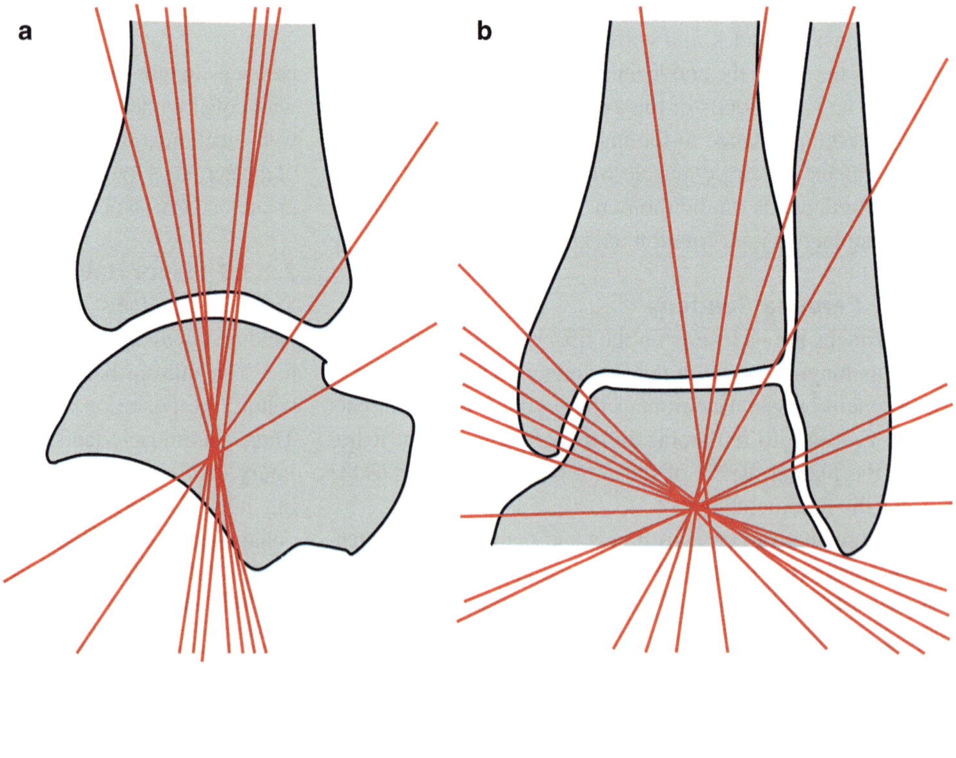

Fig. 2.12 The ankle joint: a uniaxial, modified hinge joint. These pictures show the dynamic position of the ankle joint axis in 8 healthy ankles for each 10° interval from 30° of plantarflexion to 30° of dorsiflexion, projected onto (**a**) the sagittal plane and (**b**) the coronal plane. (Modified from: Lundberg A, Svensson OK, Nemeth G, Selvik G. The axis of rotation of the ankle joint. J Bone Joint Surg Br. 1989;71(1):94–9)

Hintermann and Nigg [61] studied the rotational movements of the tibia and calcaneus that occurred with dorsiflexion-plantarflexion and axial loading in cadaver foot-leg specimens using an unconstrained testing apparatus. Independent of the foot flexion position, significant internal rotation of the tibia and eversion of the calcaneus were noted after the ankle complex was axially loaded. Independent of loading, 10° of dorsiflexion resulted in 0.1° of eversion and 2.1° of internal rotation of the tibia. Conversely, 10° of plantarflexion resulted in 1.6° of inversion and 1.3° of external rotation of the tibia. The tibia and calcaneus' induced rotational movements differed significantly between the specimens. These results suggested that the foot "axes" did not change when the ankle complex was axially loaded. They supported previous reports that the ankle complex utilizes different axes for dorsiflexion and plantarflexion [61].

2.3 Range of Motion

The ankle range of motion in humans around the globe is significantly different due to geographical and cultural differences in daily activities of life [62–65]. However, further aspects that may influence the range of motion are age, gender, the position of other joints such as the knee and hip joints, and comorbidities. Nevertheless, all movements of the ankle during normal gait—dorsiflexion, plantarflexion, supination, and pronation—occur at multiple levels and involve several hindfoot and midfoot joints [66]. For example, hindfoot movement results from a combination of movement about the tibiotalar and subtalar joints [58, 61, 67–70]. The major contributors to overall ankle motion are plantarflexion and dorsiflexion and are, therefore, particularly important for clinical evaluation. Data collected by various authors suggest that the average plantarflexion and dorsiflexion of the ankle are between 40° and 56° and 13° and 33°, respectively [58, 68–70].

During most everyday activities, such as walking on even surfaces (10°–15° plantarflexion and 10° dorsiflexion), walking upstairs (37° total range of motion), and walking downstairs (56° total range of motion), only a partial range of motion is required [71]. For elderly people to complete their daily routines, it has been suggested that only a 15°–20° range of motion is sufficient [71].

Several studies have shown that the ankle range of motion may change due to age and gender [72–74]. Nigg et al. [74] showed that in younger persons, ankle range of motion was usually greater in women; however, among older persons, the female subjects had 8° less dorsiflexion and 8° more plantarflexion than males [74]. Accordingly, Grimston et al. showed that within each gender, there is a consistent trend for a range of motion decrease with age once the maximum has been reached at age 14–16 or 17–20 in females and males, respectively [73]. These results diverge from those published by Macedo and Magee [72]. They measured ankle range of motion in 90 women aged 18 to 59 and saw that plantarflexion and dorsiflexion increased with age [72]. However, the highest age in this patient group (59 years) was lower than in the study by Nigg et al. [74], so results may not be wholly comparable.

Besides the age-related change in range of motion, Macedo and Magee [75] also looked at the differences in the range of motion between dominant and nondominant sides of the upper and lower extremities in the same cohort. They found passive dorsiflexion (2.1°; 95% CI 0.5°–3.7°), passive plantarflexion (−2.5°; 95% CI −4.6 to −0.4°), active plantarflexion (−3.4°; 95% CI −5.6° to −1.2°), and active inversion (1.5°; 95% CI −0.2° to 3.2°) to be significantly different between the dominant and nondominant leg. Ferrario et al. [76] measured the asymmetry of the active range of motion of the ankle and its coupled movements in 65 young adults. Only 20% of female and 34% of male subjects had more than a 5° difference in total range of motion between both ankles [76]. In conclusion, limb dominance and asymmetry in the actions of the lower extremities during walking and running is a common phenomenon [77]. Therefore, it is unsurprising that differences in the range of motion can be found. These differences may not have high clinical significance. Therefore, using the contralateral ankle as a reference value for pre-injury or normal range of motion is justifiable but must be considered [75, 76].

Mitchell et al. [78] addressed the effect of pelvic, hip, and knee positions on the ankle's range of motion. Their biomechanical study found that pelvic posture may not significantly influence the ankle range of motion regardless of hip and knee joint position. However, persons with hip flexion and knee extension found a significantly reduced ankle range of motion [78]. Thoms and Rome [79] measured active ankle joint dorsiflexion in 26 healthy subjects in 3 different positions and obtained 6.59° ± 4.96° for the supine position, 6.45° ± 4.64° for the prone position, and 11.67° ± 5.96° for sitting position.

The ankle's range of motion may be reduced in patients with systemic diseases. The subjects with diabetes mellitus have reduced passive range of motion of the ankle and increased stiffness compared to a control group without diabetes [80]. This may explain the pathological changes in plantar loading and the high rate of ulcer formation in patients with diabetes mellitus [80, 81].

2.4 Load Transmission in the Ankle Joint

Load transmission in the ankle occurs in contact pressure between the tibia, fibula, and talus (Fig. 2.13). The contact pressure depends on the contact area between these joints.

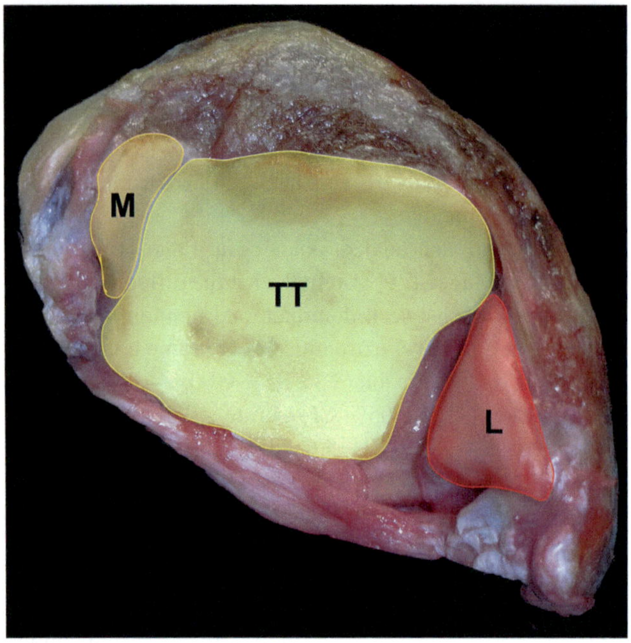

Fig. 2.13 Contact area of the ankle mortise. The ankle has a surface contact area of approximately 12 cm^2, of which the tibiotalar contact area (TT) accounts for approximately 7 cm^2 and the mediolateral contact areas (M and L) for approximately 5 cm^2

2.4.1 Contact Area of the Ankle

Numerous studies have been performed addressing measurements of the surface contact area of the ankle joint [2, 82–86]. Reports of whole ankle contact area vary from 150 to 940 mm^2, depending on load and ankle position [87]. Controversies exist about changes to the amount of contact area as a function of the flexion position [2, 88, 89], which may be attributed to differences in load, position, and measurement techniques [90]. Kura et al. [82] measured ankle contact areas in various joint positions in nine cadaveric feet. The available articular area was divided into central, medial, and lateral zones, measured in unloaded ankles as 922 ± 120 mm^2, 178 ± 66 mm^2, and 308 ± 60 mm^2, respectively. After load application of 667 N in a neutral position, the measured contact areas showed no significant changes. In plantarflexion there was a decrease in contact area [82]. Wan et al. [85] measured in vivo articular cartilage contact areas in nine healthy persons using three-dimensional models created from MRI. The average cartilage coverage area was 964.9 ± 156.1 mm^2 and 1304.8 ± 208.4 mm^2 on the tibial and talar surface. The cartilage contact areas were measured at different phases of gait—heel strike position, mid-stance position, and toe-off position. They measured the following contact areas for these three positions for tibial and talar cartilage surface areas: 28.2 ± 4.2% and 20.9 ± 3.6%, 43.7 ± 5.5% and 31.0 ± 5.0%, and 34.8 ± 4.1% and 25.8 ± 3.9%, respectively [85]. Millington et al. [84] measured the ankle joint contact area under physiological load (1000 N) in 10 cadaveric specimens in neutral and 20° dorsiflexion, supination, pronation, and plantarflexion using a stereophotography technique. The greatest tibiotalar contact area was measured in dorsiflexion with 734 ± 169 mm^2 and the smallest in plantarflexion with 439 ± 141 mm^2. The greatest talofibular contact area was measured in dorsiflexion with 202 ± 78 mm^2 and the smallest in pronation with 77 ± 49 mm^2 [84]. Calhoun et al. [2] analyzed pressure distribution in the ankle joint under multiple axial loads (490, 686, and 980 N) in different joint positions using pressure-sensitive Fuji film. Inversion or eversion of the ankle in the neutral or dorsiflexion position resulted in a decrease in total contact areas and an increase in average pressures. The total contact area was generally higher, and the average pressure was lower in dorsiflexion. The pressure distribution patterns differed in dorsiflexion and plantarflexion: the main force transmission area moved anteriorly to posteriorly on the talus during the movement from dorsiflexion to plantarflexion. The talar dome contributed the most to the load transfer, with 77% to 90% of the load [2]. These findings were confirmed later by Michelson et al. [83].

2.4.2 Load Transmission Forces at the Ankle Joint

During gait, a significant cartilage contact deformation occurs in the ankle joint. Wan et al. [91] were able to show, using a combined dual fluoroscopic and MRI technique, that the average cartilage thickness in the ankle without weight-bearing was 1.43 ± 0.15 mm and 1.42 ± 0.18 mm in the distal tibial and proximal talar cartilage layers, respectively. After applying total loading, an increase of >15% in contact strains was observed in more than 40% of the contact area. Ankle cartilage on the tibial and talar sides experienced large deformation during load transmission through the ankle joint [91].

Haraguchi et al. [92] performed discrete element analysis, a method described in detail by Benemerito et al. [93], to assess the three-dimensional contact characteristics and ligament tension in the ankle joint during the stance phase of gait. They showed that most ankle joint loading during the stance phase occurred across the articular surfaces, while stabilization due to ligament tension played an inferior role. However, the medial ligaments play a more important part than the lateral ligaments: the deep deltoid ligament transferred the most force during the stance phase (57.2%), followed by the superficial part of the deltoid ligament (26.1%) [92]. Tochigi et al. [94] identified in their biomechanical study that the integrity of articular surface geometry plays a crucial role in passive ankle stability.

Park et al. [95] measured contact pressure distribution using finite element analysis integrated with motion analysis.

The peak contact pressure of the talus cartilage was 6.6 MPa at the first peak of gait, 5.9 MPa at mid-stance, and 8.8 MPa at the second peak. For the ankle, the peak contact pressure was located at the lateral cartilage of the talus. The contact pressure distribution also confirmed that the contact region in the talus cartilage moved to the anterior area as the stance phase proceeded from the first peak to the second peak [95].

2.4.3 Load Transmission Through the Fibula

The dynamic function of the fibula has been shown to play an important role in load transmission during gait [96–98]. Lambert [99] indirectly measured that the fibula received approximately one-sixth of the load applied to the knee joint. These results were confirmed by direct measurements performed by Takebe et al. [98], who addressed the role of the fibula in 6 cadaveric specimens under the load of 60 kg (Fig. 2.14). In the neutral position, the fibula transmitted an average of 6.4% of the load. Positioned at 15° dorsiflexion, the fibula transmitted a higher load (10.4%), whereas ankles at 15° plantarflexion transmitted lower (2.3% of load) loads than at neutral [98]. Goh et al. [100] investigated the effect of fibular resection and hereby showed that an average of 7.12% of the load was transferred by the fibula with increasing load transmission in dorsiflexion and eversion. Resection of the proximal fibula led to a radical decrease in fibular load transmission from 0.62 to 0.81% [100]. Wang et al. [101] addressed the role of the fibula in weight-bearing and its contribution to ankle joint stability. Under an axial load of 1500 N, the fibula transmitted an average of 17% of the load. The dorsiflexion position of the ankle joint significantly increased the fibular load transmission. Also, the artificially created distal tibiofibular instability changed the fibular load transmission [101].

The current literature addresses the effect of fibulectomy on the load transmission and kinematics of the ankle joint [11, 102]. Bozkurt et al. [11] analyzed gait in three proximal, middle, and distal fibulectomy patients. The study revealed that the distal fibulectomy significantly alters ankle kinematics, while the proximal fibulectomy impairs knee joint stability. The middle fibulectomy with in situ remaining proximal and distal fragments has only slightly influenced the biomechanical properties of gait [11]. Similar results were observed in the biomechanical study by Pacelli et al. [102] addressing ankle instability following free fibular graft harvest. They found that only 10% of the distal fibular length was needed to maintain intrinsic ankle stability.

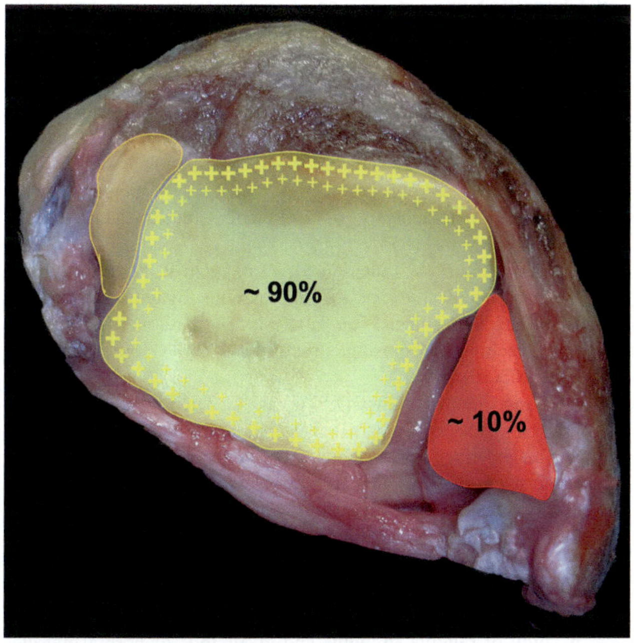

Fig. 2.14 Distribution of load transmission at the ankle joint. Force transmission at the distal fibula accounts for up to 10% of overall transmission forces at the ankle joint, depending on flexion position. Load transmission at the distal tibia occurs mainly eccentrically through the cortical rim, and there is almost no force transmission through the center of the distal tibia

2.5 Conclusions

- The ankle joint is a highly congruent and dynamic joint consisting of three bones.
- Articular surfaces and a complex ligamentous system guide talar motion within the ankle mortise and ensure stability.
- Given the talus' conically shaped surface, the ankle does not move as a pure hinge mechanism; instead, the axis of rotation changes from dorsi- to plantarflexion.
- The strength of the distal tibia is lower than that of the talus, and the load transfer occurs mainly through the circumferential cortex. In contrast, the load transfer through the fibula accounts for only approximately 10%.
- The overall range of motion at the ankle joint differs significantly among individuals, and there are also intraindividual differences; however, for most daily activities, only a partial range of motion is required.

References

1. Inman VT. The joints of the ankle. Baltimore, MD: Williams & Wilkins; 1976.
2. Calhoun JH, Li F, Ledbetter BR, Viegas SF. A comprehensive study of pressure distribution in the ankle joint with inversion and eversion. Foot Ankle Int. 1994;15(3):125–33.

3. Isman RE, Inman VT. Anthropometric studies of the human foot and ankle. Technical Report, Biomechanics Laboratory, San Francisco. 1968;58.
4. Knupp M, Ledermann H, Magerkurth O, Hinterman B. The surgical tibiotalar angle: a radiologic study. Foot Ankle Int. 2005;26(9):713–6.
5. Stufkens SA, Barg A, Bolliger L, Stucinskas J, Knupp M, Hintermann B. Measurement of the medial distal tibial angle. Foot Ankle Int. 2011;32(3):288–93.
6. Magerkurth O, Knupp M, Ledermann H, Hintermann B. Evaluation of hindfoot dimensions: a radiological study. Foot Ankle Int. 2006;27(8):612–6.
7. Frigg A, Frigg R, Hintermann B, Barg A, Valderrabano V. The biomechanical influence of tibio-talar containment on stability of the ankle joint. Knee Surg Sports Traumatol Arthrosc. 2007;15(11):1355–62.
8. Hvid I, Rasmussen O, Jensen NC, Nielsen S. Trabecular bone strength profiles at the ankle joint. Clin Orthop Relat Res. 1985;199:306–12.
9. Kofoed H. Cylindrical cemented ankle arthroplasty: a prospective series with long-term follow-up. Foot Ankle Int. 1995;16(8):474–9.
10. Bozkurt M, Tonuk E, Elhan A, Tekdemir I, Doral MN. Axial rotation and mediolateral translation of the fibula during passive plantarflexion. Foot Ankle Int. 2008;29(5):502–7.
11. Bozkurt M, Yavuzer G, Tonuk E, Kentel B. Dynamic function of the fibula. Gait analysis evaluation of three different parts of the shank after fibulectomy: proximal, middle and distal. Arch Orthop Trauma Surg. 2005;125(10):713–20.
12. Karrholm J, Hansson LI, Selvik G. Mobility of the lateral malleolus. A roentgen stereophotogrammetric analysis. Acta Orthop Scand. 1985;56(6):479–83.
13. Barnett CH, Napier JR. The axis of rotation at the ankle joint in man; its influence upon the form of the talus and the mobility of the fibula. J Anat. 1952;86(1):1–9.
14. Thordarson DB, Motamed S, Hedman T, Ebramzadeh E, Bakshian S. The effect of fibular malreduction on contact pressures in an ankle fracture malunion model. J Bone Joint Surg Am. 1997;79(12):1809–15.
15. Hayes AT, Tochigi Y, Saltzman CL. Ankle morphometry on 3D-CT images. Iowa Orthop J. 2006;26:1–4.
16. Anderson M, Blais MM, Green WT. Lengths of the growing foot. J Bone Joint Surg Am. 1956;38-A(5):998–1000.
17. Stagni R, Leardini A, Ensini A, Cappello A. Ankle morphometry evaluated using a new semi-automated technique based on X-ray pictures. Clin Biomech (Bristol, Avon). 2005;20(3):307–11.
18. Kuo CC, Lu HL, Leardini A, Lu TW, Kuo MY, Hsu HC. Three-dimensional computer graphics-based ankle morphometry with computerized tomography for total ankle replacement design and positioning. Clin Anat. 2014;27(4):659–68.
19. Athavale SA, Joshi SD, Joshi SS. Internal architecture of the talus. Foot Ankle Int. 2008;29(1):82–6.
20. Pal GP, Routal RV. Architecture of the cancellous bone of the human talus. Anat Rec. 1998;252(2):185–93.
21. Schiff A, Li J, Inoue N, Masuda K, Lidtke R, Muehleman C. Trabecular angle of the human talus is associated with the level of cartilage degeneration. J Musculoskelet Neuronal Interact. 2007;7(3):224–30.
22. Krause M, Rupprecht M, Mumme M, Puschel K, Amling M, Barvencik F. Bone microarchitecture of the talus changes with aging. Clin Orthop Relat Res. 2013;471(11):3663–71.
23. Gelberman RH, Mortensen WW. The arterial anatomy of the talus. Foot Ankle. 1983;4(2):64–72.
24. Kelly PJ, Sullivan CR. Blood supply of the talus. Clin Orthop Relat Res. 1963;30:37–44.
25. Mulfinger GL, Trueta J. The blood supply of the talus. J Bone Joint Surg Br. 1970;52(1):160–7.
26. Golano P, Vega J, de Leeuw PA, Malagelada F, Manzanares MC, Gotzens V, et al. Anatomy of the ankle ligaments: a pictorial essay. Knee Surg Sports Traumatol Arthrosc. 2010;18(5):557–69.
27. Hintermann B, Ruiz R. Foot and ankle instability—a clinical guide to diagnosis and surgical management. 1st ed. Springer International Publishing; 2021.
28. Colville MR, Marder RA, Boyle JJ, Zarins B. Strain measurement in lateral ankle ligaments. Am J Sports Med. 1990;18(2):196–200.
29. Renstrom P, Wertz M, Incavo S, Pope M, Ostgaard HC, Arms S, et al. Strain in the lateral ligaments of the ankle. Foot Ankle. 1988;9(2):59–63.
30. Sarrafian SK. Anatomy of foot and ankle. 2nd ed. Philadelphia: Lippincott Williams and Wilkins; 1993.
31. Johnson EE, Markolf KL. The contribution of the anterior talofibular ligament to ankle laxity. J Bone Joint Surg Am. 1983;65(1):81–8.
32. Rasmussen O, Tovborg-Jensen I. Mobility of the ankle joint: recording of rotatory movements in the talocrural joint in vitro with and without the lateral collateral ligaments of the ankle. Acta Orthop Scand. 1982;53(1):155–60.
33. Hollis JM, Blasier RD, Flahiff CM. Simulated lateral ankle ligamentous injury. Change in ankle stability. Am J Sports Med. 1995;23(6):672–7.
34. Boss AP, Hintermann B. Anatomical study of the medial ankle ligament complex. Foot Ankle Int. 2002;23(6):547–53.
35. Harper MC. Deltoid ligament: an anatomical evaluation of function. Foot Ankle. 1987;8(1):19–22.
36. Milner CE, Soames RW. The medial collateral ligaments of the human ankle joint: anatomical variations. Foot Ankle Int. 1998;19(5):289–92.
37. Yammine K. The morphology and prevalence of the Deltoid complex ligament of the ankle. Foot Ankle Spec. 2017;10(1): 55–62.
38. Hintermann B, Golanó P. The anatomy and function of the Deltoid ligament. Tech Foot Ankle Surg. 2014;13(2):67–72.
39. Close JR. Some applications of the functional anatomy of the ankle joint. J Bone Joint Surg Am. 1956;38-A(4):761–81.
40. Grath GB. Widening of the ankle mortise. A clinical and experimental study. Acta Chir Scand Suppl. 1960;Suppl 263:1–88.
41. Rasmussen O, Kromann-Andersen C, Boe S. Deltoid ligament. Functional analysis of the medial collateral ligamentous apparatus of the ankle joint. Acta Orthop Scand. 1983;54(1):36–44.
42. Yammine K, Jalloul M, Assi C. Distal tibiofibular syndesmosis: a meta-analysis of cadaveric studies. Morphologie. 2022;106(355):241–51.
43. Tano A, Nimura A, Tsutsumi M, Yamaguchi R, Okawa A, Akita K. Anatomical study of the interosseous ligament of the tibiofibular syndesmosis: an analysis of osseous morphology and attaching interposing structures. J Bone Joint Surg Am. 2021;103(10):905–12.
44. Bejarano-Pineda L, Guss D, Waryasz G, DiGiovanni CW, Kwon JY. The syndesmosis, part I: anatomy, injury mechanism, classification, and diagnosis. Orthop Clin North Am. 2021;52(4):403–15.
45. Hintermann B, Nigg BM, Sommer C. Foot movement and tendon excursion: an in vitro study. Foot Ankle Int. 1994;15(7):386–95.
46. Otis JC, Deland JT, Lee S, Gordon J. Peroneus brevis is a more effective evertor than peroneus longus. Foot Ankle Int. 2004;25(4):242–6.
47. Silver RL, de la Garza J, Rang M. The myth of muscle balance. A study of relative strengths and excursions of normal muscles about the foot and ankle. J Bone Joint Surg Br. 1985;67(3):432–7.
48. Wickiewicz TL, Roy RR, Powell PL, Edgerton VR. Muscle architecture of the human lower limb. Clin Orthop Relat Res. 1983;179:275–83.
49. Ruiz R, Hintermann B. Clinical appearance of medial ankle instability. Foot Ankle Clin. 2021;26(2):291–304.

50. Uchiyama I, Edama M, Yokota H, Hirabayashi R, Sekine C, Maruyama S, et al. Anatomical study of sites and surface area of the attachment region of Tibial posterior tendon attachment. Int J Environ Res Public Health. 2022;19(24).
51. Hintermann B, Ruiz R. Biomechanics of medial ankle and Peritalar instability. Foot Ankle Clin. 2021;26(2):249–67.
52. Hintermann B. Biomechanische Aspekte der Muskel-Sehnen-Funktion [Biomechanical aspects of muscle-tendon functions]. Orthopade. 1995;24(3):187–92.
53. Karauda P, Podgorski M, Paulsen F, Polguj M, Olewnik L. Anatomical variations of the tibialis anterior tendon. Clin Anat. 2021;34(3):397–404.
54. Zielinska N, Tubbs RS, Paulsen F, Szewczyk B, Podgorski M, Borowski A, et al. Anatomical variations of the tibialis anterior tendon insertion: an updated and comprehensive review. J Clin Med. 2021;10(16).
55. Deforth M, Zwicky L, Horn T, Hintermann B. The effect of foot type on the Achilles tendon moment arm and biomechanics. Foot (Edinb). 2019;38:91–4.
56. Hicks JH. The mechanics of the foot. I. The joints. J Anat. 1953;87(4):345–57.
57. Lundberg A, Svensson OK, Nemeth G, Selvik G. The axis of rotation of the ankle joint. J Bone Joint Surg Br. 1989;71(1):94–9.
58. Lundberg A, Goldie I, Kalin B, Selvik G. Kinematics of the ankle/foot complex: plantarflexion and dorsiflexion. Foot Ankle. 1989;9(4):194–200.
59. Sammarco GJ, DiRaimondo CV. Surgical treatment of lateral ankle instability syndrome. Am J Sports Med. 1988;16(5):501–11.
60. Siegler S, Chen J, Schneck CD. The three-dimensional kinematics and flexibility characteristics of the human ankle and subtalar joints—part I: kinematics. J Biomech Eng. 1988;110(4):364–73.
61. Hintermann B, Nigg BM. In vitro kinematics of the axially loaded ankle complex in response to dorsiflexion and plantarflexion. Foot Ankle Int. 1995;16(8):514–8.
62. Watanabe H, Ogata K, Amano T, Okabe T. The range of joint motions of the extremities in healthy Japanese people—the difference according to age. Nihon Seikeigekai Gakkai Zasshi. 1979;53(3):275–61.
63. Roaas A, Andersson GB. Normal range of motion of the hip, knee and ankle joints in male subjects, 30-40 years of age. Acta Orthop Scand. 1982;53(2):205–8.
64. Ahlberg A, Moussa M, Al-Nahdi M. On geographical variations in the normal range of joint motion. Clin Orthop Relat Res. 1988;234:229–31.
65. Kumar A, Charlebois SJ, Cain EL, Smith RA, Daniels AU, Crates JM. Effect of fibular plate fixation on rotational stability of simulated distal tibial fractures treated with intramedullary nailing. J Bone Joint Surg Am. 2003;85(4):604–8.
66. Kitaoka HB, Luo ZP, An KN. Three-dimensional analysis of normal ankle and foot mobility. Am J Sports Med. 1997;25(2):238–42.
67. Lundberg A, Svensson OK, Bylund C, Goldie I, Selvik G. Kinematics of the ankle/foot complex—part 2: pronation and supination. Foot Ankle. 1989;9(5):248–53.
68. Lundberg A, Svensson OK, Bylund C, Selvik G. Kinematics of the ankle/foot complex—part 3: influence of leg rotation. Foot Ankle. 1989;9(6):304–9.
69. de Asla RJ, Wan L, Rubash HE, Li G. Six DOF in vivo kinematics of the ankle joint complex: application of a combined dual-orthogonal fluoroscopic and magnetic resonance imaging technique. J Orthop Res. 2006;24(5):1019–27.
70. Imai K, Tokunaga D, Takatori R, Ikoma K, Maki M, Ohkawa H, et al. In vivo three-dimensional analysis of hindfoot kinematics. Foot Ankle Int. 2009;30(11):1094–100.
71. Stauffer RN, Chao EY, Brewster RC. Force and motion analysis of the normal, diseased, and prosthetic ankle joint. Clin Orthop Relat Res. 1977;127:189–96.
72. Macedo LG, Magee DJ. Effects of age on passive range of motion of selected peripheral joints in healthy adult females. Physiother Theory Pract. 2009;25(2):145–64.
73. Grimston SK, Nigg BM, Hanley DA, Engsberg JR. Differences in ankle joint complex range of motion as a function of age. Foot Ankle. 1993;14(4):215–22.
74. Nigg BM, Fisher V, Allinger TL, Ronsky JR, Engsberg JR. Range of motion of the foot as a function of age. Foot Ankle. 1992;13(6):336–43.
75. Macedo LG, Magee DJ. Differences in range of motion between dominant and nondominant sides of upper and lower extremities. J Manip Physiol Ther. 2008;31(8):577–82.
76. Ferrario VF, Turci M, Lovecchio N, Shirai YF, Sforza C. Asymmetry of the active nonweightbearing foot and ankle range of motion for dorsiflexion-plantar flexion and its coupled movements in adults. Clin Anat. 2007;20(7):834–42.
77. Sadeghi H, Allard P, Prince F, Labelle H. Symmetry and limb dominance in able-bodied gait: a review. Gait Posture. 2000;12(1):34–45.
78. Mitchell B, Bressel E, McNair PJ, Bressel ME. Effect of pelvic, hip, and knee position on ankle joint range of motion. Phys Ther Sport. 2008;9(4):202–8.
79. Thoms VR, K. Effect of subject position on the reliability of measurement of active ankle joint dorsiflexion. Foot Ankle. 1997;7:153–8.
80. Rao S, Saltzman C, Yack HJ. Ankle ROM and stiffness measured at rest and during gait in individuals with and without diabetic sensory neuropathy. Gait Posture. 2006;24(3):295–301.
81. Rao SR, Saltzman CL, Wilken J, Yak HJ. Increased passive ankle stiffness and reduced dorsiflexion range of motion in individuals with diabetes mellitus. Foot Ankle Int. 2006;27(8):617–22.
82. Kura H, Kitaoka HB, Luo ZP, An KN. Measurement of surface contact area of the ankle joint. Clin Biomech (Bristol, Avon). 1998;13(4–5):365–70.
83. Michelson JD, Checcone M, Kuhn T, Varner K. Intra-articular load distribution in the human ankle joint during motion. Foot Ankle Int. 2001;22(3):226–33.
84. Millington S, Grabner M, Wozelka R, Hurwitz S, Crandall J. A stereophotographic study of ankle joint contact area. J Orthop Res. 2007;25(11):1465–73.
85. Wan L, de Asla RJ, Rubash HE, Li G. Determination of in-vivo articular cartilage contact areas of human talocrural joint under weightbearing conditions. Osteoarthr Cartil. 2006;14(12):1294–301.
86. Windisch G, Odehnal B, Reimann R, Anderhuber F, Stachel H. Contact areas of the tibiotalar joint. J Orthop Res. 2007;25(11):1481–7.
87. Ward KA, Soames RW. Contact patterns at the tarsal joints. Clin Biomech (Bristol, Avon). 1997;12(7–8):496–507.
88. Beaudoin AJ, Fiore SM, Krause WR, Adelaar RS. Effect of isolated talocalcaneal fusion on contact in the ankle and talonavicular joints. Foot Ankle. 1991;12(1):19–25.
89. Macko VW, Matthews LS, Zwirkoski P, Goldstein SA. The joint-contact area of the ankle. The contribution of the posterior malleolus. J Bone Joint Surg Am. 1991;73(3):347–51.
90. Leardini A, O'Connor JJ, Catani F, Giannini S. The role of the passive structures in the mobility and stability of the human ankle joint: a literature review. Foot Ankle Int. 2000;21(7):602–15.
91. Wan L, de Asla RJ, Rubash HE, Li G. In vivo cartilage contact deformation of human ankle joints under full body weight. J Orthop Res. 2008;26(8):1081–9.
92. Haraguchi N, Armiger RS, Myerson MS, Campbell JT, Chao EY. Prediction of three-dimensional contact stress and ligament tension in the ankle during stance determined from computational modeling. Foot Ankle Int. 2009;30(2):177–85.

93. Benemerito I, Modenese L, Montefiori E, Mazza C, Viceconti M, Lacroix D, et al. An extended discrete element method for the estimation of contact pressure at the ankle joint during stance phase. Proc Inst Mech Eng H. 2020;234(5):507–16.
94. Tochigi Y, Rudert MJ, Saltzman CL, Amendola A, Brown TD. Contribution of articular surface geometry to ankle stabilization. J Bone Joint Surg Am. 2006;88(12):2704–13.
95. Park S, Lee S, Yoon J, Chae SW. Finite element analysis of knee and ankle joint during gait based on motion analysis. Med Eng Phys. 2019;63:33–41.
96. Scranton PE Jr, McMaster JG, Kelly E. Dynamic fibular function: a new concept. Clin Orthop Relat Res. 1976;118: 76–81.
97. Weinert CR Jr, McMaster JH, Ferguson RJ. Dynamic function of the human fibula. Am J Anat. 1973;138(2):145–9.
98. Takebe K, Nakagawa A, Minami H, Kanazawa H, Hirohata K. Role of the fibula in weight-bearing. Clin Orthop Relat Res. 1984;184:289–92.
99. Lambert KL. The weight-bearing function of the fibula. A strain gauge study. J Bone Joint Surg Am. 1971;53(3):507–13.
100. Goh JC, Mech AM, Lee EH, Ang EJ, Bayon P, Pho RW. Biomechanical study on the load-bearing characteristics of the fibula and the effects of fibular resection. Clin Orthop Relat Res. 1992;279:223–8.
101. Wang Q, Whittle M, Cunningham J, Kenwright J. Fibula and its ligaments in load transmission and ankle joint stability. Clin Orthop Relat Res. 1996;330:261–70.
102. Pacelli LL, Gillard J, McLoughlin SW, Buehler MJ. A biomechanical analysis of donor-site ankle instability following free fibular graft harvest. J Bone Joint Surg Am. 2003;85(4):597–603.

3 Biomechanical Considerations for Total Ankle Arthroplasty

With advances in understanding the biomechanics of the ankle, much progress has been made in total ankle arthroplasty in the last decades. This section aims to highlight the main achievements of the past years in terms of scientific knowledge and the requirements for a total ankle arthroplasty.

3.1 Biomechanical Changes in the Osteoarthritic Ankle

Patients with post-traumatic ankle (tibiotalar) osteoarthritis show significant changes in ankle joint kinematics [1–5]. Kozanek et al. [6] measured ankle kinematics in six patients [7] with unilateral post-traumatic ankle osteoarthritis using MRI and dual fluoroscopic imaging techniques. When results were compared to data from a regular cohort of a previous study [8], a significant decrease in the ankle range of motion was observed during gait and a breakdown of the normal hindfoot motion coupling [6]. Horisberger et al. [9] observed in 120 patients that plantar pressure distribution (measured using dynamic pedobarography) in patients with post-traumatic osteoarthritis was significantly different from the unaffected contralateral foot. The affected foot's maximum force and contact area were significantly lower, as pressured in the hindfoot and toe area. Furthermore, significant differences in plantar pressure distribution patterns occurred in patients with valgus and varus malalignment. No correlation was observed between plantar pressure distribution and functional outcome assessed by the AOFAS hindfoot score [9].

3.2 Kinematic Changes in Replaced Ankles

Advances in understanding the biomechanics of the ankle and improved surgical techniques of the new generation of total ankle arthroplasty have contributed to better reproducing the anatomy, physiological function, and kinematics of the ankle in total ankle arthroplasty.

Valderrabano et al. assessed kinematic changes after ankle fusion and total ankle arthroplasty about the range of motion [10], movement transfer [11], and talar movement [12]. All measurements were performed in native ankles, then in ankles with two components (Agility), then in ankles with a three-component prosthesis (Hintegra and STAR), and last but not least in fused ankles. They found near-normal kinematics after total ankle arthroplasty and significantly impaired results in fused ankles [10–12]. Komistek et al. [13] used fluoroscopy to evaluate translational and rotational motions of the hindfoot in the sagittal and frontal planes in ten subjects with a healthy ankle on one side and a total ankle arthroplasty on the opposite side (Buechel-Pappas prosthesis). The average range of motion for healthy versus replaced ankles was 37.4° and 32.3°, respectively. Comparable kinematic motion patterns were generally observed for healthy and replaced ankles [13].

The non-physiological articular surface geometry of the ankle implant will cause abnormal ankle joint kinematics and may lead to premature failure of total ankle arthroplasty [14, 15]. Most commercial ankle implants currently used in total ankle arthroplasty are non-physiological in terms of articular surface geometry adopted symmetric medial and lateral condyles and high conformity [16]. Although these ankle implants did not perform poorly in the short and medium term, the medium- and long-term results still needed to be better, compared with hip and knee arthroplasty [17]. In addition, previous studies have shown that asymmetric implants, which are more anatomically similar, such as Hintegra and Salto Talaris, can reduce the incidence of degenerative arthritis in adjacent joints and have a lower failure rate than symmetric implants [18–23]. Hintegra and Salto Talaris implants were designed with a lateral condyle radius larger than the medial condyle.

Motion recovery of the ankle joint after total ankle arthroplasty is closely related to the articular surface geometry of the implant [14, 24], and the patient with total ankle

B. Hintermann, R. Ruiz, *Total Ankle Replacement*, https://doi.org/10.1007/978-3-031-56810-7_3

arthroplasty still could not recover the best ankle functions due to the non-physiological articular surface geometry of the ankle implant [25]. Belvedere et al. [14] discovered that using natural surfaces, the talar dome with a saddle-shaped truncated cone produced mobility behavior near the ankle joint. Recently, Zhao et al. [26] designed a new anatomic talar component of total ankle arthroplasty, and the talus component was based on the 71 anatomic measurements of the Chinese talus dome. However, the detailed biomechanical differences between the anatomical articular geometry and non-physiological ankle implants are still unknown, as are the effects of variations in articular surface conformity on ankle forces, motions, and bone-implant interface interactions.

A conflicting problem remains in morphologic differences of the osteoarthritic ankle when compared to healthy controls. In a CT-based examination, Wiewiorski et al. [27] found a flattening of the talus that appeared more pronounced in the frontal aspect of the talus. The osteoarthritic talus sagittal arc radii were significantly larger than the control groups. Furthermore, the anteroposterior width and sagittal curvature of the distal tibia were significantly larger in osteoarthritic ankles than in normal ankles. However, most current ankle prostheses have been designed using morphometrics of only healthy ankles [28, 29].

3.3 Anatomical Restraints of Ankle Motion

The stability and integrity of the ankle joint depend on the articular geometry and ligamentous attachments. Ankle ligaments have a passive guiding and stabilizing effect on the ankle joint. On the medial side, the solid deep deltoid ligament is a secondary restraint against lateral and anterior talar excursion [30–32], whereas, on the lateral side, the relatively weak anterior talofibular ligament is the only restraint against anterior talar excursion [33–37]. The anterior talofibular ligament is most susceptible to injury and subsequent insufficiency [38–40], often leading to anterolateral dislocation of the talus out of the mortise and posterior dislocation of the fibula, respectively [41]. In such a case, reconstruction of the anterior talofibular ligament (or “ligament balancing”) may be advised when unconstrained prostheses are used for total ankle arthroplasty [42].

Rotation about a vertical axis occurs during gait [43, 44]. Rotatory stability is provided by the collateral ligaments, which, with their tension, compress the medial and lateral talar facets against their corresponding malleoli, and by the shape of the articular surfaces [31, 45–47]. Due to the truncated conical shape of the talus with its medially directed apex, the three lateral ligaments (anterior talofibular, posterior talofibular, and calcaneofibular ligaments) control the greater movement on the lateral side, whereas the deltoid ligament controls the lesser movement on the medial side. This has important implications for ligament balancing in total ankle arthroplasty, as non-anatomic prosthetic design and malposition of components may provoke medial ligament stress with consequent pain, posteromedial ossification, and loss of range of motion [20, 48] or lateral ligament insufficiency with consequent lateral ankle instability, respectively [41, 42].

During most activities, the ankle’s primary torsional and anteroposterior stabilizers are the soft tissues [49, 50]. In contrast, the ankle’s articulating surface geometry is the primary inversion/eversion stabilizer, with the collateral ligaments playing a secondary role (Fig. 3.1) [45, 47]. If a prosthesis does not provide intrinsic inversion and eversion stability, an unstable ankle will result, as noted by Burge and Evans [51]. They used a spherical, meniscal-bearing ankle design to observe the role of the surfaces in ankle stability. While the prosthesis provided inversion/eversion stability entirely, they found an anteroposterior laxity of 7 mm. The authors concluded that the anteroposterior restraint (as provided by the normal tibial articular surface, concave in the sagittal plane) might be lost when the surface is replaced by a flat prosthetic design. The more the geometry of the articular surfaces is changed from its physiological condition, the more the prosthesis depends upon the soft tissues for stability. A prosthesis should, therefore, be as anatomic as possible to mimic the physiological joint motion and guarantee proper ligament balancing.

The stability of the loaded ankle depends on its articular shape [31, 36, 45–47]. Stormont et al. [47] performed serial sectioning of the ankle ligaments and subjected the ankle to physiologic torque and loads. The articular surface accounted for 30% of ankle stability in rotation and 100% of ankle stability in inversion and eversion (Fig. 3.1). In a similar study, McCullough and Burge [45] found that increased ankle loading requires increased rotatory forces to cause displacement in any direction. The congruity of the articular surface of the ankle joint thus creates an inherently stable articulation with loading, and no ligamentous restraints exist in inversion and eversion. The articular surfaces provide the sole restraint of the joint under loaded conditions. This has important implications in the design of total ankle prostheses and may explain poor results with prosthetic designs that expose the ankle ligaments to eversion and inversion forces while the ankle is loaded [10]. Conversely, the ideal ankle prosthesis provides intrinsic stability against translational and rotational forces in all planes.

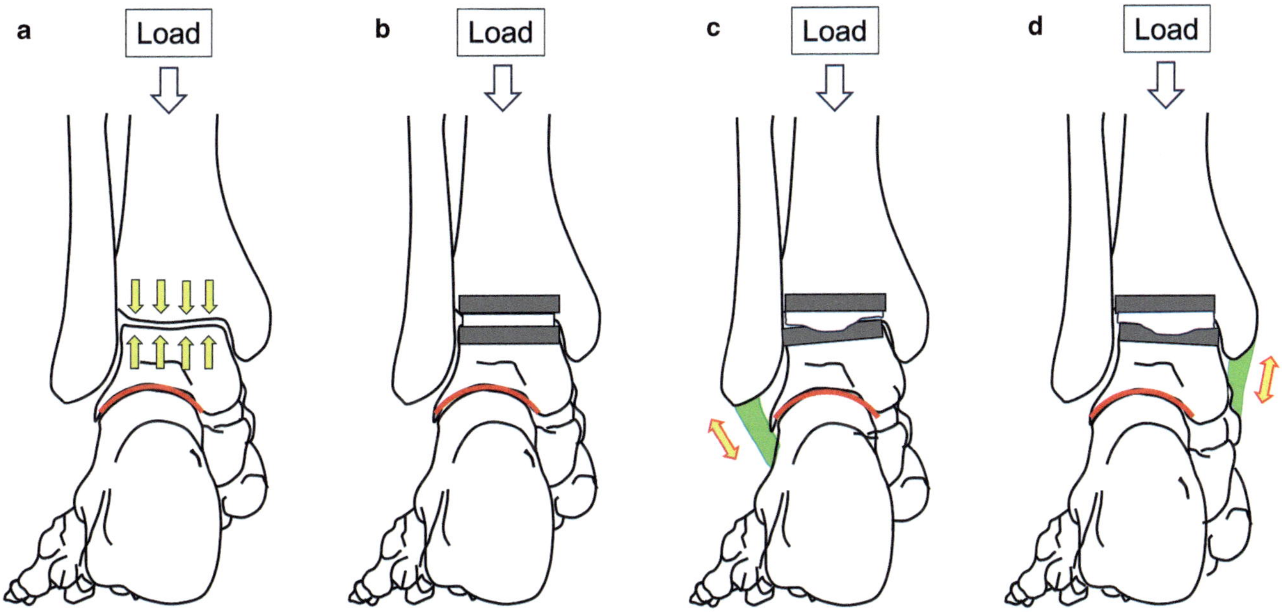

Fig. 3.1 The role of the surface in ankle stabilization, coronal plane. (**a**) Given the high congruency and the parallelism of tibiotalar articulating surface geometry, the ankle is the ankle joint's primary inversion/eversion stabilizer (see text). In contrast, the subtalar joint's rounded-shaped articular configuration does not stabilize the talus in the frontal plane. (**b**) An ankle prosthesis with parallel articulating surfaces, which imitates ankle biomechanics, will stabilize the coronal plane. A rounded articulating surface, in contrast, will permit some inversion/eversion movement at the interface and does rely on stabilization by the collateral ligaments. Therefore, when loading the foot, the lateral ligaments become stressed in a varus-type ankle (**c**), whereas the medial ligaments in a valgus-type ankle (**d**)

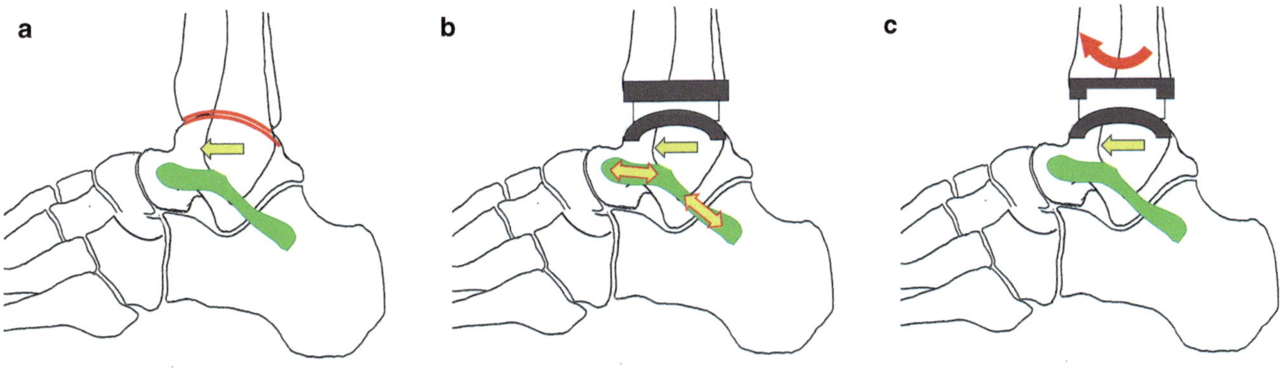

Fig. 3.2 The role of the surface in ankle stabilization, sagittal plane. (**a**) The concave articular configuration of the ankle stabilizes the talus against anterior translational forces of the talus, typically when downhill walking or during push-off by the created force of the Achilles tendon. (**b**) When replacing the ankle with a flat prosthetic surface and the inlayer is permitted to free translation, as the case for a mobile-bearing ankle, the ligaments are not protected, and they may be exposed to forces they cannot withstand, thereby overloading the peroneus brevis tendon. (**c**) In contrast, a fixed-bearing ankle provides sagittal plane stability, but the shear forces at the bone-implant interface increase, which may result in loosening

If the concave tibial surface is replaced by a flat surface analogously to total knee replacement, a forward motion of the talus no longer results in tibiotalar separation, and the stabilizing influence of joint load is absent [52]. A flat prosthetic surface does not protect the ligaments and may expose them to forces they cannot withstand (Fig. 3.2). Stauffer et al. [53] calculated an anteroposterior shear force of 70% of body weight during walking. This study shows the importance of bony and ligamentous anteroposterior restraints for the continuous neutralization of the shear force on the ankle joint. Restoration of correct soft-tissue tension is, then, mandatory with the use of unconstrained ankle prostheses, and this can only be achieved with anatomically shaped devices.

3.4 Contact Area of the Ankle

The complex geometry of the mortise and trochlea of the talus influences load characteristics [54–61]. Reports of whole ankle contact area vary from 1.5 to 9.4 cm^2, depending on load and ankle position [55, 62–67]. Calhoun et al. [55] found that contact surface area increased from plantarflexion to dorsiflexion and that force per unit area decreased proportionately. They also observed that the medial and lateral facets had the greatest contact with the malleoli in dorsiflexion. In another study using a dynamic model, progressive lateral loading with concomitant medial unloading was observed during dorsiflexion and associated external rotation [66]. Further, for load-bearing human joints, it has been widely shown that a sufficiently sized area of congruent contact is the most desirable interface condition when using a deformable surface (e.g., polyethylene) against metal [52, 68]. All these findings implicate the need to achieve a physiological joint contact area in total ankle arthroplasty with an appropriately aligned and adequately balanced hindfoot.

3.5 Axial Load, Shear, and Stress Forces at the Ankle Joint

A vertical load on the ankle is 5.2 times body weight during gait [53]. In diseased ankles, the joint load decreased to approximately three times body weight; the same values were noted in replaced ankles. Anteroposterior and lateral shear forces during gait were estimated to reach two and three times body weight levels, respectively. The vertical load transmitted to the trabecular bone at the prosthesis-bone interface may exceed the inherent trabecular bone strength reached in normal daily activities. With an interface area of 7 cm^2, the average compressive load per unit area at the interface during gait would be approximately 3.5 MPa in a patient of 700 N body weight [53]. More strenuous physical activity could result in a much higher unit load, provoking a collapse of the cancellous bone surface of the tibia. Bone remodeling, however, may increase the inherent strength of the bone. Estimations suggest that at least three times higher bone strength than the aforementioned values must be reached to meet the requirements of daily physical activities if collapse is to be prevented [69].

Ground reaction, gravitational, ligament, and muscle forces produce a mixture of three-dimensional compressive, shear, and torsional loads to the ankle joint. Therefore, one may easily assume that force is not necessarily directly perpendicular to the bone-implant interface but more angular. This introduces shear forces in addition to those of direct compression. Furthermore, force vectors on a prosthesis are not necessarily central; instead, the point of application of many force vectors is often eccentric. This might show that when an eccentric force is placed on the medial side of the tibial prosthesis, there will be a downward force vector on the medial side and a corresponding lift-off or compressive neutralizing force on the lateral side. This same phenomenon can also occur in the anteroposterior direction. The repeated contralateral force equalization might lead to micro-instability and micromotion. More than 0.15 mm micromotion will prevent bony ingrowth into a prosthetic implant [69] and could eventually lead to the loosening of the implant, especially in the early integration stage. Even after bony ingrowth, such continuous tilting stress may provoke failure of the bone-implant interface and consequent implant loosening or contiguous constraint at the implant-polyethylene interface and consequent polyethylene wear. Implant design and hindfoot alignment must accommodate the joint forces encountered during daily activities, especially walking and climbing stairs.

Generally, the bigger the ankle prosthesis, the bigger the potential joint lever arms and moments and the shear forces at the bone-implant interface are, as created, for instance, by inversion/eversion torques (Fig. 3.3). The importance of using anatomically shaped components in total ankle arthroplasty, thereby avoiding excessive contact stress on the supporting bone, has been stated by Kempson et al. [70] in an in vivo study. They found that after total ankle arthroplasty, ankle fractures occurred with 30% less force when a twisting motion was applied. Theoretically, the ideal ankle prosthesis should be small (necessitating minimal bone resection), as anatomic as possible (to mimic the physiological joint motion and guarantee proper ligament balancing), and consist of three components (to allow for unconstrained motion) [11, 71–74].

The contact stress at the bone-implant interface also depends on contact area size: the bigger the contact area, the smaller the mean contact stress. With increased contact area, however, peak stresses can increase by the prosthesis' eccentric loading (edge loading), contributing to prosthetic loosening [71]. Based on the experience and personal opinion of the authors, to minimize counterproductive joint contact stress, the ideal ankle prosthesis should have a large contact area between the contact surfaces, the point of load application should fall within the central third of the components, the ankle should be well aligned, and the ligaments should be well balanced.

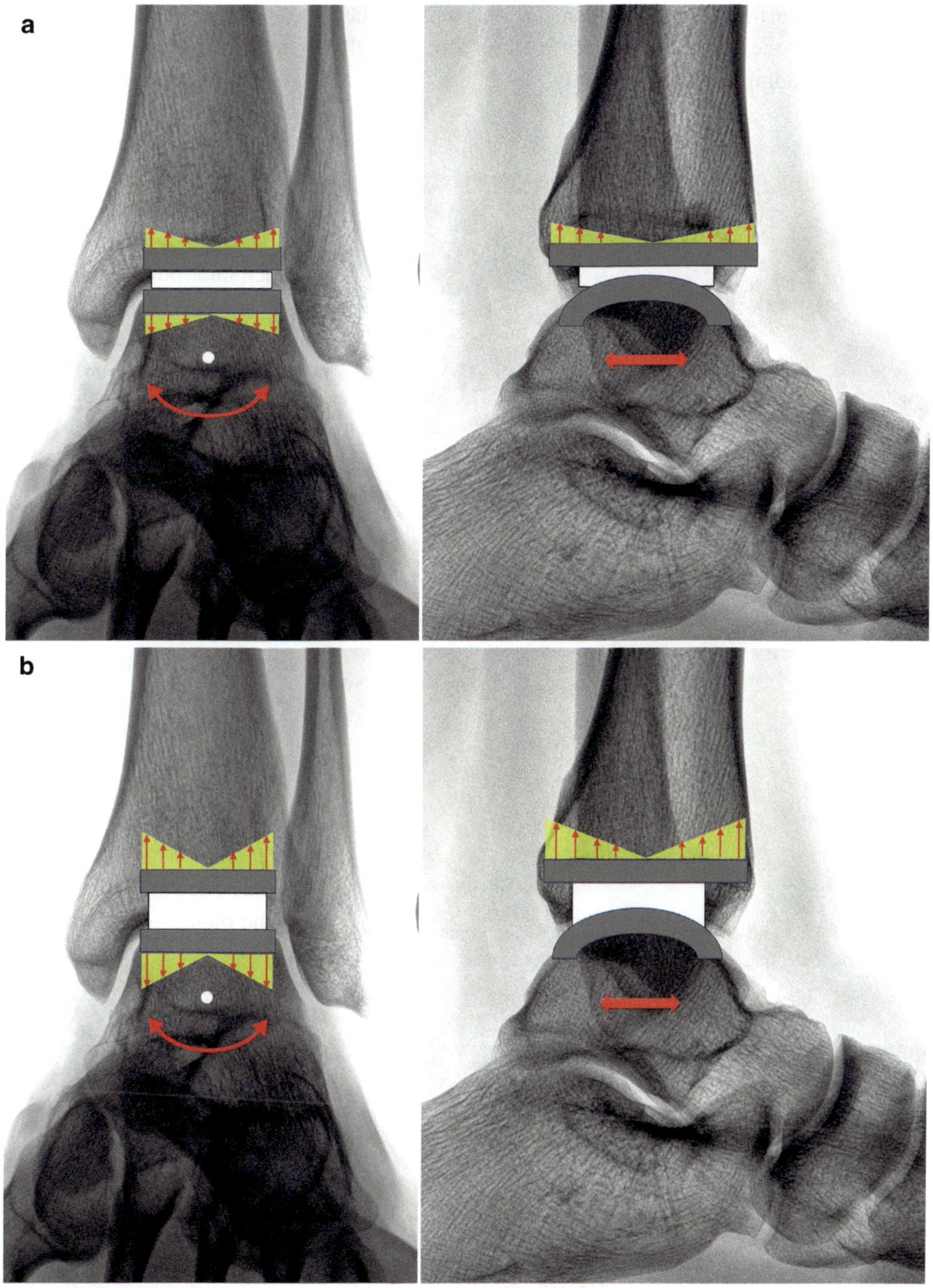

Fig. 3.3 Relationship of prosthetic size and shear forces at the bone-implant interface. The bigger the prosthesis, the bigger the created shear forces at the bone-implant interface. (**a**) Small prosthesis; (**b**) big prosthesis

3.6 Bone Support at the Ankle

Proper bone support is fundamental to the success of any prosthetic arthroplasty. Lowery [75] found that the subchondral bone of the distal tibia has an elastic modulus in the order of 300 MPa to 450 MPa. After the removal of the subchondral plate, compressive resistance decreased by a range of 30% to 50% and, with sectioning of the subchondral bone 1 cm proximal to the subchondral plate, by a range of 70–90% (Fig. 2.5). In another laboratory study, Hvid et al. [76] found the talar bone to be 40% stronger than the tibial bone.

Bone quality in the distal tibia and talus is essential to initial component stability in total ankle arthroplasty. Using measurements on axial cut CTs from 6 to 12 mm above the tibial plafond and 1–4 mm below the talar dome, Harnroongroj et al. [77] found that ankle osteoarthritis patients demonstrated greater or equal bone density in the tibia and talus compared to demographic-matched controls. In both groups, bone density decreased with increasing distance away from the articular surface, indicating that, in total ankle arthroplasty, tibial bone resection between 6 and 8 mm may provide improved initial implant stability.

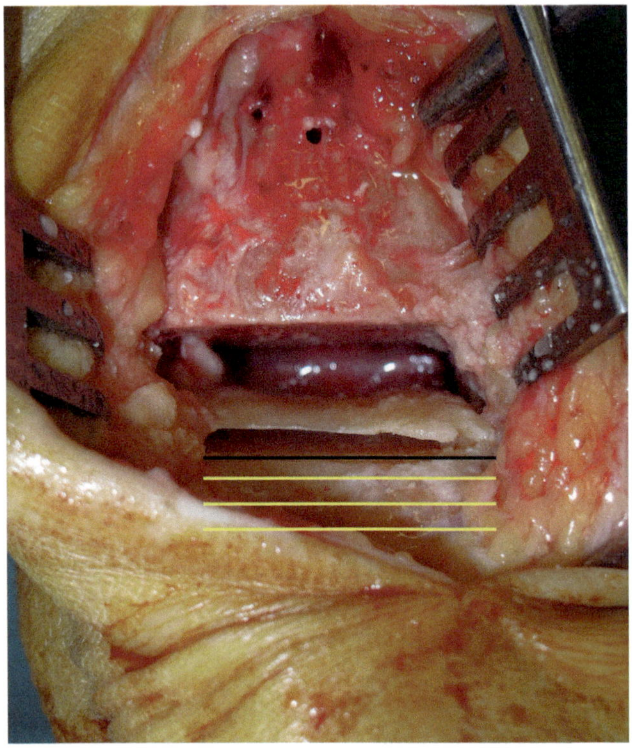

Fig. 3.4 Talar bone compressive resistance. The compressive resistance of bone decreases with the amount of bone resection on the talar body (see text)

Calderale et al. [78] found that removing part of the cortical shell of the talus placed abnormally increased stress on the remaining talar cancellous bone (Fig. 3.4). In other words, when part of the cortical shell of the talus is removed at the time of arthroplasty, the remaining bone must support a greater load than it did before arthroplasty. Ideally, the talar component of the prosthesis should be anatomically sized, fully cover the talar body, and have broad support on the talar neck. As much talar bone as possible should be saved, particularly the anterior part of the body and neck. To avoid the collapse of the bone, minimal bone resection should be performed so that the stronger superficial subchondral bone is preserved. Furthermore, conserving as much bone as possible during surgery helps ensure better support and saves bone, which may be valuable should revision become necessary [79].

Hvid et al. [76] also found an eccentricity of the area of maximal bone strength of the distal tibia that is posteromedial and not central (Fig. 2.4). This area of stiffer bone could act as a pivot point, with the risk of overloading the surrounding weaker anterolateral bone. To avoid "off-center" forces on a prosthesis and possible collapse of the weak lateral tibia, proper prosthesis alignment and adequate ligament balancing of the ankle must be achieved. In particular, valgus malalignment should be corrected.

Most ankle prostheses use anchoring features, e.g., stems and pegs, to enhance stability (Fig. 4.9). However, their effect may be limited as they extend into the weaker metaphyseal bone with reduced trabecular strength. On the contrary, if the bone is sclerotic, it may hinder complete contact with the prosthetic surface with the resection surface of the underlying bone, thus acting as a stress shield (Fig. 3.5). This was

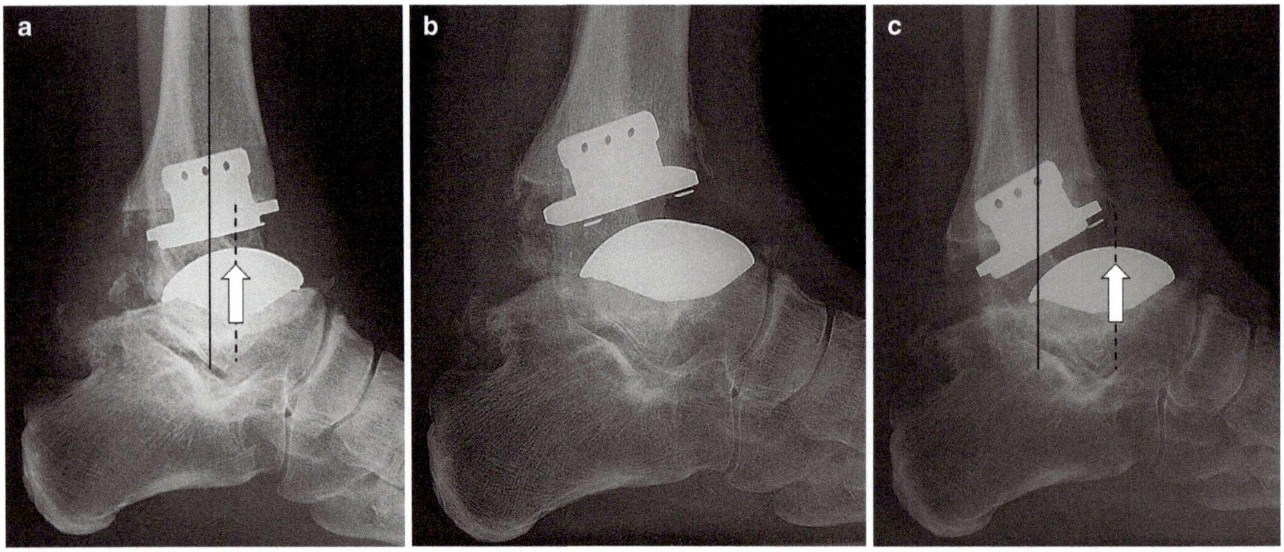

Fig. 3.5 Impact of insufficient implant-bone contact. A 62-year-old patient with post-traumatic osteoarthritis underwent total ankle arthroplasty with a Salto ankle using a fin-bar feature to anchor the tibial component. (**a**) The tibial component was not correctly inserted, leaving a significant gap between the component and the bone. (**b**) Due to a too-anterior positioning of the talar component, the primary load transfer occurred in the anterior ankle, resulting in an increasing tilt, as seen after 6 months. (**c**) Three months later, the component is seen to have tilted more and impacted into the anterior tibial plafond. The weakening of the anterior ledge of the tibia by creating a window for inserting the component may have favored this process

substantiated by the investigations of Ficklscherer et al. [80] using thermoelastic stress analysis. They demonstrated that load transmission accumulates with high maxima around the anchoring systems. Ideally, the tibial component should be anatomically sized, fully cover the tibial plafond, not weaken the cortical rim, and have broad support on the cortical rim of the distal tibia.

Total joint arthroplasties of the hip and knee have demonstrated the fundamental importance of proper bone support. The reason for many failures of joint arthroplasties was the excessive bone removal necessary to insert a bulky prosthesis. Revision surgery after removing such implants is challenging due to a large amount of bone loss at the initial surgery. Fortunately, after a failed total knee or hip arthroplasty, it is often possible to revise the arthroplasty with long-stem implants, which makes it possible to bypass the area of bone loss. In the ankle, however, a long-stem prosthesis is not an option for revision, particularly not on the talar side.

3.7 Gait Changes

In gait analysis, ankle osteoarthritis showed a significant deficiency in six of seven spatiotemporal variables, a decrease of the triplanar ankle movement, a decrease of the second active maximal vertical and the maximal medial ground reaction force, a reduction of the sagittal and transverse ankle joint moments, and a reduction of the ankle joint power [7]. Three months after total ankle arthroplasty surgery, patients experienced a worsening gait. At 12 months follow-up, all spatiotemporal variables were not different from the usual subjects (full rehabilitation); in 6 of 11 kinematic and kinetic variables, there was a partial rehabilitation [7]. Detrembleur and Leemrijse [81] addressed the effects of total ankle arthroplasty on gait disability by analyzing energetic and mechanical variables. They found that total ankle arthroplasty has a beneficial effect on locomotor function, improving the AOFAS score, speed, spatiotemporal parameters, ankle amplitude instance, and vertical center of mass displacement [81]. Brodsky et al. [82] confirmed these results in 33 patients at a mean follow-up of 7.6 years. Patients improved in multiple objective parameters of gait compared with preoperative function [82]. The gait patterns of patients following total ankle arthroplasty more closely resembled normal gait compared to the gait patterns of patients following arthrodesis, dorsal motion in the sagittal plane being primarily responsible for the differences [83–86]. When comparing differences in gait mechanics in patients with a fixed- versus mobile-bearing total ankle arthroplasty, Queen et al. [87] could demonstrate no statistically or clinically meaningful difference when examining gait mechanics and pain 1 year after total ankle arthroplasty.

Although total ankle arthroplasty did not restore gait to that of healthy controls, improvements across nearly all gait parameters have been observed, with gait function approaching that of controls [7, 83, 88]. When compared with preoperative function, total ankle arthroplasty demonstrated a marked improvement [83–85, 87, 89–91].

3.8 Conclusions

- A total ankle prosthesis should be as anatomic as possible to mimic the unique requirements of the ankle.
- The tibiotalar articulating surfaces should provide eversion and inversion stability.
- With the use of a mobile-bearing ankle, anteroposterior stability of the replaced ankle joint is provided by ligaments. Proper ligament balancing should be achieved using precise implantation techniques and anatomic surfaces.
- Bone resection should be minimal to ensure optimal support and to save the bone, which is valuable should revision become necessary.
- The high contact area between the component and the bone is the base of a complete and stable bonding; this, in turn, reduces strain shielding and micromotion.
- To minimize contact stress and to avoid edge loading, the ankle prosthesis should have a large contact area between the surfaces, the point of load application should fall within the central third of the components, the ankle should be well aligned, and the ligaments should be well balanced.
- One of the limiting factors in assessing the success of total ankle arthroplasty is differentiating improvements based on pain relief versus biomechanical changes at the joint.

References

1. Brown TD, Johnston RC, Saltzman CL, Marsh JL, Buckwalter JA. Posttraumatic osteoarthritis: a first estimate of incidence, prevalence, and burden of disease. J Orthop Trauma. 2006;20(10):739–44.
2. Demetriades L, Strauss E, Gallina J. Osteoarthritis of the ankle. Clin Orthop Relat Res. 1998;349:28–42.
3. Saltzman CL, Zimmerman MB, O'Rourke M, Brown TD, Buckwalter JA, Johnston R. Impact of comorbidities on the measurement of health in patients with ankle osteoarthritis. J Bone Joint Surg Am. 2006;88(11):2366–72.
4. Thomas RH, Daniels TR. Ankle arthritis. J Bone Joint Surg Am. 2003;85(5):923–36.
5. Zeininger A, Schmitt D, Hughes-Oliver C, Queen RM. The effect of ankle osteoarthritis and total ankle arthroplasty on center of pressure position. J Orthop Res. 2021;39(6):1245–52.
6. Kozanek M, Rubash HE, Li G, de Asla RJ. Effect of post-traumatic tibiotalar osteoarthritis on kinematics of the ankle joint complex. Foot Ankle Int. 2009;30(8):734–40.

7. Valderrabano V, Nigg BM, von Tscharner V, Stefanyshyn DJ, Goepfert B, Hintermann B. Gait analysis in ankle osteoarthritis and total ankle replacement. Clin Biomech (Bristol, Avon). 2007;22(8):894–904.
8. de Asla RJ, Wan L, Rubash HE, Li G. Six DOF in vivo kinematics of the ankle joint complex: application of a combined dual-orthogonal fluoroscopic and magnetic resonance imaging technique. J Orthop Res. 2006;24(5):1019–27.
9. Horisberger M, Hintermann B, Valderrabano V. Alterations of plantar pressure distribution in posttraumatic end-stage ankle osteoarthritis. Clin Biomech (Bristol, Avon). 2009;24(3):303–7.
10. Valderrabano V, Hintermann B, Nigg BM, Stefanyshyn D, Stergiou P. Kinematic changes after fusion and total replacement of the ankle: part 1: range of motion. Foot Ankle Int. 2003;24(12):881–7.
11. Valderrabano V, Hintermann B, Nigg BM, Stefanyshyn D, Stergiou P. Kinematic changes after fusion and total replacement of the ankle: part 2: movement transfer. Foot Ankle Int. 2003;24(12):888–96.
12. Valderrabano V, Hintermann B, Nigg BM, Stefanyshyn D, Stergiou P. Kinematic changes after fusion and total replacement of the ankle: part 3: talar movement. Foot Ankle Int. 2003;24(12):897–900.
13. Komistek RD, Stiehl JB, Buechel FF, Northcut EJ, Hajner ME. A determination of ankle kinematics using fluoroscopy. Foot Ankle Int. 2000;21(4):343–50.
14. Belvedere C, Siegler S, Ensini A, Toy J, Caravaggi P, Namani R, et al. Experimental evaluation of current and novel approximations of articular surfaces of the ankle joint. J Biomech. 2018;75:159–63.
15. Zhang Y, Chen Z, Zhao H, Zhao D, Zhang X, Ma X, et al. Comparison of joint load, motions and contact stress and bone-implant interface micromotion of three implant designs for total ankle arthroplasty. Comput Methods Prog Biomed. 2022;223:106976.
16. Gross CE, Palanca AA, DeOrio JK. Design rationale for total ankle arthroplasty systems: an update. J Am Acad Orthop Surg. 2018;26(10):353–9.
17. Currier BH, Hecht PJ, Nunley JA 2nd, Mayor MB, Currier JH, Van Citters DW. Analysis of failed ankle arthroplasty components. Foot Ankle Int. 2019;40(2):131–8.
18. Zhao D, Huang D, Zhang G, Wang X, Zhang T, Ma X. Positive and negative factors for the treatment outcomes following total ankle arthroplasty? A systematic review. Foot Ankle Surg. 2020;26(1):1–13.
19. Harston A, Lazarides AL, Adams SB Jr, DeOrio JK, Easley ME, Nunley JA 2nd. Midterm outcomes of a fixed-bearing total ankle arthroplasty with deformity analysis. Foot Ankle Int. 2017;38(12):1295–300.
20. Brunner S, Barg A, Knupp M, Zwicky L, Kapron AL, Valderrabano V, et al. The Scandinavian total ankle replacement: long-term, eleven to fifteen-year, survivorship analysis of the prosthesis in seventy-two consecutive patients. J Bone Joint Surg Am. 2013;95(8):711–8.
21. Kvarda P, Peterhans US, Susdorf R, Barg A, Ruiz R, Hintermann B. Long-term survival of HINTEGRA total ankle replacement in 683 patients: a concise 20-year follow-up of a previous report. J Bone Joint Surg Am. 2022;104:881.
22. Bonnin M, Gaudot F, Laurent JR, Ellis S, Colombier JA, Judet T. The Salto total ankle arthroplasty: survivorship and analysis of failures at 7 to 11 years. Clin Orthop Relat Res. 2011;469(1):225–36.
23. Bonnin M, Judet T, Colombier JA, Buscayret F, Graveleau N, Piriou P. Midterm results of the Salto total ankle prosthesis. Clin Orthop Relat Res. 2004;424:6–18.
24. Deleu PA, Besse JL, Naaim A, Leemrijse T, Birch I, Devos Bevernage B, et al. Change in gait biomechanics after total ankle replacement and ankle arthrodesis: a systematic review and meta-analysis. Clin Biomech (Bristol, Avon). 2020;73:213–25.
25. Lullini G, Caravaggi P, Leardini A, Ortolani M, Mazzotti A, Giannini S, et al. Retrospective comparison between a two- and three-component ankle arthroplasty: clinical and functional evaluation via gait analysis. Clin Biomech (Bristol, Avon). 2020;80:105180.
26. Zhao DH, Huang DC, Zhang GH, Fan YP, Yu J, Wang SB, et al. Talar dome investigation and Talocrural joint Axis analysis based on three-dimensional (3D) models: implications for prosthetic design. Biomed Res Int. 2019;2019:8634159.
27. Wiewiorski M, Hoechel S, Anderson AE, Nowakowski AM, DeOrio JK, Easley ME, et al. Computed tomographic evaluation of joint geometry in patients with end-stage ankle osteoarthritis. Foot Ankle Int. 2016;37(6):644–51.
28. Kakkar R, Siddique MS. Stresses in the ankle joint and total ankle replacement design. Foot Ankle Surg. 2011;17(2):58–63.
29. Kuo CC, Lu HL, Leardini A, Lu TW, Kuo MY, Hsu HC. Three-dimensional computer graphics-based ankle morphometry with computerized tomography for total ankle replacement design and positioning. Clin Anat. 2014;27(4):659–68.
30. Boss AP, Hintermann B. Anatomical study of the medial ankle ligament complex. Foot Ankle Int. 2002;23(6):547–53.
31. Harper MC. Deltoid ligament: an anatomical evaluation of function. Foot Ankle. 1987;8(1):19–22.
32. Hintermann B. Medial ankle instability. Foot Ankle Clin. 2003;8(4):723–38.
33. Stagni R, Leardini A, O'Connor JJ, Giannini S. Role of passive structures in the mobility and stability of the human subtalar joint: a literature review. Foot Ankle Int. 2003;24(5):402–9.
34. Milner CE, Soames RW. Anatomy of the collateral ligaments of the human ankle joint. Foot Ankle Int. 1998;19(11):757–60.
35. Renstrom P, Wertz M, Incavo S, Pope M, Ostgaard HC, Arms S, et al. Strain in the lateral ligaments of the ankle. Foot Ankle. 1988;9(2):59–63.
36. Hintermann B, Ruiz R. Foot and ankle instability—a clinical guide to diagnosis and surgical management. 1st ed. Springer International Publishing; 2021.
37. Hintermann B. Biomechanics of the unstable ankle joint and clinical implications. Med Sci Sports Exerc. 1999;31(7 Suppl):S459–69.
38. Baumhauer JF, Alosa DM, Renstrom AF, Trevino S, Beynnon B. A prospective study of ankle injury risk factors. Am J Sports Med. 1995;23(5):564–70.
39. Burks RT, Morgan J. Anatomy of the lateral ankle ligaments. Am J Sports Med. 1994;22(1):72–7.
40. Johnson EE, Markolf KL. The contribution of the anterior talofibular ligament to ankle laxity. J Bone Joint Surg Am. 1983;65(1):81–8.
41. Hintermann B, Ruiz R. Joint preservation strategies for managing varus ankle deformities. Foot Ankle Clin. 2022;27(1):37–56.
42. Hintermann B, Ruiz R. Total replacement of varus ankle: three-component prosthesis design. Foot Ankle Clin. 2019;24(2):305–24.
43. Close JR. Some applications of the functional anatomy of the ankle joint. J Bone Joint Surg Am. 1956;38-A(4):761–81.
44. Levens AS, Inman VT, Blosser JA. Transverse rotation of the segments of the lower extremity in locomotion. J Bone Joint Surg Am. 1948;30A(4):859–72.
45. McCullough CJ, Burge PD. Rotatory stability of the load-bearing ankle. An experimental study. J Bone Joint Surg Br. 1980;62-B(4):460–4.
46. Sommer C, Hintermann B, Nigg BM, van den Bogert AJ. Influence of ankle ligaments on tibial rotation: an in vitro study. Foot Ankle Int. 1996;17(2):79–84.
47. Stormont DM, Morrey BF, An KN, Cass JR. Stability of the loaded ankle. Relation between articular restraint and primary and secondary static restraints. Am J Sports Med. 1985;13(5):295–300.
48. Valderrabano V, Hintermann B, Dick W. Scandinavian total ankle replacement: a 3.7-year average follow-up of 65 patients. Clin Orthop Relat Res. 2004;424:47–56.
49. Cass JR, Morrey BF, Chao EY. Three-dimensional kinematics of ankle instability following serial sectioning of lateral collateral ligaments. Foot Ankle. 1984;5(3):142–9.
50. Cass JR, Settles H. Ankle instability: in vitro kinematics in response to axial load. Foot Ankle Int. 1994;15(3):134–40.

51. Burge P, Evans M. Effect of surface replacement arthroplasty on stability of the ankle. Foot Ankle. 1986;7(1):10–7.
52. Markolf KL, Bargar WL, Shoemaker SC, Amstutz HC. The role of joint load in knee stability. J Bone Joint Surg Am. 1981;63(4):570–85.
53. Stauffer RN, Chao EY, Brewster RC. Force and motion analysis of the normal, diseased, and prosthetic ankle joint. Clin Orthop Relat Res. 1977;127:189–96.
54. Beaudoin AJ, Fiore SM, Krause WR, Adelaar RS. Effect of isolated talocalcaneal fusion on contact in the ankle and talonavicular joints. Foot Ankle. 1991;12(1):19–25.
55. Calhoun JH, Li F, Ledbetter BR, Viegas SF. A comprehensive study of pressure distribution in the ankle joint with inversion and eversion. Foot Ankle Int. 1994;15(3):125–33.
56. Lundberg A, Svensson OK, Nemeth G, Selvik G. The axis of rotation of the ankle joint. J Bone Joint Surg Br. 1989;71(1):94–9.
57. Macko VW, Matthews LS, Zwirkoski P, Goldstein SA. The joint-contact area of the ankle. The contribution of the posterior malleolus. J Bone Joint Surg Am. 1991;73(3):347–51.
58. Tarr RR, Resnick CT, Wagner KS, Sarmiento A. Changes in tibiotalar joint contact areas following experimentally induced tibial angular deformities. Clin Orthop Relat Res. 1985;199:72–80.
59. Inman VT. The joints of the ankle. Baltimore, MD: Williams & Wilkins; 1976.
60. Hicks JH. The mechanics of the foot. I. The joints. J Anat. 1953;87(4):345–57.
61. Barnett CH, Napier JR. The axis of rotation at the ankle joint in man; its influence upon the form of the talus and the mobility of the fibula. J Anat. 1952;86(1):1–9.
62. Ward KA, Soames RW. Contact patterns at the tarsal joints. Clin Biomech (Bristol, Avon). 1997;12(7–8):496–507.
63. Kura H, Kitaoka HB, Luo ZP, An KN. Measurement of surface contact area of the ankle joint. Clin Biomech (Bristol, Avon). 1998;13(4–5):365–70.
64. Wan L, de Asla RJ, Rubash HE, Li G. Determination of in-vivo articular cartilage contact areas of human talocrural joint under weightbearing conditions. Osteoarthr Cartil. 2006;14(12):1294–301.
65. Millington S, Grabner M, Wozelka R, Hurwitz S, Crandall J. A stereophotographic study of ankle joint contact area. J Orthop Res. 2007;25(11):1465–73.
66. Michelson JD, Checcone M, Kuhn T, Varner K. Intra-articular load distribution in the human ankle joint during motion. Foot Ankle Int. 2001;22(3):226–33.
67. Windisch G, Odehnal B, Reimann R, Anderhuber F, Stachel H. Contact areas of the tibiotalar joint. J Orthop Res. 2007;25(11):1481–7.
68. Buechel FF, Pappas MJ, Iorio LJ. New Jersey low contact stress total ankle replacement: biomechanical rationale and review of 23 cementless cases. Foot Ankle. 1988;8(6):279–90.
69. Muhlhofer H, Ercan Y, Drews S, Matsuura M, Meissner J, Linsenmaier U, et al. Mineralisation and mechanical strength of the subchondral bone plate of the inferior tibial facies. Surg Radiol Anat. 2009;31(4):237–43.
70. Kempson GE, Freeman MA, Tuke MA. Engineering considerations in the design of an ankle joint. Biomed Eng. 1975;10(5):166–71, 80.
71. Jyoti, Mondal S, Ghosh R. Biomechanical analysis of three popular tibial designs for TAR with different implant-bone interfacial conditions and bone qualities: a finite element study. Med Eng Phys. 2022;104:103812.
72. Richter D, Krahenbuhl N, Susdorf R, Barg A, Ruiz R, Hintermann B. What are the indications for implant revision in three-component total ankle arthroplasty? Clin Orthop Relat Res. 2021;479(3): 601–9.
73. Hintermann B, Knupp M, Zwicky L, Barg A. Total ankle replacement for treatment of end-stage osteoarthritis in elderly patients. J Aging Res. 2012;2012:345237.
74. Barg A, Knupp M, Henninger HB, Zwicky L, Hintermann B. Total ankle replacement using HINTEGRA, an unconstrained, three-component system: surgical technique and pitfalls. Foot Ankle Clin. 2012;17(4):607–35.
75. Lowery RB. Fractures of the talus and os calcis. Opin Orthop. 1005;6:25–34.
76. Hvid I, Rasmussen O, Jensen NC, Nielsen S. Trabecular bone strength profiles at the ankle joint. Clin Orthop Relat Res. 1985;199:306–12.
77. Harnroongroj T, Volpert LG, Ellis SJ, Sofka CM, Deland JT, Demetracopoulos CA. Comparison of tibial and talar bone density in patients undergoing total ankle replacement vs non-ankle arthritis matched controls. Foot Ankle Int. 2019;40(12):1408–15.
78. Calderale PM, Garro A, Barbiero R, Fasolio G, Pipino F. Biomechanical design of the total ankle prosthesis. Eng Med. 1983;12(2):69–80.
79. Hintermann B, Zwicky L, Knupp M, Henninger HB, Barg A. HINTEGRA revision arthroplasty for failed total ankle prostheses. J Bone Joint Surg Am. 2013;95(13):1166–74.
80. Ficklscherer A, Wegener B, Niethammer T, Pietschmann MF, Muller PE, Jansson V, et al. Thermoelastic stress analysis to validate tibial fixation technique in total ankle prostheses—a pilot study. Ulus Travma Acil Cerrahi Derg. 2013;19(2):98–102.
81. Detrembleur C, Leemrijse T. The effects of total ankle replacement on gait disability: analysis of energetic and mechanical variables. Gait Posture. 2009;29(2):270–4.
82. Brodsky JW, Scott DJ, Ford S, Coleman S, Daoud Y. Functional outcomes of total ankle arthroplasty at a mean follow-up of 7.6 years: a prospective, 3-dimensional gait analysis. J Bone Joint Surg Am. 2021;103(6):477–82.
83. Singer S, Klejman S, Pinsker E, Houck J, Daniels T. Ankle arthroplasty and ankle arthrodesis: gait analysis compared with normal controls. J Bone Joint Surg Am. 2013;95(24):e191.
84. Flavin R, Coleman SC, Tenenbaum S, Brodsky JW. Comparison of gait after total ankle arthroplasty and ankle arthrodesis. Foot Ankle Int. 2013;34(10):1340–8.
85. Brodsky JW, Polo FE, Coleman SC, Bruck N. Changes in gait following the Scandinavian total ankle replacement. J Bone Joint Surg Am. 2011;93(20):1890–6.
86. Choi JH, Coleman SC, Tenenbaum S, Polo FE, Brodsky JW. Prospective study of the effect on gait of a two component total ankle replacement. Foot Ankle Int. 2013;34(11):1472–8.
87. Queen RM, Franck CT, Schmitt D, Adams SB. Are there differences in gait mechanics in patients with a fixed versus mobile bearing total ankle arthroplasty? A randomized trial. Clin Orthop Relat Res. 2017;475(10):2599–606.
88. Doets HC, van Middelkoop M, Houdijk H, Nelissen RG, Veeger HE. Gait analysis after successful mobile bearing total ankle replacement. Foot Ankle Int. 2007;28(3):313–22.
89. Piriou P, Culpan P, Mullins M, Cardon JN, Pozzi D, Judet T. Ankle replacement versus arthrodesis: a comparative gait analysis study. Foot Ankle Int. 2008;29(1):3–9.
90. Queen RM, De Biassio JC, Butler RJ, DeOrio JK, Easley ME, Nunley JA. J. Leonard Goldner award 2011: changes in pain, function, and gait mechanics two years following total ankle arthroplasty performed with two modern fixed-bearing prostheses. Foot Ankle Int. 2012;33(7):535–42.
91. Queen RM, Butler RJ, Adams SB Jr, DeOrio JK, Easley ME, Nunley JA. Bilateral differences in gait mechanics following total ankle replacement: a two year longitudinal study. Clin Biomech (Bristol, Avon). 2014;29(4):418–22.

4 Basic Considerations for Total Ankle Arthroplasty

There is 1 bone above the ankle and 26 bones and as many joints below it that can affect the alignment and functioning of the ankle joint. The normal soft-tissue envelope around the ankle is thin, and because of possible antecedent trauma and initial surgical repairs, this envelope is often scarred and inelastic. These same issues, combined with the post-traumatic period of immobilization, lack of physical therapy, chronic pain, and progressive periarticular bone formation, often lead to significant loss of ankle joint motion. In addition, progressive joint incongruency, destruction of the articular surfaces, and talar dislocation out of the ankle mortise may cause alteration of ankle joint mechanics, malalignment of the hindfoot, and destabilization of the ankle joint complex.

Human joint replacement design is generally subject to anatomically and functionally based expectations, mechanical and material resistance analysis, surgical and clinical requirements, and industrial and manufacturing constraints. For total ankle arthroplasty, the specific challenges are to restore the original anatomy and biomechanics, to provide stability in the coronal plane against e-/inversion and in the sagittal plane against anterior extrusion of the talus, and to be feasible because of the small dimension of bones and limited surgical exposure. As with other joint replacements, firm fixation to the bone and stable bone-component interface over time are mandatory for the success of the replacement surgery.

Another dilemma the surgeon is confronted with is between mobile- and fixed-bearing designs. Unconstrained or semi-constrained designs may provide more mobility but require incongruent contact, thereby giving rise to large contact stresses and potentially high wear rates. Conversely, congruent designs may produce large contact areas with low contact stresses but transmit undesirable constraint forces that can overload the fixation system at the bone-component interface.

In summary, though the market has progressed in total ankle arthroplasty over the last decade(s), many controversies exist in dealing with total ankle arthroplasty. This section may help guide the choice of ankle prostheses and inform future implant design, thus aiding surgeons in achieving better post-implantation outcomes through an enhanced understanding of what role geometric features of the implants play in preventing loosening.

4.1 Characteristics of Ankle (Osteo-) Arthritis

To understand the problems with total ankle arthroplasty, it is first necessary to understand the pathology and varieties of ankle arthritis. Ankle arthritis includes primary and secondary arthritis (post-traumatic osteoarthritis and systemic arthritis [neuropathic arthropathy, inflammatory arthritis, and, rarely, infectious arthritis]). Osteoarthrosis is probably a better descriptive term for primary and post-traumatic arthritis conditions, as it minimizes the inflammatory component of this disorder. However, the term osteoarthritis has been established in the current literature, and it is thus also used in this textbook.

4.1.1 Primary Osteoarthritis

Primary osteoarthritis is characterized by loss of joint cartilage and hypertrophy of bone. The exact mechanisms have not been defined, but subchondral bone injury and mechanical stress contribute to the damage [1]. The radiographic hallmarks are joint space narrowing (which correlates with loss of joint cartilage), osteophyte formation, subchondral bone cysts, and subchondral sclerosis (Fig. 4.1). There is usually an absence of juxta-articular osteoporosis in primary osteoarthrosis.

4.1.2 Post-traumatic Osteoarthritis

While hip and knee osteoarthrosis are predominantly of degenerative etiology and seen in older patients, approximately 80%

B. Hintermann, R. Ruiz, *Total Ankle Replacement*, https://doi.org/10.1007/978-3-031-56810-7_4

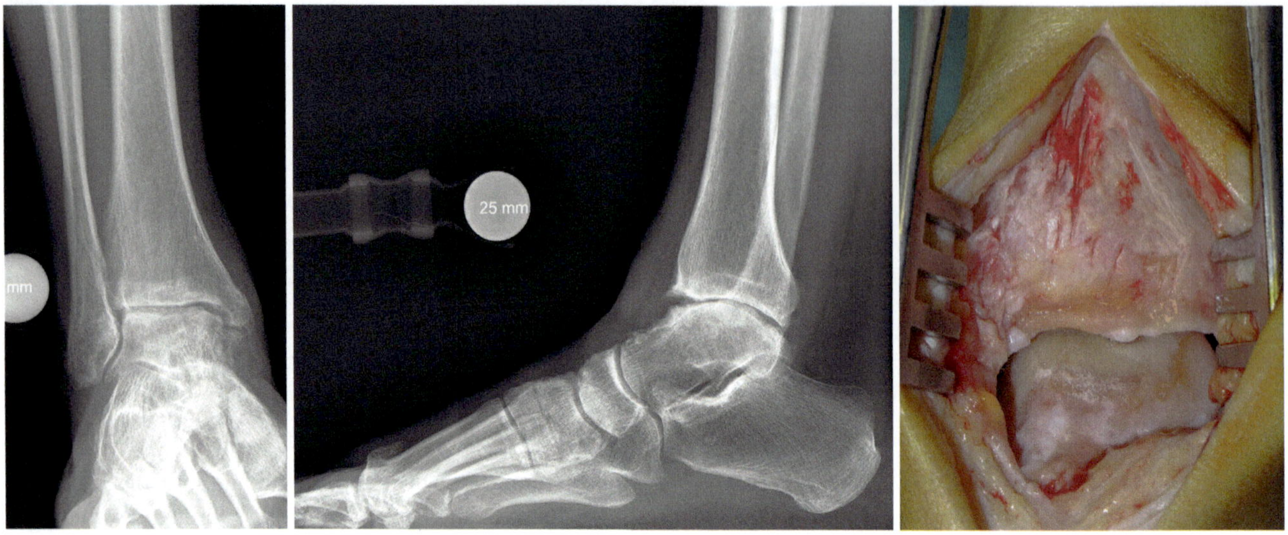

Fig. 4.1 Primary osteoarthritis. A 56-year-old male patient with primary osteoarthritis was treated by arthroscopic osteophyte resection 14 months ago, with subsequent deterioration

of ankle osteoarthritis is post-traumatic in origin [2–6] and occurs mainly in younger patients [2, 7–10]. Post-traumatic osteoarthritis usually occurs secondary to fractures, severe ligament lesions, and dislocation injuries. The soft-tissue envelope around the ankle is typically involved, often scarred and inelastic. Chronic pain and progressive periarticular formation of new bone may often lead to significant loss of ankle joint motion. In addition to joint space narrowing, osteophyte formation, subchondral bone cysts, and subchondral sclerosis, post-traumatic osteoarthritis also potentially includes joint incongruency, malalignment, and dislocation (Fig. 4.2).

4.1.3 Systemic Arthritis

Systemic or inflammatory arthritis includes the various presentations of rheumatoid arthritis, mixed connective tissue disorders, and synovial inflammatory conditions of unknown etiology [1]. Besides rheumatoid disease (Fig. 4.3) [11–13], secondary osteoarthritis has also been found to be associated with a variety of underlying diseases/pathologies, such as hemochromatosis (Fig. 4.4) [14], hemophilia (Fig. 4.5) [15–19], gout (Fig. 4.6) [20], neuropathic diseases [4, 7, 21, 22], and avascular talus necrosis, osteochondrosis dissecans, or post-infectious arthritis (Fig. 4.7) [7, 23–28].

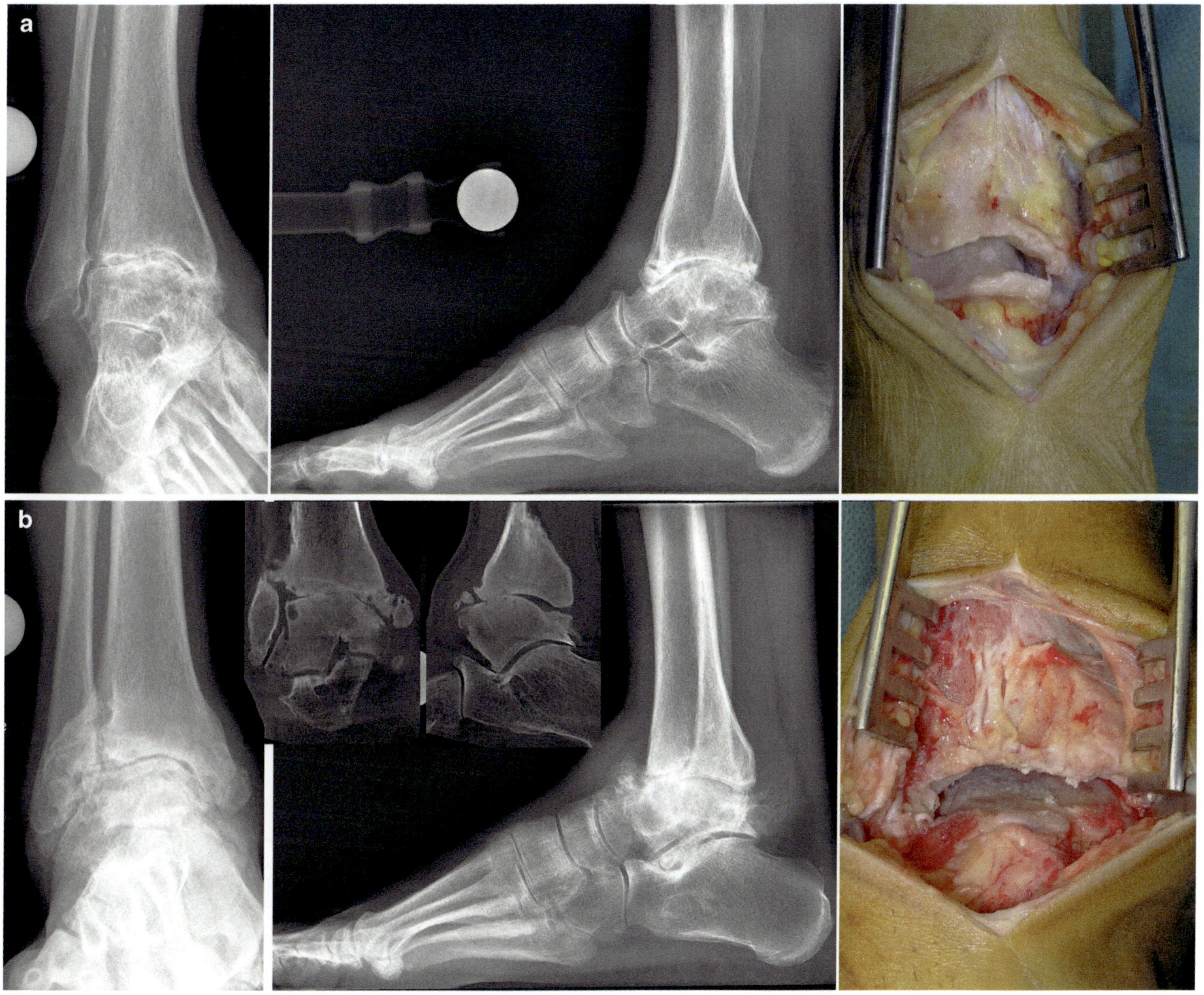

Fig. 4.2 Post-traumatic osteoarthritis. (**a**) A 61-year-old female patient over 30 years after a severe ankle sprain. (**b**) A 50-year-old former professional soccer player who sustained many injuries

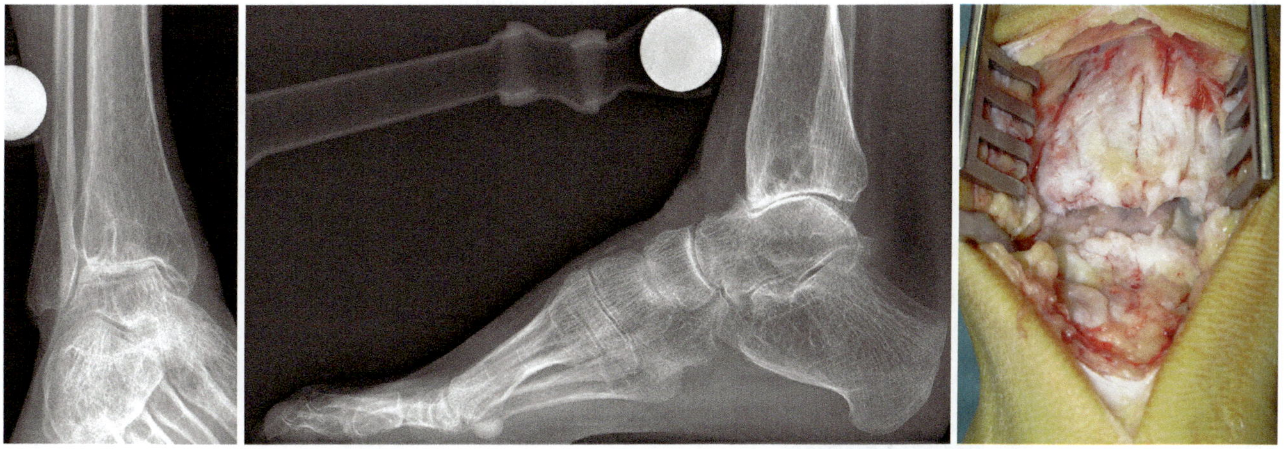

Fig. 4.3 Rheumatoid arthritis. A 47-year-old female patient suffering from rheumatoid arthritis typically shows the involvement of the other joints in the disease

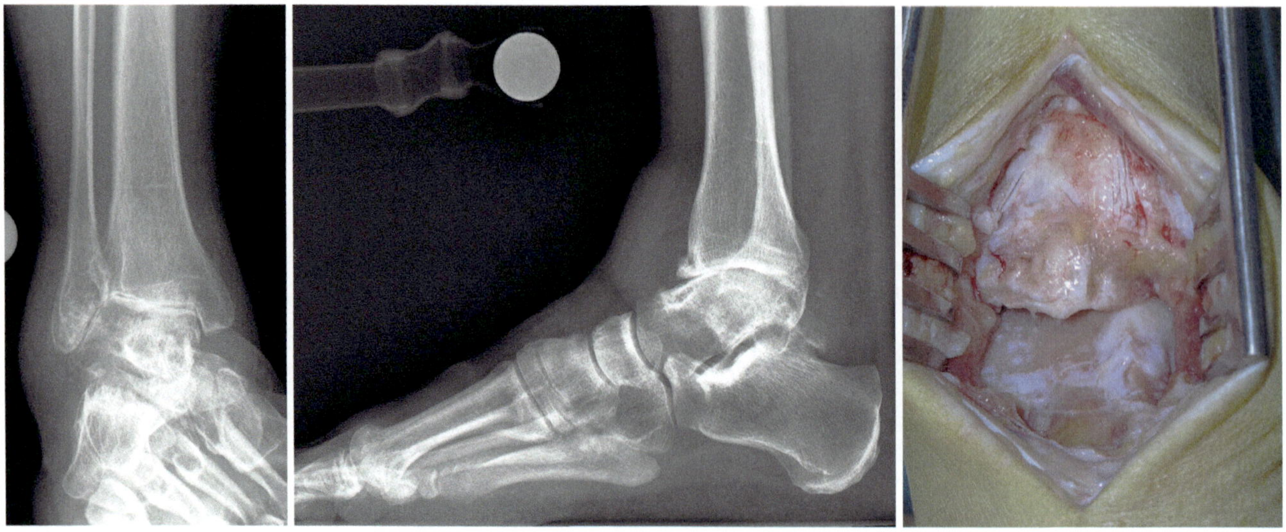

Fig. 4.4 Hemochromatosis. A 54-year-old banker in whom hemochromatosis was detected at the age of 32 years

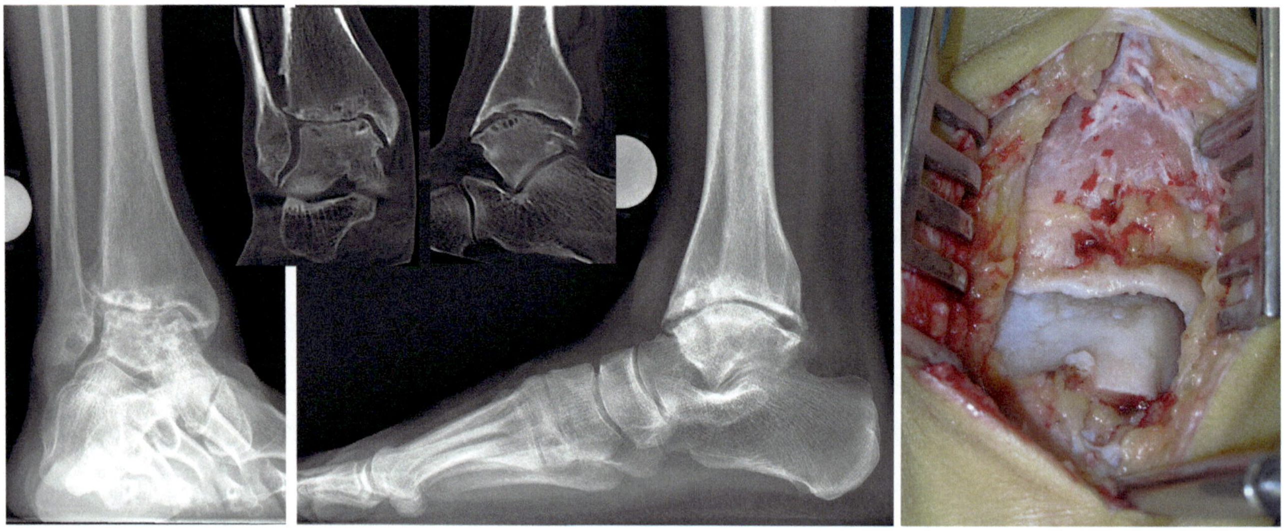

Fig. 4.5 Hemophilia. A 37-year-old professional piano player is suffering from hemophilia A

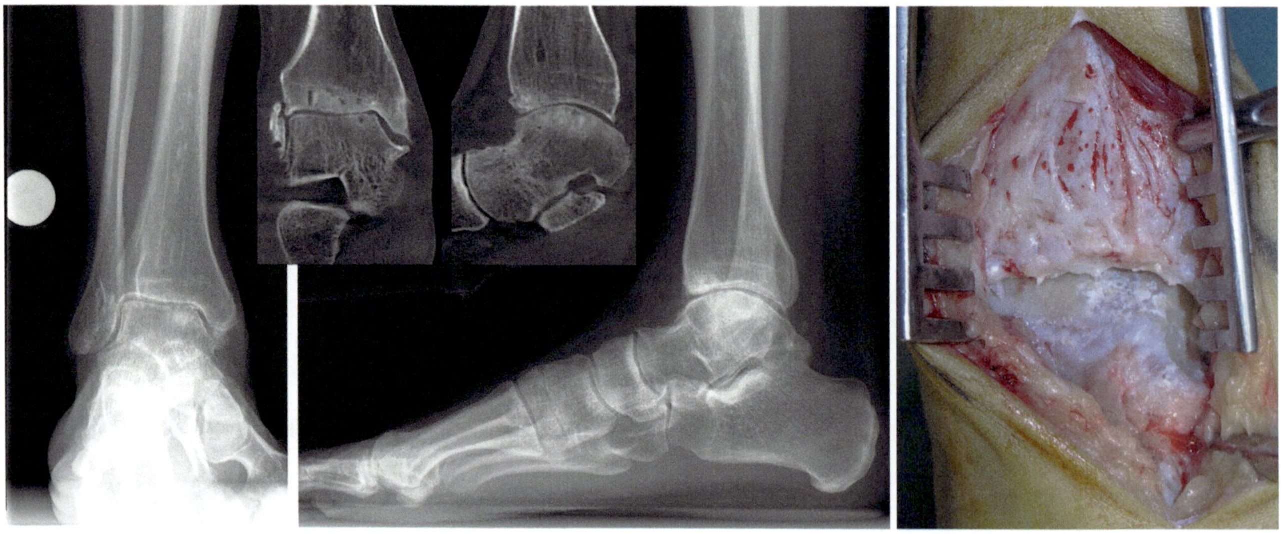

Fig. 4.6 Gout arthritis. A 51-year-old pilot is suffering from gout arthritis

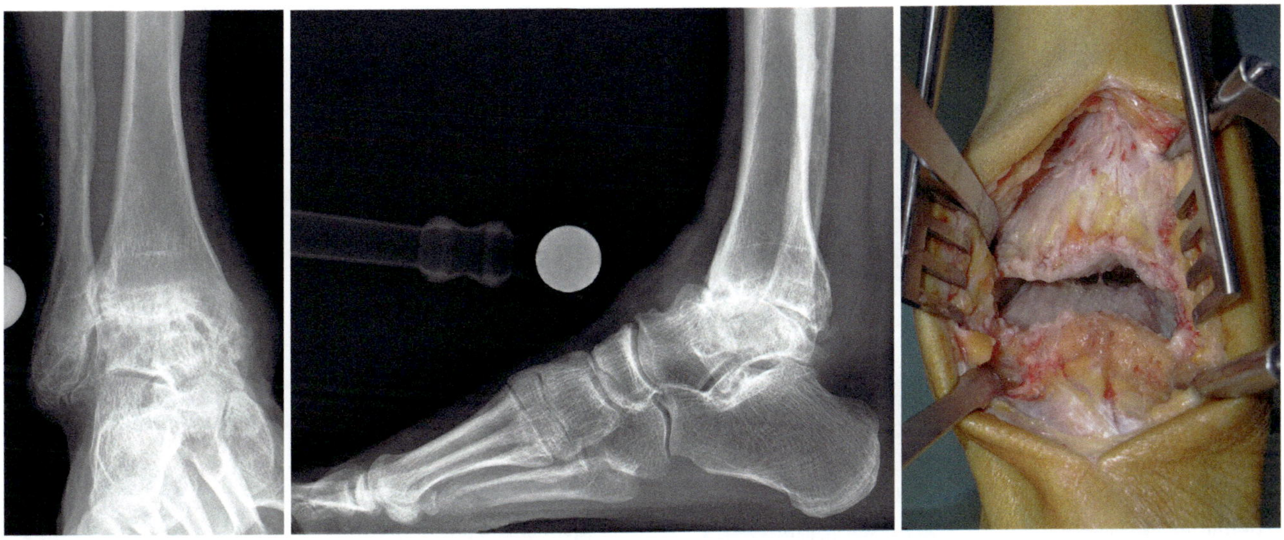

Fig. 4.7 Post-infectious arthritis. A 49-year-old former high-level tennis player suffered from septic arthritis after a cortisone injection 13 years ago that stopped his career

4.2 Prosthetic Designs

Quantitative knowledge of the ankle complex morphology is crucial for understanding implant design, replicating the joint function, and properly sizing the components [29, 30]. The radius of curvature of the talar component, for example, affects the mobility and stability of the replaced ankle [29, 31, 32]. Using implants with precisely matched sizes can substantially reduce complications and increase implant survival rates [7, 33]. A good shape match between the inner surfaces of the prosthesis and the resection surface is an essential factor for long-term fixation [21, 34–36]. Knowledge of ankle morphology is also crucial for the operative technique in total ankle arthroplasty: an optimal level and inclination of the surgical cuts, both at the tibia and talus, minimizes the amount of bone removal and saves subchondral solid bone [21, 37–39].

4.2.1 The Constraint-Conformity/Congruency Conflict

There are two design philosophies in total ankle arthroplasty: constraint type and conformity/congruency type. To understand these philosophies, the following terms must be defined:

- Constraint is the resistance of an implant to a particular degree of freedom, such as anteroposterior translation or axial rotation. Excessive constraint leads to high shear forces at the bone-implant interface and, thus, to early component loosening. Reducing constraint minimizes the transmission of shear forces at the bone-implant interface.
- Conformity and congruency are geometric measures of the closeness of fit of the articulation. Fully conforming or congruent prostheses have articular surfaces with the same sagittal radii of curvature, which results in complete articular contact. Fully conforming or congruent articulations typically have low wear rates because the polyethylene contact stress remains below its fatigue threshold for delamination and pitting. Partially conforming or incongruent articulations have a wide range of articular surfaces, from round-on-flat designs to articulations with radii of curvature that vary by only a few millimeters.

The "constraint-conformity/congruency conflict" becomes evident in fixed-bearing designs with fully conforming articulations (Fig. 4.8a, b). Such designs create high axial constraints, which results in excessive axial loosening torque. Mobile-bearing implants attempt to overcome this constraint-conformity conflict by offering two separate, fully conforming, or congruent articulations that function together to reduce axial and shear constraints at the bone-implant interface (Fig. 4.8c, d).

Theoretically, to reduce constraint, fixed-bearing ankles can be only partially conforming. As a result, they have higher wear rates because polyethylene contact stresses are increased. With less conformity, wear is typically more significant. This is particularly true when the prosthesis is not perfectly balanced. In such a case, edge loading may occur, leading to high contact stress on thin polyethylene.

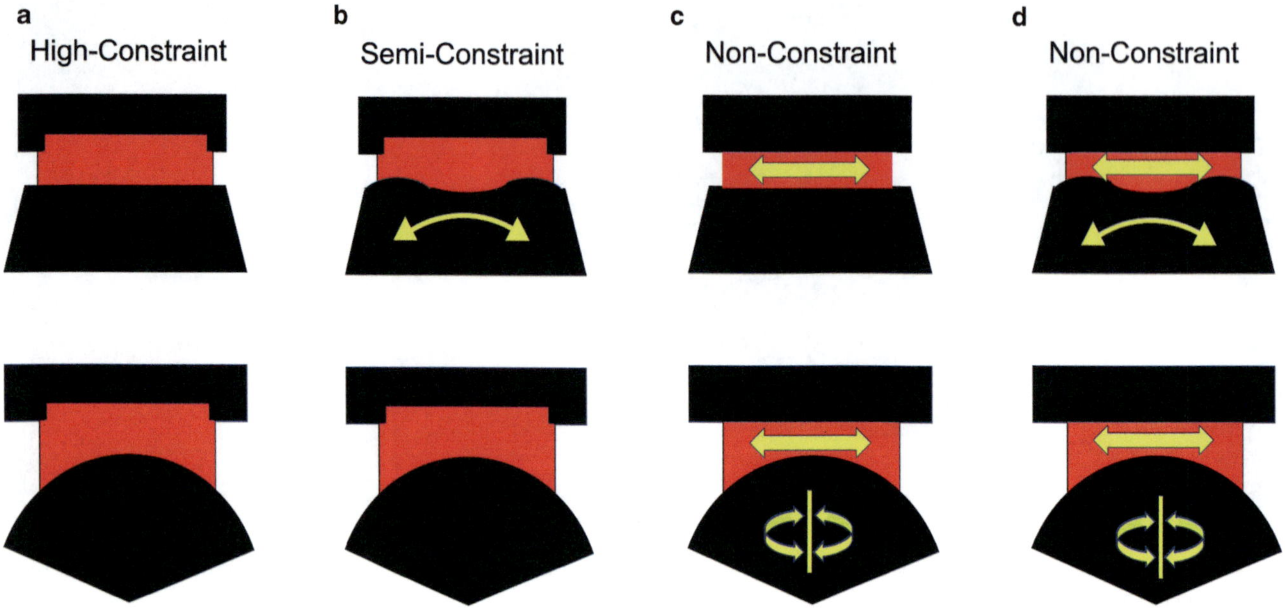

Fig. 4.8 Constraint-conformity/congruency conflict. (**a**) A fixed-bearing high-constraint prosthesis does not allow translational and rotational movement in the horizontal plane and no tilting movement in the coronal plane. (**b**) Fixed-bearing: If a non-conform rounded surface replaces the parallelism of the articulating surfaces, some additional rotational movement in the coronal plane is possible. (**c**) A mobile-bearing non-constraint prosthesis does allow translational and rotational movement in the horizontal plane. (**d**) Mobile-bearing: If a non-conform rounded surface replaces the parallelism of the articulating surfaces, some additional rotational movement in the coronal plane is possible

4.2.2 Stress-Transfer to the Bone

There has been a relative shortage of basic science laboratory research on total ankle arthroplasty and few investigations into design criteria. In one of the few laboratory investigations of total ankle arthroplasty design, Falsig et al. [40] evaluated stress transfer to the distal tibial trabecular bone for three different generic distal tibial prostheses: a polyethylene tibial component, a metal-backed polyethylene tibial component, and a long-stem metal-backed tibial component. An eccentric anterolateral load of 2100 N (approximately three times body weight) was applied to the three prostheses. Adding a metal backing reduced compressive stresses in the trabecular bone by 25%, from 20 N/mm^2 for an all-polyethylene tibial component to 15 N/mm^2 for a metal-backed component [40]. Shear stresses were herewith also reduced. For the long-stem implant, almost a complete reduction of the compressive stress in the metaphyseal trabecular bone was measured because they were transferred to the long stem, bypassing the distal tibia [40].

4.3 Fixation Configuration to the Bone

Various fixation configurations have been designed for tibial components of total ankle implants, and new implant designs are emerging. In general, stem-type implants require the highest volume of bone resection before implantation. In contrast, peg-type implants require the lowest (Fig. 4.9). Several studies have suggested that the geometry of the tibial component significantly impacts the micromotion at the bone-implant interface [41–44]. The highest micromotion was found in stem-type implants, next to keel-type implants, followed by bar-type implants, whereas the lowest micromotion was observed in peg-type geometries [41].

A stemmed tibial implant, in contrast, can help align the prosthesis and aid implant stability in the presence of bone deficit [45]. It has been shown that high initial stability can be achieved by large, deep, and wide fixation geometry anchored into cortical or high-bone-density trabecular bone proximal to the implant [41]. However, such a fixation method requires large bone volume resection. Also, from an operative perspective, the surgical preparation for the implantation of the stem-, keel-, and bar-type implants requires creating an anterior cortical tibial window for insertion, which may jeopardize the integrity of tibial cortical bone, thus may weaken the support to the tibial implant [46]. An alternative option is the use of an extended stem component that is placed with multiple cylindrical segments individually after having reamed a hole through the talus from the plantar surface of the foot; however, this is not without fear, as it may damage the subtalar joint and endanger the blood supply of the talus, thus causing talus necrosis [47].

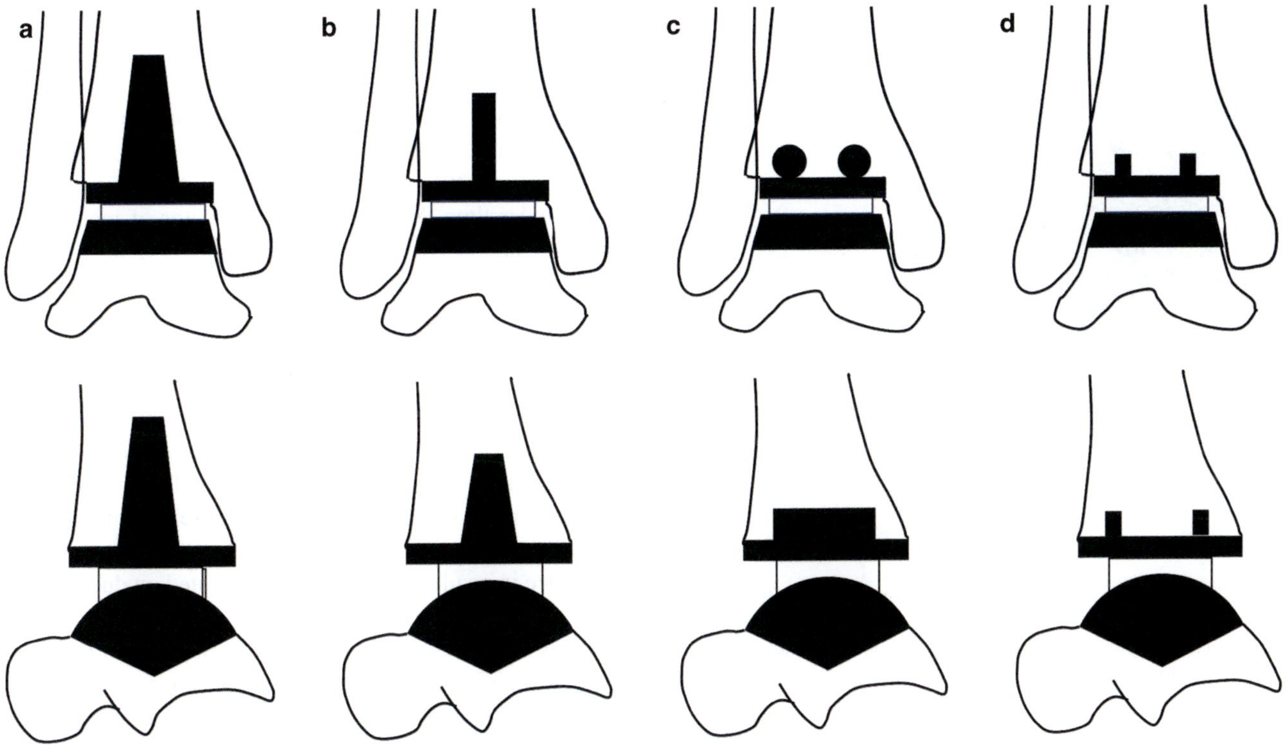

Fig. 4.9 Fixation configurations for the tibial component. (**a**) Stem type, (**b**) bar type, (**c**) keel type, and (**d**) peg type

The ideal tibial component should include the two features of decreased distal tibial bone resection and minimized disruption of the anterior tibial cortex [4, 48]. Higher distal tibial bone resection may waste large bones with high bone density, resulting in poor initial stability and difficulty for future revision surgery [49]. A recent study using finite model analysis yielded a better initial bone-implant fixation with tibial implants' low and small size [41]. The authors concluded that peg-type tibial implants that require no disruption of the anterior tibial cortex were thus suggested to be the most suitable implant design.

Fewer data about the talar component are available. Moideen et al. [50] investigated the talus-implant interface micromotion among STAR and several modified designs and found that the polka-dot design could effectively reduce micromotion. Furthermore, the 3 mm pin structure could significantly reduce the bone-implant interface micromotion on the fixation surface of the talus component of the STAR implant [50].

4.4 Effect of Micromotion at Implant-Bone Interface

The understructure of a prosthetic baseplate is essential in resisting micromotion and shear, rotatory, and eccentric forces. Volz et al. [51] studied tibial baseplate micromotion in the laboratory using four tibial baseplates of different designs. They implanted the baseplates into paired cadaveric tibias, subjected them to eccentric loads, and measured the resulting micromotion. They found four peripherally placed screws with a central peg best resisted micromotion. Others reported similar results [40]. Many of today's prosthetic designs for total knee arthroplasties have a keel on the undersurface of the tibial baseplate. In the ankle, however, because of the anatomy and limited vascularization of the talus, using a keel is difficult, if not impossible. The problem with using an implant with a stem in the distal tibia is the need to make a window for its insertion. Creating such a window may provoke a substantial weakening of the anterior tibial cortical architecture, thereby reducing its suitability to become the primary support of the prosthetic tibial baseplate.

If proper bonding is not achieved in total ankle arthroplasty due to increased implant-bone micromotion, non-physiological bone strain, or excessive strain shielding, bone resorption/remodeling may lead to implant loosening. Whether or not proper bonding can be achieved is strongly influenced by the implant design and its positioning (orientation) [52]. Reduced micromotion has also been predicted for the component designs that rely on more than a single peg to achieve fixation and have their fixation features anchored to the dense distal tibial or proximal talar bone, compared with those with a single fixation peg extending more profound into the less dense trabecular bone [53]. However, the most dominant influence on bone strain and

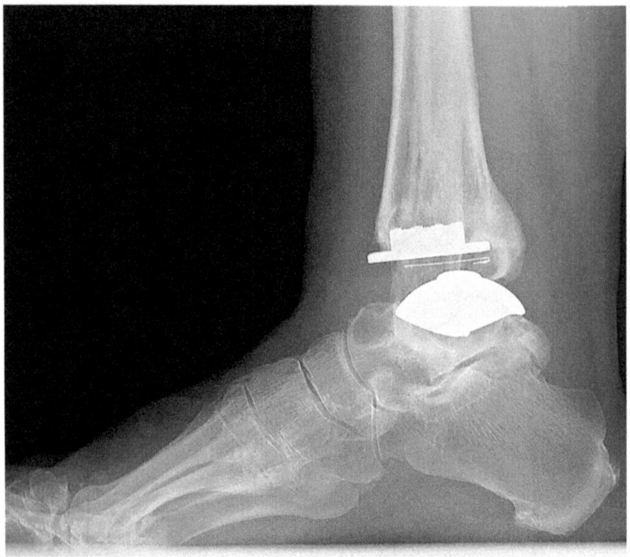

Fig. 4.10 Effect of the undersized tibial component. In this 67-year-old patient, 8 years after total ankle replacement surgery, the tibial component was found to have subsided. The too-anterior positioning of the component may have supported the subsidence by moving the main force transmission posteriorly, where the component was supported by cancellous bone only

micromotion, more so than implant design, was a gap at the fixation surface of the prosthetic device. This elevated strains and micromotion in all designs, indicating that a gap should be avoided. When forces were applied to the part of the implant not fully seated on the bone, the increase in implant-bone micromotion and bone strains was substantial, which can be attributed to the so-called "rocking horse" mechanism [54, 55].

Excessive force applied to the bone-implant interface is detrimental to the long-term stability of a prosthetic implant. Force is always measured per unit area. The surface area represents a fundamental variable of the forces acting at the ankle. If a prosthesis is undersized, it is prone to subside in the remaining soft cancellous bone (Fig. 4.10). Not only is the strongest bone removed at the time of the surgery, but the remaining bone surface is often not fully utilized for support. Expanding the prosthesis to encompass all available bone diminishes the load per unit area [37].

Finally, the amount of force and the strength of the bone support can play an essential role in implant stability. The strongest bone is likely posteromedial in the distal tibia (Fig. 2.4) [56]. This area of stiffer bone could act as a pivot point, with the risk of overloading the surrounding weaker anterolateral bone. A somewhat anterolateral placed component could aggravate this problem and increase the potential for failure.

In conclusion, optimally positioned implants can reduce the strain-shielding effect in the tibial bone, implant-bone micromotion, contact pressure, and wear depth.

4.5 (Nonpathological) Migration in Total Ankle Arthroplasty

Implant migration is the longitudinal movement of an implant to the bone in which it is embedded over time. Subsidence is the direction of the greatest translational motion over time. Migration is an indicator of mechanical loosening and is a predictor of later failure [19, 30].

In a radiostereometric analysis (RSA) of the double-coated STAR total ankle prosthesis, Carlsson et al. [57] observed a rapid initial migration for the tibial components at 6 weeks. Still, after that, all but one implant seemed stable. The migration pattern for the talar component was similar. Rotation around the three axes was observed for the tibial components at 6 weeks but not after that. The talar components became stable for rotation around the longitudinal and sagittal axes but not around the transverse axis. There was no difference in results between ankles operated on due to rheumatoid arthritis and osteoarthrosis.

Using the same technique to assess migration of the tibial component of the Buechel-Pappas total ankle prosthesis in 15 patients with rheumatoid arthritis, Nelissen et al. [58] observed increased tibial component migration during the first 3 months, which was stabilized by the 6-month follow-up. The mean lateral-medial migration was 0.8 mm, distal-proximal migration was 0.9 mm, and posteroanterior migration was −0.5 mm. The latter implies the resultant total migration was in the anterior and valgus tilting of this tibial component.

Model-based RSA analysis (MBRSA) that avoids attaching markers to the implant and positions it by its radiographic contour was used in 23 patients in whom the Mobility system was implanted [59]. The median maximum total point motion for the implants at 2 years was 1.19 (0.39–1.95) mm for the talar component and 0.90 (0.17–2.28) mm for the spherical tip of the tibial component. The general pattern for all patients was that the slope of the migration curves decreased over time. The main direction of motion for both components was that of subsidence. The median 2-year maximum total point motion inducible displacement for the talar component was 0.49 (0.27–1.15) mm, and it was 0.07 (0.03–0.68) mm for the tibial component tip.

Brigido et al. [60] investigated 20 consecutive patients who had undergone implantation with the Inbone system to evaluate implant migration after a modular stem fixed-bearing total ankle replacement implantation. However, concerns arise with their method, defining implant migration as a change in implant location from the immediate postoperative radiograph. At baseline, the average implant migration was 0.0 mm. The average implant migration was 0.7 ± 1.2 (range, 1.3–3.3) mm at 1 year and 1.0 ± 1.1 (range, 1.5–3.2) mm at 2 years. Surprisingly, implant migration was greater in males (1.2 ± 1.1 mm) than in females (0.1 ± 0.8 mm).

These findings signify that ankle implants in the noncemented construct continue to migrate for up to 2 years after implantation. This nonpathological migration or settling of the implants appears to be greater in males than in females, which greater compressive forces at the ankle could explain. Furthermore, the male anatomy tends to be larger than the female anatomy, and the larger cancellous body of the talus might allow for additional implant settling.

4.6 Fixation/Bonding to the Bone

All current ankle arthroplasty designs rely on bone ingrowth for qualitative osseointegration and implant stability. There are several significant advantages to bone ingrowth (otherwise known as cementless implantation):

- Less bone resection is required because no space is required for fixation between the bone and the implant.
- The inserted prosthesis can be kept smaller than it would be with the additional cement mantle, and the smaller the prosthesis, the smaller the moments created at the bone-implant interface.
- Inadvertent cement displacement or intra-articular spillage (which could likely cause accelerated third-body wear) is avoided.
- Bone ingrowth approaches eliminate the damage to local delicate soft tissues caused by high levels of heat released by the exothermic process of curing acrylic cement.

Today, cementless or ingrowth prostheses incorporate a porous surface at the bone interface, a calcium hydroxyapatite coating, or a combination of both (Fig. 4.11). An implant's "biologic fixation" achieves the same strength as bone cement fixation by the fourth to twelfth week, [57] and there is additional ingrowth or remodeling of the bone area for periods of up to 24 months [60]. Galante et al. [61] demonstrated that after an initial extremely tight fit of the implant onto the bone, a plateau value of the fixation strength was reached at 3 weeks. Cameron et al. [60] found that a porous-coated implant with pore sizes of up to 100 μm is similar to that with pore sizes over 100 μm. This was an important finding from a materials point of view since, for a given vol % of porosity, the smaller the pore size, the greater the number of contact points and, therefore, the more challenging the coating on the substrate. Optimizing the mechanical properties of the coating and the ingrowth capability of tissue into the porous surface layer by control of vol % of porosity and a few interparticle contact points is the design goal of porous surface layered, high load-bearing implant systems.

Hydroxyapatite coating encourages molecular bonding between the calcium hydroxyapatite crystals and the bone bed. The time required for this bonding process appears shorter than that required for ingrowth into the sole porous surface. With time, however, the hydroxyapatite coating is wholly resorbed, leaving concerns regarding the long-term fixation of the components (Fig. 4.12). The most attractive current approach is combining a porous surface with hydroxyapatite coating. Theoretically, this strategy allows for early fixation of the implant through hydroxyapatite bonding, followed later by secure ingrowth of bone within the porous, three-dimensional interstices (Fig. 4.13).

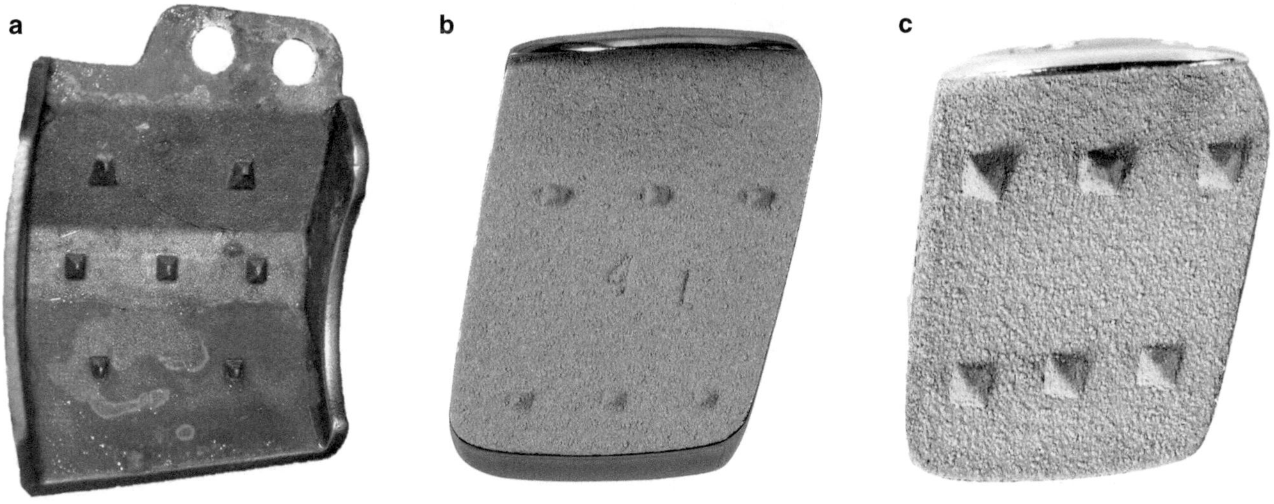

Fig. 4.11 Coating of cementless prostheses. (**a**) Component with a single hydroxyapatite coat: 6.6 years after the total ankle arthroplasty, there is a debonding from the smooth surface of the component. (**b**) Component with a porous coat of 200 μm of CoCr. (**c**) Component with a double coating with a porous coat of 200 μm and hydroxyapatite

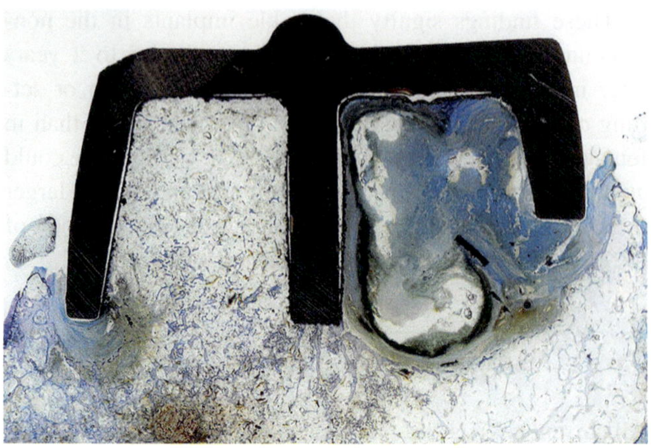

Fig. 4.12 Histologic analysis of single hydroxyapatite coating. Retrieved talar component of a STAR ankle in a 74-year-old female patient 14 years after the replacement surgery. The hydroxyapatite has only partially resorbed and mainly debonded from CoCr alloy, indicating that the bonding of the hydroxyapatite layer did not last over time

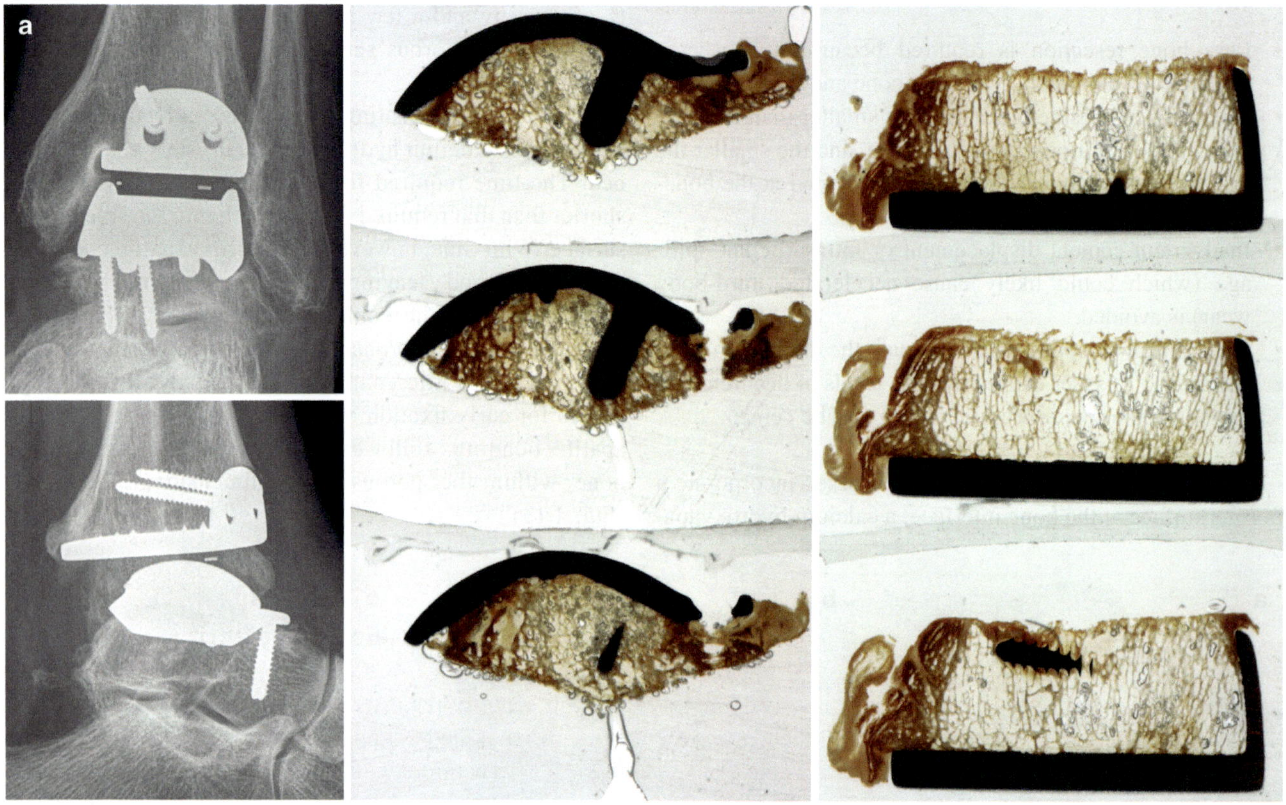

Fig. 4.13 Histologic analysis of a double coating. Retrieved H3 ankle in a 56-year-old female patient 10.5 years after the replacement surgery because of the onset of paralysis due to a disc herniation that made the conversion to an ankle fusion necessary. The patient had no pain and no limitations in her daily life. (**a**) Radiographs showing stable components at 10-year follow-up control. The prosthesis was removed with a bone block and, after freezing, sectioned, as shown for the talar and tibial components. (**b**) The histologic analysis shows a firm bonding of the trabecula to the porous-coated implant. The hydroxyapatite layer can no longer be identified, probably due to resorption. Of note, minimal stress concentration occurred at the pyramid peak site. The posterior cortex has built a solid connection to the component at its posterior margins, whereas, on the anterior side, osteointegration has occurred along the shield, and the cortex has built a solid connection at its superior border. (**c**) The detailed analysis confirms the overall solid bonding of the trabecula with the alloy with limited stress concentration around the pyramidal peaks and the pegs, though they are tinny

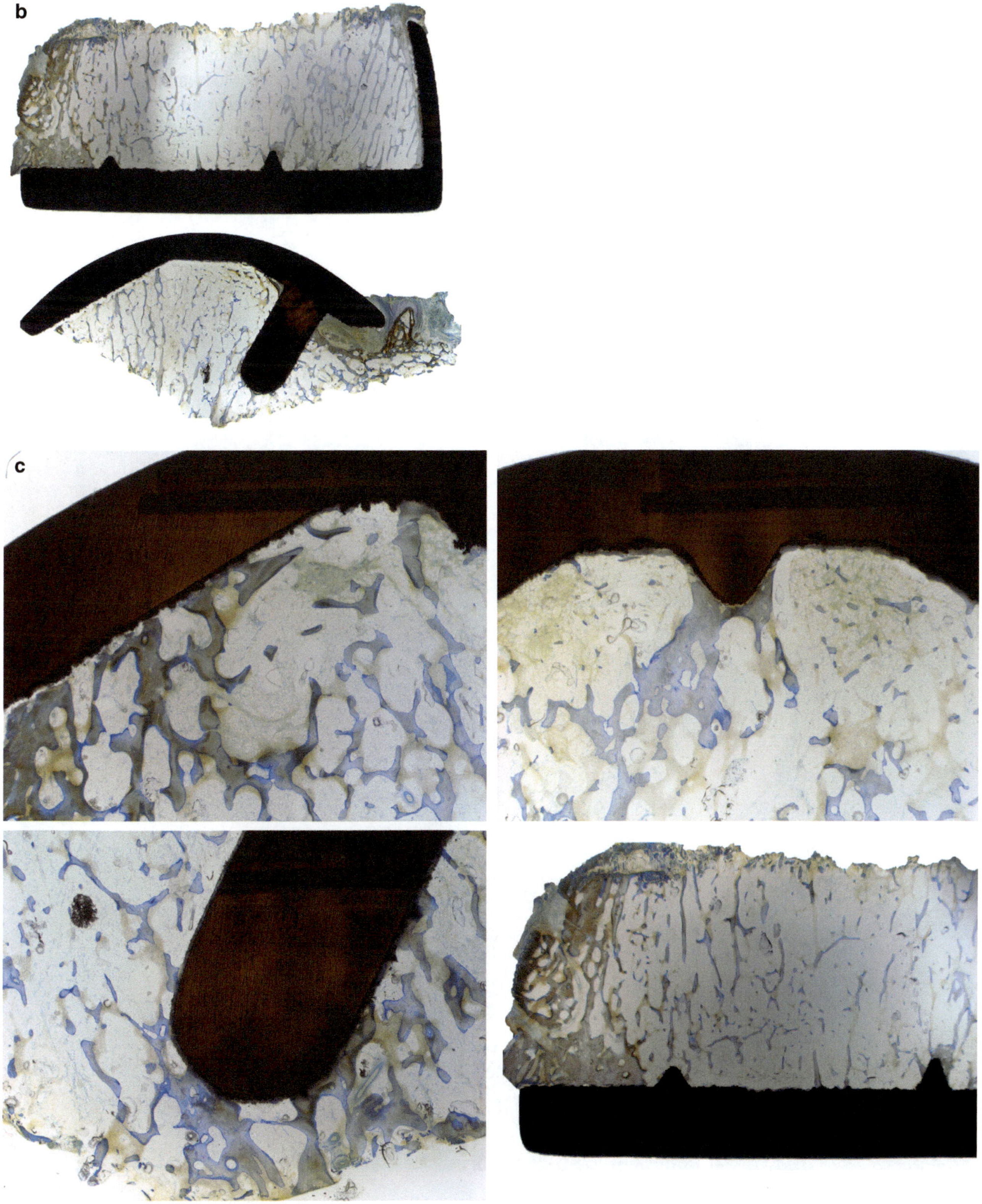

Fig. 4.13 (continued)

4.7 The Dilemma Between a Mobile- and Fixed-Bearing Ankle

In a fixed-bearing total ankle, the position of the tibial component determines the talar position and, thereby, the axis of rotation of the replaced ankle [62]. Research has shown that rotational torque [63] or translational forces [36] may be generated as the geometry of the prosthesis attempts to seek congruency, which may contribute to polyethylene wear, and potentially to early component loosening (Fig. 4.14). Using a mobile-bearing total ankle that allows free translational and rotational movement between the polyethylene and tibial

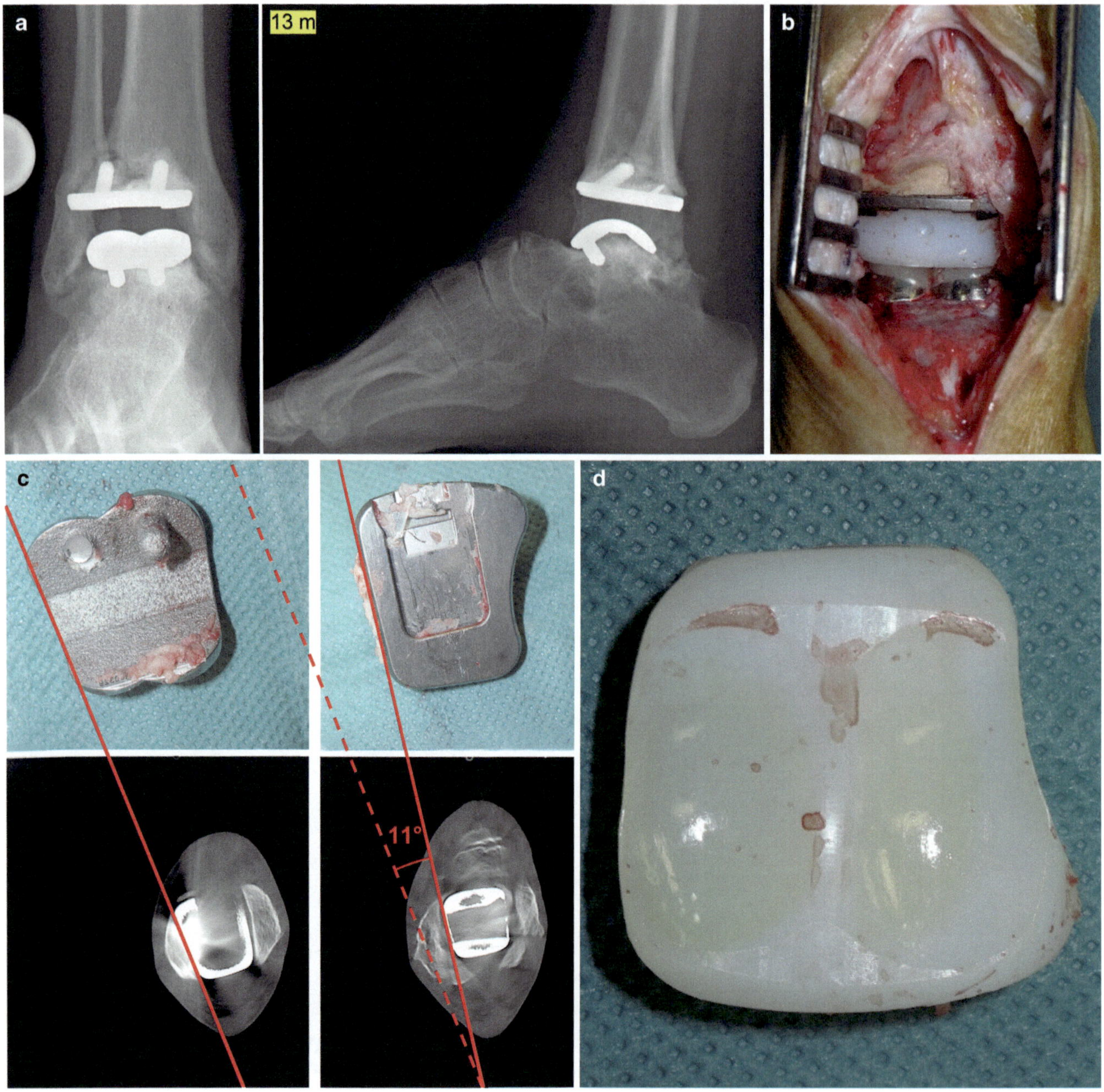

Fig. 4.14 Impact of rotational torque on polyethylene wear. A 64-year-old male patient, 13 months after total ankle arthroplasty with a fixed-bearing prosthesis, complained about pain and dysfunction of the replaced ankle. (**a**) The radiographs evidenced the loosening of the tibial component after cement fixation. (**b**) After exposure to the ankle, a prosthesis mismatch with the talar component's internal rotation can be seen. (**c**) When using the medial border of the components as the reference, an internal malrotation of 11° was calculated on preoperative weight-bearing CT scans. (**d**) The wear pattern of the articulating surfaces reflects the asymmetric wear pattern due to the changed mechanics

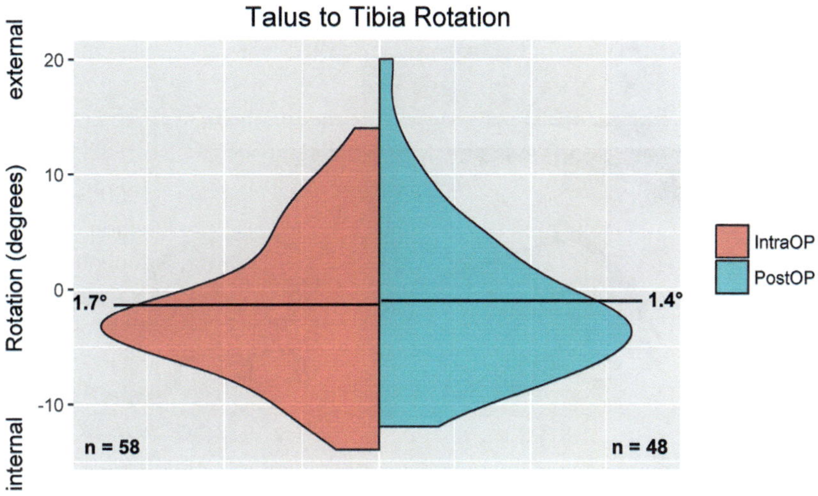

Fig. 4.15 Axial rotation of the talus to the tibia. Graph showing the axial rotation of the talus to the tibia as measured intraoperatively and postoperatively (6.3 years, by weight-bearing CT)

component (second interface) may overcome such increased forces, as the talus can adapt to the instantaneous joint geometry and soft-tissue tension (Fig. 4.8). However, other motion along the second interface in total ankle arthroplasty remains not without fear [64, 65].

Very little is known about component positioning in the axial plane, especially the mismatch in axial rotation of the talar and tibial components. Current literature fails to report whether the talar's intraoperative selected relative axial rotation to the tibial component changes over time. Hintermann et al. [66] found in a consecutive cohort of 58 patients who underwent mobile-bearing total ankle arthroplasty a relative rotation of the talar to the tibial component of 1.7° toward internal with a range as high as 28° (Fig. 4.15). Using weight-bearing CT in 48 patients after a mean of 6.3 years after total ankle arthroplasty, they found a similar relative rotation of 1.4° toward internal with a range 32° (Fig. 4.15). Intraoperative selected axial tibial rotation to the talar component in mobile-bearing total ankle arthroplasty remains stable over time. Given the wide range of measurements, the authors concluded that allowing the talus to find its position according to the individual anatomy during total ankle arthroplasty may be crucial to ensure proper axial rotational alignment in mobile-bearing total ankle arthroplasty.

Still, little is known about the effect of sagittal positioning of fixed-bearing implants on clinical outcomes. In a study with 30 patients who underwent total ankle arthroplasty using a fixed-bearing implant, Datir et al. [67] found that the lateral talar component angle significantly correlated with postoperative outcomes. However, the sagittal translation of the talar component was not evaluated. Nielsen et al. [68] investigated the Salto Talaris ankle and the Inbone II system in 71 primary total ankle arthroplasties. At the 2-year follow-up, no correlation between the postoperative anteroposterior offset ratio and functional outcome scores were observed between the two fixed-bearing implant groups.

In a study of the MAUDE database, fixed-bearing ankles were found to have a 2.8 times higher proportion of reported polyethylene wear than mobile-bearing ankles (STAR™) [69]. Predicting the talar axial position with the position of the tibial component may thus not be without risks of increased torsional deforming forces being transmitted to the polyethylene. At the same time, the prosthesis seeks congruency while the foot is loaded, leading to polyethylene wear.

A potential solution could be a prosthesis design combining the advantages of a mobile-bearing and a fixed-bearing total ankle design. Such a novel design must allow for optimal positioning of the metallic components based on the available bone stock (e.g., only minimal talar and tibial resection). Auto-aligning the polyethylene insert in the transverse plane would be required before a definitive fix to the tibial component to respect the patient's axis of ankle rotation (Fig. 4.16). Preliminary results from our institution using a novel total ankle design that allows the surgeon to convert from a mobile- to a fixed-bearing design intraoperatively after ensuring proper alignment are promising [70]. This concept may simplify total ankle arthroplasty. The question of whether it enhances implant longevity has yet to be answered.

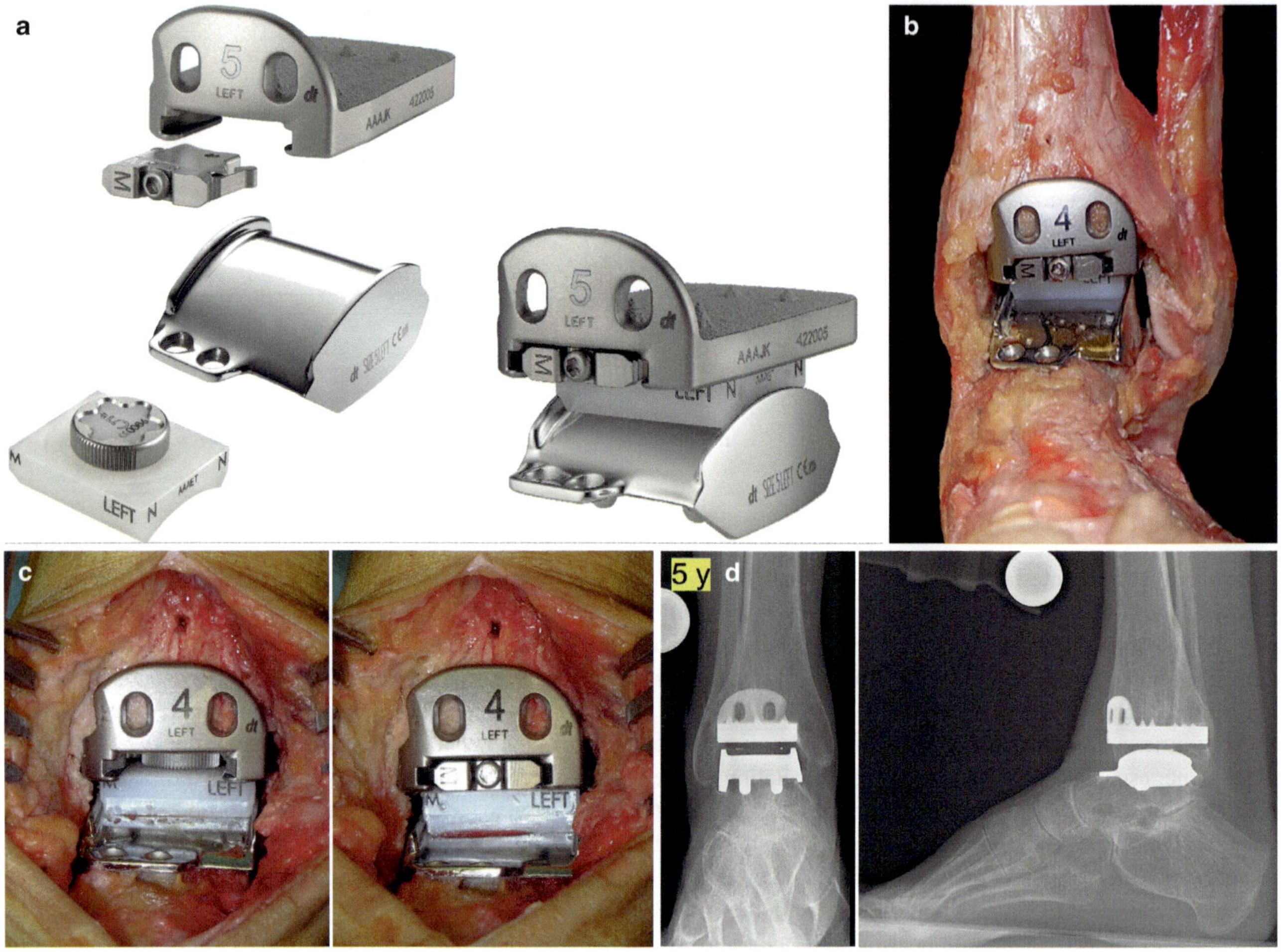

Fig. 4.16 Novel ankle design for intraoperative fixation of axial rotation. (**a**) The H2 ankle is designed to be converted from a three-component (mobile-bearing) to a two-component (fixed-bearing) prosthesis after the polyethylene has taken its position in situ. A locking device is used for the final fixation of the insert in the given position. (**b**) This example shows the malrotation of the talar to the tibial component after having it positioned best to the bony anatomy. The polyethylene insert had taken its position adapted to the axis of rotation of the ankle before it was fixed. (**c**) Anterior view of the inserted prosthesis before and after conversion to a fixed-bearing ankle. (**d**) Radiographs of the 5-year follow-up control in a 59-year-old female patient

4.8 Limitations of Polyethylene

The physical properties of polyethylene used for the mobile insert can vary according to the type of polyethylene used and how it was manufactured. The contact stresses on five total knee designs peaked between 20 and 80 MPa [71]. By rounding or dishing the polyethylene tray, the peak contact stress was reduced from 55 MPa for a round-on-flat design to 18 MPa for a design with more conforming polyethylene [72]. Increasing the conformity reduces the peak contact stress on the polyethylene. Still, it also increases stresses transferred to the bone-prosthesis interface, which can contribute to loosening. The durability of polyethylene is improved with increasing thickness [73–75]. While a minimum thickness of 4–6 mm is estimated to be needed for the hip and 6–8 mm for the knee, minimum thickness standards for the ankle have yet to be determined. Theoretically, thicker polyethylene components in the ankle may help prevent polyethylene failures, but at the expense of increasing the lever arm of forces acting at the bone-implant interface and of more generous bone cuts. However, the fundamental importance of bone conservation in the ankle has been widely recognized since the bone may be weak and the surface areas for support are small [56]. Polyethylene requirements for the ankle are, therefore, contradictory to what is necessary for conserving bone strength.

Although total ankle arthroplasty devices fail by several mechanisms, wear in the polyethylene liner constitutes one of the dominating failure modes [76, 77]. This leads to instability and loosening of the implant. Mechanisms that contribute to wear in the liners are high contact and subsurface stresses that break down the material over time (Fig. 4.17). To date, little is known about the difference in load response of polyethylene between mobile-bearing components that

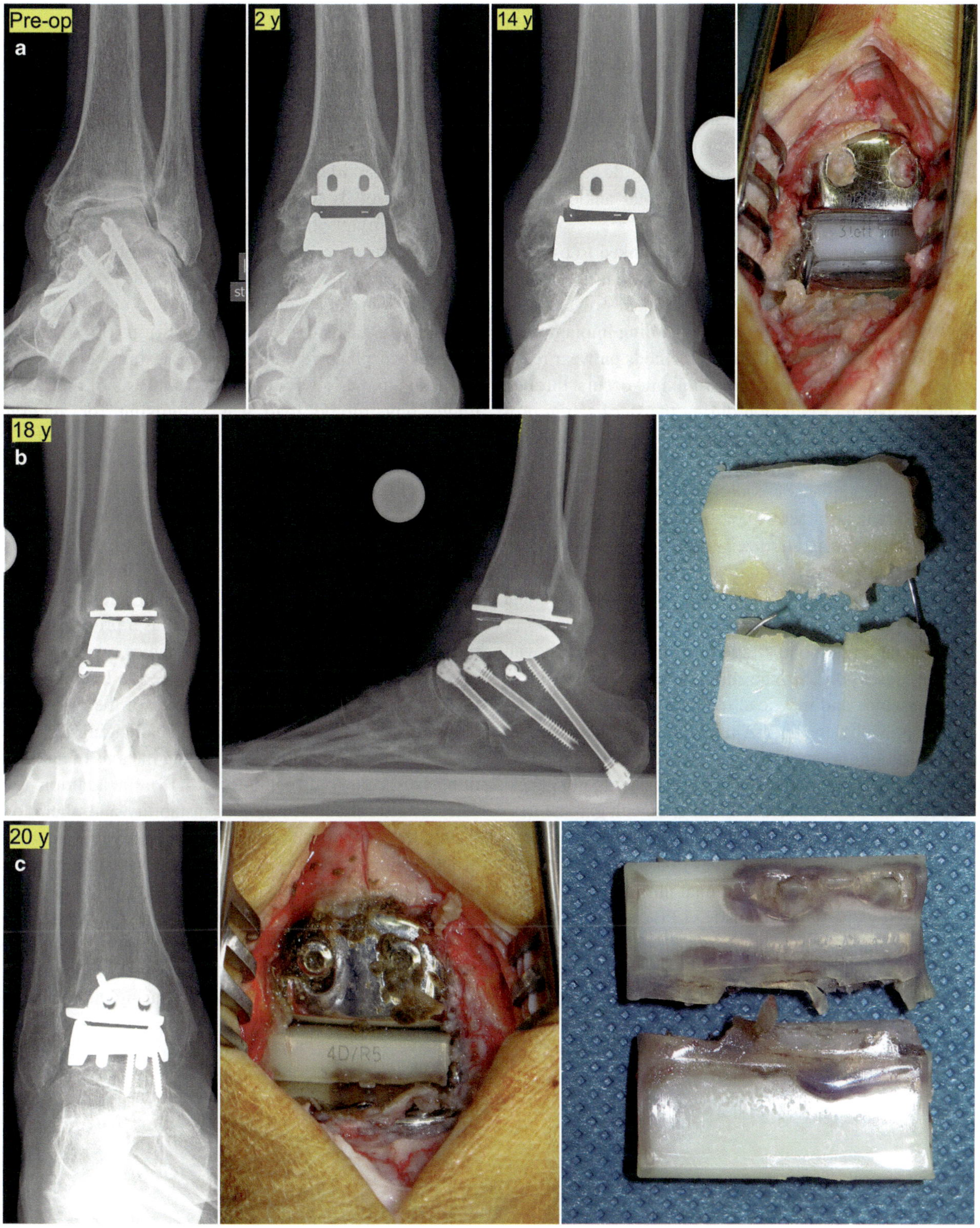

Fig. 4.17 Mechanical failure of polyethylene. (**a**) A 74-year-old farmer complained about medial pain in his left ankle for 4 months after being pain-free. He had a triple fusion with some valgus left that was not fully corrected during the replacement surgery. At a 2-year follow-up control, the ankle looked well aligned. The current X-ray, taken 14 years after the replacement surgery, evidences asymmetric polyethylene wear with a medial shift of the talus. The polyethylene insert was exchanged, and a medial sliding osteotomy was performed. The exposed ankle shows asymmetric wear. (**b**) The radiographs of a 76-year-old former postman demonstrate the fracture of the polyethylene insert 18 years after the replacement surgery. The retrieved insert shows the transverse fatigue fracture. (**c**) A 71-year-old passioned hiker reported at 20-year follow-up control that she is still delighted with her ankle, allowing her to follow all the activities. She can remember feeling a strange popping approximately 4 months ago but without pain since. The X-ray shows the fracture that was confirmed intraoperatively. There was some contact between both metallic components due to the collapse, causing the black abrasion material

can slide and rotate under the tibial component and fixed-bearing components that are fixed against the tibial component. Jiang et al. [69], who analyzed the medical device reporting in the MAUDE database, found a higher proportion of reported polyethylene fractures and a greater need for earlier revisions for polyethylene-related issues with the use of the primary mobile-bearing design (STAR ankle) as compared with fixed-bearing total ankle arthroplasty designs [69].

Polyethylene wear particles have been linked to osteolysis after total ankle arthroplasty [78, 79]. There is no consensus on the importance of highly cross-linked polyethylene (HXLPE) in total ankle arthroplasty regarding implant wear or the effect of different sterilization methods on wear resistance [80, 81]. Polyethylene cross-linking occurs through exposure to gamma irradiation during the sterilization process of manufacturing, which generates free radicals that then combine to form cross-links. Sterilization with gamma irradiation in the air causes oxidative embrittlement because residual free radicals react with absorbed oxygen. The polyethylene component is sterilized in an inert (oxygen-free) environment to reduce oxidative degradation following gamma irradiation [82]. A potential disadvantage of gamma irradiation is that, in vivo, polymer chain scission may occur after implantation in the joint due to oxygen in the synovial fluid. This causes polyethylene embrittlement, which reduces fatigue resistance and may lead to surface cracking or fracture of the polyethylene liner. Alternatives to gamma irradiation sterilization in an inert gas include sterilization in ethylene oxide or gas plasma. These processes do not generate free radicals or induce cross-linking, as with gamma irradiation [83]. Schipper et al. [84], in a laboratory study using a joint simulator, compared the wear in a semi-constrained, fixed-bearing ankle using conventional ultrahigh-molecular-weight polyethylene (CPE versus HXLPE). They found that HXLPE liners had a 3.1 times lower wear rate than CPE and produced significantly fewer and rounder particles than CPE liners, thus having more favorable wear characteristics for total ankle arthroplasty.

4.9 Positioning of the Components

Abnormal joint contact mechanics and ligament engagement patterns make correctly positioning the implants in total ankle arthroplasty difficult [85]. No validated method to accurately determine osseous landmarks to reference the ideal position of the implants has been described yet. If the tibial tuberosity is used as a reference for implant positioning, the wide range of tibial torsion is considered normal, and possible tibial bowing makes proper positioning difficult [86]. Although the tibial torsion can accurately be defined using CT, assessing the prosthesis components' position (tibial and talar) in the axial plane remains elusive. Using weight-bearing CT scans that allow for a detailed analysis of the hindfoot under physiologic load was promising for accurately assessing the prosthesis components after total ankle arthroplasty. Still, its benefit for determining the axis of rotation of the osteoarthritic ankle to be replaced remains limited [87].

The success of total ankle arthroplasty highly depends on whether the surgeon is able to balance the hindfoot (e.g., stable and neutral aligned) [64, 88]. In addition, accurate tibial and talar resection cuts, as well as a prosthesis design that restores native ankle biomechanics, were found to improve patient outcomes and enhance the longevity of the implant [89–91]. Altered biomechanics of the osteoarthritic ankle make total ankle arthroplasty challenging [5]. Due to the osteoarthritic process, determining the axis of ankle rotation is especially difficult (Fig. 4.18). In addition to the osteoarthritic process, hindfoot instability and alteration of the hindfoot alignment, which are frequently present in ankle osteoarthritis, impact on talar position [92]. Of note, it is unclear to which extent osteophyte removal, osteotomies, and release/reconstruction of periarticular ligaments can normalize the talar position during total ankle arthroplasty. Therefore, it is challenging for the surgeon to predict the axis of rotation of the ankle to be created during the replacement surgery.

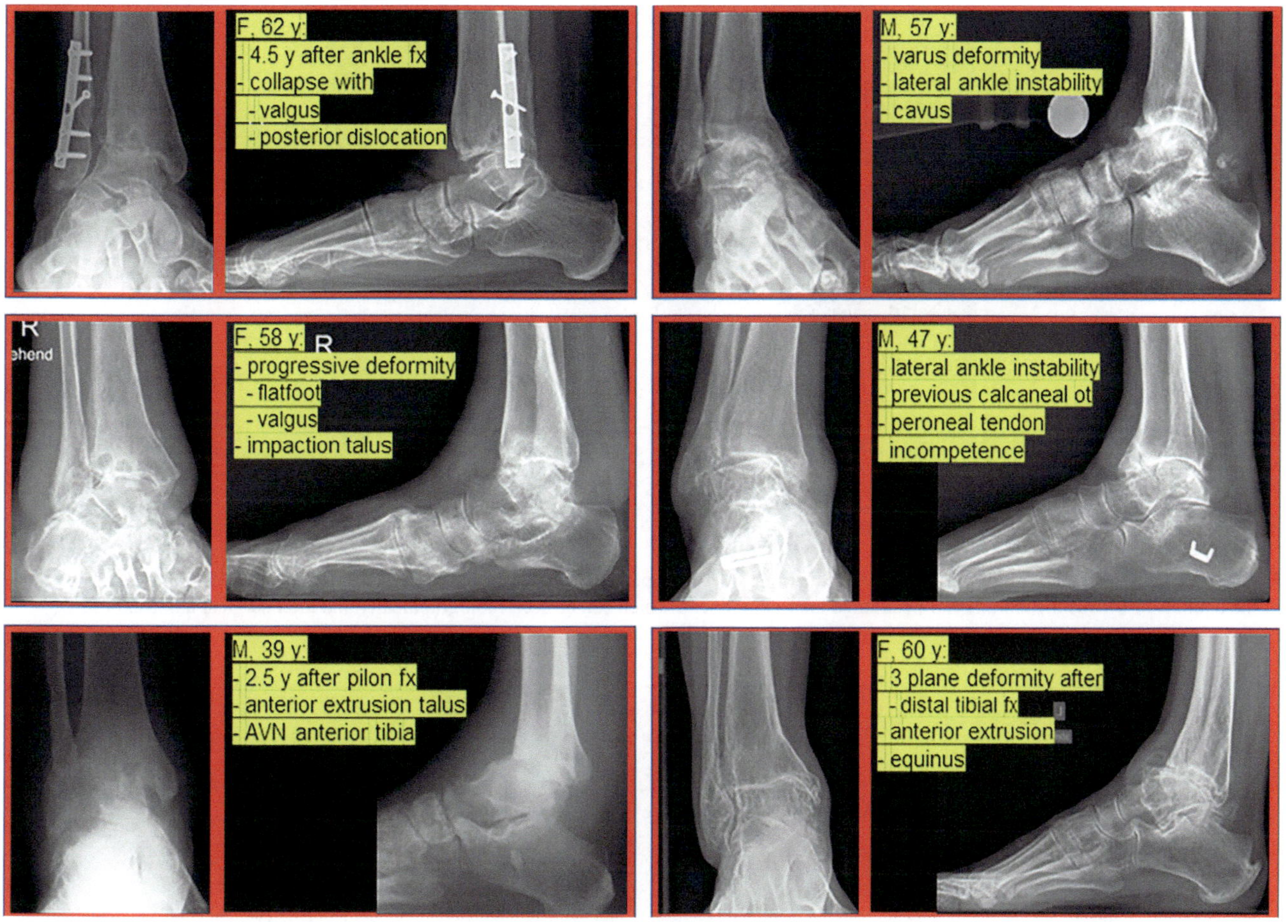

Fig. 4.18 Determination of the axis of rotation in an osteoarthritic ankle. The structural changes, particularly in posttraumatic osteoarthritis, are often significant, making determining the center of rotation difficult, if not impossible

4.10 Effect of Component Positioning on Implant-Bone Micromotion

Sopher et al. [53] investigated the effect of component positioning on implant-bone micromotion using finite element modeling. They found that any malpositioning of the implant creating a gap between it and the bone resulted in a considerable increase in micromotion and bone strains [53]. Another finite element analysis study showed that the relative debonding distance between the bone and prosthesis upon loading, as typically seen on the posterior aspect, was the main reason for the high interface micromotion between the talar component and talus bone [50]. For the tibial component, it was found that better stability can be achieved when fixed near the joint line and while relying on more than a single peg [53]. Peg-type tibial implant design may be a promising fixation method, which requires minimum bone resection volume and yields minimum micromotion under an extreme axial loading scenario [41]. Malalignment also increased peak contact stresses on the implant-bone interface [93].

4.11 Effect of Component Malposition

Total ankle arthroplasty has a steep learning curve [94, 95]. Specifically, correct positioning of the talar component is one of the most demanding steps, complicated by changes in the original center of rotation of the tibiotalar joint due to degeneration and concomitant valgus or varus hindfoot deformities. Further, the axis of rotation varies even in normal ankles and changes during the arc of motion [96]. Consequently, sagittal malposition of the talar component is a common intraoperative complication of total ankle arthroplasty (Fig. 4.19) [36, 53, 94, 97–100]. Furthermore, Lee et al. [101] have reported that malpositioning does not necessarily decrease with increased surgeon experience.

4.11.1 Sagittal Plane Malposition

Sagittal malpositioning of the talar component has biomechanical consequences on ankle motion and peak and aver-

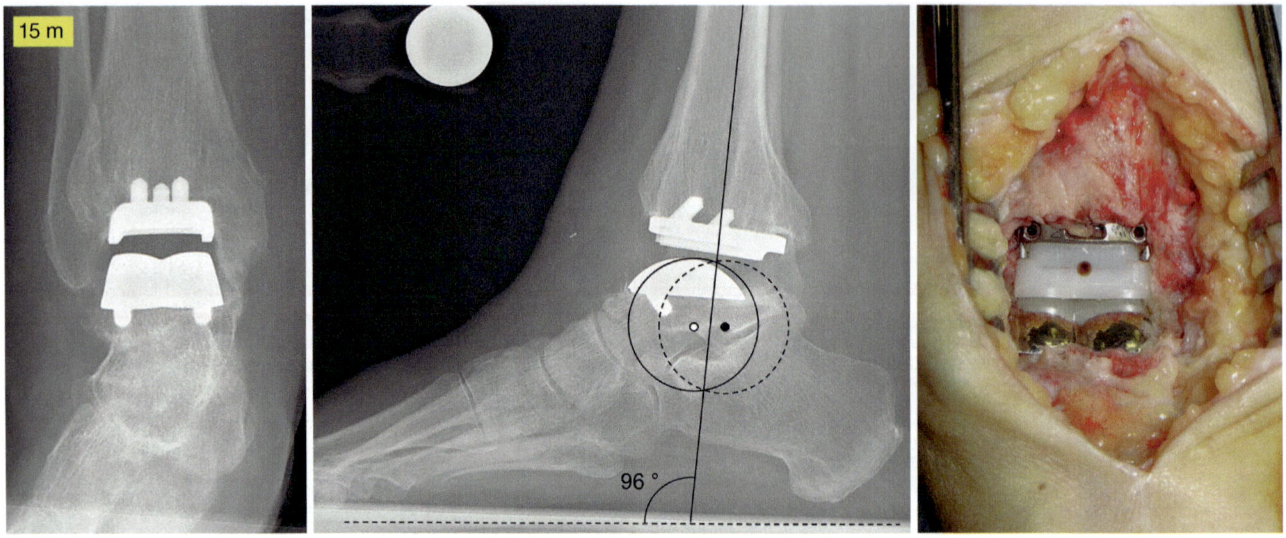

Fig. 4.19 Component malpositioning. A 61-year-old farmer's wife complained of painful stiffness in her replaced ankle 15 months ago. The cause of the equinus of 6° was the too-anterior positioned talar component, which can be seen radiographically and after surgical ankle exposure

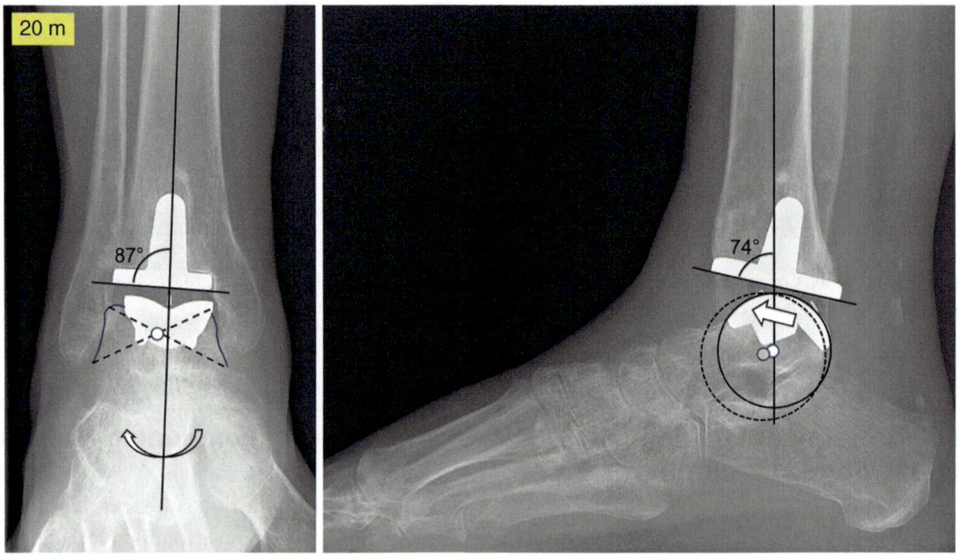

Fig. 4.20 Component malpositioning and inappropriate size. This 59-year-old patient was extremely dissatisfied 20 months after total ankle replacement with a mobile-bearing prosthesis. The pain was generated by loading the foot, and it was worse when trying to walk uphill or on the stairs. The cause of the dysfunction was the significantly increased posterior tilt of the tibial component and the too-posterior position of the talar component. The too-small and medialized talar component may have also contributed to the pain and dysfunction, as did the medial position of the talar component and the slightly valgus-positioned tibial component

age implant contact stresses (Fig. 4.20) [102, 103]. Positioning of prosthesis components, especially the talus, strongly affects resulting kinematics. Tochigi et al. [104] investigated the effect of talar component sagittal positioning on the range of motion using a specially modified STAR prosthesis. They found that anterior talar component displacement significantly decreased plantarflexion, associated with bearing lift-off, while the posterior displacement of the talar component significantly decreased dorsiflexion [104]. However, subsequent studies have failed to show a correlation between the sagittal translation of the talar component to the tibial axis (the AP offset ratio) and clinical outcomes [105, 106]. Furthermore, studies of mobile-bearing implants have shown that significant anteroposterior relocation of the talus occurs within the first 6 months, which is not likely to occur with fixed-bearing implants [90, 107].

Saltzman et al. [108] addressed the effect of ankle prosthesis malalignment on the peri-ankle ligament using an in vitro Agility prosthesis model. The anterior talofibular ligament was sensitive to transverse plane displacements,

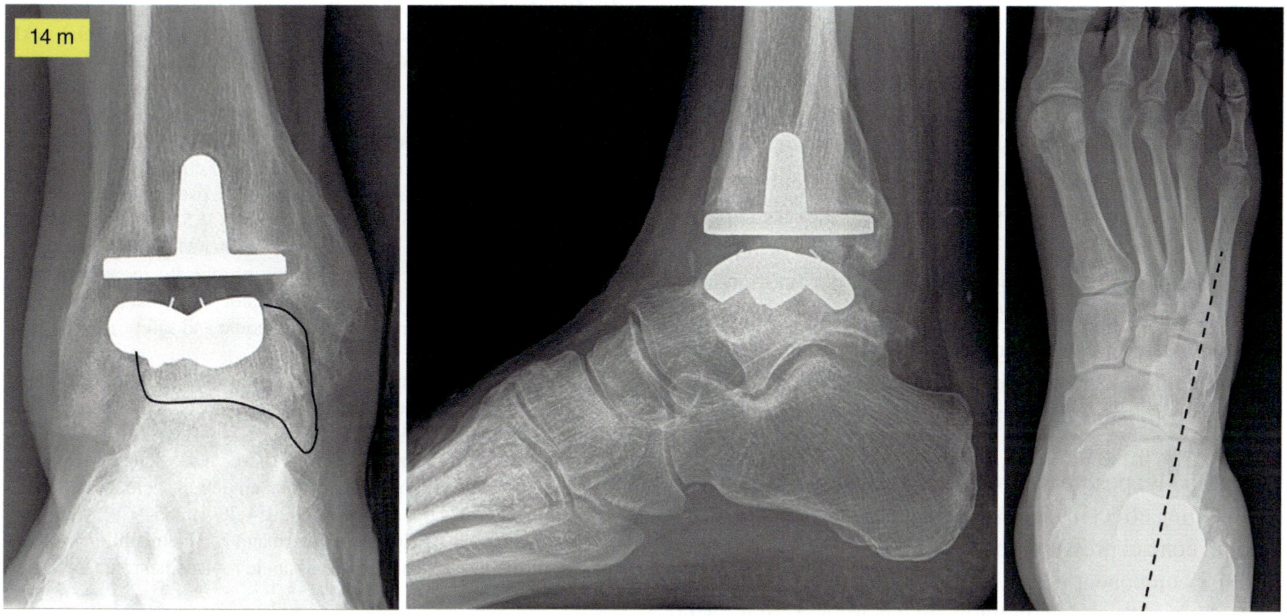

Fig. 4.21 Component malpositioning in the horizontal plane. A 52-year-old baker complained of pain medially and to a lesser extent also laterally in his replaced ankle 14 months ago. Dorsiflexion was limited to 3°. Potential causes of the pain and stiffness were too lateral and too much in external rotation malpositioned talar component. This resulted in altered mechanics of the replaced ankle and abnormal ligament strains. This may also explain the ossifications in the medial compartment

while the tibiocalcaneal ligament was sensitive to coronal plane displacements [108].

While numerous biomechanical studies have highlighted the influence of prosthetic component malalignment [63, 102, 103], only a few clinical studies describe pain relief and functional outcomes in patients with total ankle arthroplasty with various degrees of malposition [36, 98]. In a cohort of 317 patients, of which 265 (83.6%) had the preoperative diagnosis of posttraumatic osteoarthritis, Barg et al. [98] found in the group with the sagittal alignment of the talus close to the tibial axis (anteroposterior offset ratio = 0) significantly better outcome than in those with an anterior (ratio of >0) or posterior (ratio of <0) malalignment, including the pain and the range of motion. In another study on 368 ankles, the authors found the center of the tibia in 127 ankles (34.5%), anterior to the tibial axis in 136 ankles (37.0%), and posterior to the tibial axis in 105 ankles (28.5%) [36]. Most importantly, the anteroposterior ratio remained constant.

4.11.2 Horizontal Plane (Malrotation) Malposition

It has been shown that not only sagittal misalignment has a negative influence on biomechanics of the ankle but also other factors such as malrotation (Fig. 4.21) [63, 66]. Espinosa et al. [102] reported on two finite-element models of Agility and Mobility ankles. They modeled potential malalignments for the version of the tibial component, version of the talar component, and relative component rotation of the two-component design. Measured pressures consistently increased with malalignment, suggesting that accurate positioning of prosthesis components is one of the most important requirements for the procedure's success [102]. Fukuda et al. [63] reported in an in vitro study on the effect of talar component malrotation of the Agility prosthesis. They found that talar component malrotation leads to increased peak pressure, decreased contact area, and increased rotational torque, further supporting the need for accurate component placement [63].

4.11.3 Height of Joint Line

Ankle osteoarthritis often leads to an elevation of the joint line level due to subchondral bone wear and erosion of the distal tibial plafond [109, 110]. During replacement procedures, the joint line of the arthritic ankle is used as a reference point when making tibial and talar cuts. Consequently, while the ankle joint line may appear unchanged after total ankle arthroplasty, it might still be elevated compared to the non-arthritic ankle. It has not been clarified whether total ankle arthroplasty can restore the joint line to its native position and if the joint line level affects the function and clinical outcomes of the replaced ankle. However, years of adaptation, including soft-tissue contracture, bone erosion, and deformity, may not always allow the joint line to be restored to a normative value.

4.12 Conclusions

- Meticulous analysis of the osteoarthritic ankle regarding structural changes is mandatory for successful replacement surgery.
- Selected components should restore the articular surfaces as close as possible, using all available bones for support.
- Flat- and peg-type tibial implant design may be a promising fixation method with a minimum micromotion, bone resection level, and no disruption on the anterior cortical bone under an extreme axial loading scenario.
- Ankle implants in the non-cemented construct continue to migrate for up to 2 years after implantation to be afterward stable.
- Optimally positioned implants can reduce the strain-shielding effect in the tibial bone, implant-bone micromotion, contact pressure, and wear depth.
- Talar component positioning should restore the center of rotation of the ankle. Initially, malpositioned components, and therefore abnormal ligament strains, are correlated with later adverse outcomes.
- High ligament strain at implantation may restrict joint motion and reduce the motion range obtained after post-operative rehabilitation.
- There is evidence that, in a mobile-bearing ankle, abnormal talar motion within the ankle mortise, especially in the coronal plane, may cause polyethylene wear, whereas, in a fixed-bearing ankle, axial malrotation may cause asymmetric polyethylene wear.

References

1. Quill GE. An approach to the management of ankle arthritis. In: Myerson MS, editor. Foot and ankle disorders. Philadelphia/London/Toronto/Sidney: Saunders; 2000. p. 1059–84.
2. Valderrabano V, Horisberger M, Russell I, Dougall H, Hintermann B. Etiology of ankle osteoarthritis. Clin Orthop Relat Res. 2009;467(7):1800–6.
3. Saltzman CL, Salamon ML, Blanchard GM, Huff T, Hayes A, Buckwalter JA, et al. Epidemiology of ankle arthritis: report of a consecutive series of 639 patients from a tertiary orthopaedic center. Iowa Orthop J. 2005;25:44–6.
4. Hintermann B. Total ankle arthroplasty—historical overview, current concepts and future perspectives. Wien-New York: Springer; 2004. p. 195.
5. Daniels T, Thomas R. Etiology and biomechanics of ankle arthritis. Foot Ankle Clin. 2008;13(3):341–52. vii
6. Thomas RH, Daniels TR. Ankle arthritis. J Bone Joint Surg Am. 2003;85(5):923–36.
7. Easley ME, Vertullo CJ, Urban WC, Nunley JA. Total ankle arthroplasty. J Am Acad Orthop Surg. 2002;10(3):157–67.
8. Demetriades L, Strauss E, Gallina J. Osteoarthritis of the ankle. Clin Orthop Relat Res. 1998;(349):28–42.
9. Horisberger M, Valderrabano V, Hintermann B. Posttraumatic ankle osteoarthritis after ankle-related fractures. J Orthop Trauma. 2009;23(1):60–7.
10. Gaugler M, Krahenbuhl N, Barg A, Ruiz R, Horn-Lang T, Susdorf R, et al. Effect of age on outcome and revision in total ankle arthroplasty. Bone Joint J. 2020;102-B(7):925–32.
11. Kofoed H, Sorensen TS. Ankle arthroplasty for rheumatoid arthritis and osteoarthritis: prospective long-term study of cemented replacements. J Bone Joint Surg Br. 1998;80(2):328–32.
12. Cho BK, An MY, Ahn BH. Comparison of clinical outcomes after total ankle arthroplasty between end-stage osteoarthritis and rheumatoid arthritis. Foot Ankle Int. 2021;42(5):589–97.
13. Pedersen E, Pinsker E, Younger AS, Penner MJ, Wing KJ, Dryden PJ, et al. Outcome of total ankle arthroplasty in patients with rheumatoid arthritis and noninflammatory arthritis. A multicenter cohort study comparing clinical outcome and safety. J Bone Joint Surg Am. 2014;96(21):1768–75.
14. Barg A, Elsner A, Hefti D, Hintermann B. Total ankle arthroplasty in patients with hereditary hemochromatosis. Clin Orthop Relat Res. 2011;469(5):1427–35.
15. Asencio JG, Leonardi C, Biron-Andreani C, Schved JF. Short-term and mid-term outcome of total ankle replacement in haemophilic patients. Foot Ankle Surg. 2014;20(4):285–92.
16. Barg A, Elsner A, Hefti D, Hintermann B. Haemophilic arthropathy of the ankle treated by total ankle replacement: a case series. Haemophilia. 2010;16(4):647–55.
17. van der Heide HJ, Novakova I, de Waal Malefijt MC. The feasibility of total ankle prosthesis for severe arthropathy in haemophilia and prothrombin deficiency. Haemophilia. 2006;12(6):679–82.
18. Strauss AC, Goldmann G, Wessling M, Gravius S, Muller MC, Wimmer MD, et al. Total ankle replacement in patients with haemophilia and virus infections—a safe alternative to ankle arthrodesis? Haemophilia. 2014;20(5):702–8.
19. Preis M, Bailey T, Jacxsens M, Barg A. Total ankle replacement in patients with haemophilic arthropathy: primary arthroplasty and conversion of painful ankle arthrodesis to arthroplasty. Haemophilia. 2017;23(4):e301–e9.
20. Barg A, Knupp M, Kapron AL, Hintermann B. Total ankle replacement in patients with gouty arthritis. J Bone Joint Surg Am. 2011;93(4):357–66.
21. Hintermann B, Valderrabano V. Total ankle replacement. Foot Ankle Clin. 2003;8(2):375–405.
22. Morash J, Walton DM, Glazebrook M. Ankle arthrodesis versus total ankle arthroplasty. Foot Ankle Clin. 2017;22(2):251–66.
23. Guyer AJ, Richardson G. Current concepts review: total ankle arthroplasty. Foot Ankle Int. 2008;29(2):256–64.
24. Alvine FG. The agility ankle replacement: the good and the bad. Foot Ankle Clin. 2002;7(4):737–53, vi.
25. Krause FG, Schmid T. Ankle arthrodesis versus total ankle replacement: how do I decide? Foot Ankle Clin. 2012;17(4):529–43.
26. Saltzman CL. Perspective on total ankle replacement. Foot Ankle Clin. 2000;5(4):761–75.
27. Smyth NA, Kennedy JG, Parvizi J, Schon LC, Aiyer AA. Risk factors for periprosthetic joint infection following total ankle replacement. Foot Ankle Surg. 2020;26(5):591–5.
28. Clare MP, Sanders RW. Preoperative considerations in ankle replacement surgery. Foot Ankle Clin. 2002;7(4):709–20.
29. Leardini A, Moschella D. Dynamic simulation of the natural and replaced human ankle joint. Med Biol Eng Comput. 2002;40(2):193–9.
30. Stagni R, Leardini A, Ensini A, Cappello A. Ankle morphometry evaluated using a new semi-automated technique based on X-ray pictures. Clin Biomech (Bristol, Avon). 2005;20(3):307–11.
31. Leardini A, Catani F, Giannini S, O'Connor JJ. Computer-assisted design of the sagittal shapes of a ligament-compatible total ankle replacement. Med Biol Eng Comput. 2001;39(2):168–75.
32. Leardini A, O'Connor JJ, Catani F, Giannini S. Mobility of the human ankle and the design of total ankle replacement. Clin Orthop Relat Res. 2004;424:39–46.
33. Buechel FF, Pappas MJ. The New Jersey low-contact-stress knee replacement system: biomechanical rationale and review of the

first 123 cemented cases. Arch Orthop Trauma Surg (1978). 1986;105(4):197–204.
34. Kempson GE, Freeman MA, Tuke MA. Engineering considerations in the design of an ankle joint. Biomed Eng. 1975;10(5):166–71, 80.
35. Calderale PM, Garro A, Barbiero R, Fasolio G, Pipino F. Biomechanical design of the total ankle prosthesis. Eng Med. 1983;12(2):69–80.
36. Barg A, Elsner A, Chuckpaiwong B, Hintermann B. Insert position in three-component total ankle replacement. Foot Ankle Int. 2010;31(9):754–9.
37. Barg A, Knupp M, Henninger HB, Zwicky L, Hintermann B. Total ankle replacement using HINTEGRA, an unconstrained, three-component system: surgical technique and pitfalls. Foot Ankle Clin. 2012;17(4):607–35.
38. Kofoed H. Cylindrical cemented ankle arthroplasty: a prospective series with long-term follow-up. Foot Ankle Int. 1995;16(8):474–9.
39. Hintermann B, Valderrabano V, Dereymaeker G, Dick W. The HINTEGRA ankle: rationale and short-term results of 122 consecutive ankles. Clin Orthop Relat Res. 2004;424:57–68.
40. Falsig J, Hvid I, Jensen NC. Finite element stress analysis of some ankle joint prostheses. Clin Biomech (Bristol, Avon). 1986;1(2):71–6.
41. Yu J, Zhang C, Chen WM, Zhao D, Chu P, Wang S, et al. Finite-element analysis of the influence of tibial implant fixation design of total ankle replacement on bone-implant interfacial biomechanical performance. J Orthop Surg (Hong Kong). 2020;28(3):2309499020966125.
42. Zhao D, Huang D, Zhang G, Wang X, Zhang T, Ma X. Positive and negative factors for the treatment outcomes following total ankle arthroplasty? A systematic review. Foot Ankle Surg. 2020;26(1):1–13.
43. Viceconti M, Muccini R, Bernakiewicz M, Baleani M, Cristofolini L. Large-sliding contact elements accurately predict levels of bone-implant micromotion relevant to osseointegration. J Biomech. 2000;33(12):1611–8.
44. McInnes KA, Younger AS, Oxland TR. Initial instability in total ankle replacement: a cadaveric biomechanical investigation of the STAR and agility prostheses. J Bone Joint Surg Am. 2014;96(17):e147.
45. Patel AR, Barlow B, Ranawat AS. Stem length in revision total knee arthroplasty. Curr Rev Musculoskelet Med. 2015;8(4): 407–12.
46. Cracchiolo A 3rd, Deorio JK. Design features of current total ankle replacements: implants and instrumentation. J Am Acad Orthop Surg. 2008;16(9):530–40.
47. Tennant JN, Rungprai C, Pizzimenti MA, Goetz J, Phisitkul P, Femino J, et al. Risks to the blood supply of the talus with four methods of total ankle arthroplasty: a cadaveric injection study. J Bone Joint Surg Am. 2014;96(5):395–402.
48. Gross CE, Palanca AA, DeOrio JK. Design rationale for total ankle arthroplasty systems: an update. J Am Acad Orthop Surg. 2018;26(10):353–9.
49. Berkowitz MJ, Sanders RW, Walling AK. Salvage arthrodesis after failed ankle replacement: surgical decision making. Foot Ankle Clin. 2012;17(4):725–40.
50. Moideen ISM, Lim CT, Yeow RCH, Chong DYR. Finite element analysis of bone-prosthesis interface micromotion for cementless talar component fixation through critical loading conditions. Int J Numer Method Biomed Eng. 2020;36(3):e3310.
51. Volz RG, Nisbet JK, Lee RW, McMurtry MG. The mechanical stability of various noncemented tibial components. Clin Orthop Relat Res. 1988;226:38–42.
52. Mondal S, Ghosh R. Effects of implant orientation and implant material on tibia bone strain, implant-bone micromotion, contact pressure, and wear depth due to total ankle replacement. Proc Inst Mech Eng H. 2019;233(3):318–31.
53. Sopher RS, Amis AA, Calder JD, Jeffers JRT. Total ankle replacement design and positioning affect implant-bone micromotion and bone strains. Med Eng Phys. 2017;42:80–90.
54. Suarez DR, Nerkens W, Valstar ER, Rozing PM, van Keulen F. Interface micromotions increase with less-conforming cementless glenoid components. J Shoulder Elb Surg. 2012;21(4):474–82.
55. Stamatis ED, Myerson MS. How to avoid specific complications of total ankle replacement. Foot Ankle Clin. 2002;7(4):765–89.
56. Hvid I, Rasmussen O, Jensen NC, Nielsen S. Trabecular bone strength profiles at the ankle joint. Clin Orthop Relat Res. 1985;199:306–12.
57. Carlsson A, Markusson P, Sundberg M. Radiostereometric analysis of the double-coated STAR total ankle prosthesis: a 3-5 year follow-up of 5 cases with rheumatoid arthritis and 5 cases with osteoarthrosis. Acta Orthop. 2005;76(4):573–9.
58. Nelissen RG, Doets HC, Valstar ER. Early migration of the tibial component of the Buechel-Pappas total ankle prosthesis. Clin Orthop Relat Res. 2006;448:146–51.
59. Dunbar MJ, Fong JW, Wilson DA, Hennigar AW, Francis PA, Glazebrook MA. Longitudinal migration and inducible displacement of the mobility total ankle system. Acta Orthop. 2012;83(4):394–400.
60. Brigido SA, Wobst GM, Galli MM, Protzman NM. Evaluating Component Migration: Comparing Two Generations of the INBONE(®) Total Ankle Replacement. J Foot Ankle Surg. 2015;54(5):892–5.
61. Galante J, Rostoker W, Lueck R, Ray RD. Sintered fiber metal composites as a basis for attachment of implants to bone. J Bone Joint Surg Am. 1971;53(1):101–14.
62. Saito GH, Sturnick DR, Ellis SJ, Deland JT, Demetracopoulos CA. Influence of tibial component position on altered kinematics following total ankle arthroplasty during simulated gait. Foot Ankle Int. 2019;1071100719858620:873.
63. Fukuda T, Haddad SL, Ren Y, Zhang LQ. Impact of talar component rotation on contact pressure after total ankle arthroplasty: a cadaveric study. Foot Ankle Int. 2010;31(5):404–11.
64. Yi Y, Cho JH, Kim JB, Kim JY, Park SY, Lee WC. Change in talar translation in the coronal plane after mobile-bearing total ankle replacement and its association with lower-limb and Hindfoot alignment. J Bone Joint Surg Am. 2017;99(4):e13.
65. Ruiz R, Susdorf R, Krahenbuhl N, Barg A, Hintermann B. Syndesmotic overload in 3-component total ankle replacement. Foot Ankle Int. 2020;41(3):275–85.
66. Hintermann B, Susdorf R, Krahenbuhl N, Ruiz R. Axial rotational alignment in mobile-bearing total ankle arthroplasty. Foot Ankle Int. 2020;41(5):521–8.
67. Datir A, Xing M, Kakarala A, Terk MR, Labib SA. Radiographic evaluation of INBONE total ankle arthroplasty: a retrospective analysis of 30 cases. Skeletal Radiol. 2013;42(12): 1693–701.
68. Nielsen NM, Saito GH, Sanders AE, Ellis SJ, Sofka CM, Demetracopoulos CA. Sagittal tibiotalar alignment may not affect functional outcomes in fixed-bearing total ankle replacement: a retrospective cohort study. HSS J. 2020;16(Suppl 2): 300–4.
69. Jiang H, Wu L, Randsborg PH, Houck J, Sun L, Marine M, et al. Analysis of polyethylene-related revisions after total ankle replacements reported in US Food and Drug Administration medical device adverse event database. Foot Ankle Int. 2023;44(1):13–20.
70. Kvarda P, Toth L, Horn-Lang T, Susdorf R, Ruiz R, Hintermann B. How does a novel in situ fixed-bearing implant design perform in revision Ankle arthroplasty in the short term? A survival, clinical, and radiologic analysis. Clin Orthop Relat Res. 2023;481:1360.
71. Wright TM, Bartel DL. The problem of surface damage in polyethylene total knee components. Clin Orthop Relat Res. 1986;205:67–74.

72. Ewald FC, Walker PS. The current status of total knee replacement. Rheum Dis Clin N Am. 1988;14(3):579–90.
73. Bartel DL, Rawlinson JJ, Burstein AH, Ranawat CS, Flynn WF Jr. Stresses in polyethylene components of contemporary total knee replacements. Clin Orthop Relat Res. 1995;317:76–82.
74. Bartel DL, Bicknell VL, Wright TM. The effect of conformity, thickness, and material on stresses in ultra-high molecular weight components for total joint replacement. J Bone Joint Surg Am. 1986;68(7):1041–51.
75. Bartel DL, Burstein AH, Toda MD, Edwards DL. The effect of conformity and plastic thickness on contact stresses in metal-backed plastic implants. J Biomech Eng. 1985;107(3):193–9.
76. Jay Elliot B, Gundapaneni D, Goswami T. Finite element analysis of stress and wear characterization in total ankle replacements. J Mech Behav Biomed Mater. 2014;34:134–45.
77. Affatato S, Taddei P, Leardini A, Giannini S, Spinelli M, Viceconti M. Wear behaviour in total ankle replacement: a comparison between an in vitro simulation and retrieved prostheses. Clin Biomech (Bristol, Avon). 2009;24(8):661–9.
78. Dalat F, Barnoud R, Fessy MH, Besse JL, French Association of Foot Surgery AFCP. Histologic study of periprosthetic osteolytic lesions after AES total ankle replacement. A 22 case series. Orthop Traumatol Surg Res. 2013;6:285–95.
79. Schipper ON, Haddad SL, Pytel P, Zhou Y. Histological analysis of early osteolysis in total ankle arthroplasty. Foot Ankle Int. 2017;38(4):351–9.
80. Bischoff JE, Fryman JC, Parcell J, Orozco Villasenor DA. Influence of crosslinking on the wear performance of polyethylene within total ankle arthroplasty. Foot Ankle Int. 2015;36(4):369–76.
81. Bischoff JE, Dharia MA, Hertzler JS, Schipper ON. Evaluation of total ankle arthroplasty using highly crosslinked ultrahigh-molecular-weight polyethylene subjected to physiological loading. Foot Ankle Int. 2019;40(8):880–7.
82. Muratoglu OK, Merrill EW, Bragdon CR, O'Connor D, Hoeffel D, Burroughs B, et al. Effect of radiation, heat, and aging on in vitro wear resistance of polyethylene. Clin Orthop Relat Res. 2003;417:253–62.
83. White SE, Paxson RD, Tanner MG, Whiteside LA. Effects of sterilization on wear in total knee arthroplasty. Clin Orthop Relat Res. 1996;331:164–71.
84. Schipper ON, Haddad SL, Fullam S, Pourzal R, Wimmer MA. Wear characteristics of conventional ultrahigh-molecular-weight polyethylene versus highly cross-linked polyethylene in total ankle arthroplasty. Foot Ankle Int. 2018;39(11):1335–44.
85. Spirt AA, Assal M, Hansen ST Jr. Complications and failure after total ankle arthroplasty. J Bone Joint Surg Am. 2004;86-A(6):1172–8.
86. Strecker W, Keppler P, Gebhard F, Kinzl L. Length and torsion of the lower limb. J Bone Joint Surg Br. 1997;79(6):1019–23.
87. Barg A, Bailey T, Richter M, de Cesar NC, Lintz F, Burssens A, et al. Weightbearing computed tomography of the foot and ankle: emerging technology topical review. Foot Ankle Int. 2018;39(3):376–86.
88. Queen RM, Adams SB Jr, Viens NA, Friend JK, Easley ME, Deorio JK, et al. Differences in outcomes following total ankle replacement in patients with neutral alignment compared with tibiotalar joint malalignment. J Bone Joint Surg Am. 2013;95(21):1927–34.
89. Valderrabano V, Hintermann B, Nigg BM, Stefanyshyn D, Stergiou P. Kinematic changes after fusion and total replacement of the ankle: part 3: talar movement. Foot Ankle Int. 2003;24(12):897–900.
90. Lee KB, Kim MS, Park KS, Cho KJ, Primadhi A. Effect of anterior translation of the talus on outcomes of three-component total ankle arthroplasty. BMC Musculoskelet Disord. 2013;14:260.
91. Lee KJ, Wang SH, Lee GW, Lee KB. Accuracy assessment of measuring component position after total ankle arthroplasty using a conventional method. J Orthop Surg Res. 2017;12(1):115.
92. Kim JB, Yi Y, Kim JY, Cho JH, Kwon MS, Choi SH, et al. Weight-bearing computed tomography findings in varus ankle osteoarthritis: abnormal internal rotation of the talus in the axial plane. Skeletal Radiol. 2017;46(8):1071–80.
93. van Hoogstraten SWG, Hermus J, Loenen ACY, Arts JJ, van Rietbergen B. Malalignment of the total ankle replacement increases peak contact stresses on the bone-implant interface: a finite element analysis. BMC Musculoskelet Disord. 2022;23(1):463.
94. Lee KB, Cho SG, Hur CI, Yoon TR. Perioperative complications of HINTEGRA total ankle replacement: our initial 50 cases. Foot Ankle Int. 2008;29(10):978–84.
95. Saltzman CL, Amendola A, Anderson R, Coetzee JC, Gall RJ, Haddad SL, et al. Surgeon training and complications in total ankle arthroplasty. Foot Ankle Int. 2003;24(6):514–8.
96. Lundberg A, Svensson OK, Nemeth G, Selvik G. The axis of rotation of the ankle joint. J Bone Joint Surg Br. 1989;71(1): 94–9.
97. Younger A, Veljkovic A. Current update in total ankle arthroplasty: salvage of the failed total ankle arthroplasty with anterior translation of the talus. Foot Ankle Clin. 2017;22(2):301–9.
98. Barg A, Elsner A, Anderson AE, Hintermann B. The effect of three-component total ankle replacement malalignment on clinical outcome: pain relief and functional outcome in 317 consecutive patients. J Bone Joint Surg Am. 2011;93(21):1969–78.
99. Goldberg AJ, Sharp B, Cooke P. Early failure in total ankle replacements due to component malposition: a report of two cases. Foot Ankle Int. 2009;30(8):783–7.
100. Schuberth JM, Patel S, Zarutsky E. Perioperative complications of the agility total ankle replacement in 50 initial, consecutive cases. J Foot Ankle Surg. 2006;45(3):139–46.
101. Lee KT, Lee YK, Young KW, Kim JB, Seo YS. Perioperative complications and learning curve of the mobility total ankle system. Foot Ankle Int. 2013;34(2):210–4.
102. Espinosa N, Walti M, Favre P, Snedeker JG. Misalignment of total ankle components can induce high joint contact pressures. J Bone Joint Surg Am. 2010;92(5):1179–87.
103. Tochigi Y, Rudert MJ, Brown TD, McIff TE, Saltzman CL. The effect of accuracy of implantation on range of movement of the Scandinavian total ankle replacement. J Bone Joint Surg Br. 2005;87(5):736–40.
104. Tochigi Y, Suh JS, Amendola A, Saltzman CL. Ankle alignment on lateral radiographs. Part 2: reliability and validity of measures. Foot Ankle Int. 2006;27(2):88–92.
105. Braito M, Dammerer D, Reinthaler A, Kaufmann G, Huber D, Biedermann R. Effect of coronal and sagittal alignment on outcome after mobile-bearing total ankle replacement. Foot Ankle Int. 2015;36(9):1029–37.
106. Cho J, Yi Y, Ahn TK, Choi HJ, Park CH, Chun DI, et al. Failure to restore sagittal tibiotalar alignment in total ankle arthroplasty: its relationship to the axis of the tibia and the positioning of the talar component. Bone Joint J. 2015;97-B(11):1525–32.
107. Usuelli FG, Maccario C, Manzi L, Tan EW. Posterior talar shifting in mobile-bearing total ankle replacement. Foot Ankle Int. 2016;37(3):281–7.
108. Saltzman CL, Tochigi Y, Rudert MJ, McIff TE, Brown TD. The effect of agility ankle prosthesis misalignment on the peri-ankle ligaments. Clin Orthop Relat Res. 2004;424: 137–42.
109. Bischoff JE, Schon L, Saltzman C. Influence of geometry and depth of resections on bone support for total ankle replacement. Foot Ankle Int. 2017;38(9):1026–34.
110. Harnroongroj T, Hummel A, Ellis SJ, Sofka CM, Caolo KC, Deland JT, et al. Assessing the ankle joint line level before and after total ankle arthroplasty with the "joint line height ratio". Foot Ankle Orthop. 2019;4(4):2473011419884359.

Part II

Diagnosis, Planning, Surgical Procedure and Postoperative Care

Diagnostic Workup of the Osteoarthritic Ankle

5

Recognizing critical preoperative risk factors and careful preoperative planning are essential factors for limiting complications and obtaining satisfactory results. Meticulous clinical and radiological assessment is required. Clinically, the surgeon should examine and document the soft-tissue conditions, hindfoot alignment, ankle stability, foot deformities, foot vascularization, and sensibility. Lateral and anteroposterior weight-bearing foot and ankle radiographs, including an alignment view, are mandatory and may help identify possible osteoarthritis in adjacent joints and varus and valgus deformities of the hindfoot and longitudinal arch. A CT scan helps to identify bony lesions and, if done under weight-bearing, to understand deformities and instability patterns of the whole ankle joint complex, especially at the peritalar joints. MRI may also help to determine the condition of the subchondral bone, particularly for potential osteonecrosis.

5.1 Clinical Examination

Preoperative planning starts with carefully assessing patient history, including a complete study of all available medical records mentioning the previous trauma and surgical treatment. The patient should be asked about the nature and the mechanism of the trauma, surgeries, concomitant diseases, or infections in the past. In patients with ankle stiffness and/or equinus contracture, whether the stiffness and/or contracture progressed in the last months should be clarified.

The routine physical examination includes careful inspection of both lower extremities and observation of the patient while walking and standing (Fig. 5.1). Hindfoot stability should be assessed manually while the patient is sitting. Ankle alignment and range of motion are assessed while the patient is standing. Range of motion is determined clinically with a goniometer placed along the lateral border of the leg and foot for measuring sagittal plane motion (plantarflexion/dorsiflexion). Assessment of the subtalar motion (pronation/supination) and sinus tarsi palpation may help exclude subtalar osteoarthritis. Next, pain or tenderness by palpation is evaluated. The patient's neurovascular status should be evaluated; in particular, the integrity of the tibial nerve function should be proven. Muscular functional status and atrophy should be assessed. Particular attention should be paid to the soft tissues around the ankle, especially scars, flaps, possible tightness of the heel cord, and the function of plantar flexors, including the posterior tibial muscle and flexor hallucis longus muscle.

B. Hintermann, R. Ruiz, *Total Ankle Replacement*, https://doi.org/10.1007/978-3-031-56810-7_5

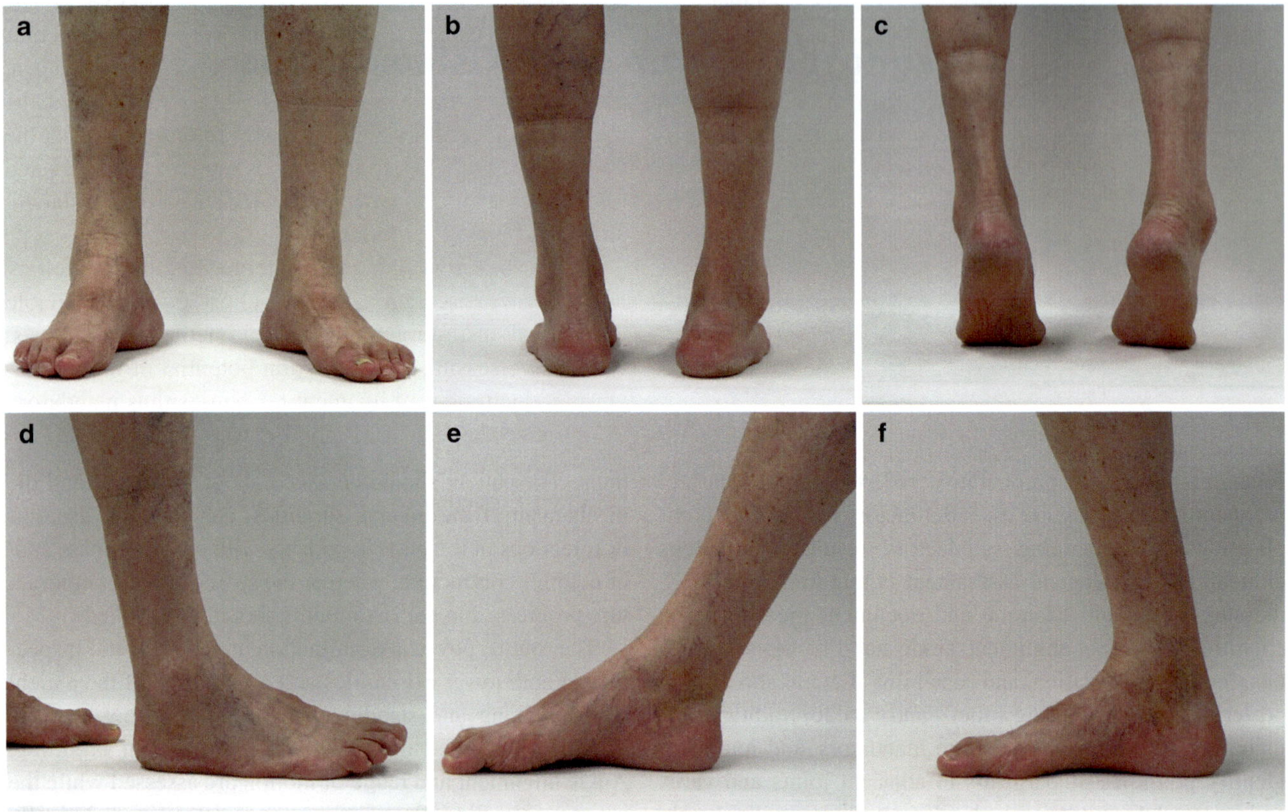

Fig. 5.1 Clinical inspection. Most deformities and functional changes of the whole foot can be seen by visual inspection. This 54-year-old sports teacher suffers from progressive medial pain in his right ankle. (**a**) The AP view evidences a unilateral cavovarus deformity. (**b**) From the posterior view, the varus is more pronounced and increases in the tiptoe position due to the plantarflexed first ray (**c**). The leg is additionally seen to rotate externally. (**d**) The lateral view shows the overload of the lateral foot. Motion at the ankle is well-preserved, as seen for plantarflexion (**e**) and dorsiflexion (**f**)

5.2 Imaging Evaluation

5.2.1 Radiographs

The routine radiographic evaluation includes bilateral weight-bearing anteroposterior and lateral views of the foot and ankle (Fig. 5.2). A hindfoot alignment view should be performed for an appropriate assessment of inframalleolar alignment [1, 2]. The radiographs should be used to identify and quantify the tibiotalar joint's degenerative changes, malposition, and deformities [3]. Furthermore, standard radiographs permit identifying and assessing possible concomitant degenerative changes and deformations in the adjacent joints of the hindfoot and midfoot.

If a deformity above the ankle is suspected, it is generally accepted that radiographic evaluation should commence with weight-bearing bilateral mortise and lateral films on long cassettes [4, 5]. However, measurements are sometimes made on only mortise images of the ankle, which do not include the tibial plateau. Stufkens et al. [6], in a study on 24 healthy volunteers, assessed the difference between the lateral distal tibial angle (LDTA) when measured on whole lower limb radiographs and mortise radiographs of the ankle. They found a mean value of 87.9 ± 2.2° in the mortise views and a mean of 85.4 ± 2.6°, the difference between both measurements accounting for up to 5°. This may be important when planning coronal deformity correction of the distal tibia or assessing the placement of total ankle replacement tibia components.

Weight-bearing radiography is the reference standard for alignment evaluation, but overlapping bones and hardware limit the evaluation of osteoarthritic bony detail.

5.2.2 Computed Tomography (CT)

Recently, we started the routine use of weight-bearing CT that correctly evaluates foot and ankle anatomical disposition under physiological standing load to assess hindfoot alignment and complexity of the degenerative changes of the hindfoot [7–11]. We have found it helpful to understand

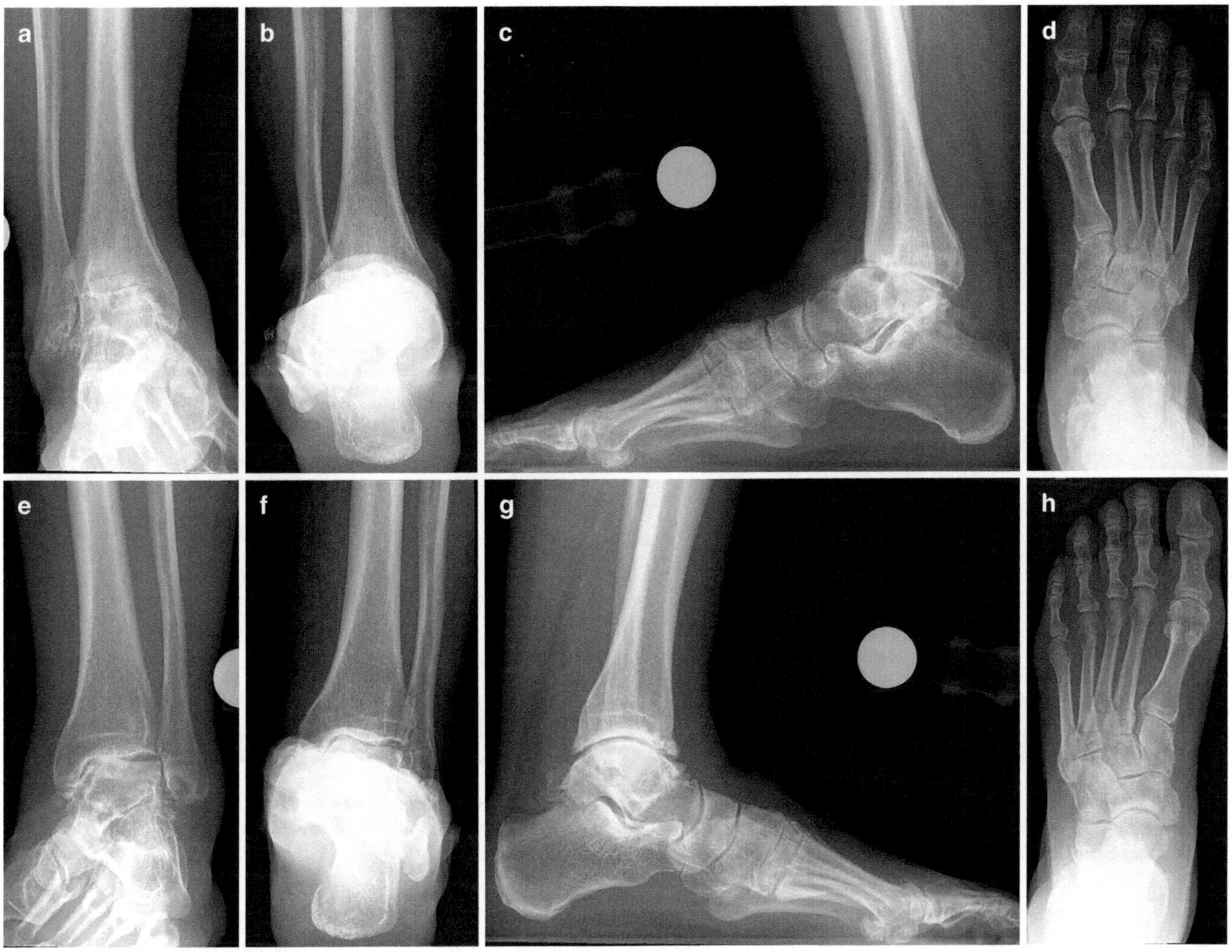

Fig. 5.2 Standard weight-bearing radiographs and alignment view. Standard weight-bearing radiographs are essential to understand the pathology and planning the surgery. This 66-year-old passioned hunter sustained recurrent sprains in both ankles but never underwent specific treatment. While the AP (**a**) and the alignment view (**b**) suggest a well-balanced and aligned ankle, the lateral view demonstrates a significant anterior extrusion of the talus with bone erosion at the talar dome and anterior tibia (**c**). (**d**) The DP view of the foot also looks average. (**e–h**) Comparison with the contralateral ankle may help better understand the pathology. In this patient, however, the left ankle is also destabilized with involvement of the peritalar joints, resulting in a varus-valgus "zig-zag" deformity, causing some forefoot supination

overall pathologic processes in the tibiotalar and peritalar joints, particularly segmental deformity (Fig. 5.3).

Auto-generated 3-D measurements of the hind- and midfoot were reliable in healthy individuals and patients with post-traumatic end-stage ankle osteoarthritis [12]. Such measurements may be crucial for a detailed understanding of the location and extent of hindfoot deformities, possibly impacting decision-making in treating end-stage ankle osteoarthritis [13].

Single-photon emission computed tomography combined with computed tomography (SPECT/CT) may aid in diagnosing periarticular arthritis/activity and thus be beneficial in decision-making whether neighboring joints of the ankle should be fused before or at the time of total ankle arthroplasty (Fig. 5.4) [14, 15].

5.2.3 Magnetic Resonance Imaging (MRI)

MRI is not routinely recommended in the preoperative assessment of end-stage ankle osteoarthritis. However, it has value in identifying and understanding the ongoing osteoarthritic process in the ankle joint (Fig. 5.5). For instance, it allows us to identify cartilage degradation and subchondral bone marrow lesions and to grade the severity of ankle osteoarthritis with a clinically helpful high degree of reproducibility [16]. MRI imaging may also help evaluate the possible tendon and muscular pathologies [17]. Furthermore, MRI may be used for detailed quantification of capsular and pericapsular thickening and scarring in patients with arthrofibrosis of the foot and ankle [18].

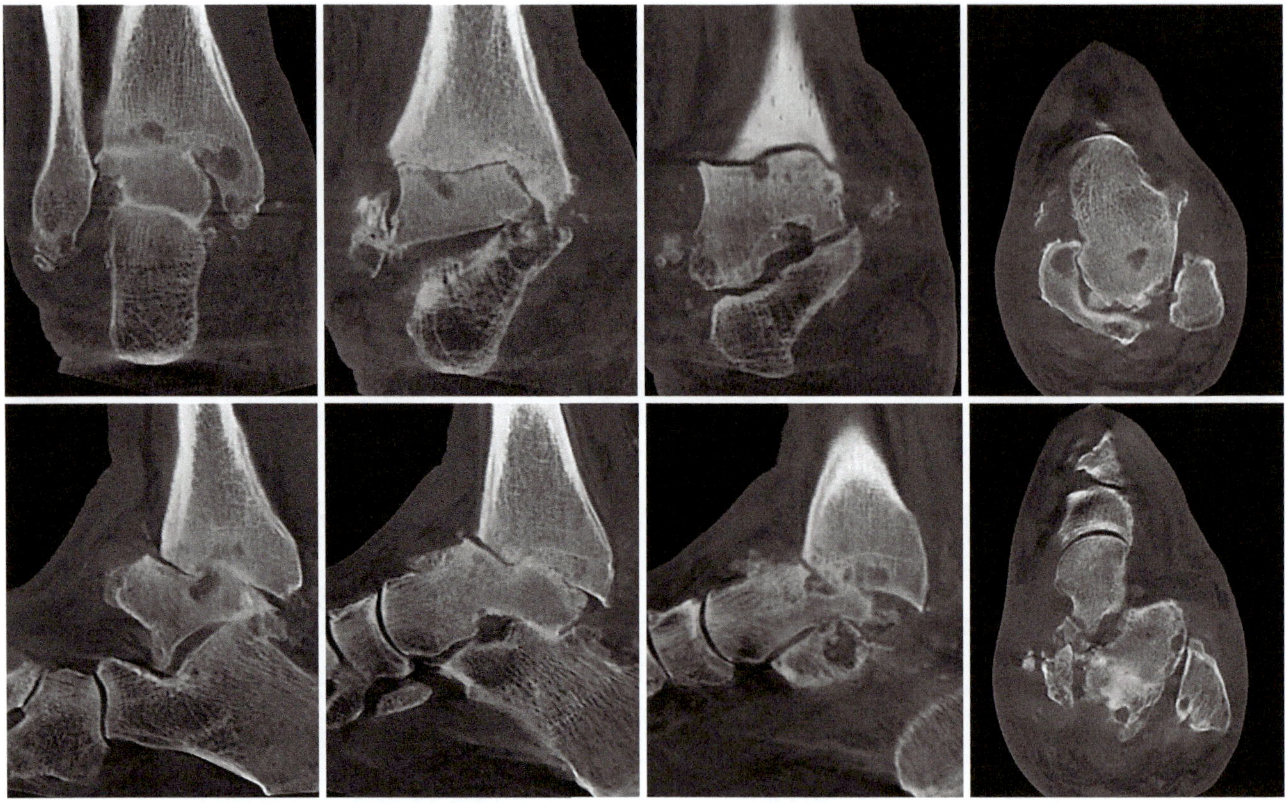

Fig. 5.3 Weight-bearing CT scan. In the same patient as Fig. 5.2, the weight-bearing CT helps better understand the osteoarthritic and destabilization process. Besides the significant defect on the talar dome with hooked-in anterior tibia, it shows that the peritalar joints are more involved in the destabilization process than expected by the radiographic analysis

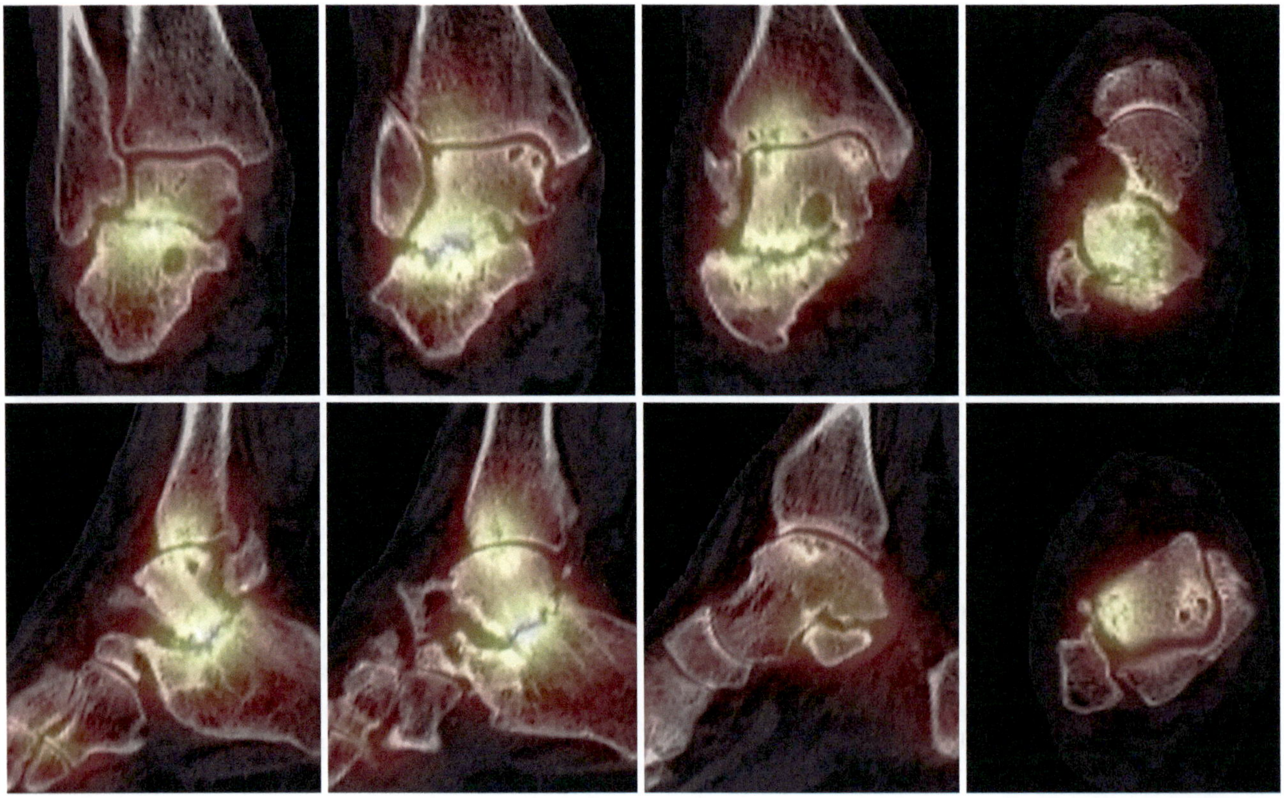

Fig. 5.4 SPECT-CT. In this 53-year-old female patient, the SPECT-CT confirms an advanced stage of osteoarthritis in both the ankle and the subtalar joint that helps to decide on a subtalar fusion during the ankle replacement surgery

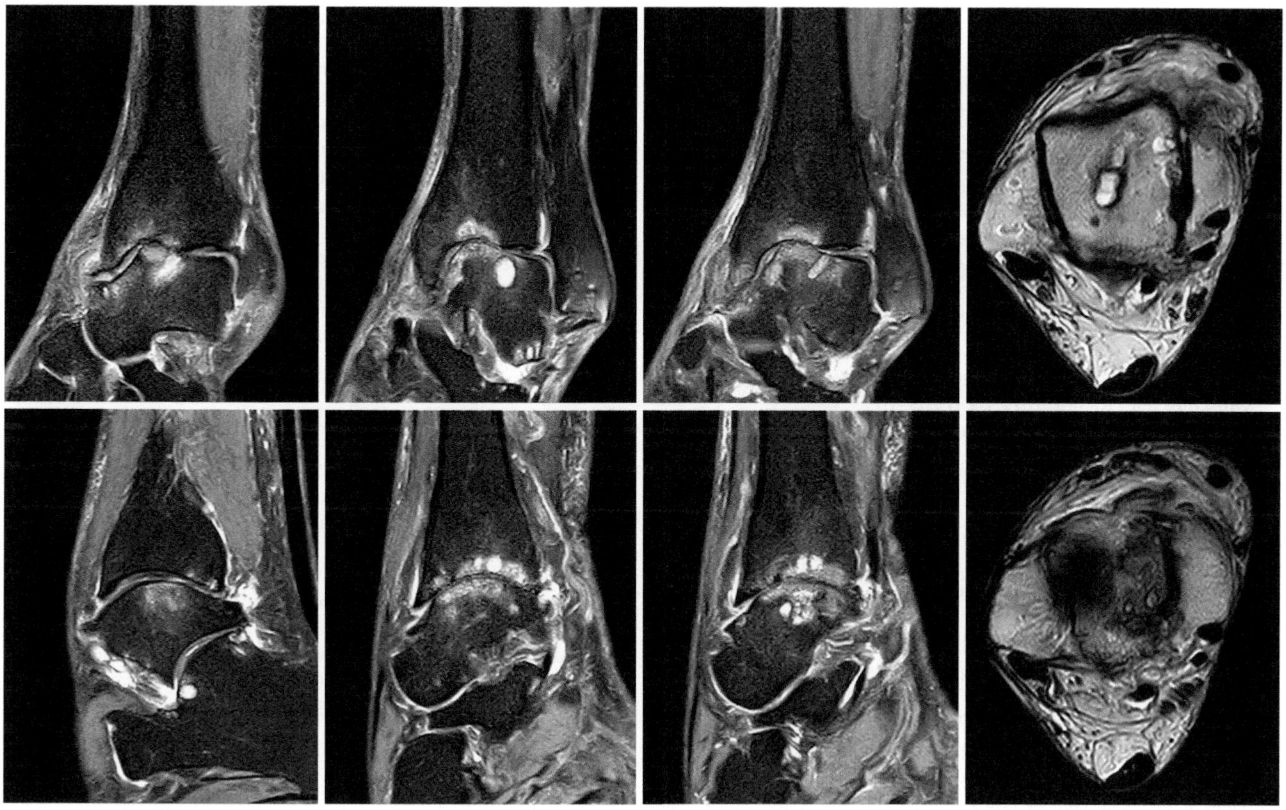

Fig. 5.5 MRI. Though to some extent helpful to understand the osteoarthritic changes in more detail, it does not provide additional information about the periarticular soft-tissue structures in this 59-year-old former high-level volleyball player patient with varus osteoarthritis

5.3 Patient's Expectations

The most crucial step in the decision-making process for total ankle arthroplasty is understanding the patient's expectations [19]. In choosing between fusion and total ankle arthroplasty, the patient with end-stage ankle osteoarthritis should know the benefits in favor of total ankle arthroplasty including restoring some ankle motion, improving gait biomechanics to a certain extent, and avoiding advanced adjacent joint degeneration more commonly seen following ankle fusion [20–24]. They should know that range of motion is the main factor determining the eventual postoperative range of motion [25].

They need to know that the gait velocity will be lower when compared with a healthy person. Still, usually, they have faster speed when compared with their preoperative arthritic ankle condition [20, 22, 23, 26]. The surgeon must clearly explain that he or she will get a more normal ankle but never a normal ankle that will allow for high-impact activities. Indeed, besides pain relief, the patient's activity may improve and allow for some sports and recreational activities [27]. Among ten patients who underwent both an ankle fusion on one side and a total ankle arthroplasty on the contralateral side, most participants preferred the increased range of motion provided by their total ankle arthroplasty, describing its flexibility or movement as "more normal" or natural and better for maintaining balance, shifting one's weight, and accommodating stairs [28].

5.4 Conclusions

- Addressing the osteoarthritic ankle is highly complex and is mainly associated with deformity, instability, and bad soft tissues.
- Careful clinical examination and thorough radiographic assessment are mandatory to anticipate potential problems and complications during the replacement surgery.
- Weight-bearing radiographs are the key elements for assessing the foot and ankle. Weight-bearing CT scans can further help to understand the thorough pathology.
- A SPECT-CT may further aid in diagnosing periarticular arthritis/activity and thus benefit decision-making.
- The most crucial step in the decision-making process for total ankle arthroplasty is understanding the patient's expectations.
- Counseling patients appropriately on expectations after total ankle arthroplasty is paramount to avoid dissatisfaction.

References

1. Barg A, Amendola RL, Henninger HB, Kapron AL, Saltzman CL, Anderson AE. Measurement of supramalleolar alignment on the anteroposterior and hindfoot alignment views: influence of ankle position and radiographic projection angle. Foot Ankle Int. 2015;36(11):1352–61.
2. Saltzman CL, El-Khoury GY. The hindfoot alignment view. Foot Ankle Int. 1995;16(9):572–6.
3. Linklater JM, Read JW, Hayter CL. Imaging of the foot and ankle. In: Coughlin MJ, Saltzman CL, Anderson RB, editors. Mann's surgery of the foot and ankle. 9th ed. Philadelphia, PA: Elsevier Saunders; 2014. p. 61–120.
4. Cadden AR. Imaging in total ankle replacement. Semin Musculoskelet Radiol. 2012;16(3):205–16.
5. Hintermann B, Ruiz R. Joint preservation strategies for managing varus ankle deformities. Foot Ankle Clin. 2022;27(1):37–56.
6. Stufkens SA, Barg A, Bolliger L, Stucinskas J, Knupp M, Hintermann B. Measurement of the medial distal tibial angle. Foot Ankle Int. 2011;32(3):288–93.
7. Colin F, Horn Lang T, Zwicky L, Hintermann B, Knupp M. Subtalar joint configuration on weightbearing CT scan. Foot Ankle Int. 2014;35(10):1057–62.
8. Krahenbuhl N, Tschuck M, Bolliger L, Hintermann B, Knupp M. Orientation of the subtalar joint: measurement and reliability using Weightbearing CT scans. Foot Ankle Int. 2016;37(1):109–14.
9. Barg A, Bailey T, Richter M, de Cesar NC, Lintz F, Burssens A, et al. Weightbearing computed tomography of the foot and ankle: emerging technology topical review. Foot Ankle Int. 2018;39(3):376–86.
10. Lintz F, de Cesar Netto C, Barg A, Burssens A, Richter M, Weight Bearing CTISG. Weight-bearing cone beam CT scans in the foot and ankle. EFORT Open Rev. 2018;3(5):278–86.
11. Richter M, de Cesar NC, Lintz F, Barg A, Burssens A, Ellis S. The assessment of ankle osteoarthritis with weight-bearing computed tomography. Foot Ankle Clin. 2022;27(1):13–36.
12. Kvarda P, Heisler L, Krahenbuhl N, Steiner CS, Ruiz R, Susdorf R, et al. 3D assessment in posttraumatic ankle osteoarthritis. Foot Ankle Int. 2021;42(2):200–14.
13. Krahenbuhl N, Siegler L, Deforth M, Zwicky L, Hintermann B, Knupp M. Subtalar joint alignment in ankle osteoarthritis. Foot Ankle Surg. 2019;25(2):7.
14. DeSutter C, Dube V, Ross A, Boyd G, Morash J, Glazebrook M. Preliminary experience with SPECT/CT to evaluate periarticular arthritis progression and the relationship with clinical outcome following ankle arthrodesis. Foot Ankle Int. 2020;41(4):392–7.
15. Pagenstert GI, Barg A, Leumann AG, Rasch H, Muller-Brand J, Hintermann B, et al. SPECT-CT imaging in degenerative joint disease of the foot and ankle. J Bone Joint Surg Br. 2009;91(9):1191–6.
16. Aboelmagd SM, Low SB, Cahir JG, Loveday D, Marshall AT, Teh J, et al. The Norwich osteoarthritis of the ankle MRI score (NOAMS): a reliability study. Clin Radiol. 2022;77(6):e449–e57.
17. Hintermann B. What the orthopaedic foot and ankle surgeon wants to know from MR imaging. Semin Musculoskelet Radiol. 2005;9(3):260–71.
18. Linklater JM, Fessa CK. Imaging findings in arthrofibrosis of the ankle and foot. Semin Musculoskelet Radiol. 2012;16(3):185–91.
19. Khilnani TK, Barth KA, Henry JK, Cororaton AD, Cody EA, Mancuso CA, et al. Association between fulfillment of preoperative expectations and diagnosis in foot and ankle surgery. Foot Ankle Int. 2023;10711007231177035:710.
20. Wu WL, Su FC, Cheng YM, Huang PJ, Chou YL, Chou CK. Gait analysis after ankle arthrodesis. Gait Posture. 2000;11(1):54–61.
21. Saltzman CL, Mann RA, Ahrens JE, Amendola A, Anderson RB, Berlet GC, et al. Prospective controlled trial of STAR total ankle replacement versus ankle fusion: initial results. Foot Ankle Int. 2009;30(7):579–96.
22. Brodsky JW, Polo FE, Coleman SC, Bruck N. Changes in gait following the Scandinavian total ankle replacement. J Bone Joint Surg Am. 2011;93(20):1890–6.
23. Valderrabano V, Nigg BM, von Tscharner V, Stefanyshyn DJ, Goepfert B, Hintermann B. Gait analysis in ankle osteoarthritis and total ankle replacement. Clin Biomech (Bristol, Avon). 2007;22(8):894–904.
24. Singer S, Klejman S, Pinsker E, Houck J, Daniels T. Ankle arthroplasty and ankle arthrodesis: gait analysis compared with normal controls. J Bone Joint Surg Am. 2013;95(24):e191. (1–10).
25. Coetzee JC, Castro MD. Accurate measurement of ankle range of motion after total ankle arthroplasty. Clin Orthop Relat Res. 2004;424:27–31.
26. Piriou P, Culpan P, Mullins M, Cardon JN, Pozzi D, Judet T. Ankle replacement versus arthrodesis: a comparative gait analysis study. Foot Ankle Int. 2008;29(1):3–9.
27. Valderrabano V, Pagenstert G, Horisberger M, Knupp M, Hintermann B. Sports and recreation activity of ankle arthritis patients before and after total ankle replacement. Am J Sports Med. 2006;34(6):993–9.
28. Conlin C, Khan RM, Wilson I, Daniels TR, Halai M, Pinsker EB. Living with both a total ankle replacement and an ankle fusion: a qualitative study from the patients' perspective. Foot Ankle Int. 2021;42(9):1153–61.

6 Indications: Contraindications for Total Ankle Replacement

No consensus exists regarding the indications and contraindications for total ankle arthroplasty. The first-generation total ankle arthroplasty indications were initially broad and included patients of all ages and diagnoses. These indications narrowed rapidly when poor intermediate-term results and high complication rates became apparent [1–6]. In general, neuroarthropathy [7–11], (diabetic) neuropathy [7, 12–14], peripheral vascular disease [7–10, 13, 15], neurologic disorders [7, 13], and active infection [7, 8, 13] were considered absolute contraindications for total ankle arthroplasty, whereas osteonecrosis [8, 16–20], loss of bone stock [7, 8, 10, 11], diabetes [21], smoking [7, 21], poor skin integrity [7, 9, 13, 15], osteoporosis [7, 9, 10, 14, 22], gross deformity [7, 8, 10, 14, 23], noncompliance [7, 13, 14], high physical demand [13, 14], high body mass index (BMI) [7, 10, 21, 24], gross ankle instability [7, 8, 25], and a history of previous joint infection [7–11, 17, 26] were considered relative contraindications. However, the scientific basis for these recommendations was scarce.

Nowadays, the number of total ankle replacements performed is tremendously increasing [27–33]. Naturally, indications are expanding [34] as surgeons are more experienced in using modern second- and third-generation arthroplasty techniques, and their confidence in the outcomes of ankle joint replacement is rising.

Proper patient selection is the most critical aspect of promoting a successful outcome (aside from intraoperative factors). The optimal patient for total ankle arthroplasty is said to be physically low-demanding [10, 11, 13, 35], non-obese [10, 21, 24], and older [11, 21, 36] with end-stage non-traumatic primary ankle arthrosis [35, 36] or multiple joint arthritis [21] with minimal deformity [10, 11, 21], good bone stock [11], no neurovascular leg impairment [11, 21], and excellent/more than two-thirds of normal range of motion [10, 36]. Unfortunately, the majority of the patients do not meet these requirements [10], and scientific evidence for these recommendations is not available [8].

In addition to patient characteristics, conflicting evidence exists on other factors, such as the prosthesis type or version used [27, 28, 37], duration of surgery [38, 39], surgeon volume [40, 41], and surgeon experience [18, 42–47], which might influence the number of complications and survival of total ankle arthroplasty.

6.1 Indications

In general, total ankle arthroplasty is indicated for severe, end-stage primary osteoarthrosis, inflammatory arthritis, and post-traumatic osteoarthrosis of the tibiotalar joint that is refractory to conservative measures (Table 6.1). A patient with bilateral ankle arthritis or ipsilateral hindfoot arthritis who has or will require a subtalar (fusion of the talocalcaneal joint) or triple arthrodesis (fusion of the talocalcaneal, talonavicular, and calcaneocuboid joints) is a particularly appropriate candidate for total ankle arthroplasty. The reason is that bilateral tibiotalar (ankle), tibiotalocalcaneal, and pantalar arthrodeses drastically reduce the physiology of the hindfoot [11, 13, 48–53] with detrimental influence on gait and patients' functional ability [54]. It has been shown that the clinical outcome of total ankle arthroplasty, when combined with hindfoot fusion, is comparable to that of ankle replacement alone [55]. For some patient groups, for example, with secondary osteoarthritis due to hemochromatosis [56] or hemophilia [57, 58], total ankle arthroplasty is incredibly beneficial and should be considered.

B. Hintermann, R. Ruiz, *Total Ankle Replacement*, https://doi.org/10.1007/978-3-031-56810-7_6

Table 6.1 Indications and contraindications of total ankle replacement

Indications:

- Primary osteoarthrosis
- Secondary/systemic osteoarthritis (i.e., inflammatory arthritis)
  - Rheumatoid arthritis
  - Hemophilia
  - Hemochromatosis
  - Mixed connective tissue disorders (i.e., scleroderma, lupus erythematosus)
  - Synovial inflammatory conditions
  - Psoriatic arthritis
  - After septic arthritis (if there is no current or active infection)
- Post-traumatic osteoarthrosis
  - After ankle fracture
  - After pilon tibial fracture
  - After talus fracture (if there is no severe dislocation)
  - After ankle sprains (chronic ankle instability)
  - Avascular osteonecrosis (AVN) (if limited to less than 25% of the talar body)

If there is:

- Good bone stock
- Normal vascular status
- No immunosuppression
- Correct hindfoot-ankle alignment
- Well-preserved ankle joint motion
- Sufficient medial and lateral ankle stability
- Low physical demand sports activities (e.g., biking, swimming, walking, golfing)

Relative contraindications:

- Previous severe trauma
  - Open fracture of the ankle
  - Fracture with dislocation of the talar body
  - With segmental bone loss (talus or tibia)
- Avascular necrosis (AVN) of the talus (of 25–50% of the talar body)
- Severe osteopenia or osteoporosis
- Long-term use of steroids (systemic, local) and/or active immunosuppression
- Demanding sports activities (e.g., tennis, jogging, alpine skiing)

Absolute contraindications:

- Neuroarthropathic degenerative disease (Charcot's ankle)
- Active or recent infection
- Avascular necrosis (AVN) of the talus (of more than 50% of the talar body)
- Severe benign joint hypermobility syndrome
- Non-reconstructable malalignment
- Severe soft-tissue problems around the ankle
- Sensory or motor dysfunction of the foot or leg
- High physical demand sports activities (e.g., contact sports)

However, the final determination of the clinical indications for total ankle arthroplasty should be pillowed by intermediate and long-term results, supported by comparing results with those of other treatment options (e.g., arthrodesis) and influenced by the feasibility of salvage after failure.

6.2 Relative Contraindications

Relative contraindications (Table 6.1) include young age [17], high physical demand, previous and successfully treated osteomyelitis of the ankle, previous severe open fracture of the ankle, previous dislocated fracture of the talus, segmental bone loss, long-term steroid use (e.g., in cases of rheumatoid arthritis, ulcerative colitis, Crohn's disease, etc.), insulin-dependent diabetes mellitus, and severe osteoporosis [12, 13, 17, 24, 59, 60]. While avascular necrosis secondary to a talus fracture may be particularly critical (Fig. 6.1), total ankle arthroplasty may be indicated for osteochondral defects after failed alternative treatments.

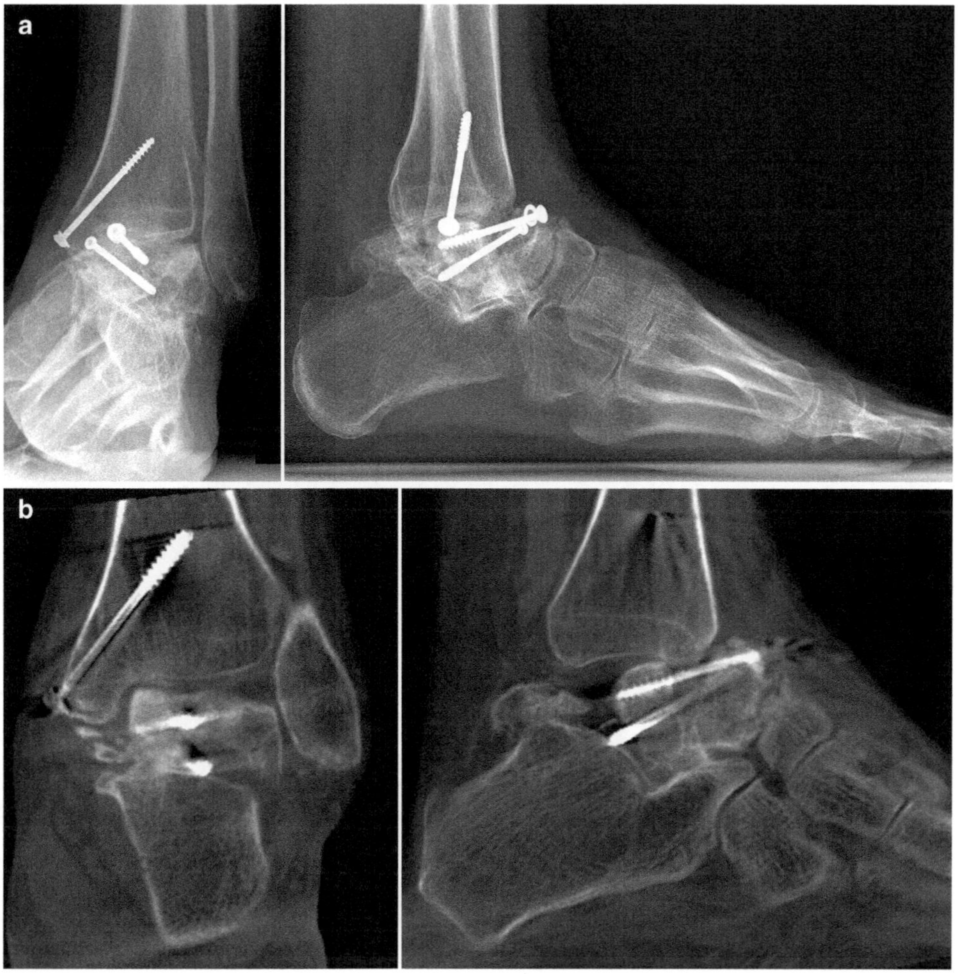

Fig. 6.1 Avascular necrosis of the talus subsequently to a talus fracture. In this ankle, 2.5 years after a talar fracture, the central part of the talar body is avascular; however, there is some viable bone on the bottom left. If a subtalar fusion is successfully healed, replacing the ankle with revision implants is an option. (**a**) Radiographs. (**b**) CT scans

6.3 Absolute Contraindications

Absolute contraindications (Table 6.1) include neuroarthropathic degenerative joint disease (Charcot's ankle), active or recent infection, significant avascular necrosis of the talus (Fig. 6.2), a compromised soft-tissue envelope around the ankle, neurological dysfunction of the foot or leg, severe non-reconstructable malalignment, and not manageable ligamentous instability of the ankle or hindfoot [11–13, 17, 59, 61].

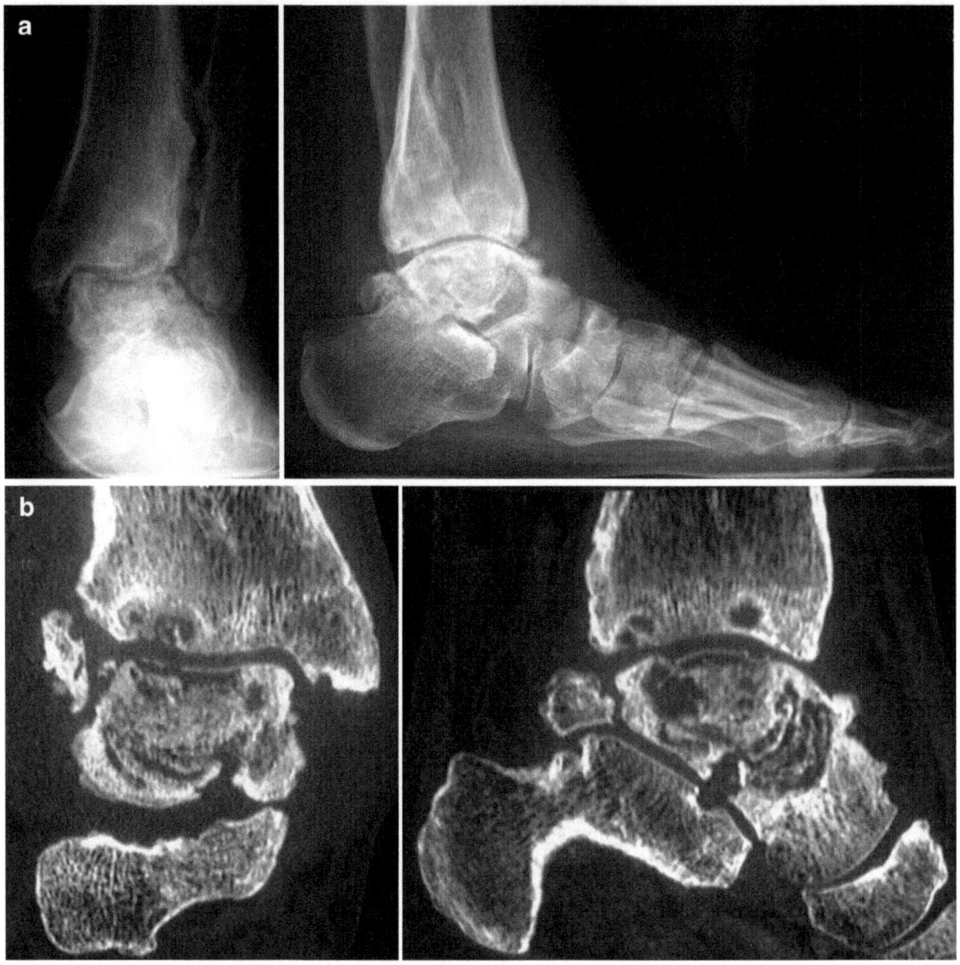

Fig. 6.2 Avascular necrosis of the talus. In this ankle, > 50% of the talar body is necrotic, making conventional total ankle arthroplasty impossible. Talar replacement with a custom-made implant might be an option as an alternative to a fusion. (**a**) Radiographs. (**b**) CT scans

6.4 General Patient Characteristics

6.4.1 Age

The ideal patient for total ankle arthroplasty is an elderly person with low physical demand. Due to the post-traumatic origin of ankle arthritis (up to 80%), patients with painful end-stage arthritis are typically younger than those with severe hip or knee arthritis [7, 62–65].

Previous studies have suggested an increased risk of implant failure in younger patients with post-traumatic osteoarthrosis. Kitaoka and Patzer [2] reported, at an average follow-up of 9 years after total ankle arthroplasty, a failure rate of 43% in patients younger than 57 years of age and of 26% in patients over 57 years of age. Stauffer and Segal [4], based on their outcome analyses, proposed that total ankle arthroplasty should not be considered in patients under 60 years of age with post-traumatic osteoarthrosis, and Alvine [66] recommended the procedure only for patients over 55 years of age.

Spirt et al. [67] reported that each 1-year increase in age at implantation of the Agility prosthesis resulted in a 3.5% decrease in failure hazard. Patients aged ≤54 years at implantation had a 2.65 times greater risk of failure than those aged ≥55. The estimated survival rate at 61 months with failure as the endpoint was 0.74 (0.60–0.91) for the younger group, compared to a survival rate at 47 months of 0.89 (0.80–0.99) for the older group [67].

Barg et al. [37] found age under 70 to be an independent predictor of failure of the Hintegra ankle prosthesis at an average follow-up of 6.3 years. In an epidemiological study by Seaworth et al. [30], younger age at implantation was also found to be a risk factor for failure. These results are in accordance with further studies by other authors showing low age at implantation to be a risk factor for revision [68, 69]. Based on 780 total ankle arthroplasties from the Swedish Ankle Register [28], patients with primary or post-traumatic osteoarthritis under 60 years of age had a 1.8 higher chance of revision than older patients. This relationship was not found for patients with rheumatoid arthritis and was only statistically significant in women [28].

On the other hand, no relation between age and survival was found in the Norwegian [27], Finnish [70], and New Zealand Ankle Register [38]. Supporting these findings, several authors have shown that age is not a risk factor for revision. Kofoed and Lundberg-Jensen [71] reported at a follow-up of 6 years an implant survival rate of 75% in patients younger than 50 years of age (*n* = 30; median age, 46 years [range, 22–49 years]) and of 81% in patients older than 50 years of age (*n* = 70; median age, 63 years [range, 51–83 years]). This difference in implant survival was not significant. The authors did not find a statistical difference in the clinical outcome, the frequency of revision procedures, and conversion to ankle arthrodesis between the two age groups. Others have also found lower age at implantation not to be a significant risk factor for revision [42, 72–79].

Recently, Gaugler et al. [65], in a consecutive series of 813 ankles (789 patients) with the use of the Hintegra ankle, found a significant improvement in the AOFAS hindfoot score and pain relief between the preoperative assessment and the last follow-up at 6.1 (0.0–15.7) years, independent of age (<50 versus ≥50 years). Age even had a positive effect on pain relief. The risk for a minor or major revision was 28.7% at a mean follow-up of 5.4 years and 11.0% at a mean follow-up of 6.9 years, respectively. The hazard of revision was not affected by age [65]. Other reports also indicated that total ankle arthroplasty in younger patients results in similar outcomes to older patients [75, 76, 80, 81].

The longevity of an implant is related to the amount of loading it is exposed to [11, 80]. Younger, more active patients typically want to resume more vigorous activities after total ankle arthroplasty than older, more sedentary patients [5, 12, 17]. Therefore, younger patients should be counseled appropriately on activity restrictions after total ankle arthroplasty. The problem remains, however, that the only alternative to total ankle arthroplasty is ankle arthrodesis. When counseling a younger patient on the potential long-term effects of ankle arthrodesis, it should be clearly stated that if the patient lives long enough, he or she can expect to develop symptomatic secondary osteoarthrosis in the adjacent joints of the hind- and midfoot [48, 50].

The Authors' Approach

When discussing arthrodesis versus *total ankle arthroplasty with a younger patient who suffers from painful end-stage ankle arthritis, one should clearly explain that total ankle arthroplasty may be a viable option for an initial period. If the implant fails over time, and revision arthroplasty is not feasible anymore, then conversion to ankle arthrodesis can be performed. This "two-stage approach" to ankle arthrodesis may effectively preserve the adjacent joints from overuse and secondary osteoarthrosis. We cannot emphasize enough, however, how important it is only to use total ankle implants that require minimal bone resection, thereby saving bone for further revisions or, if necessary, an isolated ankle joint fusion at a later time point. Implants that (because of the extended bone resection) require tibiotalocalcaneal fusion once they have failed should not be considered for younger patients.*

6.4.2 Gender

The possible influence of gender on outcome and revision rates has not yet been studied explicitly. By results from other reports [68, 72], no influence of gender on total ankle arthroplasty survival was found in registry studies [27–29, 38, 70]. In a national database study, male gender was found to be a statistically significant risk factor for the occurrence of one or more complications within 30 days after surgery [82]. Using the National Inpatient Sample database for patients who underwent total ankle arthroplasty between 2016 and 2019, females demonstrated significantly higher risks of medical and surgical complications [33]. Female gender was also a significant risk factor for wound-healing problems; however, after correcting for confounding variables, it was no longer a predictor for disturbed wound healing [83].

6.4.3 Weight/Body Mass Index Restrictions

The specific configuration of the ankle joint, with its considerable surface area of contact, can tolerate joint reactive forces of four to six times body weight during gait [60, 84–86]. Patients with arthritic changes at the ankle joint tend to alter their gait to compensate for the decreased range of motion, thereby decreasing forces across the ankle to three times body weight. This has been shown to remain constant up to 1 year after total ankle arthroplasty [4]. However, since stiffness usually increases with arthritic ankle and hindfoot joint changes, rotational and shear forces are suggested to be higher in patients with foot and ankle arthritis. Theoretically, the greater the individual's body weight, the greater the forces transmitted to the implants after ankle replacement. However, the body mass index (BMI) to implant size ratio is even more important than weight alone, especially for potential subsidence of the talar component [87]. On the other hand, the few studies that have included patient weight in outcome evaluation after total ankle arthroplasty have failed to show a correlation between patient weight and implant failure or pain [88].

Barg et al. [89] reported a survival rate of 93% at 6-year follow-up in a group of 123 obese patients who had undergone Hintegra total ankle arthroplasty. This is comparable to the results of a total cohort consisting of 722 Hintegra prostheses, where obesity was not associated with failure of the total ankle arthroplasty [37]. In a study of 39 total ankle arthroplasties (Mobility, Hintegra, and STAR) in obese patients (BMI $\geq$30 kg/m^2), Bouchard et al. [88], at an average of 3.8 years of follow-up, found no differences about the functional outcome, patients' satisfaction, complications, and revisions between non-obese and obese patients. These findings were in accordance with those of others [90, 91].

With longer follow-up (8 years) of the Agility prosthesis, however, Schipper et al. [24] found obese patients to have a 2.8 times higher chance of revision than non-obese patients. Especially obese patients with idiopathic osteoarthritis were at risk.

In a Medicare database study, obese patients had a significantly higher chance of complications, including revision, within 90 days than the non-obese group [92]. In another study, obese patients demonstrated a substantially enhanced risk of medical adversities [33].

The Authors' Approach

A high BMI (within reasonable limits) should not be considered a contraindication for total ankle arthroplasty. However, obese patients with comorbidities are not ideal candidates for total ankle arthroplasty.

6.4.4 Activity Level

Implant longevity is related to the loading history placed on an ankle prosthesis [93]. Vigorous, repetitive, impact-type loading will likely result in an early mechanical failure of the implant. Shear forces in the sagittal and coronal planes have been estimated to reach up to two times body weight during gait and even higher with more strenuous activities [60, 85, 86, 94]. With some ankle designs, the vertical loads applied to the trabecular bone at the bone-implant interface during normal daily activities may exceed the inherent strength of the bone. Although bone remodeling may occur over time, thereby increasing the inherent trabecular strength, it must increase to at least three times the applied load to prevent the collapse of the components [95] (see Sect. 3.6).

Valderrabano et al. [96] found no harmful influence of an increased activity level on the revision rate at an average of 2.8 years of follow-up in 152 Hintegra total ankle arthroplasties. Naal et al. [97], in an investigation of 101 total ankle arthroplasties (Mobility [n = 54] and Buechel-Pappas [n = 47]) at 3.7 years, found no relationship between physical activity level and the incidence of periprosthetic lucencies. Similar findings were observed for the Salto prosthesis by Bonnin et al. [98], who found no relationship between activity level and adverse effects.

Despite the absence of sound scientific evidence, guidelines for sports activities after total ankle arthroplasty have been proposed [96]. These were confirmed in a recent survey among foot and ankle surgeons regarding sports activities after total ankle arthroplasty [99].

There is consensus in the literature that total ankle arthroplasty is designed to support the stress associated with daily life activities and is not intended to enable the resumption of high-impact, strenuous exercise [17, 100]. Patients should, therefore, be generally restricted from any high-impact or stop-and-go exercises, including jogging, competitive sports, and heavy lower-body weightlifting [13]. However, low-impact or sedentary activities such as walking, swimming, golfing, and biking are permitted.

The Authors' Approach

When counseling a patient for total ankle arthroplasty, the patient's aspired activity level and types of physical activity should be considered. The patient should be well informed on which sports activities are possible for him/her to perform in the future without causing harm to the prosthesis. The authors generally permit patients to participate in low-impact activities, such as downhill and cross-country skiing (classical technique only), not having observed any related problems thus far.

6.4.5 Smoking

Although little is reported in the literature regarding the success rates for total ankle arthroplasty in smokers when compared to nonsmokers, it is generally thought that smoking may indirectly influence outcomes since smoking increases the immediate perioperative risks. The systemic vasoconstrictive effects of nicotine are known to inhibit wound healing. Delayed wound healing and necrosis are common complications of ankle replacement surgery (up to 40% in some series) [1, 4, 21, 66, 101]. The continued presence of nicotine can also adversely affect bony ingrowth into uncemented components. Finally, nicotine significantly increased the risk of nonunion in arthrodeses in smokers compared to nonsmokers [102]. These matters should be remembered and are of utmost importance when considering total ankle prostheses that rely on syndesmotic fusion or need additional, complex hindfoot reconstruction, including osteotomies and arthrodeses of other joints.

In a retrospective review of 642 Inbone, Salto Talaris, and STAR total ankle arthroplasties, smoking increased wound breakdown significantly [103]. Infections and (non-)revision surgery were not significantly different between groups.

In other studies, <12 pack years of smoking was not found to be a significant risk factor for wound-healing problems or infection in a combined cohort of primary and revision arthroplasties [15, 83, 104]. This is in accordance with results from others [73, 105].

The Authors' Approach
With the current knowledge of the disadvantageous effects of smoking on bone and soft-tissue healing and the benefits of (temporary) perioperative cessation, asking patients to abstain from smoking before their high-risk total ankle arthroplasty surgery seems reasonable.

6.5 Comorbidities

6.5.1 Diabetes

Patients with diabetes have approximately twice the likelihood of developing osteoarthritis compared to patients without diabetes. Additionally, they are considered more complex due to the pathophysiology of the disease and the frequent presence of other comorbidities [11, 70, 75, 105–110]. Maintaining mobility and independence is of heightened importance in patients with diabetes, as diabetes is already associated with fewer steps per day, an increased risk of experiencing cardiovascular morbidity, and overall mortality [111–113]. Diabetes has historically been a relative contraindication for total ankle arthroplasty due to the probability of having more comorbidities and poor surgical outcomes compared with nondiabetics [11, 21, 70, 75, 105–110]. However, patients with diabetes may stand to gain quality of life from a total ankle arthroplasty due to the ability to maintain joint motion and, in turn, promote more steps per day and continued mobility and encourage functional independence [112].

A current meta-analysis including 14 articles published between 2010 and 2020 suggests no significant differences in major adverse events between patients with or without diabetes having undergone total ankle arthroplasty or ankle arthrodesis [114]. However, a primary concern was that the severity of diabetes was not well defined. Of the 14 citations, only two discussed HbA_{1c} levels, whereas another classified diabetes as controlled or uncontrolled.

At an average of 5 years of follow-up of 173 Hintegra total ankle arthroplasties, clinical failure defined as an AOFAS hindfoot score of 79 or less was significantly higher in the diabetic group (21%), compared to the nondiabetic group (15%). However, the number of revisions was similar between groups. The rate of delayed wound healing was not significantly different between groups except when comparing uncontrolled diabetics to nondiabetics [115]. Raikin et al. [83] also found diabetes to be a risk factor for minor wound-healing problems (solvable with local wound care and oral antibiotics) in well-controlled diabetics. A relationship with major wound-healing problems requiring surgery was not observed. Whalen et al. [15] did not find a relationship between diabetes and wound breakdown. Delayed wound healing and diabetes were found to be risk factors for infection in a retrospective review of a cohort of primary and revision total ankle arthroplasties by Patton et al. [104]. In a national database study, after correcting for confounding variables, diabetes was found to be independently associated with in-hospital (general) complications (relative risk 4.1) but not with surgical debridement [116]. Regardless of diabetes type, patients with uncontrolled diabetes mellitus exhibited significantly increased odds of surgical and systemic complications, higher mortality, and increased length of stay during the index hospitalization following lower extremity total joint arthroplasty [117].

The Authors' Approach
The notion of diabetes being a contraindication for primary total ankle arthroplasty is not univocally supported by the current literature, except for uncontrolled diabetes. As it preserves anatomical movement compared to arthrodesis, retaining the functionality of the joint by performing a total ankle arthroplasty becomes an important consideration when electing which therapy should be applied. However, it is advised to have diabetic patients counseled preoperatively to optimize their diabetic control before performing surgery.

6.5.2 Neuro(arthro)pathy and Vascular Insufficiency

There is no literature regarding the influence of neuroarthropathy and vascular insufficiency on the results of total ankle arthroplasty, most probably since these conditions are still considered absolute contraindications for total ankle arthroplasty. Whalen et al. [15], in an analysis of total ankle arthroplasties, found wound breakdown in 16 cases, with 4 progressing to deep infection. Three of these were later shown to have an occluded or absent anterior tibial artery, leading the authors to recommend preoperative vascular studies in patients with known risk factors for cardiovascular disease.

6.5.3 Bilateral Ankle Osteoarthritis

Though contrary reports can be found [118, 119], bilateral ankle fusion is said to impair gait and function considerably [120, 121]. Therefore, patients with bilateral ankle osteoarthritis should be especially considered for total ankle arthroplasty [11, 122]. In a series of 16 patients with total ankle arthroplasty on one side and contralateral ankle arthrodesis, patients were equally satisfied with each ankle [119]. While comparing the result of 23 patients who had undergone simultaneous sequential bilateral total ankle arthroplasty to 46 patients with unilateral total ankle arthroplasty, Barg et al. [54] found significantly less pain relief and a lower SF-36 physical component summary score, after 4 months, for the bilateral group. However, after 2 years, the outcome of both groups was comparable. This indicates that simultaneous bilateral total ankle arthroplasty needs a prolonged recovery period.

6.6 Factors Related to the Ankle Joint

6.6.1 Etiology of Arthritis

Approximately 1% of the world's adult population is affected by painful ankle osteoarthritis with dysfunction and impaired mobility [63]. It has been shown that the mental and physical disability associated with end-stage ankle osteoarthritis is at least as severe as that associated with end-stage hip osteoarthritis [123]. While the etiology of hip and knee osteoarthritis is well understood and widely highlighted in numerous clinical studies, research on ankle osteoarthritis is limited in the current literature [123]. The knowledge and exact analysis of the underlying etiology is essential for selecting the best treatment strategy and is vital to achieving satisfactory long-term results and avoiding postoperative complications.

Unlike the hip and knee, the ankle joint is rarely affected by primary osteoarthritis. Instead, numerous clinical and epidemiologic studies have identified previous trauma as the most common origin for ankle osteoarthritis, showing that patients with post-traumatic osteoarthritis are younger than patients with primary osteoarthritis [5, 13, 63, 124, 125]. Saltzman et al. [124] evaluated 639 patients presenting with painful end-stage ankle osteoarthritis (Kellgren grade 3 or 4). In this patient cohort, 445 patients (70%) had post-traumatic, 76 patients (12%) had rheumatoid, and 46 (7%) had primary ankle osteoarthritis. While rotational ankle fractures were identified as the most common reason for post-traumatic ankle osteoarthritis (164 patients), previous ligamental injuries were also found as a reason for ankle osteoarthritis in 126 patients. These trends were confirmed by a study performed by Valderrabano et al. [63], who evaluated etiologies of ankle osteoarthritis in 390 consecutive patients (406 ankles) with painful end-stage ankle osteoarthritis. As much as 78% of patients presented with post-traumatic osteoarthritis. In their study, malleolar fractures were the most common reason for degenerative changes in the ankle joint (157 patients), followed by ankle ligament lesions (60 patients). Only 31 patients were affected by primary osteoarthritis, while secondary osteoarthritis was considered the more common etiology of end-stage ankle osteoarthritis (46 patients) [63]. Secondary osteoarthritis has also been found to be associated with a variety of underlying diseases/pathologies, such as rheumatoid disease [126–128], hemochromatosis [56], hemophilia [57, 58, 129–131], gout [132], instability [133], neuropathic diseases [7, 12–14], avascular talus necrosis, osteochondritis dissecans, or post-infectious arthritis [7–11, 17, 26].

Survival of total ankle arthroplasty was not influenced by the etiology of arthritis in the Norwegian Arthroplasty Register [27], in the New Zealand Ankle Registry [38], in the Finnish Arthroplasty Register [70], and others [37, 67, 68, 74, 134–136]. Contrary to these findings, the Swedish register estimated that survival at 10 years of follow-up was 72% for patients with rheumatoid arthritis, 68% in primary osteoarthritis, and 66% in post-traumatic osteoarthritis [28]. Barg et al. [37] also found lower survival in patients with primary osteoarthritis (71%) and post-traumatic osteoarthritis (84%), compared to other etiologies (94%) at >10 years of follow-up. Most recently, Megerian et al. [137] reported that 55 patients with post-traumatic osteoarthritis had a markedly higher complication rate after total ankle arthroplasty than 44 patients with primary osteoarthritis, at higher risk of failure requiring prosthesis explant. Post-traumatic osteoarthritis was also markedly associated with preoperative valgus malalignment, an identified risk factor in this series for revision surgery and prosthesis explant. The authors also suggested that pilon fractures may represent a group at risk of complications related to talar implant subsidence and loosening compared with malleolar fractures.

The relationship between etiology and survival of total ankle arthroplasty may be confounded by activity level, with, for instance, patients suffering from the inflammatory joint disease being less active due to the nature of their disease with multiple joints affected. This might explain the absence of differences in survival between varying etiologies at shorter follow-ups, whereas more prolonged follow-up survival in inflammatory joint disease patients might be better [138]. This would be in accordance with the findings of Hurowitz et al. [73], who found that patients with the inflammatory joint disease were younger at implantation but showed better survival.

The Authors' Approach

According to the literature, we did not find evidence that the underlying etiology influences the survival of total ankle arthroplasty. However, there is a need for careful patient selection, and total ankle arthroplasty should be performed cautiously in patients who are taking immunosuppressive agents.

6.6.2 Deformity

A majority of osteoarthritic ankles present with a coronal plane deformity. In an analysis of 390 patients (406 ankles) with end-stage ankle (osteo)arthritis, Valderrabano et al. [63] found a varus deformity (defined as the angle between the tibial shaft and the talar dome being <90°) in 55%. In contrast, 8% presented a valgus deformity (the angle between the tibial shaft and the talar dome being >99°). Coronal plane deformities of >10° were considered absolute contraindications for total ankle arthroplasty in the early stages of total ankle arthroplasty implantation [72]. With advances in implants and techniques, coronal plane deformities are not considered a limit anymore [139–142]. However, the importance of deformity correction before or during total ankle arthroplasty has been recognized [36, 143–146], and many surgical techniques have been described to correct these deformities [139, 144, 147–156].

Differentiating between symmetrical and asymmetrical deformities is paramount, as asymmetrical deformities indicate a loss of ligamentous support resulting in a disbalanced ankle, whereas, in symmetrical deformities, the ankle remains somehow balanced [45, 148, 157–159]. While symmetrical coronal plane deformities can be addressed by supramalleolar and inframalleolar correcting osteotomies alone [158, 160], asymmetrical deformities may need additional ligament reconstruction and tendon transfers [139, 161–163]. Contract varus ankles can be reliably corrected through a medial malleolar osteotomy as described by Doets et al. [147], with a vertical osteotomy or with an open wedge flip osteotomy described by Hintermann et al. [139]. Valgus ankles, in contrast, are primarily associated with a floppy hindfoot and can be successfully addressed using the prosthesis as a spacer, thereby tightening the loose ligaments [13, 149, 162]. However, when the deep deltoid ligament (the prime stabilizer of the ankle joint) has become insufficient, valgus ankles pose a more complex problem. They tend to relapse into valgus with maltracking of the talus, especially when associated with an incompetent medial arch progressive collapsing foot deformity [164, 165].

Karantana et al. [166] did not observe any differences in functional outcome and prosthesis component survivorship between the patients with or without preoperative deformities if the deformity was addressed at the time of prosthesis implantation. Daniels et al. [167] demonstrated that correction of moderate to severe varus deformities is possible and results in good functional outcomes and stability of prosthesis components. Kim et al. [168] reported that the clinical outcome of total ankle arthroplasty performed in ankles with preoperative varus deformity of more than 10° is comparable with that of neutrally aligned ankles. However, simultaneous surgical procedures addressing the preoperative deformity are necessary to achieve good results.

The Authors' Approach

Considering the scientific evidence, it seems safe to assume that deformity is no longer a contraindication for total ankle arthroplasty as long as the surgeon can adequately balance and stabilize the ankle joint.

6.6.3 Hindfoot-Ankle Instability

Ligamentous ankle instability can be managed simultaneously or staged through soft-tissue reconstruction. Valgus deformity associated with an incompetent deltoid-spring ligament complex is generally considered to be far more technically challenging than a varus deformity and may be a contraindication for ankle arthroplasty [60, 78]. Varus deformity associated with lateral ligamentous instability can be managed with direct anatomic lateral reconstruction, with or without the medial release of the deltoid ligament, particularly for long-standing instability [139, 151, 169]. Results after total ankle arthroplasty in patients with ligamentous instability have been somewhat unpredictable, and those who have a clinically deficient deltoid ligament are at higher risk for subsequent failure of total ankle arthroplasty [7, 8, 17, 25].

The Authors' Approach

*In the case of mild but relevant pathology of the anterior talofibular ligament (*e.g.*, elongation or partial tear), this ligament may be reconstructed anatomically with local structures, if possible (the Broström technique). In the case of anterior subluxation of the talus (*e.g.*, with total loss of anterior talofibular ligament function), augmentation with a tendon graft or internal brace is necessary.*

6.6.4 Prior Procedures

Either contract skin scars or unstable chronic wound problems may be encountered in post-traumatic cases or those with previous surgeries. From a cohort of 619 primary and 347 revision total ankle arthroplasties, 29 (15 primaries, 14 revisions) were diagnosed with the deep infection. The number of prior surgeries in the infected group was 2.3, compared to 1.1 in the matched control group [104]. These results are in accordance with the findings from other authors [39]. Hurowitz et al. [73] and Whalen et al. [15], on the other hand, found no significant influence of previous surgery on survival and wound breakdown, respectively.

Early referral to a plastic surgeon and competent examination of the cutaneous soft tissues may be of prophylactic importance and may prevent unexpected postoperative exacerbations. In such cases, evaluation of macro- and microcirculation, sensitivity, neurological functions, and soft-tissue elasticity, both clinically and with imaging techniques, represents the golden standard.

6.6.5 Osteopenia and Osteoporosis

The primary concern with total ankle arthroplasty in patients with osteopenia or osteoporosis is inadequate bony fixation and early subsidence of the components, particularly the tibial component. Previous studies by Hvid et al. [95] have emphasized that the tibial bone is up to 40% weaker than the corresponding talar bone and that, after removing only 5 mm of bone, there is a tremendous loss of trabecular strength in the distal tibia. Theoretically, this problem can be solved using a larger implant with a larger corresponding surface area of contact, as with the Agility ankle [66]. This prosthesis, however, also requires tibiofibular fusion and the removal of more bone, including the subchondral plate.

In a consecutive series of 683 Hintegra ankles, which requires a minimal bone resection, uses an anatomically shaped large implant, and requires a flat cut that does not weaken the cortical architecture of the distal tibia, no subsidence was observed in any patient, including a few patients with osteoporosis despite allowing weight-bearing immediately postoperatively [136]. Nevertheless, severe osteopenia or osteoporosis should generally be considered a relative contraindication to total ankle arthroplasty [17, 35, 36, 61].

6.6.6 Avascular Talar Necrosis

Avascular necrosis of the talus causes considerable morbidity to the talar bone, and the treatment options are limited [20, 170]. In several studies, avascular necrosis of the talus has been identified as an absolute contraindication for total ankle arthroplasty [8, 16, 17]. Of the nine cases reported by Lee et al. [19], five had collapsed at 2–5 years of follow-up, and three more had complications. They also reported two cases where a Hintegra ankle was implanted for avascular necrosis after establishing talar revascularization with magnetic resonance imaging and radionuclide bone scanning. These two patients had AOFAS scores of 91 and 85 at 30 and 24 months of follow-up.

Devalia et al. [171] reported results of seven patients treated with a two-stage procedure, consisting of subtalar arthrodesis for revascularization of the talus, followed by total ankle arthroplasty on average 10 months later. At 3 years of follow-up, the AOFAS score was 78. In two patients, radiological signs of talar subsidence were noted at 1-year follow-up without progression or deterioration of clinical scores at 3 years.

Replacing part or all of the talus with a customized prosthesis has been developed for the treatment of a range of pathologies affecting the talus, including avascular necrosis or osteonecrosis following trauma, progressive bone cysts with possible collapse after total ankle arthroplasty, medications, autoimmune conditions, and tumors (Fig. 6.3) [170, 172, 173]. Results of total talar replacement have only been reported in a few case series/reports. In the first year after implantation, these patients seem to go well [174]. Isolated talar body replacement (without replacing the distal tibia) with a metal component has been very successful at 10–36 years of follow-up. Twenty-eight of 33 were still in place at the latest follow-up, with an average AOFAS score of 75 [175]. At 53 months of follow-up of 55 ceramic total talar replacements, 0 needed revision, and scores on foot and ankle questionnaires had significantly improved [176, 177]. Though short-term results were a promising alternative to tibiotalocalcaneal fusion, further studies are required to ensure reliable outcomes.

6.6.7 Bone Defects

Bone defects after failed total ankle arthroplasty are common [114, 178–180]. As long as enough genuine bone is left to support the talar component firmly, the defect can be filled with autograft or allograft bone. Some current total ankle systems offer particular revision components to compensate for bone loss [178]. Another option is using bone cement to fill the defect and screws to fix the cement plumb to the underlying original bone firmly.

6.6.8 Adjacent Joint (Osteo)Arthritis

The management of adjacent joint (osteo)arthritis in the presence of an arthritic ankle is still a matter of considerable debate. The surgeon must first determine the severity of the involvement of the adjacent joints and must identify any deformity that may be present throughout these joints. Ankle arthrodesis is said to increase osteoarthritis in neighboring joints [48, 50, 83], and therefore, total ankle arthroplasty should be considered in patients with concomitant ankle and peritalar osteoarthritis [181]. A causal relationship has yet to be definitively established [182, 183]. Treatment options for combined ankle and subtalar osteoarthritis are total ankle arthroplasty with subtalar arthrodesis (either as a staged procedure or simultaneous) or tibiotalocalcaneal fusion [184].

Some surgeons propose to proceed with total ankle arthroplasty before subtalar or triple arthrodesis, mainly if there is no evidence of structural or rigid deformity [59]. On occasion, because of the procedure, the affected joints (especially the subtalar and midfoot joints) will realign themselves during prosthesis implantation due to the tension in the ankle and lengthening of the medial column. Sometimes, especially in the post-traumatic population, even though significant radiographic changes are present, and patients may lose range of motion, the adjacent joints no longer seem symptomatic once the ankle is replaced. This may be due to the stress reduction that results from restoring some motion at

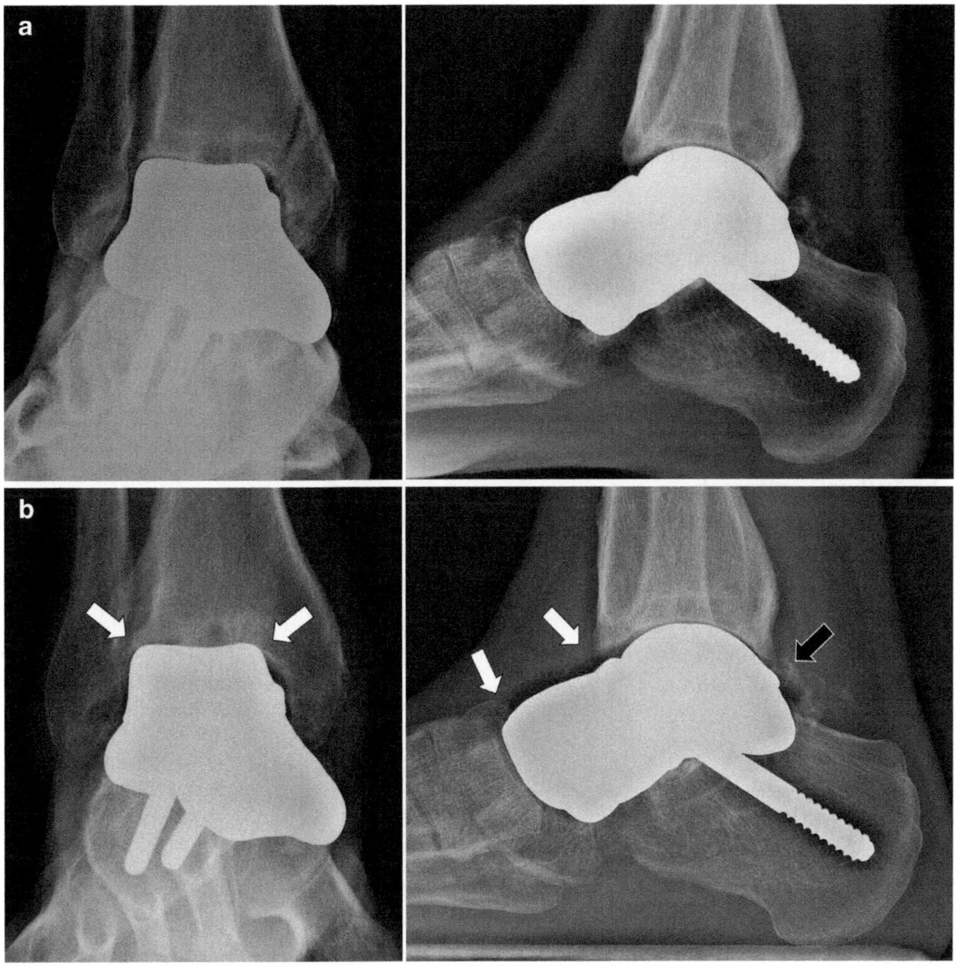

Fig. 6.3 Talar replacement with a customized implant. This 42-year-old patient underwent talar replacement surgery with a customized implant for secondary osteoarthritis due to avascular necrosis of the talar body. (**a**) Postoperative radiographs show a regular position of the implant. (**b**) 3.2 years later, the patient experiences pain while loading the foot and complained of progressive loss of motion. The radiographs evidence ongoing signs of subsidence of the implant (white arrows) and periarticular ossifications (black arrow)

the ankle [185]. Conversely, some surgeons propose to proceed with subtalar or triple arthrodesis before total ankle arthroplasty to obtain a rigid plantigrade foot, particularly in fixed deformities or rheumatoid patients [59].

In a consecutive series of 1001 total ankle arthroplasties, 26 patients subsequently required a hind- or midfoot fusion. The fusion rate was 93%, and the complication rate was 12%. SF-36 score was 56 at an average of 71 months of follow-up [186]. This fusion rate is similar to the 92% reported by Usuelli et al. [187] in 25 patients undergoing simultaneous total ankle arthroplasty with subtalar fusion. No further major complications were reported. At 12 months of follow-up, the average SF-12 physical health score was 44, the mental health component was 51, and the visual analog pain score was 2.

Kim et al. [55] compared the results of 60 patients with total ankle arthroplasty and pre-, per-, or postoperative hindfoot fusions to those of a control group with isolated total ankle arthroplasty consisting of the remainder of the same cohort. Patient satisfaction, complication, and survival rates were not different between groups.

The Authors' Approach

If there is no fixed deformity in post-traumatic patients, total ankle arthroplasty may be done first. Additional fusions should be considered during the same surgery if this does not result in a properly aligned foot. If the foot is well aligned and stable after total ankle arthroplasty, additional alignment surgery can be considered later. Such potential secondary surgeries are seldom necessary (estimated to be less than 5%). A subtalar or triple arthrodesis is done first in rheumatoid patients, mainly if a fixed deformity exists. If there are no notable compromises, especially about the soft-tissue envelope, total ankle arthroplasty is performed subsequently during the same surgery.

6.6.9 Infection and Post-infectious Ankle Osteoarthritis

There is consensus that active or recent infection is a contraindication for total ankle arthroplasty or arthroplasty in general. While many authors suggest that previous ankle infection is an absolute contraindication for total ankle arthroplasty [5, 8, 15, 188], others do not share this opinion [13, 189–191]. However, there needs to be more discussion in the orthopedic literature on ankle replacement in patients with previous infections of the ankle joint or the surrounding soft tissues.

Shi et al. [191] reported 22 arthroplasties in patients who were symptom-free for an average of 9 years after prior septic arthritis or osteomyelitis of the ankle. While none was afflicted by deep infection, 14% required reoperation (two subtalar arthrodeses, one cyst grafting). AOFAS, SF-36, and VAS scores all improved significantly. Others supported these results [26, 37, 189, 192].

The Authors' Approach

Carefully evaluating patients with previous infection or predisposing factors, including a thorough history, physical examination, and overlying skin and soft-tissue assessment, is mandatory when planning the treatment with total ankle arthroplasty. However, the sparse literature does not support post-infectious osteoarthritis as a contraindication for total ankle arthroplasty.

6.7 Conclusions

- Knowledge of the indications, as well as both relative and absolute contraindications, is of great importance.
- Many factors historically considered contraindications for total ankle arthroplasty should no longer be considered contraindications based on scientific evidence, especially younger age.
- Malalignment, in particular, should no longer be considered a contraindication as long as it is corrected before or at replacement surgery.
- There is no scientific evidence that body mass index, activity level, diabetes, and previous infection are contraindications; nevertheless, total ankle arthroplasty should be considered with caution, and the surgeon should try to judge the patient as a whole when choosing between total ankle arthroplasty and ankle arthrodesis.

References

1. Bolton-Maggs BG, Sudlow RA, Freeman MA. Total ankle arthroplasty. A long-term review of the London hospital experience. J Bone Joint Surg Br. 1985;67(5):785–90.
2. Kitaoka HB, Patzer GL. Clinical results of the Mayo total ankle arthroplasty. J Bone Joint Surg Am. 1996;78(11):1658–64.
3. McGuire MR, Kyle RF, Gustilo RB, Premer RF. Comparative analysis of ankle arthroplasty versus ankle arthrodesis. Clin Orthop Relat Res. 1988;226:174–81.
4. Stauffer RN, Segal NM. Total ankle arthroplasty: four years' experience. Clin Orthop Relat Res. 1981;160:217–21.
5. Thomas RH, Daniels TR. Ankle arthritis. J Bone Joint Surg Am. 2003;85(5):923–36.
6. Wynn AH, Wilde AH. Long-term follow-up of the Conaxial (Beck-Steffee) total ankle arthroplasty. Foot Ankle. 1992;13(6):303–6.
7. Easley ME, Vertullo CJ, Urban WC, Nunley JA. Total ankle arthroplasty. J Am Acad Orthop Surg. 2002;10(3):157–67.
8. Guyer AJ, Richardson G. Current concepts review: total ankle arthroplasty. Foot Ankle Int. 2008;29(2):256–64.
9. Alvine FG. The agility ankle replacement: the good and the bad. Foot Ankle Clin. 2002;7(4):737–53. vi
10. Krause FG, Schmid T. Ankle arthrodesis versus total ankle replacement: how do I decide? Foot Ankle Clin. 2012;17(4):529–43.
11. Saltzman CL. Perspective on total ankle replacement. Foot Ankle Clin. 2000;5(4):761–75.
12. Hintermann B, Valderrabano V. Total ankle replacement. Foot Ankle Clin. 2003;8(2):375–405.
13. Hintermann B. Total ankle arthroplasty—historical overview, current concepts and future perspectives. Wien-New York: Springer; 2004. p. 195.
14. Morash J, Walton DM, Glazebrook M. Ankle arthrodesis versus total ankle arthroplasty. Foot Ankle Clin. 2017;22(2):251–66.
15. Whalen JL, Spelsberg SC, Murray P. Wound breakdown after total ankle arthroplasty. Foot Ankle Int. 2010;31(4):301–5.
16. Anderson T, Montgomery F, Carlsson A. Uncemented STAR total ankle prostheses. J Bone Joint Surg Am. 2004;86-A Suppl 1(Pt 2):103–11.
17. Clare MP, Sanders RW. Preoperative considerations in ankle replacement surgery. Foot Ankle Clin. 2002;7(4):709–20.
18. Myerson MS, Won HY. Primary and revision total ankle replacement using custom-designed prostheses. Foot Ankle Clin. 2008;13(3):521–38. x
19. Lee KB, Cho SG, Jung ST, Kim MS. Total ankle arthroplasty following revascularization of avascular necrosis of the talar body: two case reports and literature review. Foot Ankle Int. 2008;29(8):852–8.
20. Gross CE, Haughom B, Chahal J, Holmes GB Jr. Treatments for avascular necrosis of the talus: a systematic review. Foot Ankle Spec. 2014;7(5):387–97.
21. Gougoulias NE, Khanna A, Maffulli N. History and evolution in total ankle arthroplasty. Br Med Bull. 2009;89:111–51.
22. Cody EA, Lachman JR, Gausden EB, Nunley JA 2nd, Easley ME. Lower bone density on preoperative computed tomography predicts Periprosthetic fracture risk in total ankle arthroplasty. Foot Ankle Int. 2019;40(1):1–8.
23. Wood PL. Experience with the STAR ankle arthroplasty at Wrightington Hospital, UK. Foot Ankle Clin. 2002;7(4):755–64. vii
24. Schipper ON, Denduluri SK, Zhou Y, Haddad SL. Effect of obesity on total ankle arthroplasty outcomes. Foot Ankle Int. 2016;37(1):1–7.
25. van der Plaat LW, Haverkamp D. Patient selection for total ankle arthroplasty. Orthop Res Rev. 2017;9:63–73.
26. Smyth NA, Kennedy JG, Parvizi J, Schon LC, Aiyer AA. Risk factors for periprosthetic joint infection following total ankle replacement. Foot Ankle Surg. 2020;26(5):591–5.
27. Fevang BT, Lie SA, Havelin LI, Brun JG, Skredderstuen A, Furnes O. 257 ankle arthroplasties performed in Norway between 1994 and 2005. Acta Orthop. 2007;78(5):575–83.
28. Henricson A, Nilsson JA, Carlsson A. 10-year survival of total ankle arthroplasties: a report on 780 cases from the Swedish ankle register. Acta Orthop. 2011;82(6):655–9.
29. Tomlinson M, Harrison M. The New Zealand joint registry: report of 11-year data for ankle arthroplasty. Foot Ankle Clin. 2012;17(4):719–23.

30. Seaworth CM, Do HT, Vulcano E, Mani SB, Lyman SL, Ellis SJ. Epidemiology of total ankle arthroplasty: trends in New York state. Orthopedics. 2016;39(3):170–6.
31. Karzon AL, Kadakia RJ, Coleman MM, Bariteau JT, Labib SA. The rise of total ankle arthroplasty use: a database analysis describing case volumes and incidence trends in the United States between 2009 and 2019. Foot Ankle Int. 2022;43(11):1501–10.
32. Law TY, Sabeh KG, Rosas S, Hubbard Z, Altajar S, Roche MW. Trends in total ankle arthroplasty and revisions in the Medicare database. Ann Transl Med. 2018;6(7):112.
33. Sambandam S, Senthil T, Serbin P, Viswanathan VK, Mounasamy V, Wukich D. Analysis of baseline characteristics, length of stay, cost of care, complications and subgroup analysis of patients undergoing total ankle arthroplasty-a large database study. J Foot Ankle Surg. 2023;62(2):310–6.
34. Hsu AR, Haddad SL. Will total ankle arthroplasty become the new standard for end-stage ankle arthritis? Orthopedics. 2014;37(4):221–3.
35. Maffulli N, Longo UG, Locher J, Romeo G, Salvatore G, Denaro V. Outcome of ankle arthrodesis and ankle prosthesis: a review of the current status. Br Med Bull. 2017;124(1):91–112.
36. Conti SF, Wong YS. Complications of total ankle replacement. Clin Orthop Relat Res. 2001;391:105–14.
37. Barg A, Zwicky L, Knupp M, Henninger HB, Hintermann B. HINTEGRA total ankle replacement: survivorship analysis in 684 patients. J Bone Joint Surg Am. 2013;95(13):1175–83.
38. Hosman AH, Mason RB, Hobbs T, Rothwell AG. A New Zealand national joint registry review of 202 total ankle replacements followed for up to 6 years. Acta Orthop. 2007;78(5):584–91.
39. Kessler B, Sendi P, Graber P, Knupp M, Zwicky L, Hintermann B, et al. Risk factors for periprosthetic ankle joint infection: a case-control study. J Bone Joint Surg Am. 2012;94(20):1871–6.
40. Basques BA, Bitterman A, Campbell KJ, Haughom BD, Lin J, Lee S. Influence of surgeon volume on inpatient complications, cost, and length of stay following total ankle arthroplasty. Foot Ankle Int. 2016;37(10):1046–51.
41. Pinar N, Vernet E, Bizot P, Brilhault J. Total ankle arthroplasty—total ankle arthroplasty in Western France: influence of volume on complications and clinical outcome. Orthop Traumatol Surg Res. 2012;98(4 Suppl):S26–30.
42. Anderson T, Montgomery F, Carlsson A. Uncemented STAR total ankle prostheses. Three to eight-year follow-up of fifty-one consecutive ankles. J Bone Joint Surg Am. 2003;85(7):1321–9.
43. Clement RC, Krynetskiy E, Parekh SG. The total ankle arthroplasty learning curve with third-generation implants: a single surgeon's experience. Foot Ankle Spec. 2013;6(4):263–70.
44. Schuberth JM, Patel S, Zarutsky E. Perioperative complications of the agility total ankle replacement in 50 initial, consecutive cases. J Foot Ankle Surg. 2006;45(3):139–46.
45. Haskell A, Mann RA. Perioperative complication rate of total ankle replacement is reduced by surgeon experience. Foot Ankle Int. 2004;25(5):283–9.
46. Myerson MS, Mroczek K. Perioperative complications of total ankle arthroplasty. Foot Ankle Int. 2003;24(1):17–21.
47. Schimmel JJ, Walschot LH, Louwerens JW. Comparison of the short-term results of the first and last 50 Scandinavian total ankle replacements: assessment of the learning curve in a consecutive series. Foot Ankle Int. 2014;35(4):326–33.
48. Coester LM, Saltzman CL, Leupold J, Pontarelli W. Long-term results following ankle arthrodesis for post-traumatic arthritis. J Bone Joint Surg Am. 2001;83(2):219–28.
49. Thomas R, Daniels TR, Parker K. Gait analysis and functional outcomes following ankle arthrodesis for isolated ankle arthritis. J Bone Joint Surg Am. 2006;88(3):526–35.
50. Fuchs S, Sandmann C, Skwara A, Chylarecki C. Quality of life 20 years after arthrodesis of the ankle. A study of adjacent joints. J Bone Joint Surg Br. 2003;85(7):994–8.
51. Cao L, Kyung MG, Park GY, Hwang IU, Kang HW, Lee DY. Foot and ankle motion after Tibiotalocalcaneal arthrodesis: comparison with Tibiotalar arthrodesis using a multi-segment foot model. Clin Orthop Surg. 2022;14(4):631–44.
52. Chopra S, Crevoisier X. Bilateral gait asymmetry associated with tibiotalocalcaneal arthrodesis versus ankle arthrodesis. Foot Ankle Surg. 2021;27(3):332–8.
53. Hintermann B, Nigg BM. Influence of arthrodeses on kinematics of the axially loaded ankle complex during dorsiflexion/plantarflexion. Foot Ankle Int. 1995;16(10):633–6.
54. Barg A, Knupp M, Hintermann B. Simultaneous bilateral versus unilateral total ankle replacement: a patient-based comparison of pain relief, quality of life and functional outcome. J Bone Joint Surg Br. 2010;92(12):1659–63.
55. Kim BS, Knupp M, Zwicky L, Lee JW, Hintermann B. Total ankle replacement in association with hindfoot fusion: outcome and complications. J Bone Joint Surg Br. 2010;92(11):1540–7.
56. Barg A, Elsner A, Hefti D, Hintermann B. Total ankle arthroplasty in patients with hereditary hemochromatosis. Clin Orthop Relat Res. 2011;469(5):1427–35.
57. Barg A, Elsner A, Hefti D, Hintermann B. Haemophilic arthropathy of the ankle treated by total ankle replacement: a case series. Haemophilia. 2010;16(4):647–55.
58. van der Heide HJ, Novakova I, de Waal Malefijt MC. The feasibility of total ankle prosthesis for severe arthropathy in haemophilia and prothrombin deficiency. Haemophilia. 2006;12(6):679–82.
59. Gould JS, Alvine FG, Mann RA, Sanders RW, Walling AK. Total ankle replacement: a surgical discussion. Part I. Replacement systems, indications, and contraindications. Am J Orthop (Belle Mead NJ). 2000;29(8):604–9.
60. Neufeld SK, Lee TH. Total ankle arthroplasty: indications, results, and biomechanical rationale. Am J Orthop (Belle Mead NJ). 2000;29(8):593–602.
61. Clough TM, Alvi F, Majeed H. Total ankle arthroplasty: what are the risks?: a guide to surgical consent and a review of the literature. Bone Joint J. 2018;100-B(10):1352–8.
62. Demetriades L, Strauss E, Gallina J. Osteoarthritis of the ankle. Clin Orthop Relat Res. 1998;349:28–42.
63. Valderrabano V, Horisberger M, Russell I, Dougall H, Hintermann B. Etiology of ankle osteoarthritis. Clin Orthop Relat Res. 2009;467(7):1800–6.
64. Horisberger M, Valderrabano V, Hintermann B. Posttraumatic ankle osteoarthritis after ankle-related fractures. J Orthop Trauma. 2009;23(1):60–7.
65. Gaugler M, Krahenbuhl N, Barg A, Ruiz R, Horn-Lang T, Susdorf R, et al. Effect of age on outcome and revision in total ankle arthroplasty. Bone Joint J. 2020;102-B(7):925–32.
66. Alvine FG. Total ankle arthroplasty. In: Myerson MS, editor. Foot and ankle disorders. Philadelphia-London-Toronto-Sydney: Saunders; 2000. p. 1085–102.
67. Spirt AA, Assal M, Hansen ST Jr. Complications and failure after total ankle arthroplasty. J Bone Joint Surg Am. 2004;86(6):1172–8.
68. Brunner S, Barg A, Knupp M, Zwicky L, Kapron AL, Valderrabano V, et al. The Scandinavian total ankle replacement: long-term, eleven to fifteen-year, survivorship analysis of the prosthesis in seventy-two consecutive patients. J Bone Joint Surg Am. 2013;95(8):711–8.
69. Dhawan R, Turner J, Sharma V, Nayak RK. Tri-component, mobile bearing, total ankle replacement: mid-term functional outcome and survival. J Foot Ankle Surg. 2012;51(5):566–9.
70. Skytta ET, Koivu H, Eskelinen A, Ikavalko M, Paavolainen P, Remes V. Total ankle replacement: a population-based study of

515 cases from the Finnish arthroplasty register. Acta Orthop. 2010;81(1):114–8.
71. Kofoed H, Lundberg-Jensen A. Ankle arthroplasty in patients younger and older than 50 years: a prospective series with long-term follow-up. Foot Ankle Int. 1999;20(8):501–6.
72. Doets HC, Brand R, Nelissen RG. Total ankle arthroplasty in inflammatory joint disease with use of two mobile-bearing designs. J Bone Joint Surg Am. 2006;88(6):1272–84.
73. Hurowitz EJ, Gould JS, Fleisig GS, Fowler R. Outcome analysis of agility total ankle replacement with prior adjunctive procedures: two to six year followup. Foot Ankle Int. 2007;28(3):308–12.
74. Claridge RJ, Sagherian BH. Intermediate term outcome of the agility total ankle arthroplasty. Foot Ankle Int. 2009;30(9):824–35.
75. Rodrigues-Pinto R, Muras J, Martin Oliva X, Amado P. Total ankle replacement in patients under the age of 50. Should the indications be revised? Foot Ankle Surg. 2013;19(4):229–33.
76. Demetracopoulos CA, Adams SB Jr, Queen RM, DeOrio JK, Nunley JA 2nd, Easley ME. Effect of age on outcomes in total ankle arthroplasty. Foot Ankle Int. 2015;36(8):871–80.
77. Valderrabano V, Hintermann B, Dick W. Scandinavian total ankle replacement: a 3.7-year average followup of 65 patients. Clin Orthop Relat Res. 2004;424:47–56.
78. Wood PL, Deakin S. Total ankle replacement. The results in 200 ankles. J Bone Joint Surg Br. 2003;85(3):334–41.
79. Hintermann B, Knupp M, Zwicky L, Barg A. Total ankle replacement for treatment of end-stage osteoarthritis in elderly patients. J Aging Res. 2012;2012:345237.
80. Lee GW, Seon JK, Kim NS, Lee KB. Comparison of intermediate-term outcomes of total ankle arthroplasty in patients Younger and older than 55 years. Foot Ankle Int. 2019;40(7):762–8.
81. Tenenbaum S, Bariteau J, Coleman S, Brodsky J. Functional and clinical outcomes of total ankle arthroplasty in elderly compared to younger patients. Foot Ankle Surg. 2017;23(2):102–7.
82. Zhou H, Yakavonis M, Shaw JJ, Patel A, Li X. In-patient trends and complications after total ankle arthroplasty in the United States. Orthopedics. 2016;39(1):e74–9.
83. Raikin SM, Kane J, Ciminiello ME. Risk factors for incision-healing complications following total ankle arthroplasty. J Bone Joint Surg Am. 2010;92(12):2150–5.
84. Deland JT, Morris GD, Sung IH. Biomechanics of the ankle joint. A perspective on total ankle replacement. Foot Ankle Clin. 2000;5(4):747–59.
85. Nigg BMH, B. Biomechanics of the ankle joint complex and the shoe. In: Nordin M, Andersson G, Pope MH, editors. Muskuloskeletal disorders in the workplace—principles and practice. Louis Baltimore Boston: Mosby; 1996. p. 558–69.
86. Stauffer RN, Chao EY, Brewster RC. Force and motion analysis of the normal, diseased, and prosthetic ankle joint. Clin Orthop Relat Res. 1977;127:189–96.
87. Doets HC, van Middelkoop M, Houdijk H, Nelissen RG, Veeger HE. Gait analysis after successful mobile bearing total ankle replacement. Foot Ankle Int. 2007;28(3):313–22.
88. Bouchard M, Amin A, Pinsker E, Khan R, Deda E, Daniels TR. The impact of obesity on the outcome of total ankle replacement. J Bone Joint Surg Am. 2015;97(11):904–10.
89. Barg A, Knupp M, Anderson AE, Hintermann B. Total ankle replacement in obese patients: component stability, weight change, and functional outcome in 118 consecutive patients. Foot Ankle Int. 2011;32(10):925–32.
90. Baker JF, Perera A, Lui DF, Stephens MM. The effect of body mass index on outcomes after total ankle replacement. Ir Med J. 2009;102(6):188–90.
91. Gross CE, Lampley A, Green CL, DeOrio JK, Easley M, Adams S, et al. The effect of obesity on functional outcomes and complications in total ankle arthroplasty. Foot Ankle Int. 2016;37(2):137–41.
92. Werner BC, Burrus MT, Looney AM, Park JS, Perumal V, Cooper MT. Obesity is associated with increased complications after operative management of end-stage ankle arthritis. Foot Ankle Int. 2015;36(8):863–70.
93. Espinosa N, Walti M, Favre P, Snedeker JG. Misalignment of total ankle components can induce high joint contact pressures. J Bone Joint Surg Am. 2010;92(5):1179–87.
94. Singh JA, Ramachandaran R. Does rural residence impact total ankle arthroplasty utilization and outcomes? Clin Rheumatol. 2016;35(2):381–6.
95. Hvid I, Rasmussen O, Jensen NC, Nielsen S. Trabecular bone strength profiles at the ankle joint. Clin Orthop Relat Res. 1985;199:306–12.
96. Valderrabano V, Pagenstert G, Horisberger M, Knupp M, Hintermann B. Sports and recreation activity of ankle arthritis patients before and after total ankle replacement. Am J Sports Med. 2006;34(6):993–9.
97. Naal FD, Impellizzeri FM, Loibl M, Huber M, Rippstein PF. Habitual physical activity and sports participation after total ankle arthroplasty. Am J Sports Med. 2009;37(1):95–102.
98. Bonnin MP, Laurent JR, Casillas M. Ankle function and sports activity after total ankle arthroplasty. Foot Ankle Int. 2009;30(10):933–44.
99. Macaulay AA, VanValkenburg SM, DiGiovanni CW. Sport and activity restrictions following total ankle replacement: a survey of orthopaedic foot and ankle specialists. Foot Ankle Surg. 2015;21(4):260–5.
100. Schuh R, Hofstaetter J, Krismer M, Bevoni R, Windhager R, Trnka HJ. Total ankle arthroplasty versus ankle arthrodesis. Comparison of sports, recreational activities and functional outcome. Int Orthop. 2012;36(6):1207–14.
101. Lee JJ, Patel R, Biermann JS, Dougherty PJ. The musculoskeletal effects of cigarette smoking. J Bone Joint Surg Am. 2013;95(9):850–9.
102. Cobb TK, Gabrielsen TA, Campbell DC 2nd, Wallrichs SL, Ilstrup DM. Cigarette smoking and nonunion after ankle arthrodesis. Foot Ankle Int. 1994;15(2):64–7.
103. Lampley A, Gross CE, Green CL, DeOrio JK, Easley M, Adams S, et al. Association of cigarette use and complication rates and outcomes following total ankle arthroplasty. Foot Ankle Int. 2016;37(10):1052–9.
104. Patton D, Kiewiet N, Brage M. Infected total ankle arthroplasty: risk factors and treatment options. Foot Ankle Int. 2015;36(6):626–34.
105. Cody EA, Bejarano-Pineda L, Lachman JR, Taylor MA, Gausden EB, DeOrio JK, et al. Risk factors for failure of total ankle arthroplasty with a minimum five years of follow-up. Foot Ankle Int. 2019;40(3):249–58.
106. Gross CE, Green CL, DeOrio JK, Easley M, Adams S, Nunley JA 2nd. Impact of diabetes on outcome of total ankle replacement. Foot Ankle Int. 2015;36(10):1144–9.
107. Nasell H, Ottosson C, Tornqvist H, Linde J, Ponzer S. The impact of smoking on complications after operatively treated ankle fractures—a follow-up study of 906 patients. J Orthop Trauma. 2011;25(12):748–55.
108. Lee JW, Im WY, Song SY, Choi JY, Kim SJ. Analysis of early failure rate and its risk factor with 2157 total ankle replacements. Sci Rep. 2021;11(1):1901.
109. Rushing CJ, Zulauf E, Hyer CF, Berlet GC. Risk factors for early failure of fourth generation total ankle arthroplasty prostheses. J Foot Ankle Surg. 2021;60(2):312–7.
110. Escudero MI, Le V, Barahona M, Symes M, Wing K, Younger A, et al. Total ankle arthroplasty survival and risk factors for failure. Foot Ankle Int. 2019;40(9):997–1006.
111. Halter JB, Musi N, McFarland Horne F, Crandall JP, Goldberg A, Harkless L, et al. Diabetes and cardiovascular disease in

older adults: current status and future directions. Diabetes. 2014;63(8):2578–89.
112. Hirvensalo M, Rantanen T, Heikkinen E. Mobility difficulties and physical activity as predictors of mortality and loss of independence in the community-living older population. J Am Geriatr Soc. 2000;48(5):493–8.
113. Iglay K, Hannachi H, Joseph Howie P, Xu J, Li X, Engel SS, et al. Prevalence and co-prevalence of comorbidities among patients with type 2 diabetes mellitus. Curr Med Res Opin. 2016;32(7):1243–52.
114. Tarricone A, Gee A, Chen S, De La Mata K, Muser J, Axman W, et al. A systematic review and meta-analysis of total ankle arthroplasty or ankle arthrodesis for treatment of osteoarthritis in patients with diabetes. Foot Ankle Orthop. 2022;7(3):24730114221112955.
115. Choi WJ, Lee JS, Lee M, Park JH, Lee JW. The impact of diabetes on the short- to mid-term outcome of total ankle replacement. Bone Joint J. 2014;96-B(12):1674–80.
116. Schipper ON, Jiang JJ, Chen L, Koh J, Toolan BC. Effect of diabetes mellitus on perioperative complications and hospital outcomes after ankle arthrodesis and total ankle arthroplasty. Foot Ankle Int. 2015;36(3):258–67.
117. Marchant MH Jr, Viens NA, Cook C, Vail TP, Bolognesi MP. The impact of glycemic control and diabetes mellitus on perioperative outcomes after total joint arthroplasty. J Bone Joint Surg Am. 2009;91(7):1621–9.
118. Vaughan P, Gordon D, Goldberg A, Cullen N, Singh D. Patient satisfaction and function after bilateral ankle arthrodeses. Foot Ankle Surg. 2015;21(3):160–3.
119. Henricson A, Kamrad I, Rosengren B, Carlsson A. Bilateral arthrodesis of the ankle joint: self-reported outcomes in 35 patients from the Swedish ankle registry. J Foot Ankle Surg. 2016;55(6):1195–8.
120. Wang Y, Wong DW, Tan Q, Li Z, Zhang M. Total ankle arthroplasty and ankle arthrodesis affect the biomechanics of the inner foot differently. Sci Rep. 2019;9(1):13334.
121. Chen J, Wu S, Li Y, Chen Y, Liu X, Qin B, et al. Simultaneous total ankle replacement and contralateral ankle arthrodesis for bilateral ankle osteoarthritis: a retrospective study focused on clinical outcomes and cost-effectiveness. Orthop Surg. 2022;14(8): 1808–16.
122. Desai SJ, Glazebrook M, Penner MJ, Wing KJ, Younger AS, Pinsker E, et al. Quality of life in bilateral vs. unilateral end-stage ankle arthritis and outcomes of bilateral vs. unilateral total ankle replacement. J Bone Joint Surg Am. 2017;99(2):133–40.
123. Glazebrook M, Daniels T, Younger A, Foote CJ, Penner M, Wing K, et al. Comparison of health-related quality of life between patients with end-stage ankle and hip arthrosis. J Bone Joint Surg Am. 2008;90(3):499–505.
124. Saltzman CL, Salamon ML, Blanchard GM, Huff T, Hayes A, Buckwalter JA, et al. Epidemiology of ankle arthritis: report of a consecutive series of 639 patients from a tertiary orthopaedic center. Iowa Orthop J. 2005;25:44–6.
125. Daniels T, Thomas R. Etiology and biomechanics of ankle arthritis. Foot Ankle Clin. 2008;13(3):341–52. vii
126. Kofoed H, Sorensen TS. Ankle arthroplasty for rheumatoid arthritis and osteoarthritis: prospective long-term study of cemented replacements. J Bone Joint Surg Br. 1998;80(2):328–32.
127. Cho BK, An MY, Ahn BH. Comparison of clinical outcomes after total ankle arthroplasty between end-stage osteoarthritis and rheumatoid arthritis. Foot Ankle Int. 2021;42(5):589–97.
128. Pedersen E, Pinsker E, Younger AS, Penner MJ, Wing KJ, Dryden PJ, et al. Outcome of total ankle arthroplasty in patients with rheumatoid arthritis and noninflammatory arthritis. A multicenter cohort study comparing clinical outcome and safety. J Bone Joint Surg Am. 2014;96(21):1768–75.
129. Asencio JG, Leonardi C, Biron-Andreani C, Schved JF. Short-term and mid-term outcome of total ankle replacement in haemophilic patients. Foot Ankle Surg. 2014;20(4):285–92.
130. Strauss AC, Goldmann G, Wessling M, Gravius S, Muller MC, Wimmer MD, et al. Total ankle replacement in patients with haemophilia and virus infections—a safe alternative to ankle arthrodesis? Haemophilia. 2014;20(5):702–8.
131. Preis M, Bailey T, Jacxsens M, Barg A. Total ankle replacement in patients with haemophilic arthropathy: primary arthroplasty and conversion of painful ankle arthrodesis to arthroplasty. Haemophilia. 2017;23(4):e301–e9.
132. Barg A, Knupp M, Kapron AL, Hintermann B. Total ankle replacement in patients with gouty arthritis. J Bone Joint Surg Am. 2011;93(4):357–66.
133. Nieuwe Weme RA, van Solinge G, Doornberg JN, Sierevelt I, Haverkamp D, Doets HC. Total ankle replacement for post-traumatic arthritis. Similar outcome in postfracture and instability arthritis: a comparison of 90 ankles. Acta Orthop. 2015;86(4):401–6.
134. Mann JA, Mann RA, Horton E. STAR ankle: long-term results. Foot Ankle Int. 2011;32(5):S473–84.
135. Schutte BG, Louwerens JW. Short-term results of our first 49 Scandinavian total ankle replacements (STAR). Foot Ankle Int. 2008;29(2):124–7.
136. Kvarda P, Peterhans US, Susdorf R, Barg A, Ruiz R, Hintermann B. Long-term survival of HINTEGRA total ankle replacement in 683 patients: a concise 20-year follow-up of a previous report. J Bone Joint Surg Am. 2022;104:881.
137. Megerian MF, Harlow ER, LaTulip SM, Zhao C, Ina JG, Sattar A, et al. Total ankle arthroplasty for posttraumatic fracture versus primary osteoarthritis: an analysis of complications, revisions, and prosthesis survival. J Am Acad Orthop Surg. 2023;31(14):727–37.
138. Mousavian A, Baradaran A, Schon LC, Daniel J, Pedowitz D, Kachooei AR. Total ankle replacement outcome in patients with inflammatory versus noninflammatory arthritis: a systematic review and meta-analysis. Foot Ankle Spec. 2022;16:19386400221136591.
139. Hintermann B, Ruiz R. Total replacement of Varus ankle: three-component prosthesis design. Foot Ankle Clin. 2019;24(2):305–24.
140. Joo SD, Lee KB. Comparison of the outcome of total ankle arthroplasty for osteoarthritis with moderate and severe varus malalignment and that with neutral alignment. Bone Joint J. 2017;99-B(10):1335–42.
141. Sung KS, Ahn J, Lee KH, Chun TH. Short-term results of total ankle arthroplasty for end-stage ankle arthritis with severe varus deformity. Foot Ankle Int. 2014;35(3):225–31.
142. Trajkovski T, Pinsker E, Cadden A, Daniels T. Outcomes of ankle arthroplasty with preoperative coronal-plane varus deformity of 10 degrees or greater. J Bone Joint Surg Am. 2013;95(15):1382–8.
143. Greisberg J, Hansen ST Jr. Ankle replacement: management of associated deformities. Foot Ankle Clin. 2002;7(4):721–36. vi
144. Stamatis ED, Myerson MS. How to avoid specific complications of total ankle replacement. Foot Ankle Clin. 2002;7(4): 765–89.
145. Wood PL, Sutton C, Mishra V, Suneja R. A randomised, controlled trial of two mobile-bearing total ankle replacements. J Bone Joint Surg Br. 2009;91(1):69–74.
146. de Asla RJ, Ellis S, Overley B, Parekh S, Brigido S. Total ankle arthroplasty in the setting of valgus deformity. Foot Ankle Spec. 2014;7(5):398–402.
147. Doets HC, van der Plaat LW, Klein JP. Medial malleolar osteotomy for the correction of varus deformity during total ankle arthroplasty: results in 15 ankles. Foot Ankle Int. 2008;29(2):171–7.
148. Choi WJ, Kim BS, Lee JW. Preoperative planning and surgical technique: how do I balance my ankle? Foot Ankle Int. 2012;33(3):244–9.

149. Barg A, Pagenstert GI, Leumann AG, Muller AM, Henninger HB, Valderrabano V. Treatment of the arthritic valgus ankle. Foot Ankle Clin. 2012;17(4):647–63.
150. Knupp M, Bolliger L, Barg A, Hintermann B. Total ankle replacement for varus deformity. Orthopade. 2011;40(11):964–70.
151. Roukis TS. Modified Evans peroneus brevis lateral ankle stabilization for balancing varus ankle contracture during total ankle replacement. J Foot Ankle Surg. 2013;52(6):789–92.
152. Shock RP, Christensen JC, Schuberth JM. Total ankle replacement in the varus ankle. J Foot Ankle Surg. 2011;50(1):5–10.
153. Valderrabano V, Frigg A, Leumann A, Horisberger M. [Total ankle arthroplasty in valgus ankle osteoarthritis]. Orthopade. 2011;40(11):971–4, 6–7.
154. Ryssman D, Myerson MS. Surgical strategies: the management of varus ankle deformity with joint replacement. Foot Ankle Int. 2011;32(2):217–24.
155. Schuberth JM, Christensen JC, Seidenstricker CL. Total ankle replacement with severe valgus deformity: technique and surgical strategy. J Foot Ankle Surg. 2017;56(3):618–27.
156. Hobson SA, Karantana A, Dhar S. Total ankle replacement in patients with significant pre-operative deformity of the hindfoot. J Bone Joint Surg Br. 2009;91(4):481–6.
157. Knupp M, Stufkens SA, Bolliger L, Barg A, Hintermann B. Classification and treatment of supramalleolar deformities. Foot Ankle Int. 2011;32(11):1023–31.
158. Hintermann B, Knupp M, Barg A. Supramalleolar osteotomies for the treatment of ankle arthritis. J Am Acad Orthop Surg. 2016;24(7):424–32.
159. Hintermann B, Ruiz R. Joint preservation strategies for managing Varus ankle deformities. Foot Ankle Clin. 2022;27(1):37–56.
160. Knupp M, Horisberger M, Hintermann B. A new Z-shaped calcaneal osteotomy for 3-plane correction of severe Varus deformity of the hindfoot. Tech Foot Ankle Surg. 2008;7(2):90–5.
161. Kim BS, Lee JW. Total ankle replacement for the varus unstable. Foot Ankle Tech. 2010;9:157–67.
162. Brunner S, Knupp M, Hintermann B. Total ankle replacement for the valgus unstable osteoarthritic ankle. Foot Ankle Tech. 2010;9(4):174–9.
163. Kilger R, Knupp M, Hintermann B. Peroneus longus to peroneus brevis tendon transfer. Tech Foot Ankle Surg. 2009;8(3):146–9.
164. Steiner CS, Gilgen A, Zwicky L, Schweizer C, Ruiz R, Hintermann B. Combined subtalar and naviculocuneiform fusion for treating adult acquired flatfoot deformity with medial arch collapse at the level of the naviculocuneiform joint. Foot Ankle Int. 2019;40(1):42–7.
165. Deland JT, Ellis SJ, Day J, de Cesar NC, Hintermann B, Myerson MS, et al. Indications for deltoid and spring ligament reconstruction in progressive collapsing foot deformity. Foot Ankle Int. 2020;41(10):1302–6.
166. Karantana A, Hobson S, Dhar S. The scandinavian total ankle replacement: survivorship at 5 and 8 years comparable to other series. Clin Orthop Relat Res. 2010;468(4):951–7.
167. Daniels TR, Cadden AR, Lim K. Correction of varus talar deformities in ankle joint replacement. Oper Tech Orthop. 2008;18:282–6.
168. Kim BS, Choi WJ, Kim YS, Lee JW. Total ankle replacement in moderate to severe varus deformity of the ankle. J Bone Joint Surg Br. 2009;91(9):1183–90.
169. Gould JS, Alvine FG, Mann RA, Sanders RW, Walling AK. Total ankle replacement: a surgical discussion. Part II. The clinical and surgical experience. Am J Orthop (Belle Mead NJ). 2000;29(9):675–82.
170. Jennison T, Dalgleish J, Sharpe I, Davies M, Goldberg A. Total talus replacements. Foot Ankle Orthop. 2023;8(1):24730114221151068.
171. Devalia KL, Ramaskandhan J, Muthumayandi K, Siddique M. Early results of a novel technique: hindfoot fusion in talus osteonecrosis prior to ankle arthroplasty: a case series. Foot (Edinb). 2015;25(4):200–5.
172. Kurokawa H, Taniguchi A, Morita S, Takakura Y, Tanaka Y. Total ankle arthroplasty incorporating a total talar prosthesis: a comparative study against the standard total ankle arthroplasty. Bone Joint J. 2019;101-B(4):443–6.
173. Taniguchi A, Takakura Y, Sugimoto K, Hayashi K, Ouchi K, Kumai T, et al. The use of a ceramic talar body prosthesis in patients with aseptic necrosis of the talus. J Bone Joint Surg Br. 2012;94(11):1529–33.
174. Lampert C. Ankle joint prosthesis for bone defects. Orthopade. 2011;40(11):978–83.
175. Harnroongroj T, Harnroongroj T. The Talar body prosthesis: results at ten to thirty-six years of follow-up. J Bone Joint Surg Am. 2014;96(14):1211–8.
176. Taniguchi A, Takakura Y, Tanaka Y, Kurokawa H, Tomiwa K, Matsuda T, et al. An alumina ceramic total talar prosthesis for osteonecrosis of the talus. J Bone Joint Surg Am. 2015;97(16):1348–53.
177. Tsukamoto S, Tanaka Y, Maegawa N, Shinohara Y, Taniguchi A, Kumai T, et al. Total talar replacement following collapse of the talar body as a complication of total ankle arthroplasty: a case report. J Bone Joint Surg Am. 2010;92(11):2115–20.
178. Hintermann B, Zwicky L, Knupp M, Henninger HB, Barg A. HINTEGRA revision arthroplasty for failed total ankle prostheses. J Bone Joint Surg Am. 2013;95(13):1166–74.
179. Arcangelo J, Guerra-Pinto F, Pinto A, Grenho A, Navarro A, Martin Oliva X. Peri-prosthetic bone cysts after total ankle replacement. A systematic review and meta-analysis. Foot Ankle Surg. 2019;25(2):96–105.
180. Singh G, Reichard T, Hameister R, Awiszus F, Schenk K, Feuerstein B, et al. Ballooning osteolysis in 71 failed total ankle arthroplasties. Acta Orthop. 2016;87(4):401–5.
181. Bonasia DE, Dettoni F, Femino JE, Phisitkul P, Germano M, Amendola A. Total ankle replacement: why, when and how? Iowa Orthop J. 2010;30:119–30.
182. Sheridan BD, Robinson DE, Hubble MJ, Winson IG. Ankle arthrodesis and its relationship to ipsilateral arthritis of the hind- and mid-foot. J Bone Joint Surg Br. 2006;88(2):206–7.
183. van der Plaat LW, van Engelen SJ, Wajer QE, Hendrickx RP, Doets KH, Houdijk H, et al. Hind- and midfoot motion after ankle arthrodesis. Foot Ankle Int. 2015;36(12):1430–7.
184. Marx RCM, W. C. The role of arthroplasty in combined hind foot and ankle arthritis. Sem Arthrop. 2010;21:303–9.
185. Sokolowski M, Krahenbuhl N, Wang C, Zwicky L, Schweizer C, Horn Lang T, et al. Secondary subtalar joint osteoarthritis following total ankle replacement. Foot Ankle Int. 2019;40(10):1122–8.
186. Gross CE, Lewis JS, Adams SB, Easley M, DeOrio JK, Nunley JA 2nd. Secondary arthrodesis after total ankle arthroplasty. Foot Ankle Int. 2016;37(7):709–14.
187. Usuelli FG, Maccario C, Manzi L, Gross CE. Clinical outcome and fusion rate following simultaneous subtalar fusion and total ankle arthroplasty. Foot Ankle Int. 2016;37(7):696–702.
188. van den Heuvel A, Van Bouwel S, Dereymaeker G. Total ankle replacement. Design evolution and results. Acta Orthop Belg. 2010;76(2):150–61.
189. Eichinger S, Forst R, Kindervater M. Indications and alternatives for arthroplasty in young patients. Orthopade. 2007;36(4):311–24.
190. Espinosa N, Klammer G. Treatment of ankle osteoarthritis: arthrodesis versus total ankle replacement. Eur J Trauma Emerg Surg. 2010;36(6):525–35.
191. Shi GG, Huh J, Gross CE, Adams SB Jr, Easley ME, DeOrio JK, et al. Total ankle arthroplasty following prior infection about the ankle. Foot Ankle Int. 2015;36(12):1425–9.
192. Senneville EP, Aiyer A, Smyth N. What are the important risk factors that predispose a patient to infection after total ankle arthroplasty (TAA)? Foot Ankle Int. 2019;40(1_suppl):2S–3S.

7 Planning of a Primary Total Ankle Arthroplasty

In addition to joint space narrowing, osteophyte formation, subchondral bone cysts, and subchondral sclerosis, ankle osteoarthritis also potentially includes joint incongruency, malalignment, and dislocation, which are elusive on the weight-bearing standard radiographs, making it for the surgeon impossible to determine the center of rotation for a successful replacement of the osteoarthritic ankle. Radiographic overlays in 0 and 10% magnification for both the anterior-posterior and lateral profile of the prosthesis may be helpful in preoperative planning. However, determining the height of tibial resection can, in most instances, not be predicted accurately. Moreover, during ankle replacement surgery, the placement of the tibial prosthesis is mainly based on fluoroscopy during the operation. In contrast, a small controllable range due to a small diameter of the lower tibia and intraoperative fluoroscopy is unsatisfactory because of significant perspective errors. Another challenge is the involvement of the peritalar joints in the overall collapsing process of the ankle joint complex. At the same time, the talus is tilted into the varus or valgus, which may result in a contradictory compensatory movement of the calcaneus at the subtalar joint.

7.1 Understanding the Ankle to Be Replaced

Standard weight-bearing radiographs are mandatory for careful analysis of the osteoarthritic ankle (Fig. 7.1). Comparison with the contralateral unaffected ankle may help, especially in the case of severe changes due to incongruency, malalignment, and dislocation. Determining the longitudinal axis of the tibia and fibula and the center of the talar body with the aid of a circle may help to understand the malposition and to calculate the correction needed (Fig. 7.2). For instance, a posterior position of the fibula may indicate an anterolateral extrusion of the talus subsequently to an incompetent anterior tibiofibular ligament. A peritalar instability can be seen in the AP and lateral views: a talar tilt associated with a tilt of calcaneus in the opposite direction may result in a neutral heel alignment but indicate that the ankle joint complex has collapsed (Fig. 7.3). Such a "zig-zag" [1–3] or "ping-pong" [4] deformity may be corrected by the distraction of the tibiotalar joint if the subtalar joint is mobile, indicating that less bone resection may be

B. Hintermann, R. Ruiz, *Total Ankle Replacement*, https://doi.org/10.1007/978-3-031-56810-7_7

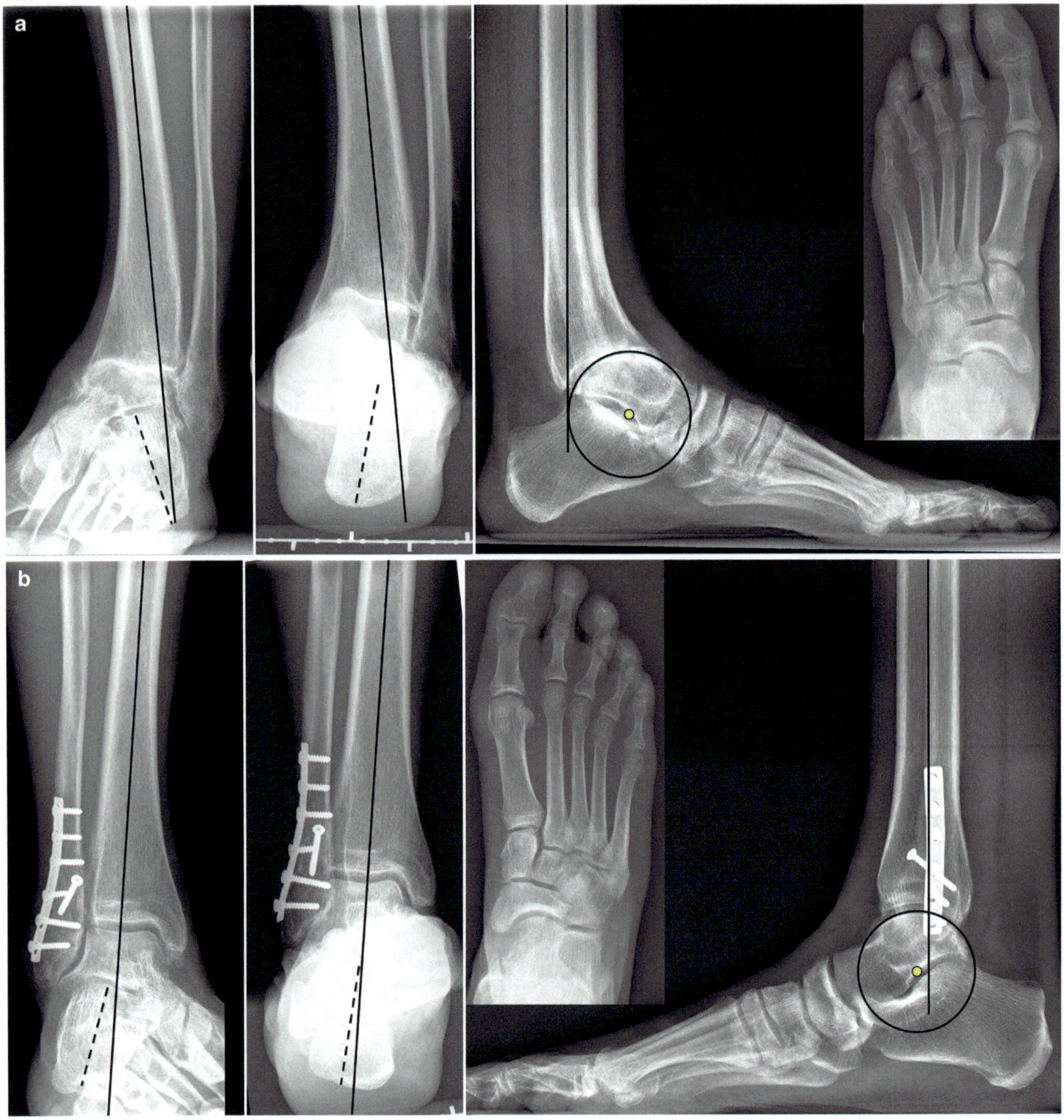

Fig. 7.1 Radiographic analysis of the osteoarthritic ankle. (**a**) Weight-bearing standard radiographs assess the osteoarthritic ankle's malalignment, incongruency, and dislocation. (**b**) Comparison with the contralateral unaffected ankle may help, especially in post-traumatic ankles

needed during the replacement surgery. Furthermore, incompetence of the syndesmotic ligaments can also be recognized on AP view and indicate that a stabilization procedure of the distal tibiofibular joint will be needed (Fig. 7.4). Radiographs in maximal dorsi- and plantarflexion may provide more information about the soft-tissue contractures and the expected range of motion after total ankle arthroplasty (Fig. 7.5).

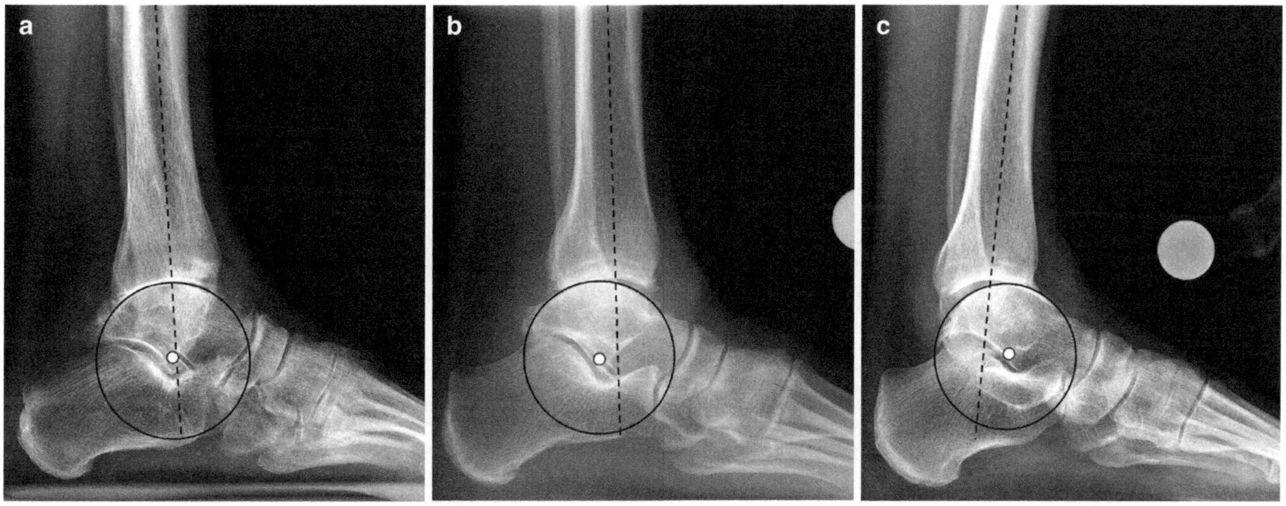

Fig. 7.2 Radiographic determination of the sagittal malalignment. Determining the longitudinal axis of the tibia and fibula and the center of the talar body with a circle may help understand the malposition and calculate the necessary correction. (**a**) Well-centralized ankle, (**b**) retro dislocation of the talus, and (**c**) anterior extrusion of the talus

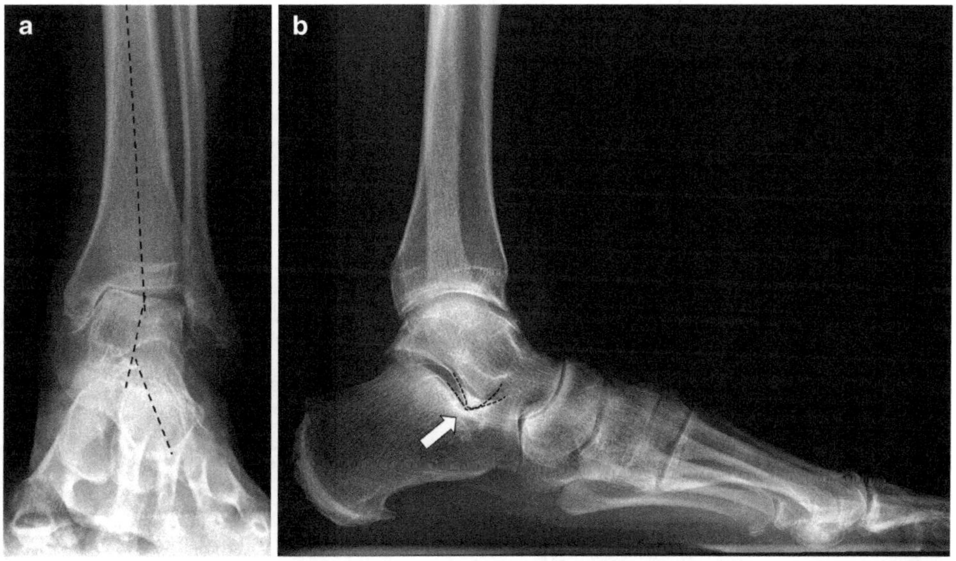

Fig. 7.3 Radiographic assessment of peritalar instability. (**a**) The AP view of this 53-year-old patient shows a talar tilt into the varus associated with a tilt of calcaneus in the opposite direction. (**b**) In the lateral view, a sinus tarsi impingement (arrow) can typically be seen, indicating that the varus tilt of the talus is corrected by maximal pronation at the subtalar joint. This explains the lateral pain in his ankle

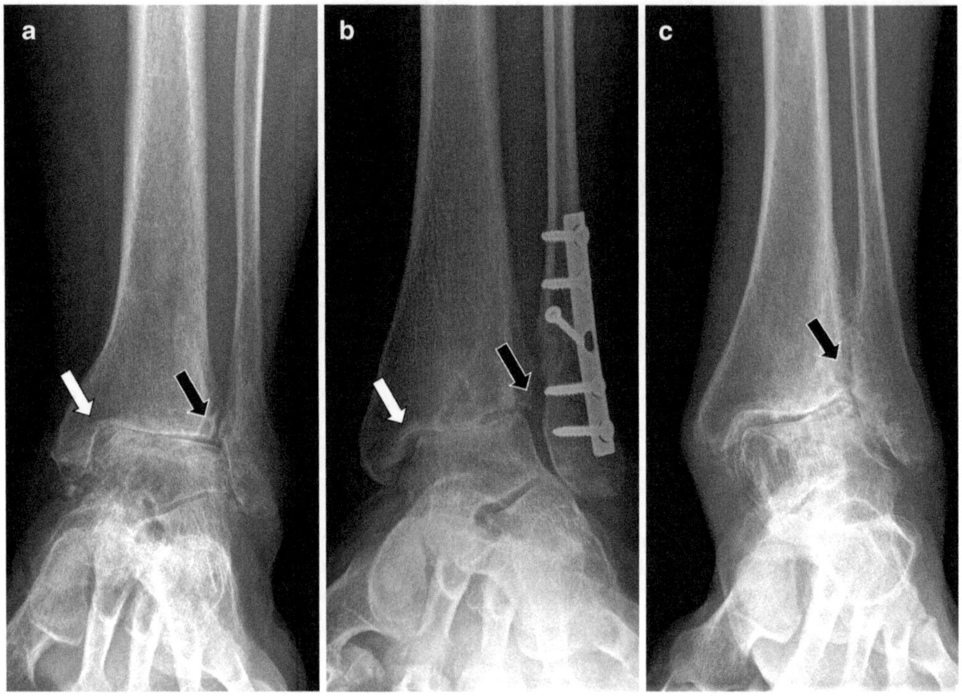

Fig. 7.4 Radiographic assessment of syndesmotic stability. The incompetence of syndesmotic ligaments can be detected on the AP view of the ankle. (**a**) Post-traumatic varus deformity of the distal tibia in a 59-year-old female patient demonstrating a widening of medial (white arrow) and lateral (black arrow) clear space. (**b**) Post-traumatic valgus deformity in a 59-year-old female patient caused by avascular necrosis of lateral tibial plafond and subsequent impaction of the talus and widening of the distal tibiofibular joint. Widening of medial (white arrow) and lateral clear space (black arrow). (**c**) Post-traumatic valgus ankle after conservatively treated mid-shaft fracture of the fibula in a 66-year-old male patient; apparently, the syndesmosis remained stable due to synostosis (black arrow) at the distal tibiofibular joint which kept the talus in place

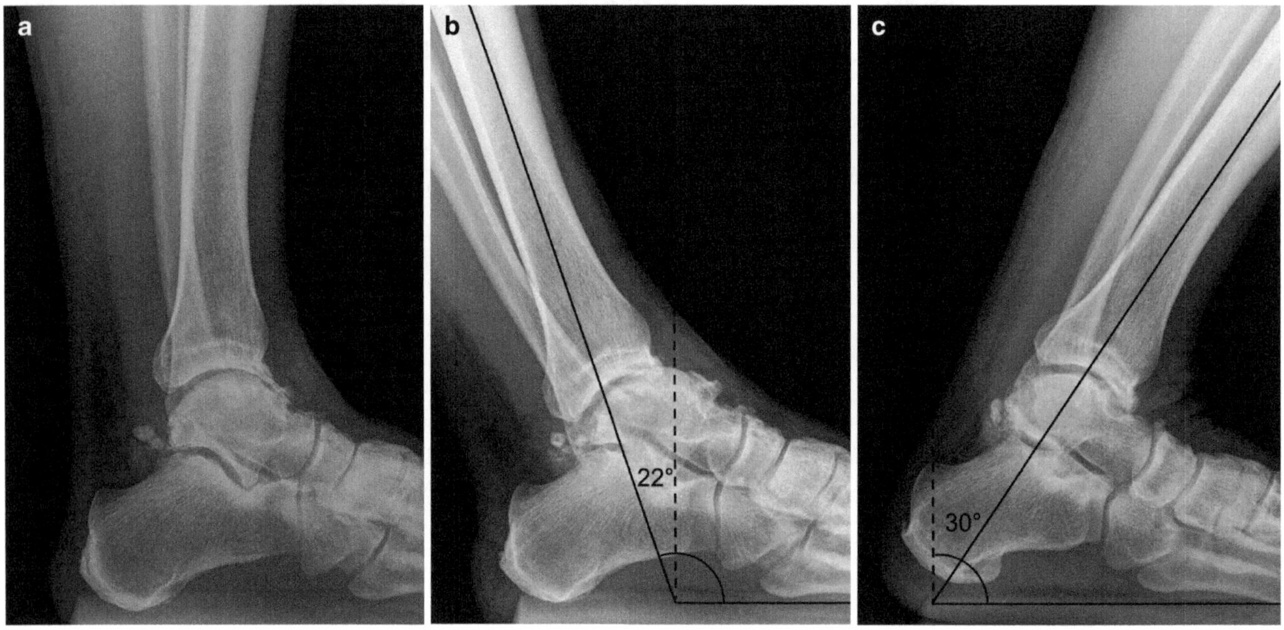

Fig. 7.5 Radiographic assessment of range of motion. Lateral views of the foot and ankle: (**a**) neutral position, (**b**) maximal plantarflexion position, and (**c**) maximal dorsiflexion position

7.2 Coronal and Sagittal Plane Alignment

The literature on the subject has shown that proper implant positioning and alignment are necessary for achieving good results in total ankle arthroplasty. Even the malpositioning of a miniature implant component has a relevant impact on motion and contact pressure, which may lead to failure [5].

7.2.1 Planning with Standard Referencing

Traditional preoperative planning methods for total ankle arthroplasty are based on anteroposterior and lateral weight-bearing radiographs (Figs. 7.1 and 7.6). A weight-bearing CT scan may provide additional information about the segmental changes within the ankle joint complex (Fig. 7.7). The standard technique uses the tibial tuberosity as a point of reference and is based on the principle that the mechanical axis of the tibia should equal the anatomical axis of the tibia (Fig. 7.8) [6].

When using a traditional system, the main parameter considered for the tibial cutting block is represented by the tibial tuberosity as the proximal reference and the middle of the anterior border of the tibiotalar joint as the distal reference. The talar resection is performed with the foot in a visually neutral position. This technique allows an experienced surgeon to adopt a good implant positioning; however, many other factors should be considered to fully re-establish gait symmetry and natural ankle motion [7]. Alternatively, some

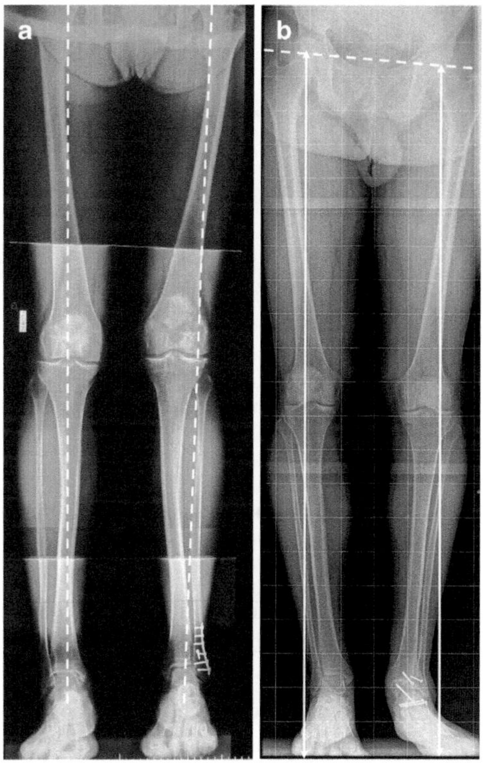

Fig. 7.6 Assessment of leg deformities. Full-plane AP radiographs can assess coronal plane deformities and leg length discrepancy. (**a**) A 62-year-old patient with post-traumatic ankle osteoarthritis of his left ankle with lateral pain due to a valgus deformity at the knee level. (**b**) A 54-year-old patient with left leg shortening after a talar fracture and end-stage ankle osteoarthritis

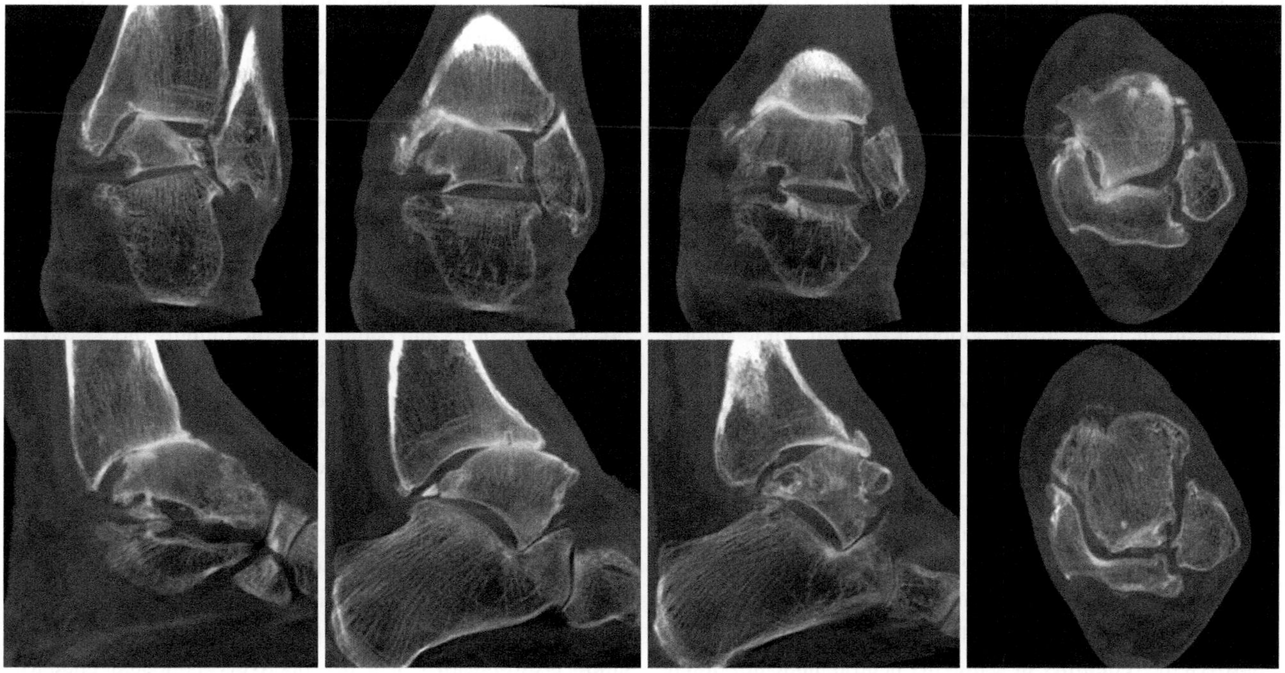

Fig. 7.7 Assessment with weight-bearing CT scan: A 64-year-old patient with a varus osteoarthritis of his left ankle showing an anterolateral extrusion of the talus with the erosion of medial tibial plafond and subsequent impaction of the talus

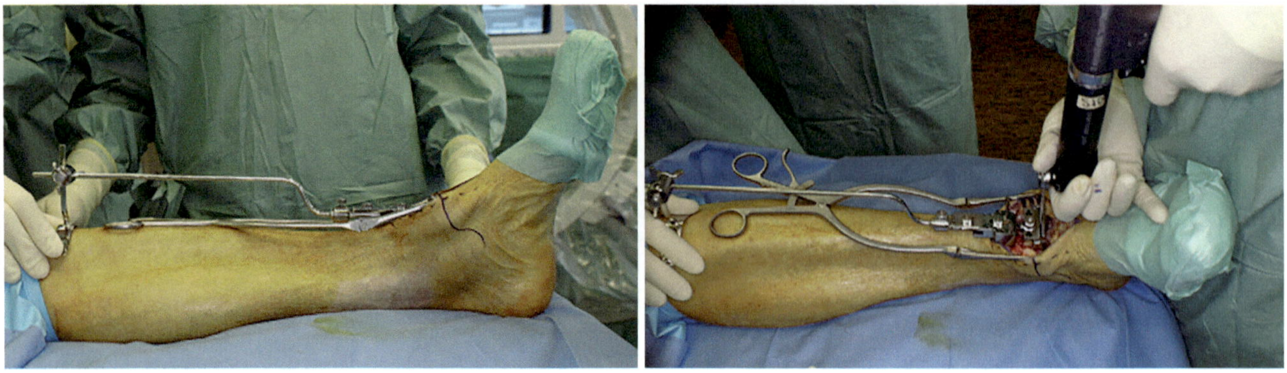

Fig. 7.8 References for alignment of tibial resection block. The references for the jig are the tibial tuberosity and the mechanical axis of the tibia (see text)

ankle replacement systems use an alignment frame with pin fixation of the tibia and the foot to guide the resection cuts under fluoroscopic control.

In a retrospective analysis, Veljkovic et al. [8] found in 60.4% of osteoarthritic ankles an anterior talar station to the tibial axis preoperatively; of these 70.7% shifted to less anterior after total ankle arthroplasty. They calculated that a 1.1 mm change in the lateral talar station (LTS) is recommended for every 1° of closing anterior distal tibial articular angle (ADTAA) change to translate anteriorly positioned preoperative ankles to a neutral postoperative position in fixed-bearing prosthetics. Conversely, a 0.6 mm change in LTS is recommended for every 1° opening ADTAA change to translate posteriorly positioned preoperative ankles to a neutral postoperative position. The authors concluded that the sagittal distal tibial cut may be one of the components in planning total ankle arthroplasty that should be customized to the individual patient based on the preoperative LTS and ADTAA measurements [8].

7.2.2 The Use of Preoperative Computer-Assisted Guidance

The recent increase in the adoption of total ankle arthroplasty reflects the improvements in implant designs and surgical techniques, including preoperative navigation systems and patient-specific instrumentation, such as custom-made cutting guides. Cutting guides are customized for each patient's anatomy based on preoperative ankle computed tomography scans, and they drive the saw intraoperatively to improve the accuracy of bone resection and implant positioning. Despite some promising results, the main queries in the literature are whether patient-specific instrumentation improves the reliability of achieving neutral ankle alignment and more accurate implant sizing, whether it is superior to standard techniques, and whether it is cost-effective.

Preoperative computer-assisted guidance has led to a better understanding of the three-dimensional ankle anatomy and associated deformities and allows for reproducible, anatomic placement of the total ankle arthroplasty components [9]. Berlet et al. [10], who evaluated the repeatability of tibia and talus patient-specific guide placement and deviation between the preoperative plan and actual implant placement in a vitro study on 15 cadaveric legs, found a deviation of fewer than 2° in all angular degrees of freedom of final implant placement from the preoperative plan. In 42 consecutive total arthroplasty cases using preoperative CT scan-derived patient-specific plans and guides, Hsu et al. [11] found that final coronal and sagittal alignments were within 3° of the predicted surgical plans and sizing was accurate within one implant size. When comparing patient-specific instrumentation with the standard referencing guide on a retrospective analysis of 99 Infinity total ankle arthroplasties, Saito et al. [12] reported that the absolute variation of the tibial component from the intended alignment was 1.6 ± 1.2° in the coronal plane and 1.9 ± 1.5° in the sagittal plane. These findings were in accordance with the reports of others [12–17].

In a review of their 50 total ankle arthroplasty patients, Biela et al. [18] found that "perfect" radiographic alignment was not consistently achieved, and the accuracy of component prediction was modest. Furthermore, the authors stated that preoperative plans and patient-specific pinning blocks did not simplify the complexity of their operations since the operative time, intraoperative image intensification time, and radiation dose per case all exceeded published historical total ankle arthroplasty controls. Ultimately, they could not support the purported benefits of this CT scan-based, engineer-provided alignment plan and patient-specific pinning blocks for this manufacturer's primary total ankle arthroplasty systems.

To determine the potential benefit of patient-specific instrumentation, Hamid et al. [19] evaluated 87 primary total ankle arthroplasties in a prospectively collected database. They found a 34 min shorter surgery time using patient-specific instrumentation compared with standard referencing, and, based on time-driven activity-based costing and associated sensitivity analysis, they calculated a cost-savings threshold of $863 at their institution.

Preoperative CT scan-derived patient-specific surgical plans and guides can help provide accurate and reproducible total ankle arthroplasty radiographic alignments. However, based on available suggestions, surgeons must continue to rely on their own surgical planning and experience to achieve optimum radiographic alignment rather than depending on engineer-based recommendations or "surface-matched" pinning blocks. Future studies are warranted to investigate the clinical and functional implications of patient-specific total ankle arthroplasty and the overall cost-effectiveness of this technique.

7.3 Height of Tibial Resection

During ankle replacement surgery, the height of resection for placement of the tibial component is arbitrary and mainly based on necessitated bone resection for receiving the component. Besides available references, the surgeon must mainly rely on instrumentation and fluoroscopy (Fig. 7.9). However, there is a small controllable range due to the small diameter of the lower tibia, and intraoperative fluoroscopy is unsatisfactory because of significant perspective errors. Though a too-extensive resection of tibial bone can be compensated with the use of a thicker polyethylene insert, it is at the expense of unnecessary bone loss, a weakening of the medial shoulder of the tibia, and loss of bone strength at the tibial side (Fig. 7.10). It also carries the risk of the created joint line being too high, which may disbalance the collateral ankle ligaments (Fig. 7.11).

Weight-bearing CT and computer navigation technology may improve resection accuracy but are often unavailable in medical institutions. An overall meticulous analysis, including assessing the distraction potential of the tibiotalar joint due to loss of ligament tension, is thus mandatory to optimize the height of tibial resection. As a rule, the more contract the osteoarthritic ankle is, the more tibial resection is needed to accommodate the tibial component

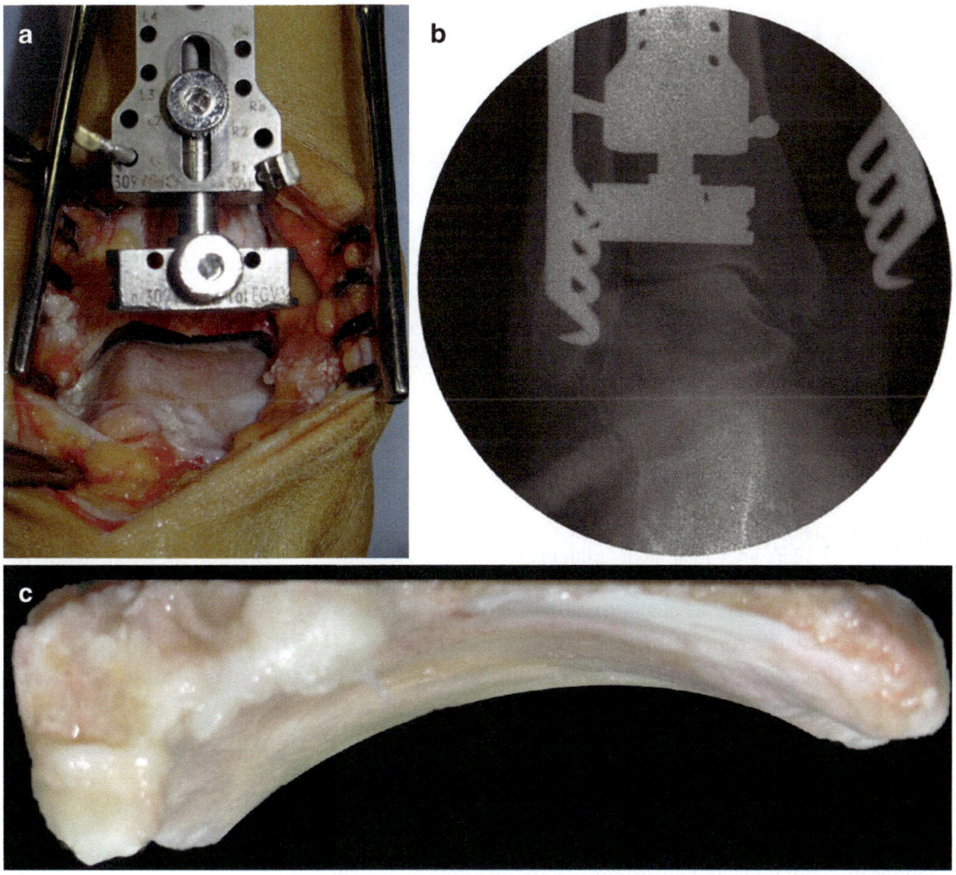

Fig. 7.9 Determination of the height of tibial resection. The amount of resection depends on the necessitated space for receiving the tibial component. (**a**) As a rule, less bone resection is needed in a lax ankle. This can best be determined with the distraction of the joint and visualization of the tibial plafond. (**b**) This is not possible in most cases; thus, the surgeon must rely on fluoroscopy. (**c**) Usually, there is a need for 3–5 mm bone resection as calculated from the apex of the tibial plafond, which also depends on the thickness of the tibial component

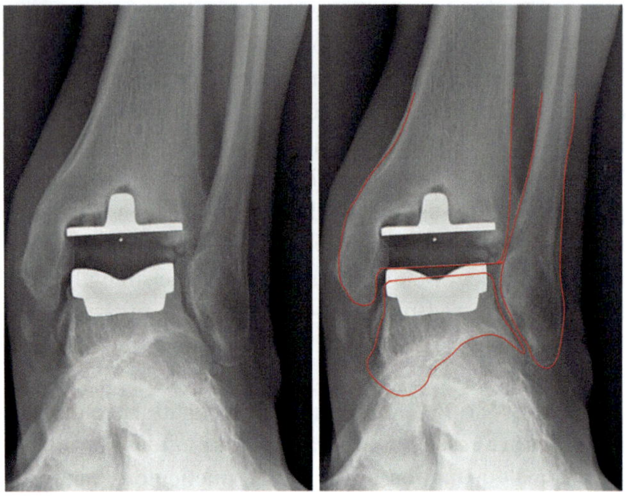

Fig. 7.10 Too high tibial resection. AP view of a 71-year-old patient 20 months after total ankle arthroplasty. The surgeon compensated for the too-extensive tibial resection with a thicker polyethylene insert. The tibial component failed after that to get firm anchorage in the weak tibial metaphysis. Notice that with the increased size of the prosthesis, the stress forces at the bone-implant interface have increased

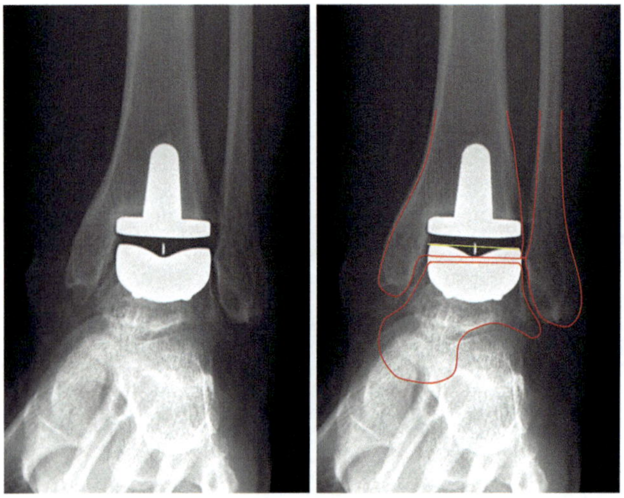

Fig. 7.11 Cranialization of the created joint line. AP view of a 63-year-old patient 3.5 years after total ankle arthroplasty. Though the ankle shows a satisfactory function, the patient is dissatisfied with the situation because of pain and swelling at the medial and lateral malleolus that increases with physical activities

as given by its thickness, including that of the predicted polyethylene insert.

7.4 Size of Components

The implant design of the talar component for total ankle arthroplasty should match the surface morphology of the talus and, with this, its size so that the replaced ankle can restore the natural motion of the tibiotalar joint and may reduce postoperative complications.

Fitting the medial and lateral surfaces of the talar trochlea with two spheres is a good way to approximate the surface of the talar trochlea (Fig. 7.12). However, with the osteoarthritic changes of the ankle, this is often very difficult when possible (Fig. 7.13). Analogously, the width of the trochlea that was measured to be posterior less than anterior by 2.4 ± 1.3 mm, with a range of 0–6 mm in normal ankles [20], can often not be predicted on plane radiographs in an osteoarthritic ankle. A CT scan may help, but anterolateral extrusion of the talus may make precise measuring inaccurate. Using an oversized component may hinder the appropriate position of the talus within the mortise and cause an overload of the ligamentous system, especially of syndesmotic ligaments [21]. Therefore, selecting a smaller talar component has generally been accepted [22]. Appropriate talar component sagittal plane positioning is also essential for a balanced ankle (Fig. 7.14).

The importance of using anatomically shaped components in total ankle arthroplasty, thereby avoiding excessive contact stress on the supporting bone, has been stated by Kempson et al. [23] in an in vivo study. This is especially important for the tibial implant that does not use a stem for fixation. They should get bony support from the overall cortical bone, as the compressive resistance of the center of the tibia is much lower (Fig. 7.15) [24, 25]. Therefore, the surgeon should select the bigger size when in doubt between two sizes based on the measuring device [22].

In fear of weakening the polyethylene subsequently to wear, using a bigger polyethylene insert is not without risks. Theoretically, thicker polyethylene components in the ankle

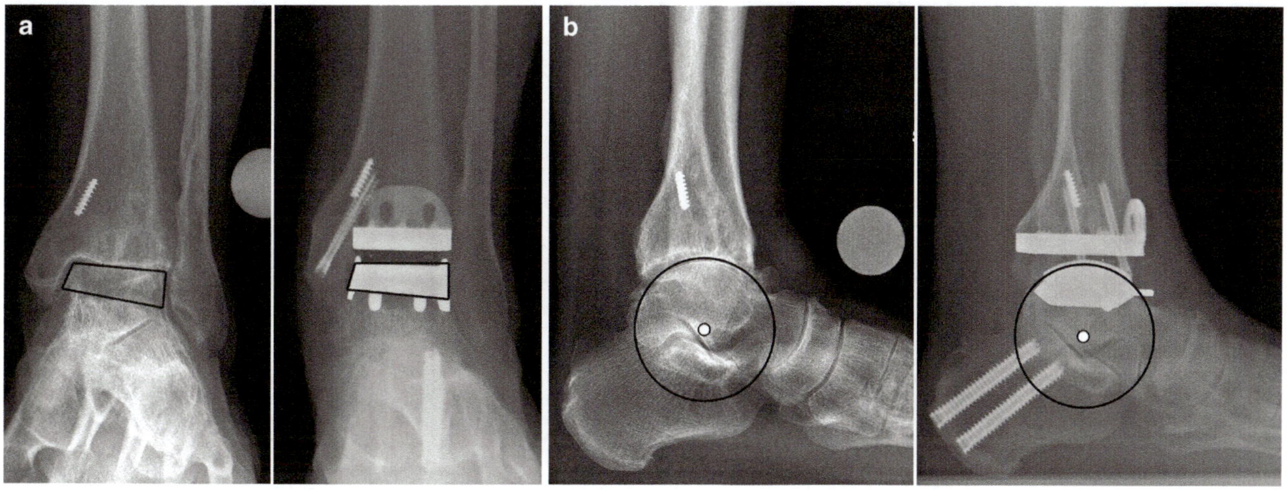

Fig. 7.12 Size of components. In this 46-year-old patient with post-traumatic ankle osteoarthritis, the component size fits well to the original articular surfaces, resulting in a close restoration of the axis of rotation. (**a**) AP view. (**b**) Lateral view

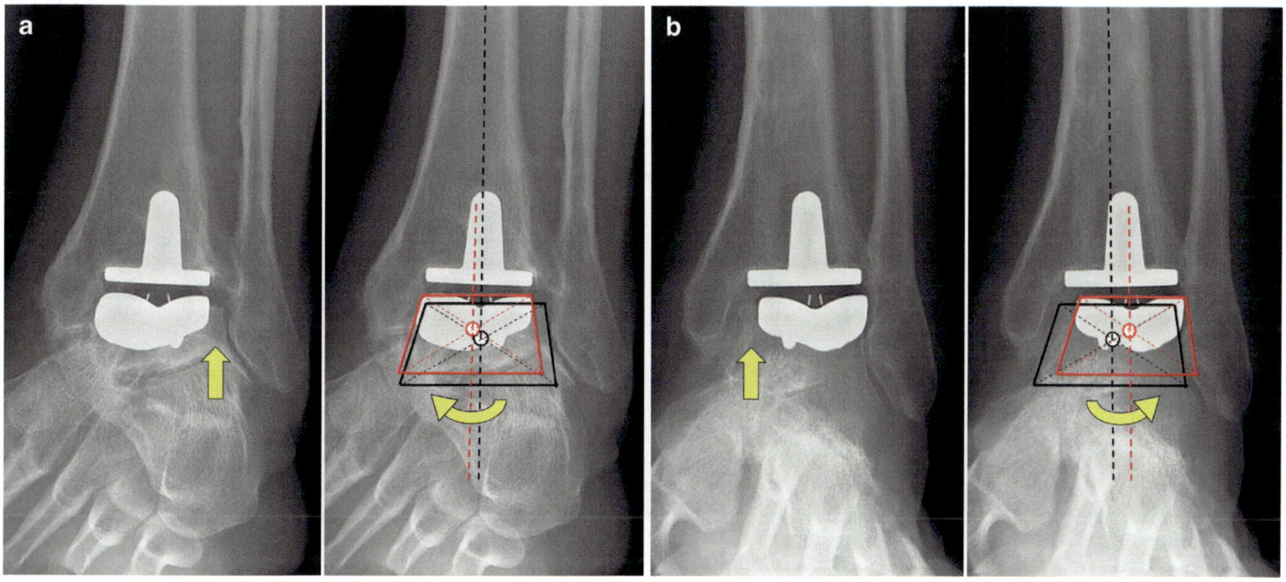

Fig. 7.13 Effect of undersized talar components in the coronal plane. Undersized talar components may result in asymmetric medial or lateral positioning, thus changing the load transmission to the talus, which may cause a tilting moment. This is especially problematic in ankle designs that do not provide intrinsic coronal plane stability, allowing for some e-/inversion. (**a**) A too-medial position causes a tilting force into the varus, whereas (**b**) a too-lateral position causes a tilting force into the valgus

may help prevent polyethylene failures, but at the expense of increasing the lever arm of forces acting at the bone-implant interface and of more generous bone cuts (Fig. 7.10). However, the fundamental importance of bone conservation in the ankle has been widely recognized since the bone may be weak and the surface areas for support small [25]. Polyethylene requirements for the ankle are, therefore, contradictory to what is necessary for conserving bone strength. Most current ankle designs use a minimal thickness of 5 mm. The few available data did not show a higher incidence of polyethylene failure with thinner inserts [26, 27], even not in obese patients [28, 29].

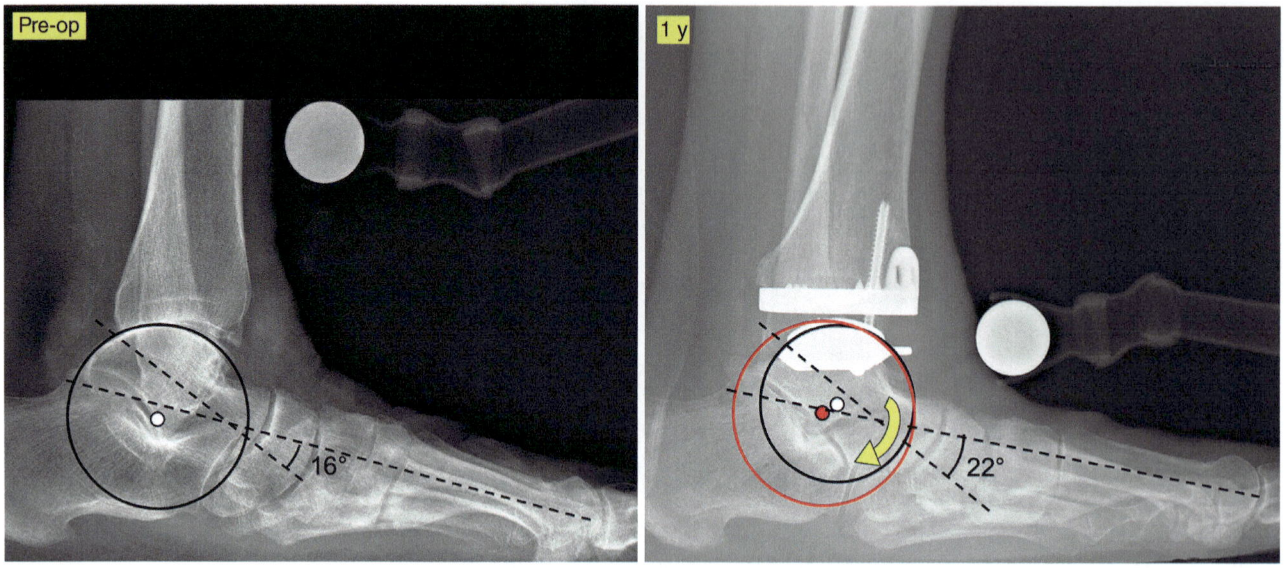

Fig. 7.14 Effect of undersized talar components in the sagittal plane. An undersized talar component creates an incongruency of the joint, which results in an asymmetric load of collateral ligaments. A too-anterior positioning of the talar component may relax the anterior portion of (anterior) deltoid-spring ligament complex in the range from neutral to dorsiflexed foot position. In contrast, a too-posterior positioning destabilizes the ankle in the plantarflexion. This may explain why, in this 66-year-old female patient, a significant increase in the talo-first metatarsal angle was seen at 1-year follow-up control despite the ankle ligaments being markedly tightened during the replacement surgery

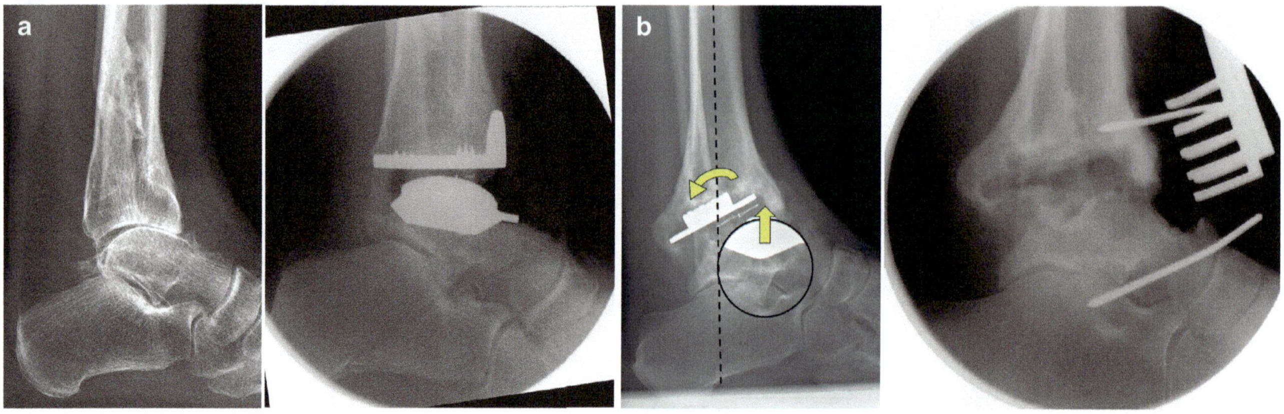

Fig. 7.15 Effect of an undersized tibial component. (**a**) The tibial component should get bony support by overall cortical bone, as the compressive resistance of the center of the tibia is much lower. (**b**) If the tibial component is undersized, it can subside into the tibial metaphysis; if it has no cortical bone support at this anterior aspect, it might break into the tibial metaphysis, especially if the talar component is too anteriorly positioned, which creates an asymmetrical load transfer to the tibial component. Notice that the anterior cortex is preserved after component removal

7.5 Malalignment Correction

One of the main challenges in replacement surgery for the osteoarthritic ankle is the correction of any deformity found proximal and distal to the ankle joint and in the ankle joint. The malalignment can be in the coronal or sagittal plane or both. Present deformities must be recognized, and sound judgment must be made to balance the ankle joint with procedures before, during, or after total ankle implantation (Fig. 7.16). Clinical and radiographic angular deformity of the ankle from the mechanical axis of the leg that is less than 5° is generally accepted as being within reasonable limits to be addressed by correcting cuts and soft-tissue procedures [1, 30–33]. There is some debate as to the level of deformity that is acceptable, with some authors who do not see any limitations for the varus ankle as long as the surgeon can bal-

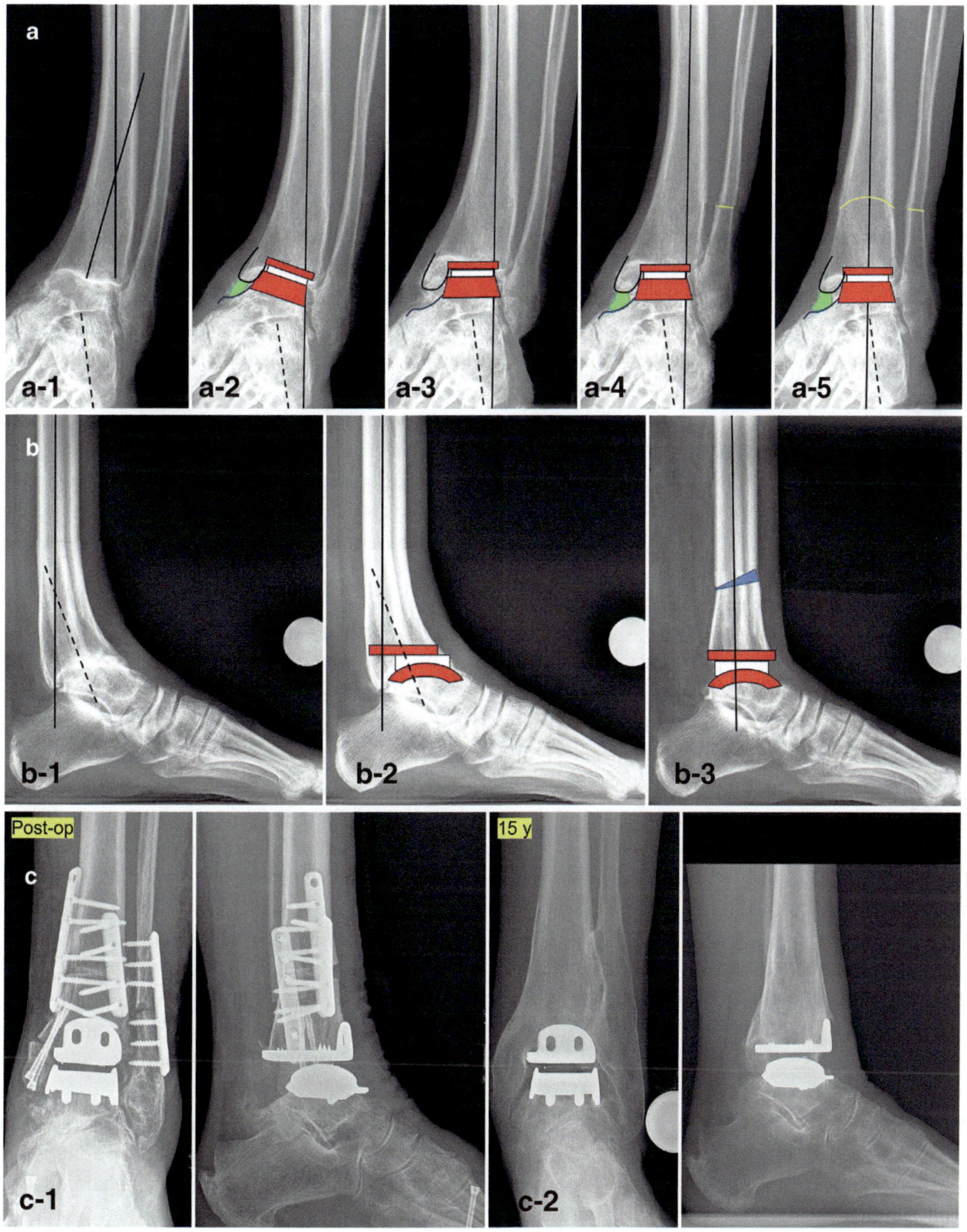

Fig. 7.16 Total ankle arthroplasty in complex three-plane deformities. A 56-year-old, active female patient with post-traumatic ankle osteoarthritis associated with a severe three-plane deformity, the CORA being extraarticular (approximately 6 cm above the ankle joint). (**a**) Coronal plane and (**b**) sagittal plane. The horizontal plane is not shown (internal malrotation of 8°, as verified by CT scan). (**a-2**) In the coronal plane, an in situ joint replacement would preserve the congruity of the joint but result in a non-balanced ankle. A correcting tibial resection associated with a medial release of the ankle (**a-3**) or a shortening osteotomy of the fibula (**a-4**) would not sufficiently balance the ankle as the translational deformity (malalignment) is not addressed. (**a-5**) A tibial and a fibular osteotomy will correct the angular deformity and translational malalignment, thus appropriately balancing the ankle. (**b-2**) In the sagittal plane, a correcting osteotomy of the tibia would address the angular deformity but not the translational malalignment, thus not balancing the ankle. (**b-3**) An open wedge osteotomy of the tibia, in contrast, would address both the angular deformity and the malalignment and thus balance the ankle. (**c**) The solution was an open wedge osteotomy of the tibia that was opened at its anterior aspect to insert an allograft; simultaneously, 10° of external rotation was performed at the osteotomy site before plate fixation. A plate fixed the fibula in the spontaneously corrected position. Besides this, a flip osteotomy of medial malleolus was made to address the intraarticular deformity, and a plantarflexing osteotomy of the first ray was made to address the forefoot pronation. (**c-1**) Radiographs postoperative and (**c-2**) at follow-up control after 15 years. The hardware was removed 1 year after surgery

ance the ankle properly by osteotomies and soft-tissue procedures [1, 33–36]. While a congruent valgus deformity can be successfully addressed by a correcting osteotomy, a valgus tilt of >10° of the talus is critical for total ankle arthroplasty [22, 37–39].

The sagittal plane deformity may be either apex anterior (procurvatum) or apex posterior (recurvatum). The deformity has a more pronounced effect the more proximal it occurs. Recurvatum deformity typically produces erosion of the anterior tibial plafond and some degrees of anterior subluxation of the talus, and it is often accompanied by functional equinus contracture. According to others [31], the authors recommend addressing sagittal plane deformities >5° when located >3 cm above the ankle.

Axial plane alignment must still be better understood and challenging to determine on two-dimensional radiographs. CT is generally regarded as the most accurate [40]. Tibial torsion is defined as the angle between the line connecting both posterior condyles of the tibia (proximal posterior condylar axis) and the line bisecting the medial and lateral malleolus, also known as the transmalleolar axis [41]. Najefi et al. [6], who found a wide range of tibial torsion (11.8–62.0°) in patients with ankle osteoarthritis, as between the medial gutter line and the medial axis of the tibia, advocated that surgeon designers and implant manufacturers should develop consistent methods to guide surgeons as to the appropriate axial rotation of their implant.

7.6 Additional Surgeries

Ligament balancing is an essential step during total ankle arthroplasty to optimize the mechanical stability of the ankle replacement.

7.6.1 Varus Ankle

A medial soft-tissue release is essential for balancing the ankle in an incongruent varus deformity [22]. Inadequate soft-tissue release about the ankle is usually associated with either instability or recurrence of deformity postoperatively. An overzealous release may produce instability on the contracted side of the joint or an increased joint space, which may lead to ankle instability of an implant or dislocation of the polyethylene due to exceeding the tibiotalar gap.

If there is residual talar tilt with lateral opening even after adequate medial release, or if there is minimal contracture on the medial side but laxity on the lateral side, then lateral ligament reconstruction is required [1, 42]. In the case of additional incompetence of the peroneus longus tendon, mainly seen in long-standing varus-supination deformities, a peroneus longus transfer to the base of the fifth metatarsal is considered [43]. This procedure effectively stabilizes the lateral soft tissue laxity, reduces the first metatarsal plantarflexion force, and is easy to combine with total ankle arthroplasty.

In a congruent varus deformity, the talus is tilted along with the varus inclined tibial plafond, yielding a talar tilt angle of fewer than 5°. In such cases, a neutralizing tibial cut must follow the medial release. A tibial bone cut at the most proximal bony defect level is required to achieve a neutrally aligned articular surface. Sometimes, we prefer a fibular shortening osteotomy to avoid too-extended medial release and destabilize the medial ankle [1].

Patients with varus ankle deformities often have limited ankle dorsiflexion after inserting the prosthesis, as it acts as a spacer. Heel cord lengthening is indicated if less than 10° of ankle dorsiflexion is achieved. Depending on the results of the Silfverskiold test, either gastrocnemius recession or percutaneous Achilles tendon lengthening is indicated.

7.6.2 Valgus Ankle

A valgus ankle is typically associated with a fibular malunion after an ankle fracture or a progressive collapsing foot deformity.

In the case of a malunited ankle, the main problem is a deviation of the anatomical axis of the ankle joint and the alteration of load distribution. The correction spectrum includes the correction of the fibular malunion and the altered relationship between the tibia, fibula, and talus to regain a correct anatomical axis and articular shape, allowing a more physiologic load distribution. An additional medial sliding osteotomy is, in general, necessary to achieve this goal [44]. If the syndesmotic ligaments are incompetent, a distal tibiofibular fusion should be considered, especially with a mobile-bearing ankle design [21].

In case of a progressive collapsing foot deformity that is typically associated with a peritalar subluxation, a subtalar and talonavicular corrective fusion should be considered [45–47]. To adequately address the associated collapsed medial arch, we prefer a subtalar fusion in combination with a navicular-cuneiform I–III fusion [48, 49]. These procedures aim to shift the heel contact point from lateral to medial and to plantarflex the first ray to get a plantigrade, balanced, and stable foot.

7.7 Conclusions

- Appropriate understanding of the ankle to be replaced is paramount for a successful total ankle arthroplasty.
- Standard radiographs are mandatory to assess deformities and osteoarthritic changes in adjacent joints.

- A CT scan, if possible under weight-bearing, may enhance the diagnosis; in particular, it provides additional information about segmental and osteoarthritic changes in the adjacent joints.
- Preoperative measurement combined with intraoperative fluoroscopy can further improve the accuracy of prosthesis placement.
- Computer navigation technology may improve the accuracy of ankle joint implantation.
- Addressing associated deformities by osteotomies or resection cuts and appropriately sizing the implants are mandatory for getting a balanced ankle.
- Care should be taken not to leave the joint gaps unbalanced or to leave the patient with residual soft tissue contracture or coronal and sagittal plane deformity.
- In a varus ankle, additional ligamentous work is often necessary for releases or reconstruction to obtain a stable and balanced ankle.
- In a valgus ankle, a medial sliding osteotomy and hind- and midfoot arthrodeses are often necessary to obtain a stable and balanced ankle and to prevent recurrences of the deformity.

References

1. Hintermann B, Ruiz R. Total replacement of varus ankle: three-component prosthesis design. Foot Ankle Clin. 2019;24(2):305–24.
2. Hintermann B, Knupp M, Barg A. Peritalar instability. Foot Ankle Int. 2012;33(5):450–4.
3. Hintermann B, Ruiz R. Joint preservation strategies for managing varus ankle deformities. Foot Ankle Clin. 2022;27(1):37–56.
4. Dodd A, Daniels TR. Total ankle replacement in the presence of talar varus or valgus deformities. Foot Ankle Clin. 2017;22(2):277–300.
5. Cenni F, Leardini A, Cheli A, Catani F, Belvedere C, Romagnoli M, et al. Position of the prosthesis components in total ankle replacement and the effect on motion at the replaced joint. Int Orthop. 2012;36(3):571–8.
6. Najefi AA, Malhotra K, Goldberg A. Mechanical and anatomical axis of the lower limb in total ankle arthroplasty. Foot (Edinb). 2020;44:101666.
7. Mazzotti A, Arceri A, Zielli S, Bonelli S, Viglione V, Faldini C. Patient-specific instrumentation in total ankle arthroplasty. World J Orthop. 2022;13(3):230–7.
8. Veljkovic A, Norton A, Salat P, Abbas KZ, Saltzman C, Femino JE, et al. Sagittal distal Tibial articular angle and the relationship to Talar subluxation in total ankle arthroplasty. Foot Ankle Int. 2016;37(9):929–37.
9. Waly FJ, Yeo NE, Penner MJ. Computed navigation guidance for ankle replacement in the setting of ankle deformity. Clin Podiatr Med Surg. 2018;35(1):85–94.
10. Berlet GC, Penner MJ, Lancianese S, Stemniski PM, Obert RM. Total ankle arthroplasty accuracy and reproducibility using preoperative CT scan-derived, patient-specific guides. Foot Ankle Int. 2014;35(7):665–76.
11. Hsu AR, Davis WH, Cohen BE, Jones CP, Ellington JK, Anderson RB. Radiographic outcomes of preoperative CT scan-derived patient-specific total ankle arthroplasty. Foot Ankle Int. 2015;36(10):1163–9.
12. Saito GH, Sanders AE, O'Malley MJ, Deland JT, Ellis SJ, Demetracopoulos CA. Accuracy of patient-specific instrumentation in total ankle arthroplasty: a comparative study. Foot Ankle Surg. 2019;25(3):383–9.
13. Giardini P, Di Benedetto P, Mercurio D, Gisonni R, Molinari M, Causero A, et al. Infinity ankle arthroplasty with traditional instrumentation and PSI prophecy system: preliminary results. Acta Biomed. 2020;91(14-S):e2020021.
14. Heisler L, Vach W, Katz G, Egelhof T, Knupp M. Patient-specific instrumentation vs standard referencing in total ankle arthroplasty: a comparison of the radiologic outcome. Foot Ankle Int. 2022;43(6):741–9.
15. Thompson MJ, Consul D, Umbel BD, Berlet GC. Accuracy of Weightbearing CT scans for patient-specific instrumentation in total ankle arthroplasty. Foot Ankle Orthop. 2021;6(4):24730114211061493.
16. Daigre J, Berlet G, Van Dyke B, Peterson KS, Santrock R. Accuracy and reproducibility using patient-specific instrumentation in total ankle arthroplasty. Foot Ankle Int. 2017;38(4):412–8.
17. Umbel BD, Hockman T, Myers D, Sharpe BD, Berlet GC. Accuracy of CT-derived patient-specific instrumentation for total ankle arthroplasty: the impact of the severity of preoperative Varus ankle deformity. Foot Ankle Spec. 2022;7:19386400211068262.
18. Biela G, Piraino J, Roukis TS. An analysis of 50 consecutive total ankle replacements undergoing preoperative computerized tomography scan-based, engineer-provided planning from a single noninventor, nonconsultant surgeon. J Foot Ankle Surg. 2023;62(2):228–36.
19. Hamid KS, Matson AP, Nwachukwu BU, Scott DJ, Mather RC 3rd, DeOrio JK. Determining the cost-savings threshold and alignment accuracy of patient-specific instrumentation in total ankle replacements. Foot Ankle Int. 2017;38(1):49–57.
20. Inman VT. The joints of the ankle. Baltimore, MD: Williams & Wilkins; 1976.
21. Ruiz R, Susdorf R, Krahenbuhl N, Barg A, Hintermann B. Syndesmotic overload in 3-component total ankle replacement. Foot Ankle Int. 2020;41(3):275–85.
22. Hintermann B. Total ankle arthroplasty—historical overview, current concepts and future perspectives. Wien-New York: Springer; 2004. p. 195.
23. Kempson GE, Freeman MA, Tuke MA. Engineering considerations in the design of an ankle joint. Biomed Eng. 1975;10(5):166–71, 80.
24. Lowery RB. Fractures of the talus and os calcis. Opin Orthop. 1005;6:25–34.
25. Hvid I, Rasmussen O, Jensen NC, Nielsen S. Trabecular bone strength profiles at the ankle joint. Clin Orthop Relat Res. 1985;199:306–12.
26. Barg A, Zwicky L, Knupp M, Henninger HB, Hintermann B. HINTEGRA total ankle replacement: survivorship analysis in 684 patients. J Bone Joint Surg Am. 2013;95(13):1175–83.
27. Kvarda P, Peterhans US, Susdorf R, Barg A, Ruiz R, Hintermann B. Long-term survival of HINTEGRA total ankle replacement in 683 patients: a concise 20-year follow-up of a previous report. J Bone Joint Surg Am. 2022;104:881.
28. Barg A, Knupp M, Anderson AE, Hintermann B. Total ankle replacement in obese patients: component stability, weight change, and functional outcome in 118 consecutive patients. Foot Ankle Int. 2011;32(10):925–32.
29. Schipper ON, Denduluri SK, Zhou Y, Haddad SL. Effect of obesity on total ankle arthroplasty outcomes. Foot Ankle Int. 2016;37(1):1–7.
30. Choi WJ, Kim BS, Lee JW. Preoperative planning and surgical technique: how do I balance my ankle? Foot Ankle Int. 2012;33(3):244–9.

31. Gauvain TT, Hames MA, McGarvey WC. Malalignment correction of the lower limb before, during, and after total ankle arthroplasty. Foot Ankle Clin. 2017;22(2):311–39.
32. Gould JS, Alvine FG, Mann RA, Sanders RW, Walling AK. Total ankle replacement: a surgical discussion. Part I. Replacement systems, indications, and contraindications. Am J Orthop (Belle Mead NJ). 2000;29(8):604–9.
33. Kim BS, Choi WJ, Kim YS, Lee JW. Total ankle replacement in moderate to severe varus deformity of the ankle. J Bone Joint Surg Br. 2009;91(9):1183–90.
34. Sung KS, Ahn J, Lee KH, Chun TH. Short-term results of total ankle arthroplasty for end-stage ankle arthritis with severe varus deformity. Foot Ankle Int. 2014;35(3):225–31.
35. Ryssman D, Myerson MS. Surgical strategies: the management of varus ankle deformity with joint replacement. Foot Ankle Int. 2011;32(2):217–24.
36. Usuelli FG, Di Silvestri CA, D'Ambrosi R, Orenti A, Randelli F. Total ankle replacement: is pre-operative varus deformity a predictor of poor survival rate and clinical and radiological outcomes? Int Orthop. 2019;43(1):243–9.
37. Brunner S, Knupp M, Hintermann B. Total ankle replacement for the valgus unstable osteoarthritic ankle. Foot Ankle Tech. 2010;9:174–9.
38. Kofoed H. Cylindrical cemented ankle arthroplasty: a prospective series with long-term follow-up. Foot Ankle Int. 1995;16(8):474–9.
39. Wood PL, Deakin S. Total ankle replacement. The results in 200 ankles. J Bone Joint Surg Br. 2003;85(3):334–41.
40. Davids JR, Davis RB. Tibial torsion: significance and measurement. Gait Posture. 2007;26(2):169–71.
41. Lee SH, Chung CY, Park MS, Choi IH, Cho TJ. Tibial torsion in cerebral palsy: validity and reliability of measurement. Clin Orthop Relat Res. 2009;467(8):2098–104.
42. Kim BS, Lee JW. Total ankle replacement for the varus unstable. Foot Ankle Tech. 2010;9:157–67.
43. Kilger R, Knupp M, Hintermann B. Peroneus longus to peroneus brevis tendon transfer. Tech Foot Ankle Surg. 2009;8(3):146–9.
44. Stufkens SA, Knupp M, Hintermann B. Medial displacement calcaneal osteotomy. Tech Foot Ankle Surg. 2009;8(2):85–90.
45. Knupp M, Schuh R, Stufkens SA, Bolliger L, Hintermann B. Subtalar and talonavicular arthrodesis through a single medial approach for the correction of severe planovalgus deformity. J Bone Joint Surg Br. 2009;91(5):612–5.
46. Rohm J, Zwicky L, Horn Lang T, Salentiny Y, Hintermann B, Knupp M. Mid- to long-term outcome of 96 corrective hindfoot fusions in 84 patients with rigid flatfoot deformity. Bone Joint J. 2015;97-B(5):668–74.
47. Knupp M, Zwicky L, Lang TH, Rohm J, Hintermann B. Medial approach to the subtalar joint: anatomy, indications, technique tips. Foot Ankle Clin. 2015;20(2):311–8.
48. Steiner CS, Gilgen A, Zwicky L, Schweizer C, Ruiz R, Hintermann B. Combined subtalar and naviculocuneiform fusion for treating adult acquired flatfoot deformity with medial arch collapse at the level of the Naviculocuneiform joint. Foot Ankle Int. 2019;40(1):42–7.
49. Hintermann B, Deland JT, de Cesar Netto C, Ellis SJ, Johnson JE, Myerson MS, et al. Consensus on indications for isolated subtalar joint fusion and naviculocuneiform fusions for progressive collapsing foot deformity. Foot Ankle Int. 2020;41(10):1295–8.

8 Surgical Technique and Postoperative Care

Proper incision technique and careful handling of the soft-tissue mantle are of utmost importance for successful total ankle arthroplasty. With a few exceptions, current total ankle systems use an anterior approach between the anterior tibial and extensor hallucis longus tendons. Once the arthritic ankle joint is exposed, the osteophytes must be removed, and the fibrotic capsule sufficiently released to make the ankle joint as normal as possible. This makes it possible to recognize potential malalignment and instability and to address such concomitant problems before or after the ankle replacement. Respecting the individual anatomy in all planes is extremely important for bone resection cuts. Heel cord lengthening is seldom necessary when the entire fibrotic capsule has been removed.

The replaced ankle should be protected postoperatively against uncontrolled movements to promote wound healing and to permit stable bone ingrowth to the implants. Most implants allow for weight-bearing, as tolerated, within 1–2 weeks after surgery. As a principle, the main rehabilitation program starts after 6 weeks, including stretching exercises, lymphatic drainage, active range-of-motion exercises, and exercises to improve muscular strength and muscular control of foot movement, with a gradual return to complete activities as tolerated. Regular clinical and radiological controls help to identify problems at an early stage and thus prevent failures. A standardized clinical and radiographic examination is recommended.

8.1 Anesthesia

General or regional anesthesia can be used for total ankle arthroplasty.

8.2 Patient Positioning

The patient is placed in a supine position with the feet on the edge of the table (Fig. 8.1). The ipsilateral hip of the patient is lifted until a strictly upward position of the whole lower extremity is obtained. A pneumatic tourniquet is applied to the ipsilateral thigh. In most cases, a pressure of 320 mmHg is sufficient, and a total tourniquet time of 2 h should not be exceeded.

If the significant deformity is to be corrected, the unaffected lower extremity should also be draped.

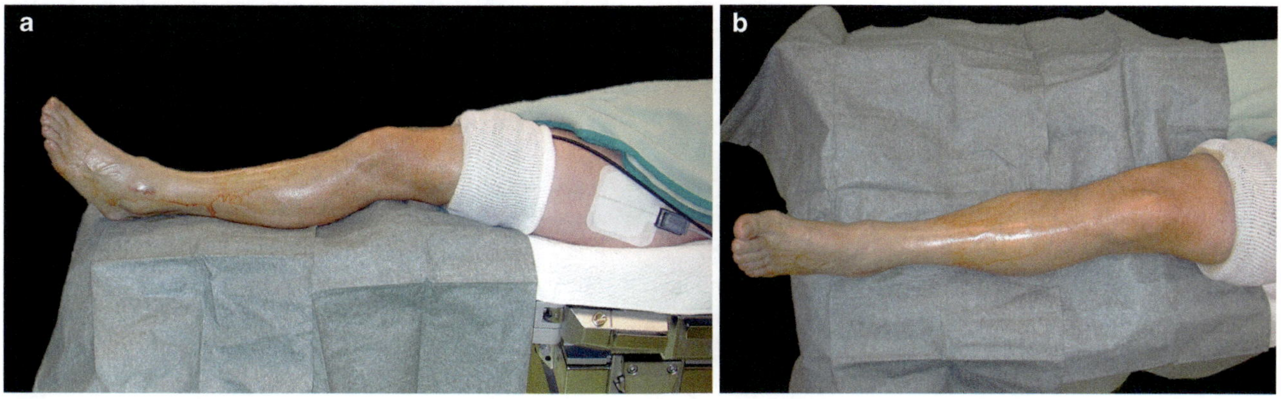

Fig. 8.1 Positioning of the patient. The patient is supine with the heel of the foot on the table's edge (**a**) and supports beneath the ipsilateral thigh to get the foot upright (**b**)

B. Hintermann, R. Ruiz, *Total Ankle Replacement*, https://doi.org/10.1007/978-3-031-56810-7_8

8.3 Surgical Approach to the Ankle

8.3.1 Anterior Approach

The standard total ankle arthroplasty technique uses an anterior approach to access and prepare the joint, correct deformities of the distal tibia, and insert the prosthesis. The anterior approach allows for adequate debridement of the medial gutter and rebalancing of soft-tissue structures in the medial and lateral aspects of the ankle. At the same time, it offers a more familiar view to the surgeon for addressing coronal plan deformities [1, 2], and correction of significant sagittal plane deformities can be challenging, however [3, 4].

A 12–15 cm longitudinal skin incision is made over the center of the ankle, taking care to identify and retract the medial branch of the superficial peroneal nerve (Fig. 8.2). The extensor retinaculum is dissected longitudinally between the extensor hallucis longus and anterior tibial tendons, through the tendon sheet of the extensor hallucis longus [5, 6] or of the anterior tibial tendon [2, 7, 8]. Once the distal tibia is exposed just beneath the anterior tibial tendon ("safety area"), the soft tissues are pushed sideways using a raspatory subperiosteally. Then, the neurovascular bundle is retracted laterally and kept away with a Hohmann retractor. A self-retaining retractor is inserted, and the Hohmann retractors are removed (Fig. 8.3a). The now fully exposed

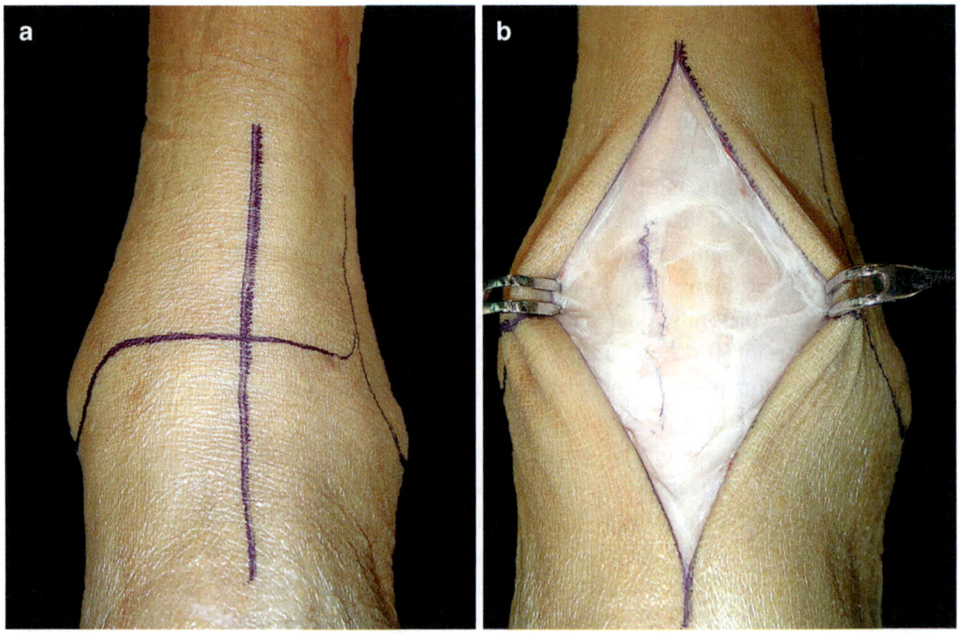

Fig. 8.2 Skin incision. A 12–15 cm long incision is made (**a**), exposing the extensor retinaculum (**b**)

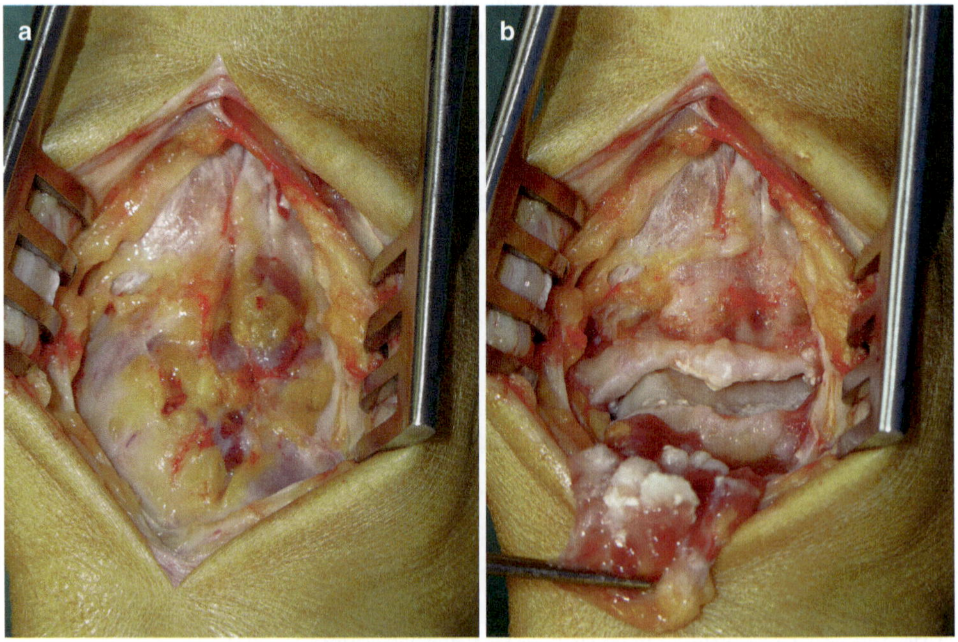

Fig. 8.3 Arthrotomy. (**a**) After a self-retaining retractor is inserted, the capsule is exposed (**a**), followed by an arthrotomy and, if necessary, partial resection of the anterior capsule (**b**)

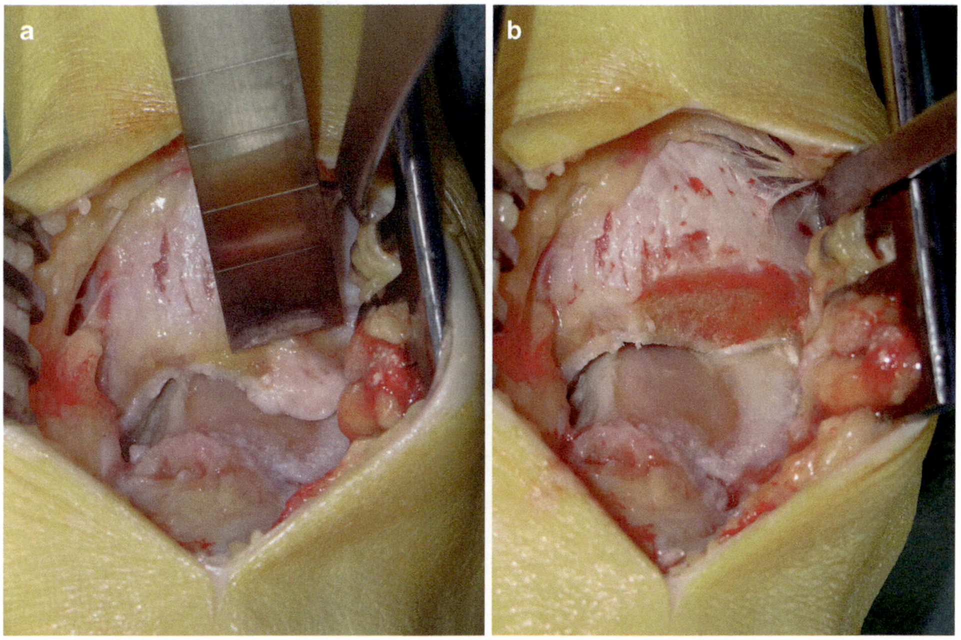

Fig. 8.4 Osteophyte removal on the tibia. (**a**) Osteophytes on the tibial side are removed to visualize the medial malleolus and the tibiotalar joint line (**b**)

capsule is vertically dissected over the midpoint of the ankle and, if necessary, partially resected to gain good exposure to the joint (Fig. 8.3b). The anterior osteophytes of the tibia are removed to expose the extent of the depression in the tibial plafond (Fig. 8.4a) and to expose the anterior aspect of the medial malleolus at the level of the tibial plafond ("anteromedial corner") (Fig. 8.4b). Similarly, the anterior osteophytes of the talus are removed, and the medial and lateral sides of the talus are cleared of any fibrosis and osteophytes (Fig. 8.5).

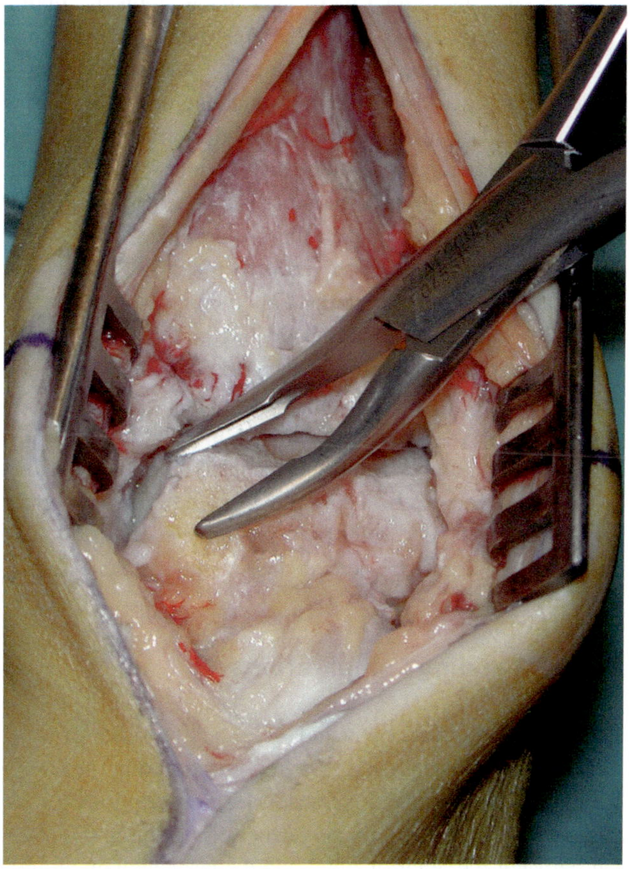

Fig. 8.5 Osteophyte removal on the talus. Osteophytes on the talar side are removed to make the joint as normal as possible. It will also facilitate the adjustment of the resection blocs

8.3.2 Lateral Transfibular Approach

The alternative lateral transfibular approach for total ankle arthroplasty has the theoretical advantage of allowing better correction of significant sagittal plane deformities [9, 10]. This is done by providing direct visualization of the center of rotation of the ankle joint, by access to the frequently contracted posterior joint capsule, and by removing the rigid lateral strut using the needed fibular osteotomy (Fig. 8.6) [11]. This technique also has the added benefit of being able to lengthen and shorten the fibula to correct the overall ankle deformity further [9]. Still, this relatively new technique has yet to be thoroughly tested in its ability to correct overall alignment and deformity, especially in the coronal plane [3]. This approach is not without fear of resulting in an incompetent distal tibiofibular construct, especially in an under-corrected valgus malalignment.

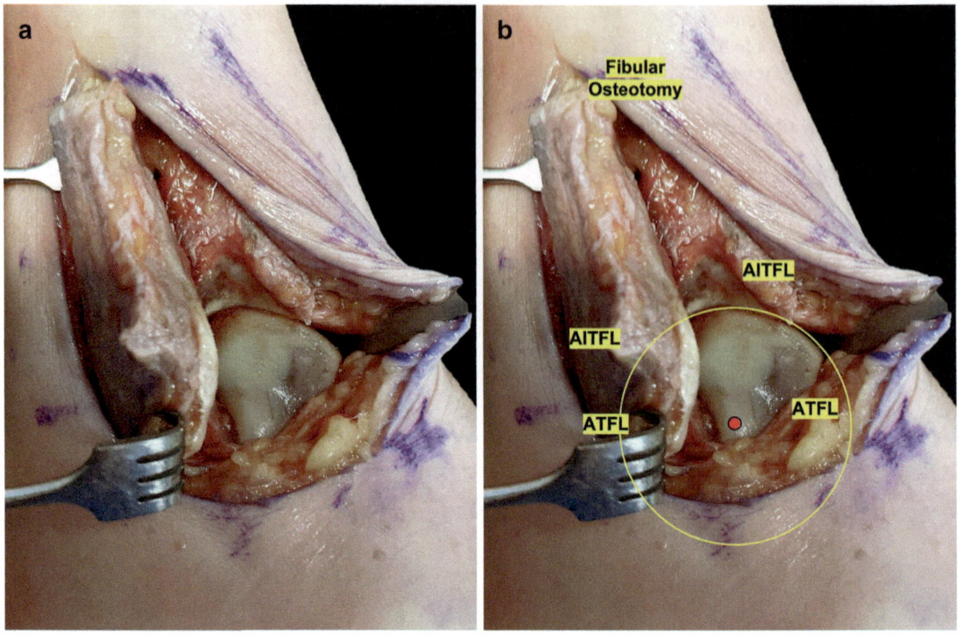

Fig. 8.6 Lateral approach. This cadaveric dissection shows the lateral approach to the ankle joint. (**a**) After exposure of the distal fibula, the anterior inferior tibiofibular ligament (AITFL) and the anterior talofibular ligament (ATFL) are dissected. The fibular segment is reflected after an oblique osteotomy of the fibula 6–7 cm proximal to the joint line was performed. (**b**) A significant advantage of this approach is that the surgeon can identify the center of rotation of the ankle (red circle)

A 15 cm longitudinal incision is made along the fibula, curved under its tip to reach the sinus tarsi. Subperiosteal dissection of the fibula and the anterior side of the tibia is made to have a full view of the joint line and the anterior osteophytes. The anterior talofibular and anterior inferior tibiofibular ligaments are identified and sectioned. After that, an extended oblique fibular osteotomy is made, starting 6–7 cm proximal to the joint line on the posterolateral side of the fibula and ending 2 cm proximal to the joint line on the anterolateral side of the fibula. This type of oblique osteotomy allows for the shortening or lengthening of the distal fibula to correct deformities in the coronal plane. The distal fibular segment is reflected and secured to the calcaneus with a K-wire to expose the lateral ankle fully. In the case of a posterior contracture, the posterior capsule is released with a periosteal elevator. A heel cord release is required if a neutral position cannot be obtained. A second medial incision is made to release and debride the medial gutter if necessary.

8.3.3 Avoiding Complications

Incisional complications include releasing the anterior tibial tendon from its sheath and scarring or transecting the superficial or deep peroneal nerves. Most descriptions of an anterior approach recommend deeper dissection in the interval between the anterior tibial and extensor hallucis longus tendons. Some surgeons even prefer to perform the deeper dissection more laterally and purposely take the extensor hallucis longus tendon out of its sheath to preserve the restraints of the anterior tibial tendon [5]. Immediately below this lies the deep peroneal nerve, which must be identified and retracted during the incision of the capsule.

The Authors' Experience

Even though we open its sheath or are disrupted during surgery, we rarely see problems with the anterior tibial tendon. Thus, we recommend using a more medial approach to prevent injuries to the neurovascular bundle.

8.4 Surgical Preparation of the Ankle

The step-by-step preparation of the ankle is given by the instrumentation and provided by the distributing company. In most ankle designs, the tibial resection is done first. In general, the jig uses the tibial tuberosity or the anterior iliac crest in patients with significant lower leg deformities as the proximal reference and the middle of the anterior border of the tibiotalar joint as the distal reference for adjustment in the coronal plane (Fig. 8.7). Parallelism to the tibia's anterior crest is attempted for sagittal plane alignment. The slope of the tibial plafond is given by the cutting block.

After exposing the ankle through an anterior approach, a distractor is mounted on the medial side to get an optimal view of the joint and to tension the collateral ankle ligaments (Fig. 8.8). The tibial resection block is positioned at the medial edge of the tibiotalar joint and then aligned regarding the proximal tibial tuberosity and anterior tibial crest. The height of resection is given by the prosthetic design; usually, 2–4 mm less than the size of the tibial component plus the polyethylene layer is aimed to be resected of

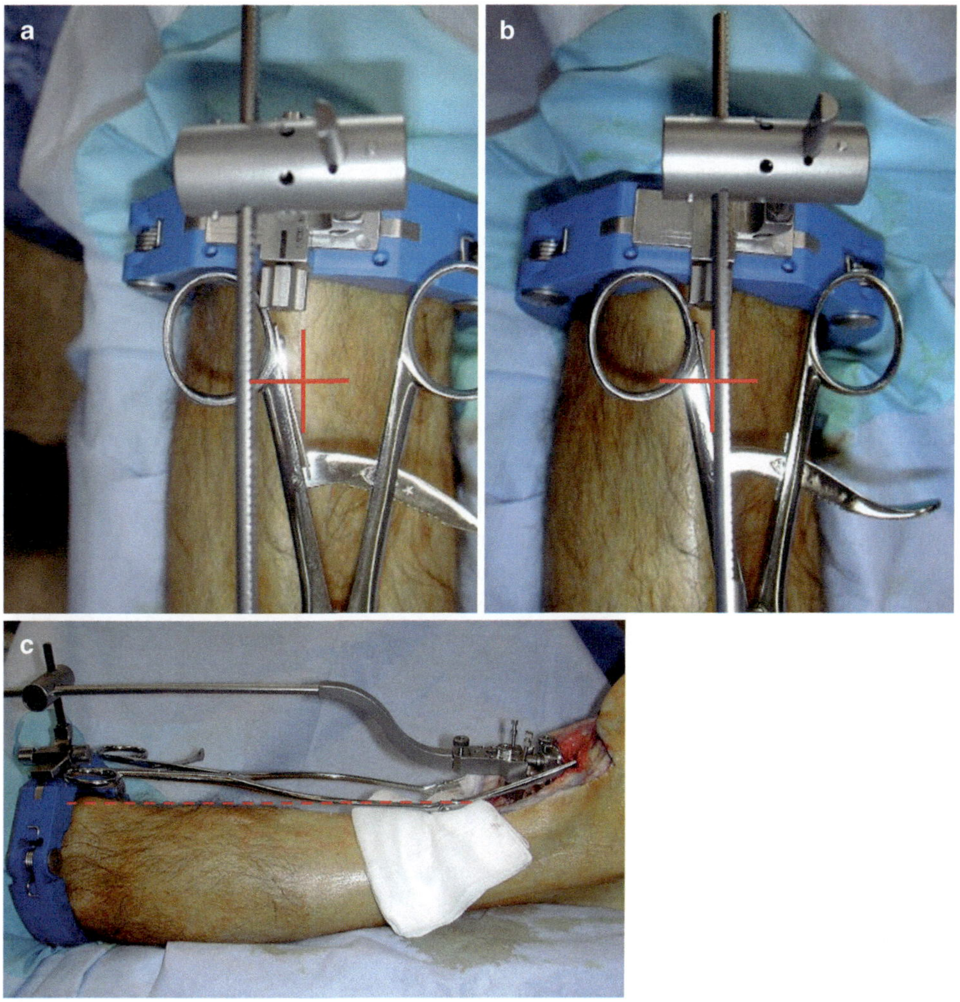

Fig. 8.7 Referencing the jig of the tibial resection bloc. The tibial tuberosity serves as the reference for the coronal plane adjustment. (**a**) Not adjusted. (**b**) Adjusted. (**c**) Parallelism to the tibia's anterior crest is attempted for sagittal plane alignment

the tibial plafond, depending on the amount of wear of the tibia and ligament laxity. The height of the intended resection is determined visually and checked under fluoroscopy (Fig. 8.9). The tibial osteotomy is done with a saw, and the articular fragment is resected. Most importantly, the talus must now be properly aligned. This is achieved by the distraction of the tibiotalar joint and tightening of the ligaments, respectively (Fig. 8.10). This allows an appropriate resection of the talus parallel to its articular surface (Fig. 8.11). A spacer of the minimal thickness of the prosthesis can be inserted to check the achieved alignment and ligament tension (Fig. 8.12). Additional bone resection or soft-tissue release must be considered if it cannot be inserted. The achieved alignment of the heel can best be checked while the foot is elevated (Fig. 8.13a). Often, it has changed to the preoperative situation because of ligament tensioning (Fig. 8.13b). The talar resection cuts are done according to the needs of the design.

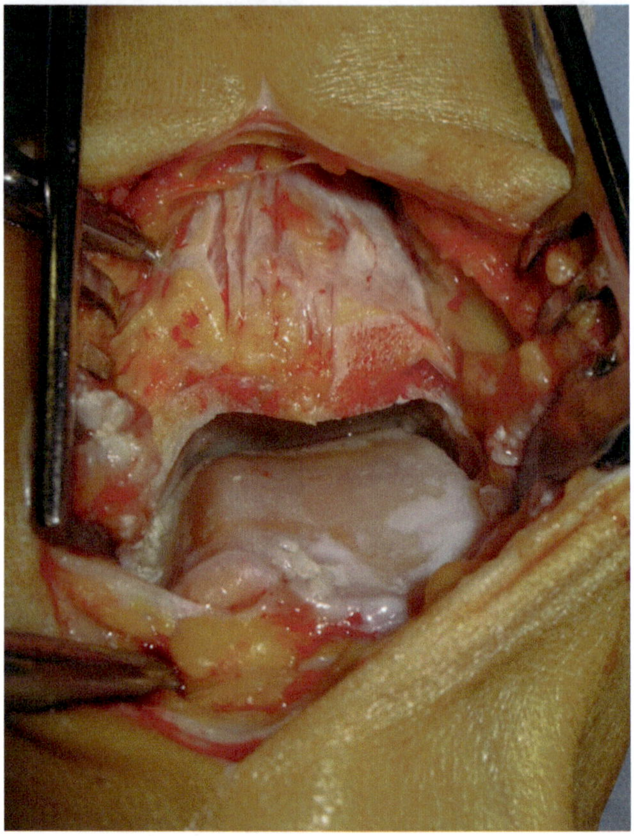

Fig. 8.8 Distraction of the ankle joint. Distraction is applied on the anteromedial aspect of the ankle joint to two K-wires to get insight into the joint and to tension the collateral ligaments, thereby realigning the hindfoot. In most cases, this allows total joint exposure and assesses the tibial plafond depth

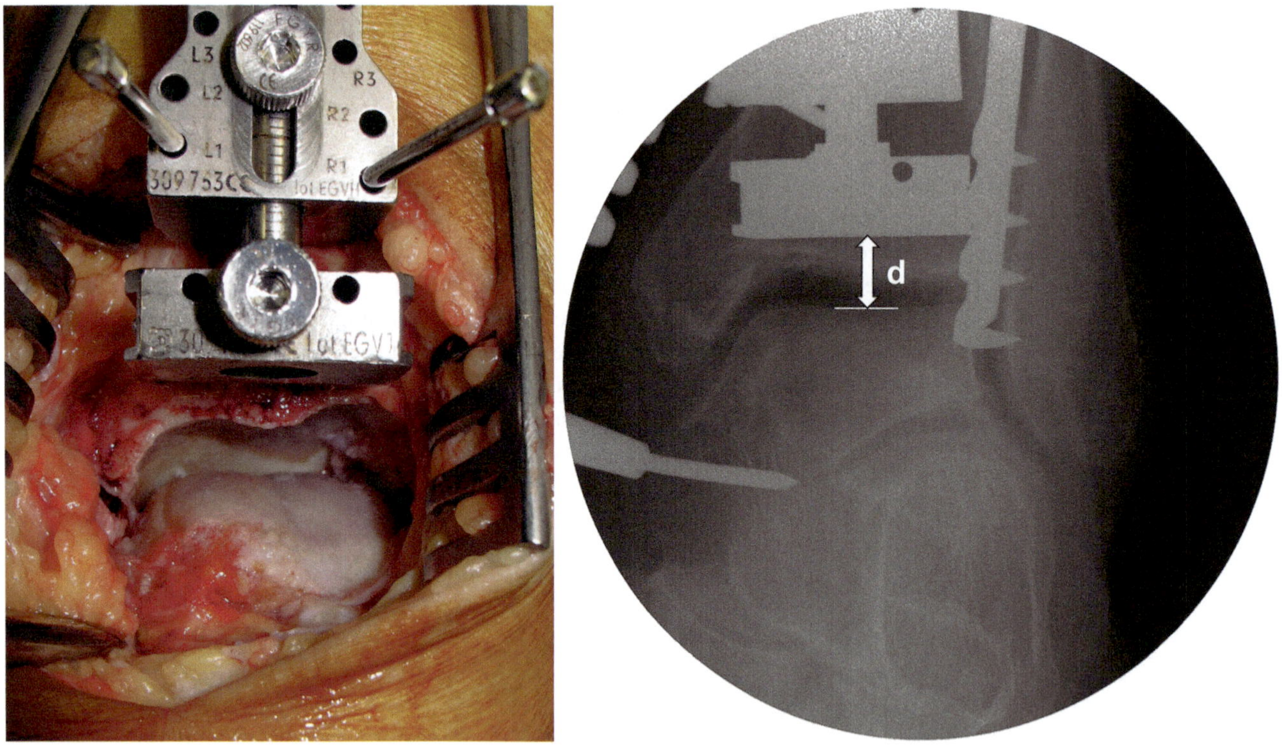

Fig. 8.9 Tibial resection. The tibial resection block is positioned regarding the medial corner and then moved upwards until the desired resection height is achieved, as checked visually and by fluoroscopy. The distance d, as indicated by the undersurface of the resection bloc and the articular surface of the talus, should account for the thickness of the tibial component and the minimal thickness of the polyethylene insert

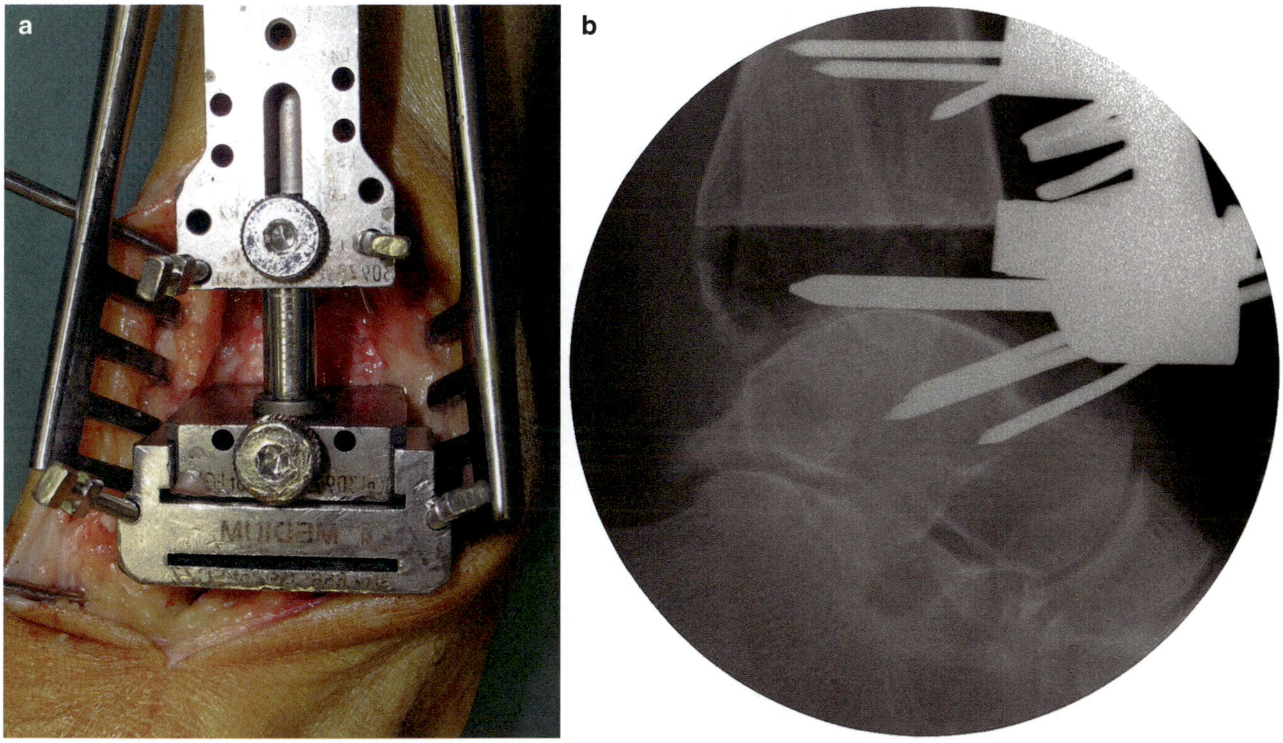

Fig. 8.10 Talar positioning for resection. (**a**) Most importantly, a distraction force to the talus must be applied to get it into the appropriate neutral position. The distraction at the anteromedial aspect of the ankle is thus removed and replaced with a distraction to the free talus while holding the foot in a neutral plantigrade position. The depicted prosthesis system uses a tongue at the talar resection block to achieve this goal. (**b**) Fluoroscopy showing the aimed position of the talus

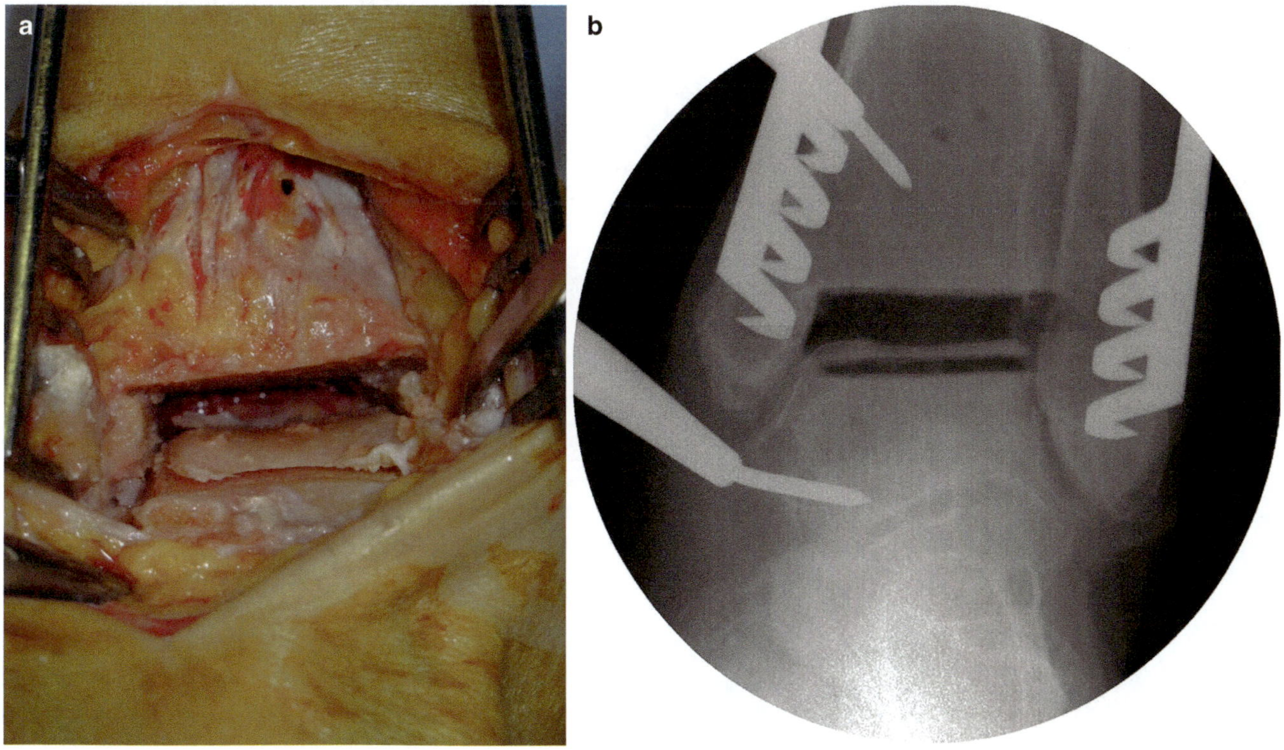

Fig. 8.11 Talar resection. The talar resection cut is done with an oscillating saw, paying attention not to hitting the malleoli. After removing the resection bloc, the parallelism of the cut to the articular surface is seen visually (**a**) and by fluoroscopy (**b**)

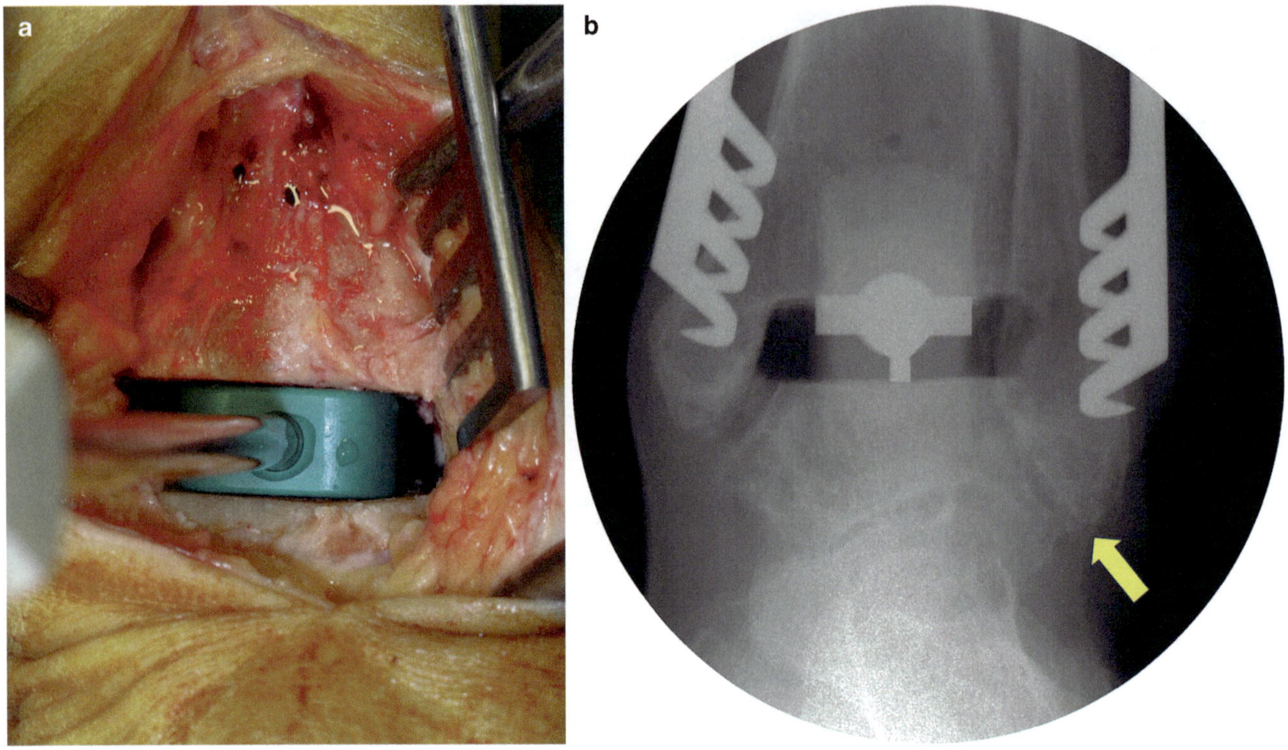

Fig. 8.12 Check with a spacer. (**a**) A spacer accounting for the minimal size of the prosthesis is inserted in the created joint space. It allows us to check the alignment and stability. (**b**) Fluoroscopy can be used to check whether the ankle is overstuffed, as best seen on the gap of the talofibular joint. In this case, there is a regular distance between the distal fibula and the talus (arrow), indicating an appropriate distraction of the joint

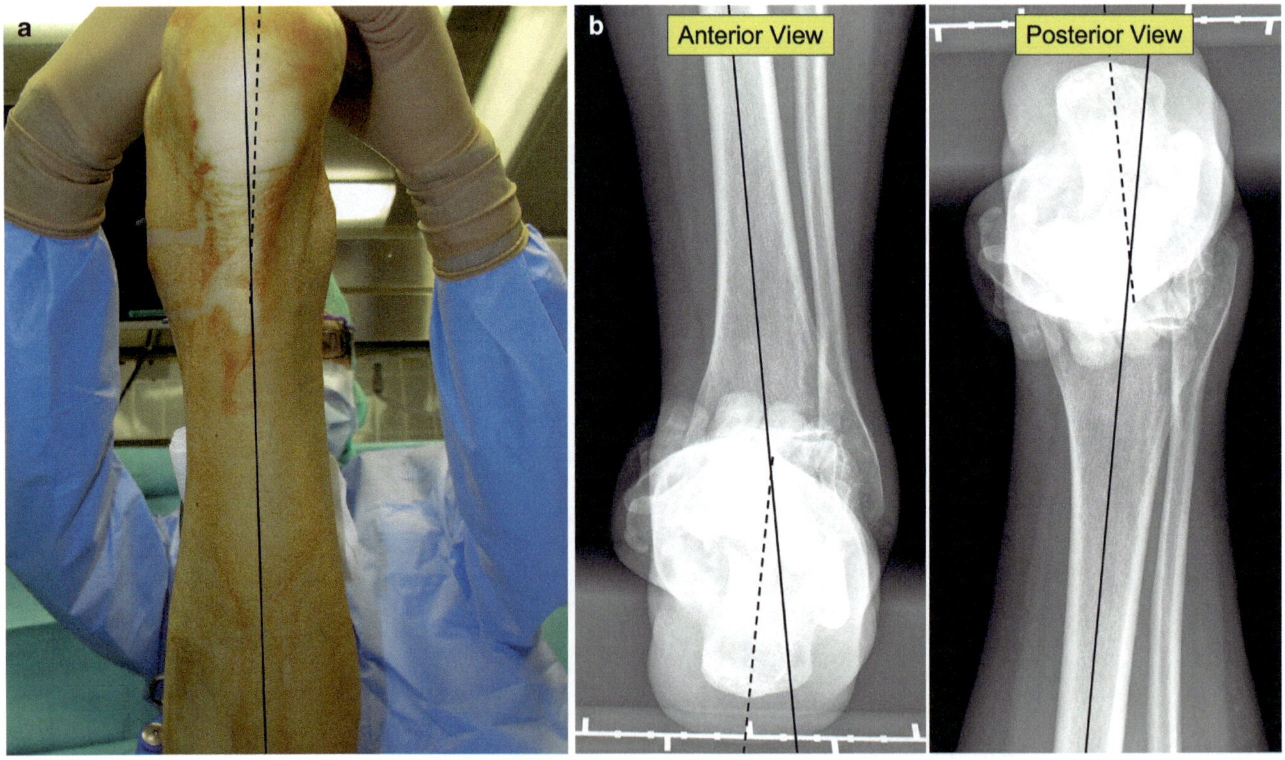

Fig. 8.13 Check of hindfoot alignment. With the spacer left in place, the leg is elevated while the foot is held in a neutral flexion position. (**a**) The hindfoot alignment is checked visually. (**b**) Notice that the hindfoot alignment can change with the distraction of the ankle joint and tensioning of the ligament, respectively, as shown in this case. Preoperatively, the talus was tilted into a varus due to erosion of the medial tibial plafond. The heel has moved slightly valgus by repositioning the talus into a neutral position

8.5 Component Insertion

The components are inserted after having prepared the tibia and talus resection surfaces. Usually, the talar component is inserted first, and the tibial component is inserted after that. In a mobile-bearing ankle, the polyethylene bearing is inserted. The stability and motion of the replaced ankle are checked clinically. The achieved alignment, stability, and joint motion are checked clinically, and the component position is checked by image intensification.

Most importantly, the foot is manually forced into maximal dorsiflexion (Fig. 8.14). With this maneuver, the components are maximally pressed against the bone, and contract fibers and scars on the posterior aspect of the ankle are released. A heel cord release procedure should be considered if a dorsiflexion of less than 10° is achieved.

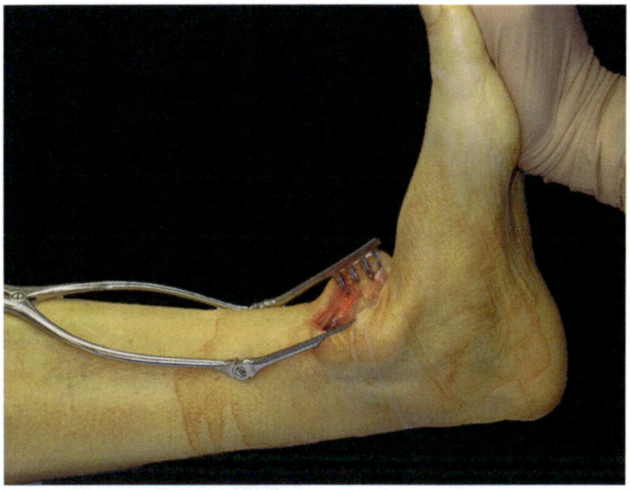

Fig. 8.14 Release of posterior contracture. After the total ankle arthroplasty, the foot is moved into the maximal dorsiflexion position; thereby, the remaining contractures of posterior soft tissues are released. By this maneuver, compression force will be applied to the components against the bone, enhancing the fit of the inserted components to the resected bony surfaces

8.6 Wound Closure

Using an anterior approach to the ankle, the retinaculum and tendon sheet are closed, and the skin is closed using interrupted sutures (Fig. 8.15). For the lateral transfibular approach, the fibula is repositioned and fixed with a plate in the desired position. The anterior talofibular ligament is reattached to the fibula, and the wound is closed step-by-step. A drain can be left intraarticularly to avoid hematoma for the first 24 h; however, it is advised not to use suction [12].

The incision is covered with a compressive dressing, and a well-padded short leg splint is used to keep the foot in a neutral position (Fig. 8.16).

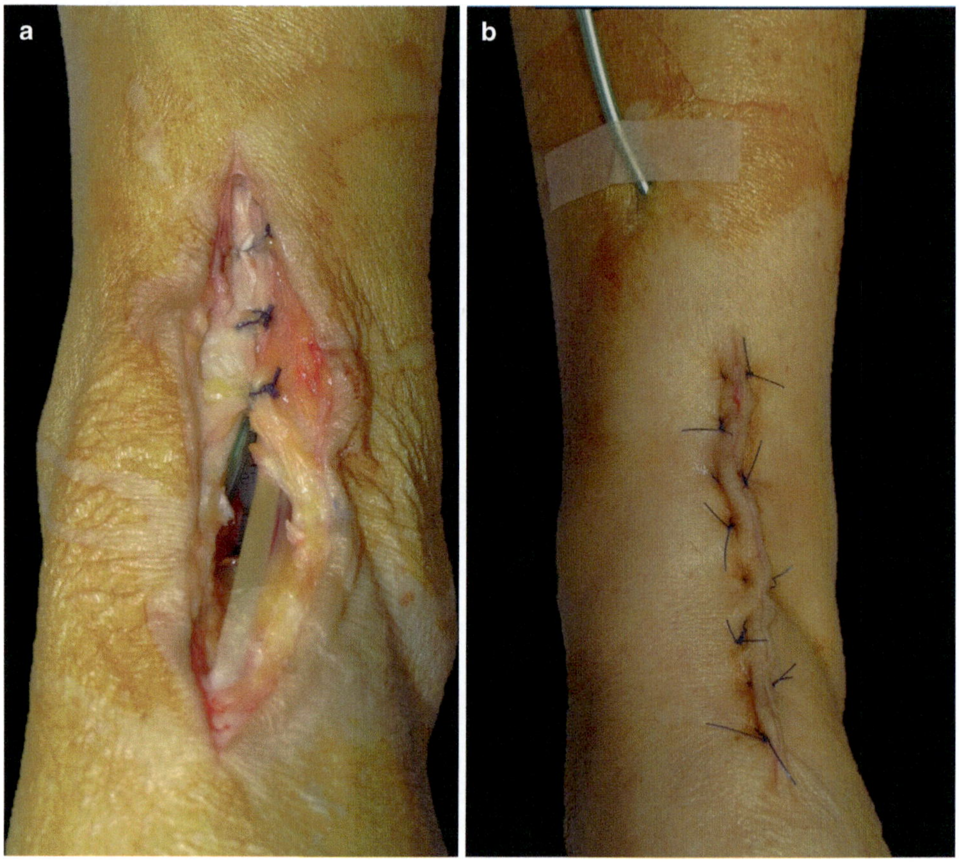

Fig. 8.15 Wound closure. (**a**) The extensor retinaculum is closed with interrupted sutures, followed by the closure of the wound (**b**)

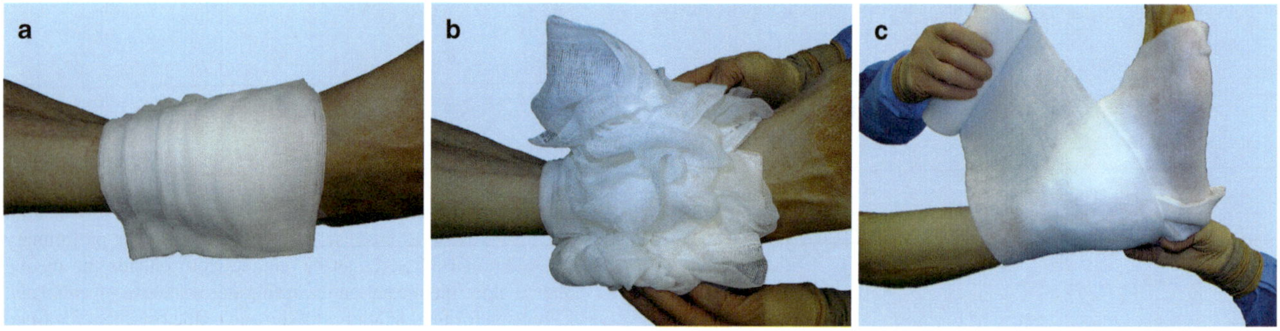

Fig. 8.16 Dressing and splint. (**a**–**b**) Compresses, (**c**–**d**) cotton bandage, (**e**–**f**) absorbent bandage, (**g**–**h**) elastic bandage, and (**i**–**j**) splint

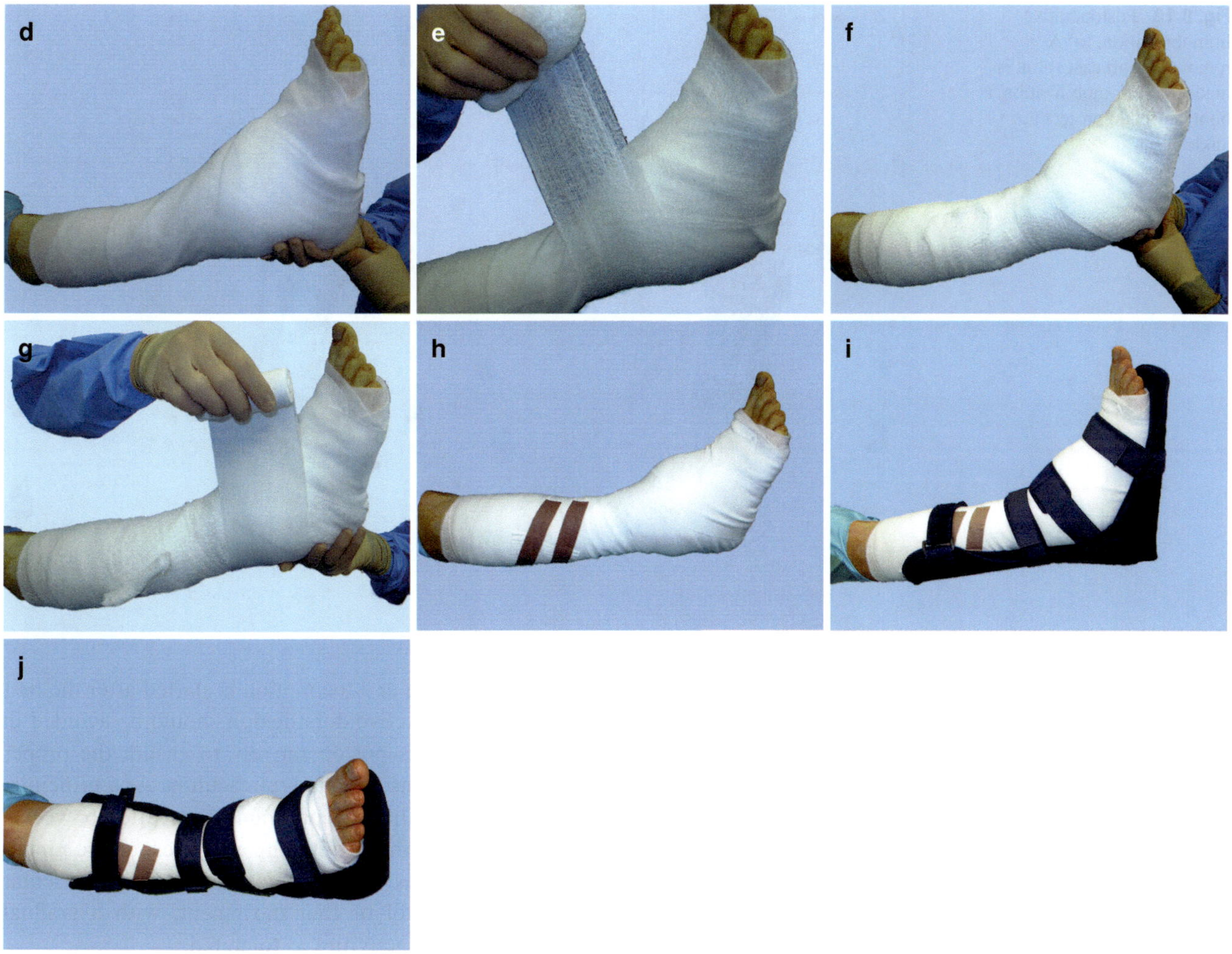

Fig. 8.16 (continued)

8.7 Aftercare

The dressing and splint are removed and changed on the second postoperative day (Fig. 8.17), and a removable soft cast is made (Fig. 8.18a). When the wound conditions are appropriate (dry wound, no secretion), the foot is placed in a stabilizing walker or cast for 6–8 weeks (Fig. 8.18b); in patients with additional procedures (e.g., fusion of adjacent joint or corrective osteotomies), the immobilization is, in general, 2 weeks longer. Weight-bearing is allowed as tolerated except for patients who underwent additional corrective osteotomies above the ankle [13, 14].

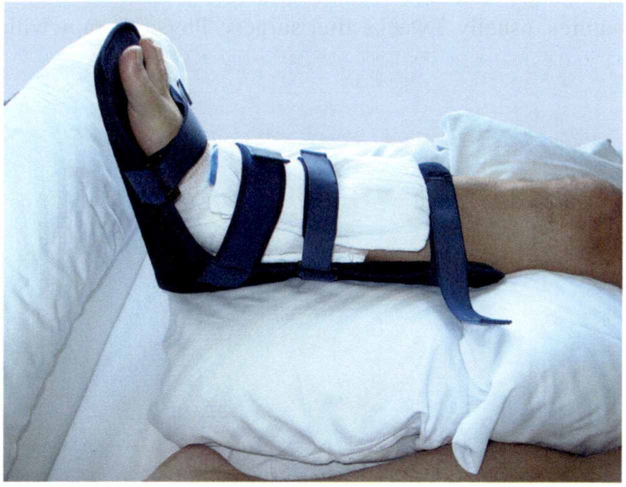

Fig. 8.17 Dressing change and wound protection. The dressing is changed on the second day while the foot is kept in the splint. Ice may be used for cooling

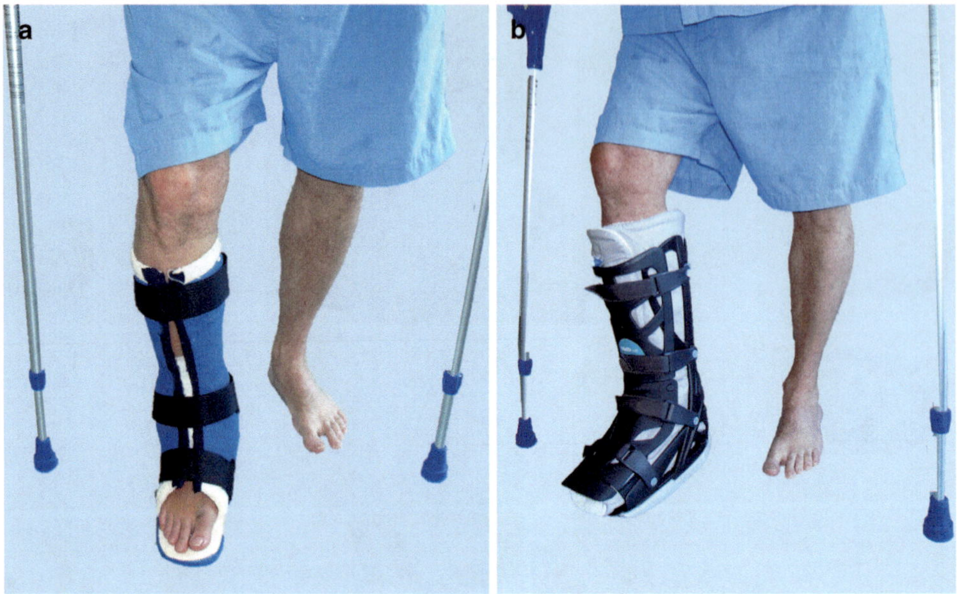

Fig. 8.18 Postoperative immobilization. (**a**) A removable soft cast splint is made. (**b**) For mobilization, a boot is used to protect the ankle

8.8 Rehabilitation Program

The replaced ankle should be protected postoperatively against uncontrolled movements to promote wound healing and to permit stable bone ingrowth to the implants. Most implants allow for weight-bearing, as tolerated, within 1–2 weeks after surgery. A stretching program is commenced immediately after surgery. The patient is asked to bear as much load as possible on the operated foot and then to bring the knee successively anterior-ward until the heel starts to lift off the floor (Fig. 8.19). The patient is advised to perform this exercise once or twice a day. Lymphatic drainage is started after the removal of the sutures, usually 2 weeks after surgery. Physiotherapy with lymphatic drainage and toe motion is started after the first dressing change. Active dorsiflexion should be avoided in the first 3–4 weeks postoperatively to ensure the proper healing of the extensor tendon retinaculum. As a principle, the leading rehabilitation program starts after 6 weeks, including gait training, stretching exercises, active range-of-motion exercises, and exercises to improve muscular strength and control of foot movement, with a gradual return to complete activities as tolerated.

In patients with persistent swelling, compression stockings are recommended. An average level (e.g., hiking, swimming, biking, golfing) and a low level (e.g., tennis, downhill skiing) of sports activities are allowed. Contact sports or activities involving jumping should be avoided [15].

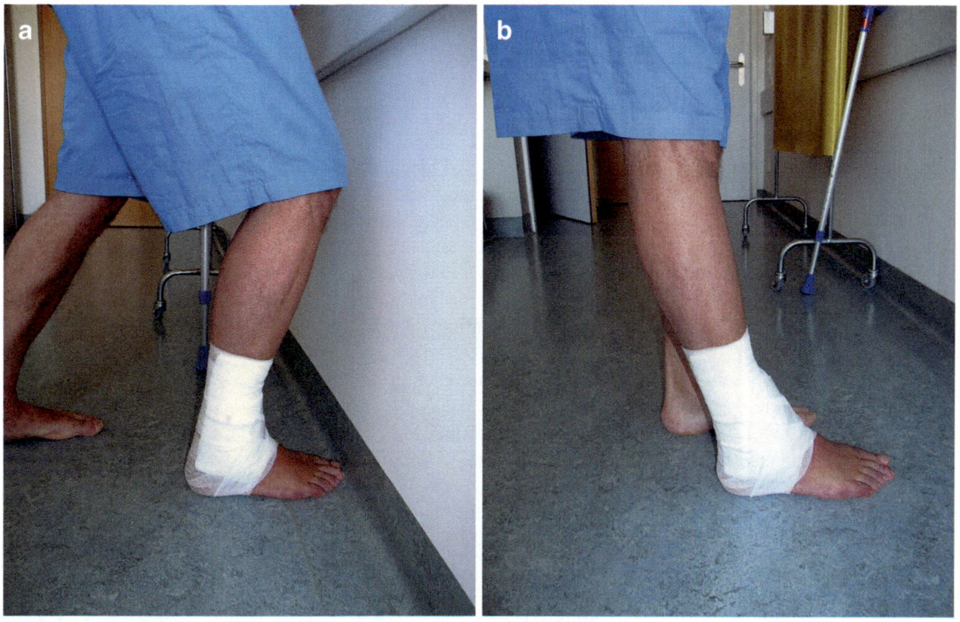

Fig. 8.19 Passive mobilization/stretching program. As soon as the wound condition permits it, passive mobilization is started. This is strictly done in a standing position and under weight-bearing. The patient is asked to make slow movements and stay for 5–10 s in extreme dorsi- and plantarflexion positions, stretching the counteracting soft tissues. Passive mobilization of the ankle by traction is strictly prohibited, as it could destroy the integrity of the prosthesis. (**a**) Extreme dorsiflexion position. (**b**) Extreme plantarflexion position

8.9 Follow-Up Examinations

Regular clinical and radiological controls help to identify problems at an early stage and thus prevent failures. At the authors' institution, the postoperative patients are seen at 6 weeks, at 4 months, at 1 year, at 2 years, at 5 years, and thereafter every 5 years for clinical and radiological control. An extensive standardized protocol is used for each control for 1 year and later.

8.9.1 Clinical Assessment

Patients should be asked to indicate their current level of function (as compared with preoperative function) in activities of daily living and specific activities (e.g., sports and climbing stairs) (Table 8.1), as well as their level of satisfaction with the procedure.

The clinical examination is based on preoperative assessment. It should include a careful assessment of the alignment of the ankle with the patient standing and the range of motion and stability of the ankle with the patient sitting and standing. Alignment, stability, and motion can be compared with the uninvolved side. All data should be recorded for the assessment of functional outcome scores. Patient-reported outcome measures (PROMs) have recently been proposed for foot and ankle surgery [16–21]. Subjective PROMs and objective biomechanical outcomes were found complementary in the assessment of surgical outcomes and, combined, helped to address the dilemma of the confounding effect of other lower extremity pathologies on PROMs, however [23]. Concerns about their use for specific procedure outcome measurement still need to be addressed [22].

The Authors' Experience

The timeline for maximal objective outcome improvement following total ankle arthroplasty is usually between 1 and 2 years. Mainly, it takes longer in ankles after previous trauma and surgeries, indicating that the condition of the soft-tissue mantle around the ankle may significantly determine the healing process. In a systematic review, however, the maximal subjective outcome improvement was found to be by 1 year postoperatively [23].

8.9.2 Radiographic Assessment

Postoperative radiographic examinations are best taken with fluoroscopy to obtain both components' standardized and accurate anteroposterior and lateral views. This allows the evaluation of migration or loosening on serial radiographs (Fig. 8.20).

Lateral views under fluoroscopy can measure true foot and ankle motion while the patient is standing on a footplate. The footplate is plantar flexed and dorsiflexed as much as possible until the tibia tends to follow foot motion.

A CT scan can assess cyst formation and degenerative diseases of neighboring joints.

Table 8.1 Clinical score

Grade	Pain	Limitation of recreational activities	Limitation of daily activities	Requirement for support	Wearing of fashionable shoes
Excellent	None	None	None	None	Yes
Good	Mild, occasional	Yes	None	None	Some
Fair	Moderate, frequent	Some	Yes	One cane	None
Poor	Severe, nearly always	Severe	Severe	Walker or brace	Orthopedic shoes

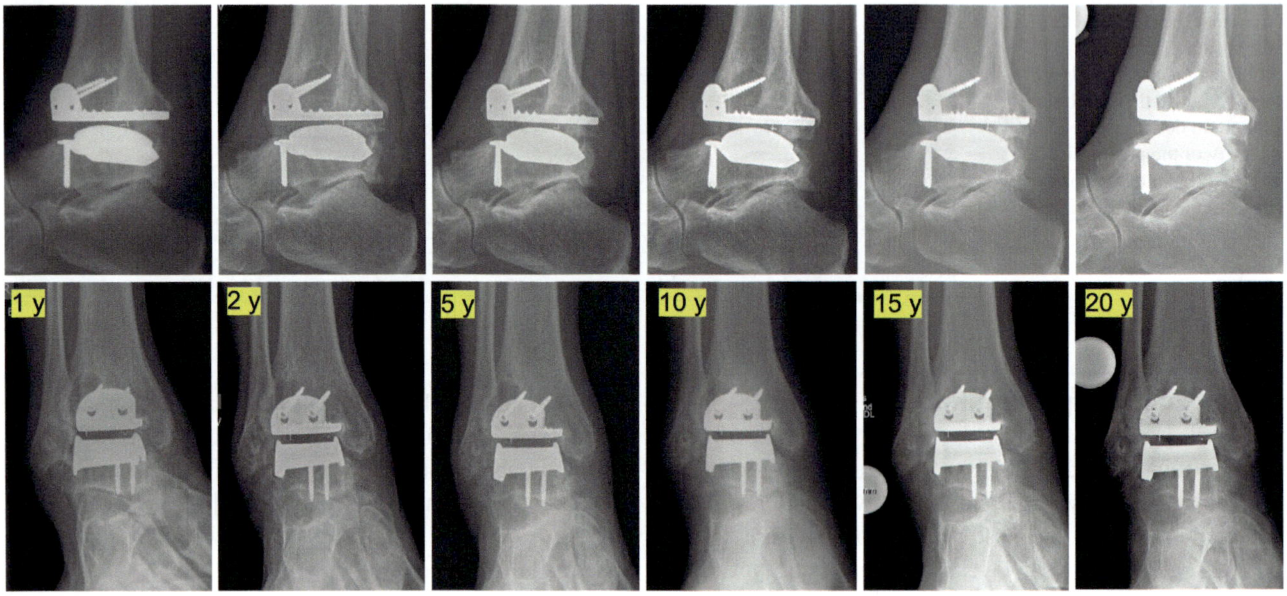

Fig. 8.20 Radiographic follow-up controls. Series of standard radiographs taken under fluoroscopic control in a 54-year-old female patient followed over 20 years

8.10 Conclusions

- Proper incision technique and careful handling of the soft-tissue mantle are of utmost importance for successful total ankle arthroplasty.
- Once the arthritic ankle joint is exposed, the osteophytes must be removed, and the fibrotic capsule sufficiently released to make the ankle joint as normal as possible.
- Respecting the individual anatomy in all planes is extremely important for bone resection cuts.
- Restoring the joint line as close as possible to the original one and correctly positioning the talar component in the sagittal plane is mandatory to achieve a well-balanced ankle after replacement.
- Before considering a heel cord lengthening, the posterior capsule should be removed and the remaining soft tissues released.
- The replaced ankle should be protected postoperatively against uncontrolled movements to promote wound healing and to permit stable bone ingrowth to the implants.
- The main rehabilitation program starts after 6 weeks, with a gradual return to complete activities as tolerated.
- Regular clinical and radiological controls help to identify problems at an early stage and thus prevent failures.

References

1. Hintermann B, Ruiz R. Total replacement of varus ankle: three-component prosthesis design. Foot Ankle Clin. 2019;24(2):305–24.
2. Hintermann B. Total ankle arthroplasty—historical overview, current concepts and future perspectives. Wien-New York: Springer; 2004. p. 195.
3. Halai MM, Pinsker E, Mann MA, Daniels TR. Should 15 degrees of valgus coronal-plane deformity be the upper limit for a total ankle arthroplasty? Bone Joint J. 2020;102-B(12):1689–96.
4. Lintz F, Mast J, Bernasconi A, Mehdi N, de Cesar NC, Fernando C, et al. 3D, weightbearing topographical study of periprosthetic cysts and alignment in total ankle replacement. Foot Ankle Int. 2020;41(1):1–9.
5. Conti SF, Wong YS. Complications of total ankle replacement. Clin Orthop Relat Res. 2001;391:105–14.

6. Wood PL. Experience with the STAR ankle arthroplasty at Wrightington Hospital, UK. Foot Ankle Clin. 2002;7(4):755–64, vii.
7. Hintermann B, Valderrabano V. Total ankle replacement. Foot Ankle Clin. 2003;8(2):375–405.
8. Barg A, Knupp M, Henninger HB, Zwicky L, Hintermann B. Total ankle replacement using HINTEGRA, an unconstrained, three-component system: surgical technique and pitfalls. Foot Ankle Clin. 2012;17(4):607–35.
9. Tan EW, Maccario C, Talusan PG, Schon LC. Early complications and secondary procedures in transfibular total ankle replacement. Foot Ankle Int. 2016;37(8):835–41.
10. VandeLune C, Barbachan Mansur NS, Iehl C, Tazegul T, Ahrenholz SJ, de Carvalho KAM, et al. Deformity correction in ankle osteoarthritis using a lateral trans-fibular total ankle replacement: a weight-bearing CT assessment. Iowa Orthop J. 2022;42(2): 36–46.
11. Barg A, Bettin CC, Burstein AH, Saltzman CL, Gililland J. Early clinical and radiographic outcomes of trabecular metal total ankle replacement using a transfibular approach. J Bone Joint Surg Am. 2018;100(6):505–15.
12. Moncman TG, Fliegel B, Massaglia J, Raikin SM, O'Neil JT, Pedowitz DI, et al. Comparison between closed suction drainage and no drainage following total ankle arthroplasty. Foot Ankle Int. 2022;43(9):1227–31.
13. Hintermann B, Knupp M, Barg A. Supramalleolar osteotomies for the treatment of ankle arthritis. J Am Acad Orthop Surg. 2016;24(7):424–32.
14. Knupp M, Stufkens SA, Bolliger L, Barg A, Hintermann B. Classification and treatment of supramalleolar deformities. Foot Ankle Int. 2011;32(11):1023–31.
15. Valderrabano V, Pagenstert G, Horisberger M, Knupp M, Hintermann B. Sports and recreation activity of ankle arthritis patients before and after total ankle replacement. Am J Sports Med. 2006;34(6):993–9.
16. Sierevelt IN, Zwiers R, Schats W, Haverkamp D, Terwee CB, Nolte PA, et al. Measurement properties of the most commonly used foot- and ankle-specific questionnaires: the FFI, FAOS and FAAM. A systematic review. Knee Surg Sports Traumatol Arthrosc. 2018;26(7):2059–73.
17. Coster MC, Bremander A, Nilsdotter A. Patient-reported outcome for 17,648 patients in 5 different Swedish orthopaedic quality registers before and 1 year after surgery: an observational study. Acta Orthop. 2023;94:1–7.
18. Gajebasia S, Jennison T, Blackstone J, Zaidi R, Muller P, Goldberg A. Patient reported outcome measures in ankle replacement versus ankle arthrodesis—a systematic review. Foot (Edinb). 2022;51:101874.
19. Clifton LJ, Kingman A, Rushton PRP, Murty A, Kakwani R, Coorsh J, et al. The Hintegra total ankle replacement: survivorship, failure modes and patient reported outcomes in seventy consecutive cases with a minimum five year follow-up. Int Orthop. 2021;45(9):2331–6.
20. Shah NS, Umeda Y, Suriel Peguero E, Erwin JT, Laughlin R. Outcome reporting in total ankle arthroplasty: a systematic review. J Foot Ankle Surg. 2021;60(4):770–6.
21. Allport J, Ramaskandhan J, Alkhreisat M, Siddique MS. Patient-reported outcome measures and radiological outcomes in mobile-bearing total ankle arthroplasty with varus or valgus deformity. Foot Ankle Int. 2021;42(2):176–82.
22. Al-Mohrej OA, Petrisor B. Foot and ankle outcome instruments: missing the target. Curr Rev Musculoskelet Med. 2023;16:246.
23. Agarwalla A, Gowd AK, Cody EA, Johnson PK, Yao K, Nunley JA 2nd, et al. Timeline for maximal subjective outcome improvement following total ankle arthroplasty. Foot Ankle Surg. 2021;27(3):305–10.

Balancing and Stabilizing the Ankle

9

The success of total ankle arthroplasty depends on to which extent the surgeon can balance and stabilize the ankle. Primary problems include deformities, osteoarthritic changes of adjacent joints, and post-traumatic changes. As a rule, supramalleolar malalignment and concomitant osteoarthritis of hindfoot joints are generally considered to be addressed before prosthetic implantation, whereas inframalleolar correcting osteotomies, ligament reconstructions, tendon transfers, and heel cord lengthening are considered at the end of the ankle replacement surgery. This section presents solutions for balancing and stabilizing a replaced ankle.

9.1 Deformity Correction

If deformities of any kind at the hip, femur, and knee are noted that may be influencing the alignment of the ankle and foot, it is recommended that these should be addressed first. The reasoning pertains to the propensity for the proximal joint alignment and length to have a higher degree of impact on more distal manipulations. In addition, distal alignment is generally based on proximal references. On the other hand, should the deformity require later correction, the implanted ankle may no longer assume the desired alignment because of the alteration of the mechanical axis after a later arthroplasty of the hip, or especially of the knee.

Although coronal plane angulation is a more commonly discussed topic [1–3], sagittal plane deformity can exist as well, either independently or as part of a multiplanar malalignment. It must be addressed for successful total ankle arthroplasty [3–9]. The deformity may occur anywhere along the tibia but has a more pronounced effect on the ankle when it occurs in the distal one-third [10]. Sagittal plane deformity of 15° (either anterior or posterior) in the distal one-third of the tibia can yield changes in ankle joint contact pressures of 40% [11]. Recurvatum deformity typically produces erosion of the anterior tibial plafond and some degree of subluxation of the talus anteriorly. It is often accompanied by functional equinus contracture driven by the proximal deformity as the foot finds the ground.

It is generally accepted that coronal deformity greater than 5° should be corrected to avoid edge loading [1, 12]. In sagittal plane deformity, the authors recommend correction of deformity if the longitudinal axis of the tibia is projected >10 mm posterior to the imaginary center of rotation.

Alternatively, to correcting osteotomies, osteoplasty using distraction osteogenesis principles can realign the tibia in any plane needed without unwanted translation or lengthening. This procedure is challenging and requires extended time in a frame [13].

9.1.1 Preoperative Analysis and Planning

Preoperative measurement includes the following angles (Fig. 9.1):

1. Coronal Plane: the distal tibial articular surface forms the lateral distal tibial angle (LDTA) and the anatomical axis of the tibia in the coronal plane (normal values 89° ± 3°).
2. The tibia's mechanical axis forms the anterior distal tibial angle (ADTA) and the ankle's joint orientation line in the sagittal plane (normal values 80° ± 3°).
3. The tibial-talar angle (α) is defined by the ankle joint's tibial and talar articular surfaces; if it measures >5°, the joint is defined as incongruent.

A meticulous analysis is mandatory to determine the origin of the deformity. The center of rotation of angulation (CORA) concept applies to any deformity (Fig. 9.2).

The following types of malalignment must be differentiated, as each type requires specific correcting surgery:

1. Diaphyseal or metaphyseal tibial malalignment (supramalleolar deformity):

B. Hintermann, R. Ruiz, *Total Ankle Replacement*, https://doi.org/10.1007/978-3-031-56810-7_9

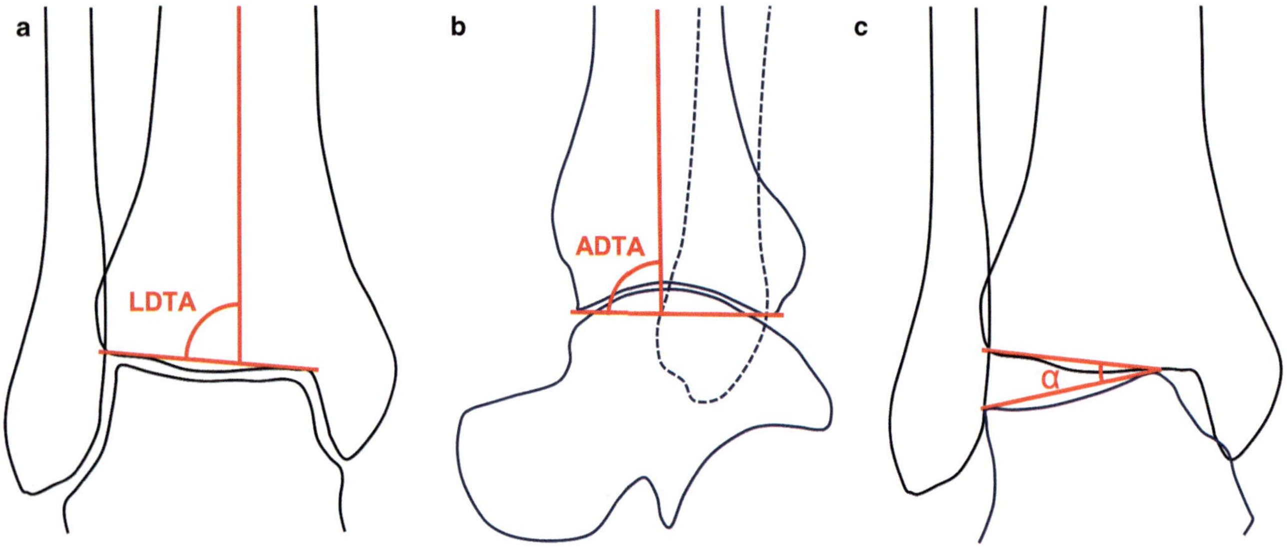

Fig. 9.1 Angle measurements. (**a**) The lateral distal tibial angle (LDTA), (**b**) the anterior distal tibial angle (ADTA), and (**c**) the tibial-talar angle (α) (see text)

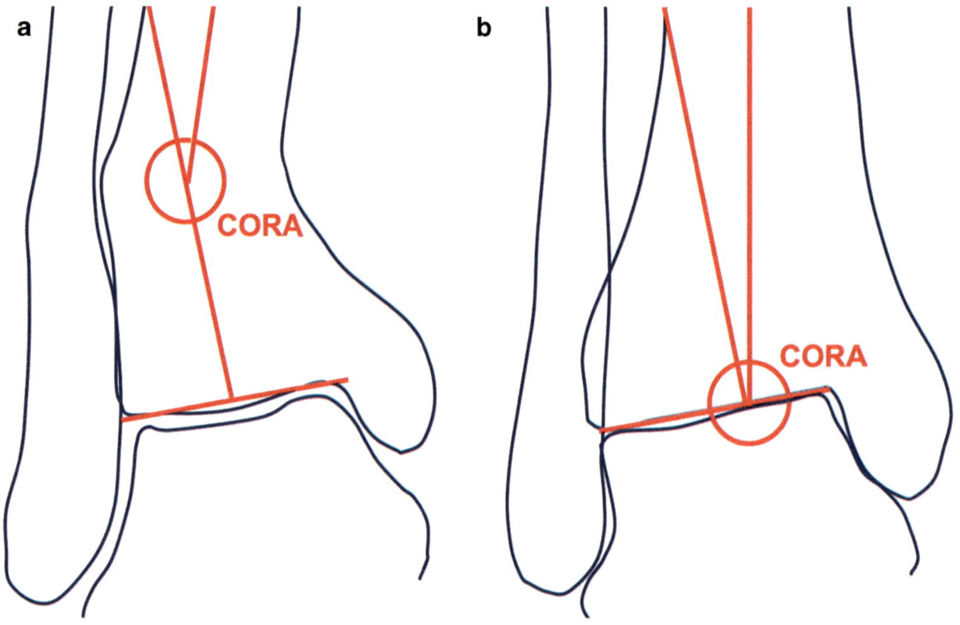

Fig. 9.2 Determination of the center of rotation and angulation (CORA). (**a**) CORA in an extraarticular deformity. (**b**) CORA in an intraarticular deformity

Characteristics. Due to previous tibial fractures which result in diaphyseal or metaphyseal tibial malalignment, either in the coronal (Fig. 9.3) or sagittal (Fig. 9.4) plane or in both (Fig. 9.5); they can also result in malrotation (Fig. 9.6).

Treatment Strategy. Diaphyseal or metaphyseal tibial malalignment must be addressed with osteotomy before considering total ankle arthroplasty. Only in cases of minimal LDTA or ADTA changes (<5°) and the CORA close to the ankle joint line (<1–2 cm) can realignment be performed with the ankle replacement tibial cut.

2. Malalignment in the ankle joint (intraarticular deformity):

   Characteristics. Due to ankle joint pathologies that include distal tibial articular surface malalignment (Figs. 9.7 and 9.8), talar tilt due to ligamentous instability (Fig. 9.9), or both (Fig. 9.10).

   Treatment Strategy. Minimal changes of LDTA or ADTA (<5°) can be addressed with the ankle replacement tibial cut but may need an additional correcting osteotomy of the fibula or the medial malleolus. In most instances, soft-tissue procedures, including soft-tissue releases, ligament reconstruction, and tendon transfers, are necessary for appropriately balancing the replaced ankle.

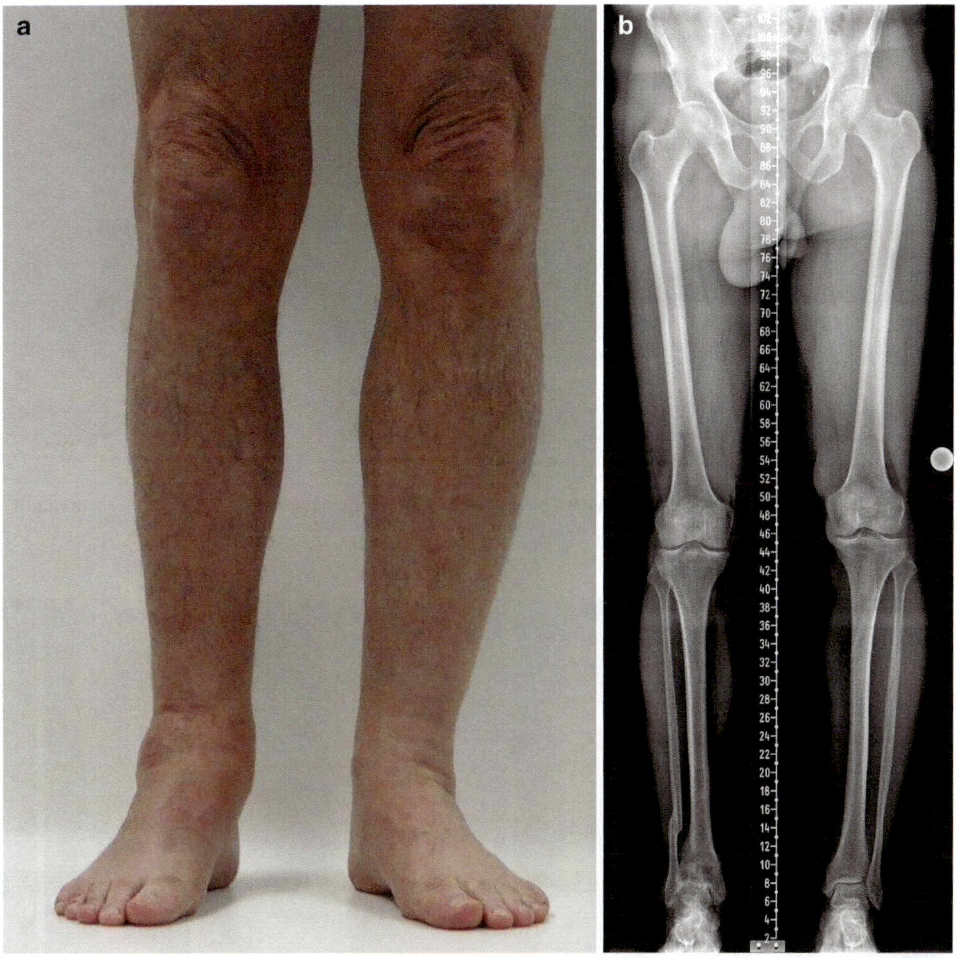

Fig. 9.3 Coronal plane deformity. A 68-year-old patient 24 years after a conservatively treated open tibial fracture. (**a**) AP view shows an abduction deformity. (**b**) Long-standing radiographs show the tibial malunion with external rotation and valgus deformity with leg shortening

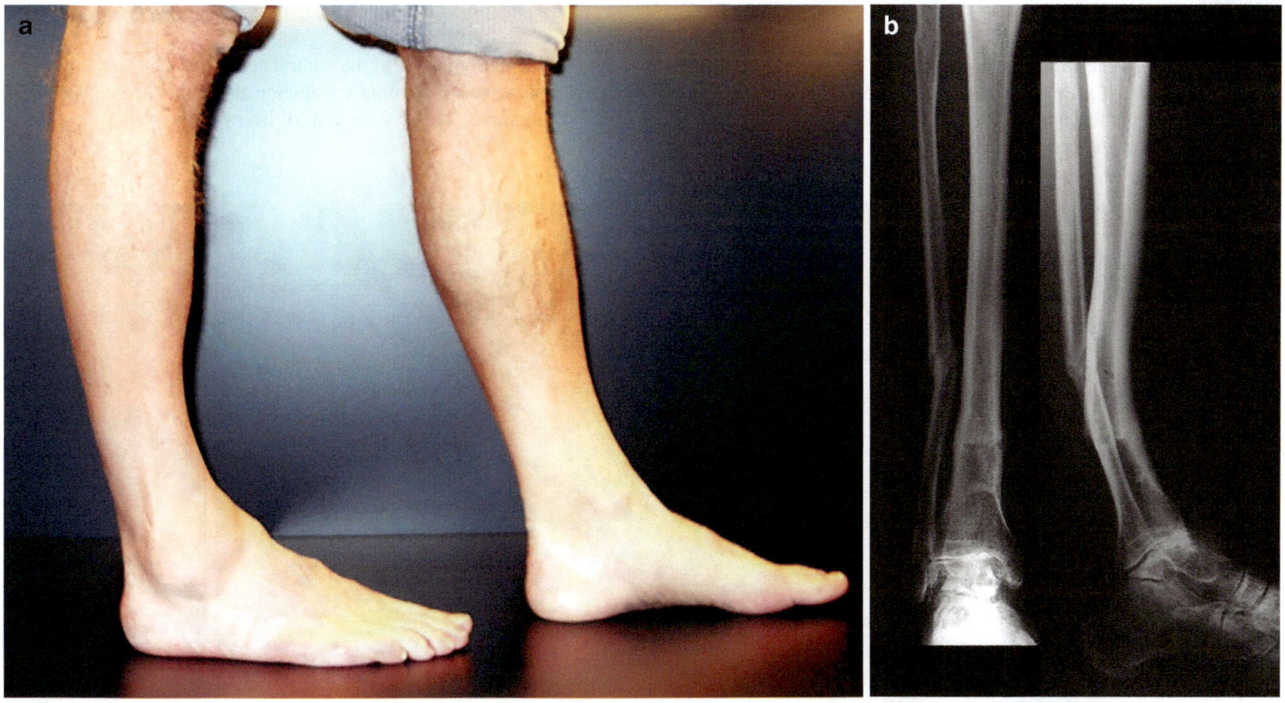

Fig. 9.4 Sagittal plane deformity. A 62-year-old former downhill ski racer 36 years after a tibial fracture with a subsequent infection that stopped his career. (**a**) The recurvatum deformity resulted in a progressive equinus that he is trying to compensate for with a hyperextension at his knee. (**b**) Radiograph showing the equinus position of his ankle with anterior extrusion of the talus

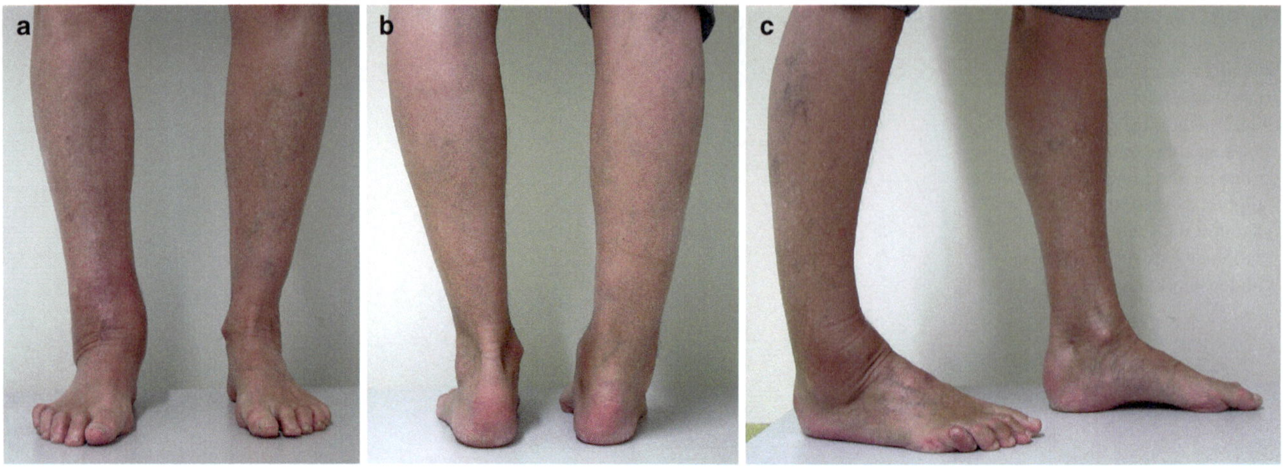

Fig. 9.5 Bi-planar deformity. Clinical views of a 57-year-old female patient showing a varus-recurvatum deformity 22 years after a distal tibial fracture. (**a**) AP view, (**b**) posterior view, and (**c**) lateral view

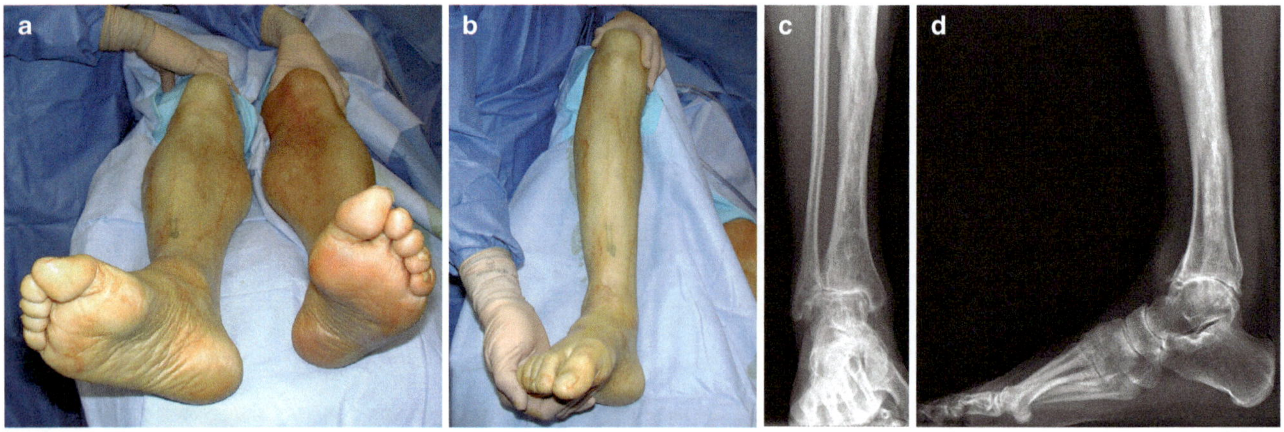

Fig. 9.6 Malrotation deformity. Right leg after a conservatively treated mid-shaft fracture of the tibia at the age of 13 years. The fracture healed after 9 months of extension treatment, with a lengthening of the tibia of 2 cm. (**a**) While the knees are held parallel, the external malrotation of >20° is evident compared to the contralateral side. (**b**) The ankle contours are preserved, indicating a malunion above the metaphysis of the tibia. Radiographs, (**c**) AP view and (**d**) lateral view

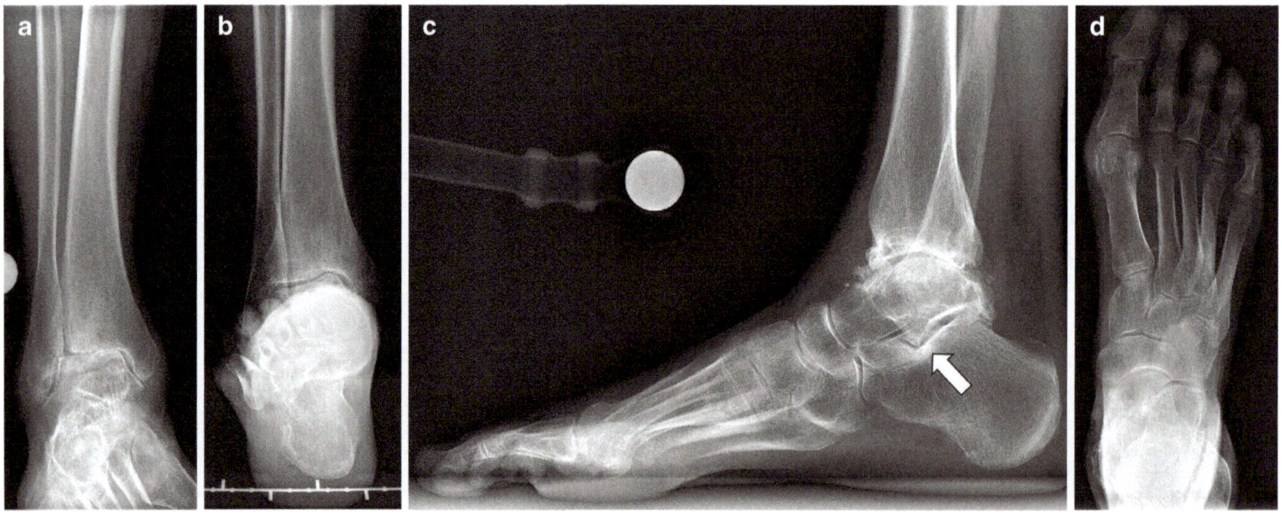

Fig. 9.7 Intraarticular varus deformity. Ankle series of a 71-year-old patient suffering from end-stage varus ankle osteoarthritis. (**a**) The AP view shows a distal tibial articular surface malalignment that is even more pronounced in the alignment view, indicating that the primary pathology is in the anteromedial part of the tibial plafond (**b**); besides distinct compensatory pronation at the subtalar joint (with typical closure of sinus tarsi, arrow), no pathologies are seen in the lateral (**c**) and DP views (**d**) of the foot

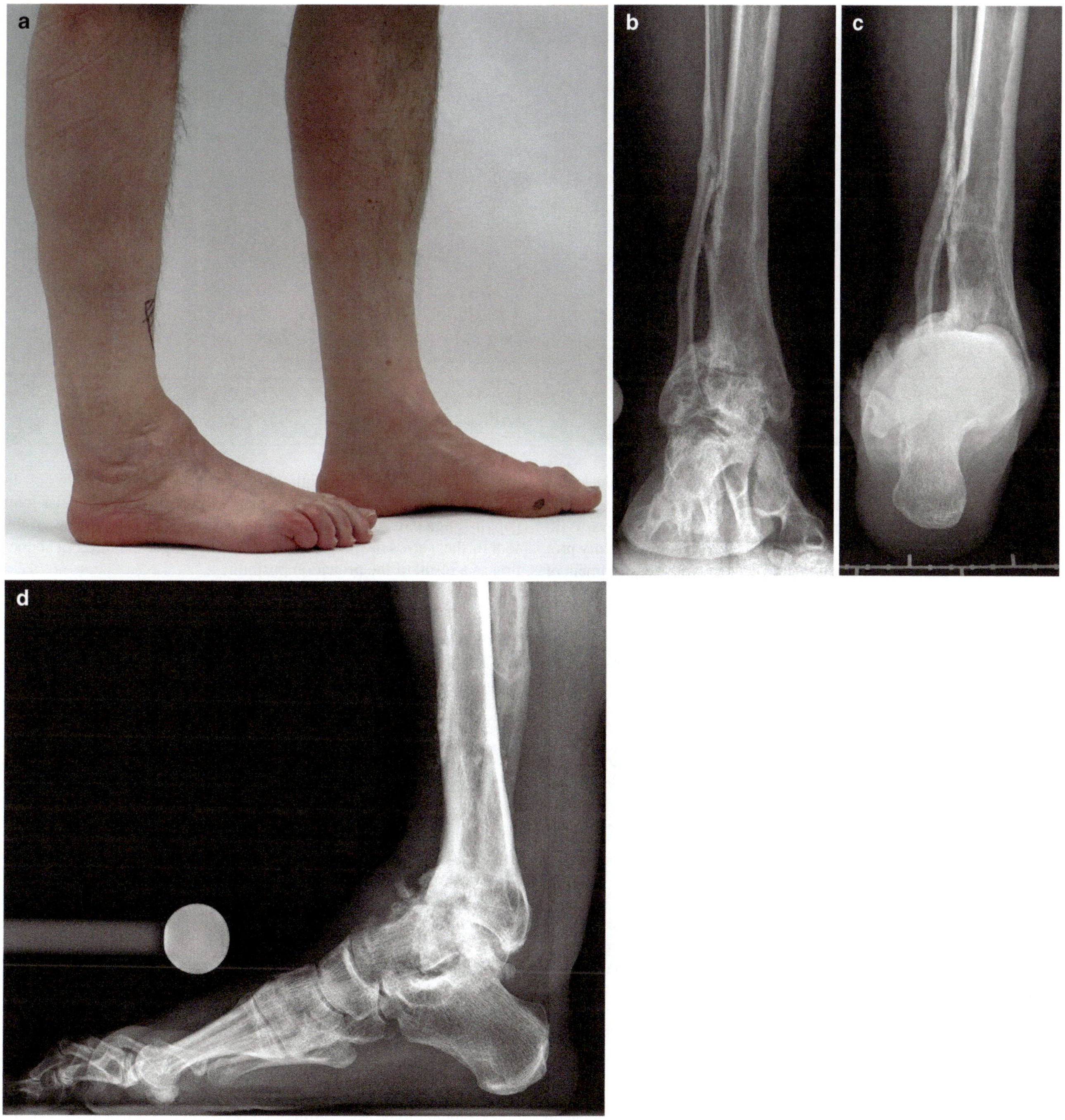

Fig. 9.8 Intraarticular valgus and recurvatum deformity. Ankle series of a 62-year-old farmer with a sagittal distal tibial articular surface malalignment 9 years after a complex ankle fracture. (**a**) The lateral view of the foot evidences the posterior dislocated position of the tibia with shortening of the heel and anterior extrusion of the talus, respectively. (**b–d**) Standard radiographs showing a complex three-plane deformity of the distal tibial articular surface with posterior tilt associated with a valgus tilt and shortening of the fibula

3. In varus or valgus hindfoot malalignment (inframalleolar deformity):

   Characteristics. Due to multi-articular degeneration of the hindfoot involving the subtalar and midtarsal joints, which can result in varus (Fig. 9.11) or valgus (Fig. 9.12) malalignment.

   Treatment Strategy. In the case of varus/valgus hindfoot malalignment without joint degeneration, calcaneal osteotomies are usually sufficient to correct the deformity. If varus/valgus hindfoot malalignment is due to multi-articular degeneration, hindfoot arthrodesis is usually advised to correct the deformity, and it can be combined with calcaneal osteotomies.

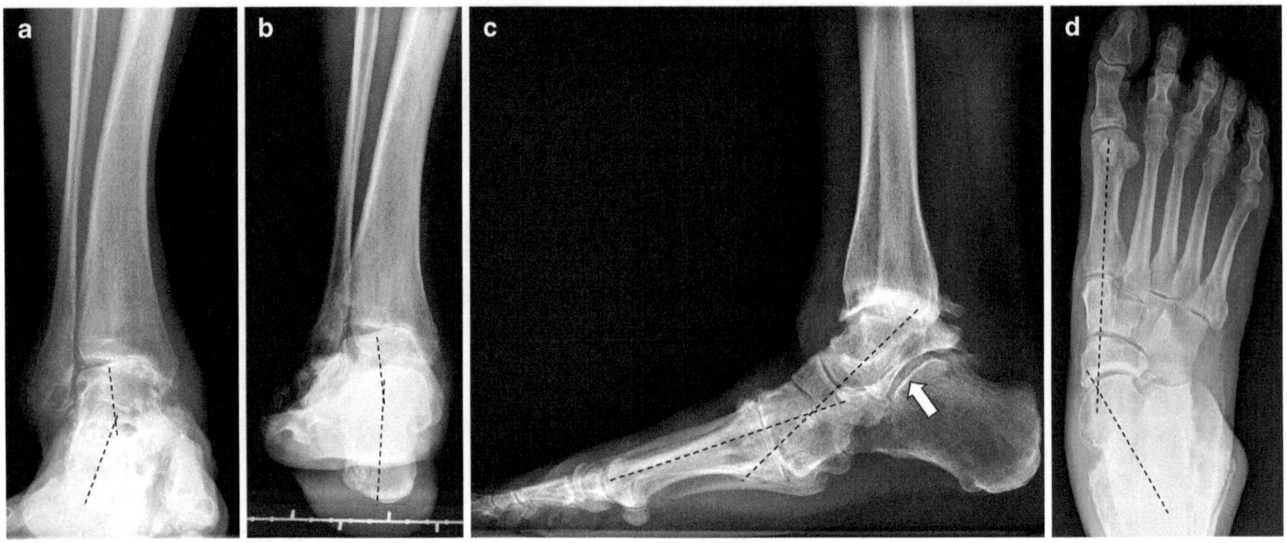

Fig. 9.9 Intraarticular varus deformity in a globally unstable ankle. Ankle series of a 56-year-old former soccer player with a globally unstable ankle after multiple sprains. (**a**) The AP view shows a varus tilt of the talus within the ankle mortise associated with compensatory pronation at the subtalar joint, which minimizes the varus malalignment of the heel (**b**); (**c**) the underlying peritalar instability can be seen best in the lateral view with the talus in a plantarflexed position, subtalar joint gapping, and closure of sinus tarsi (arrow); and (**d**) the DP view of the foot further shows the increased talocalcaneal angle and forefoot abduction as a result of the pronation position

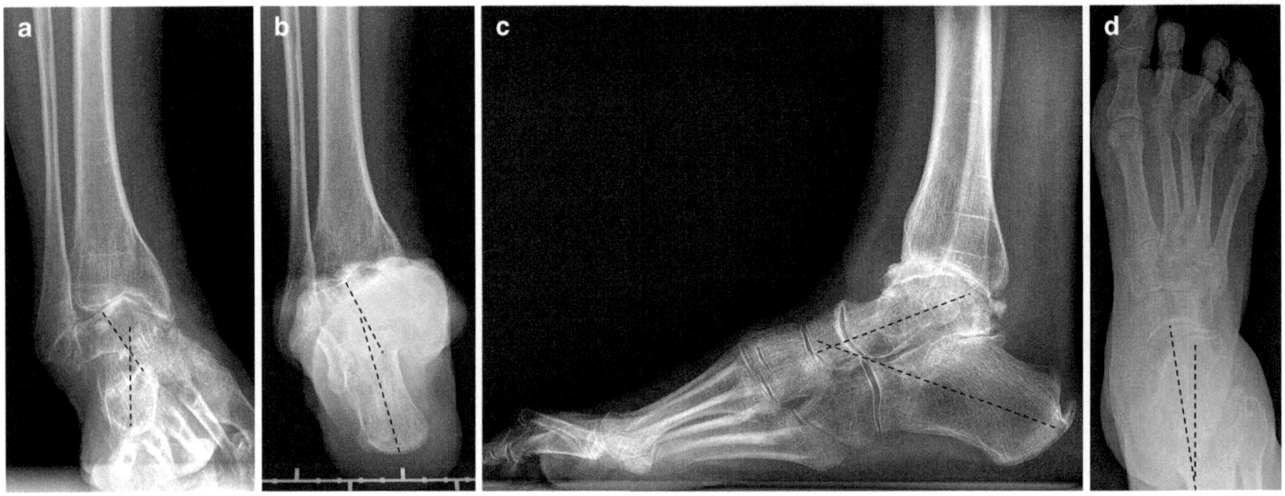

Fig. 9.10 Intraarticular varus malunion deformity. Ankle series of a 61-year-old female patient with an intraarticular varus malunion after a crush injury to the ankle at 13 years, suffering from progressive lateral ankle instability and medial ankle osteoarthritis. (**a**) The AP view shows an asymmetric varus ankle with gapping of the lateral compartment originating from the distal tibial articular surface malalignment. (**b**) The heel moment arm is slightly reduced due to the compensatory pronation at the subtalar joint. As a result of the varus-supination deformity of the foot, the talocalcaneal angle has changed in the lateral (**c**) and DP views (**d**)

9.1.2 Supramalleolar Osteotomies

Deformities originating at tibial diaphysis and higher are generally complex, often including the three planes and malrotation. A meticulous diagnostic workup is mandatory for fully understanding and defining appropriate solutions (Fig. 9.13).

The correction of tibial malalignment is made by osteotomy, which may be a closing wedge (Fig. 9.14), opening wedge (Fig. 9.15), or dome shape (Fig. 9.16). Wedge osteotomies either shorten (closing wedge) or lengthen (opening wedge) the limb and may require intraoperative translation to maintain alignment. Opening wedge osteotomies may require bone grafting to heal as well. Dome osteotomies correct angular deformity without lengthening and provide the greatest contact surface, and they do not need bone grafting. The osteotomy site is exposed as preoperatively determined regarding CORA. Under fluoroscopic

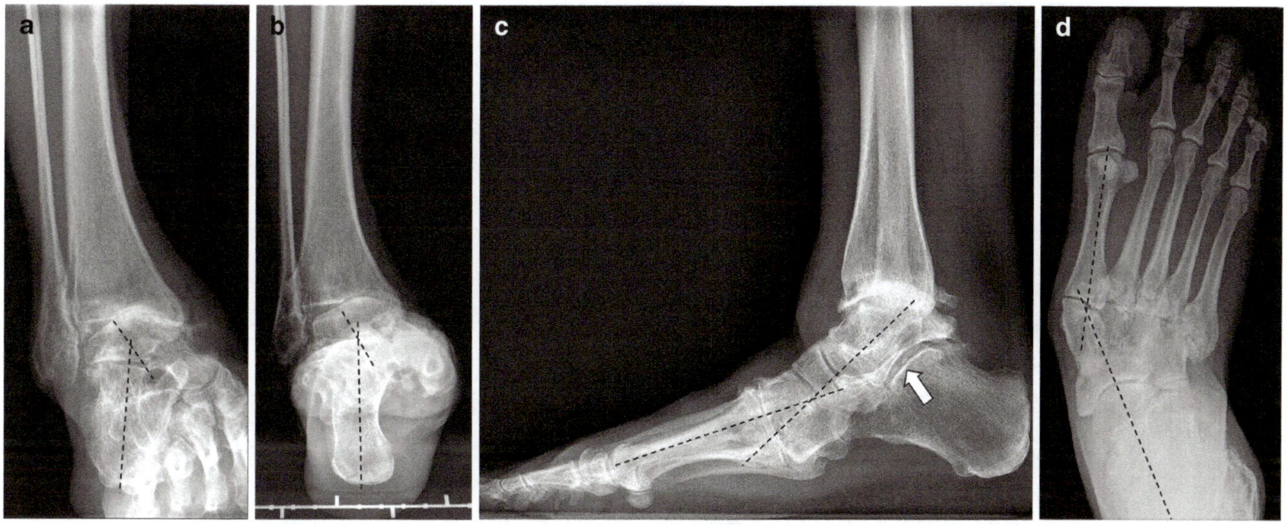

Fig. 9.11 Varus deformity with destabilization of the foot. Ankle series of a 64-year-old female patient suffering from end-stage varus osteoarthritis of her right ankle associated with multi-articular degeneration of the tarsometatarsal joints. (**a**) The AP view shows the varus-valgus deformity with gapping of the lateral compartment, whereas the heel moment arm is only slightly increased due to compensatory pronation at the subtalar joint (**b**). (**c**) The lateral view shows the breakdown at the tarsometatarsal joints associated with a peritalar subluxation (arrow) and an abduction deformity as seen in the DP view (**d**)

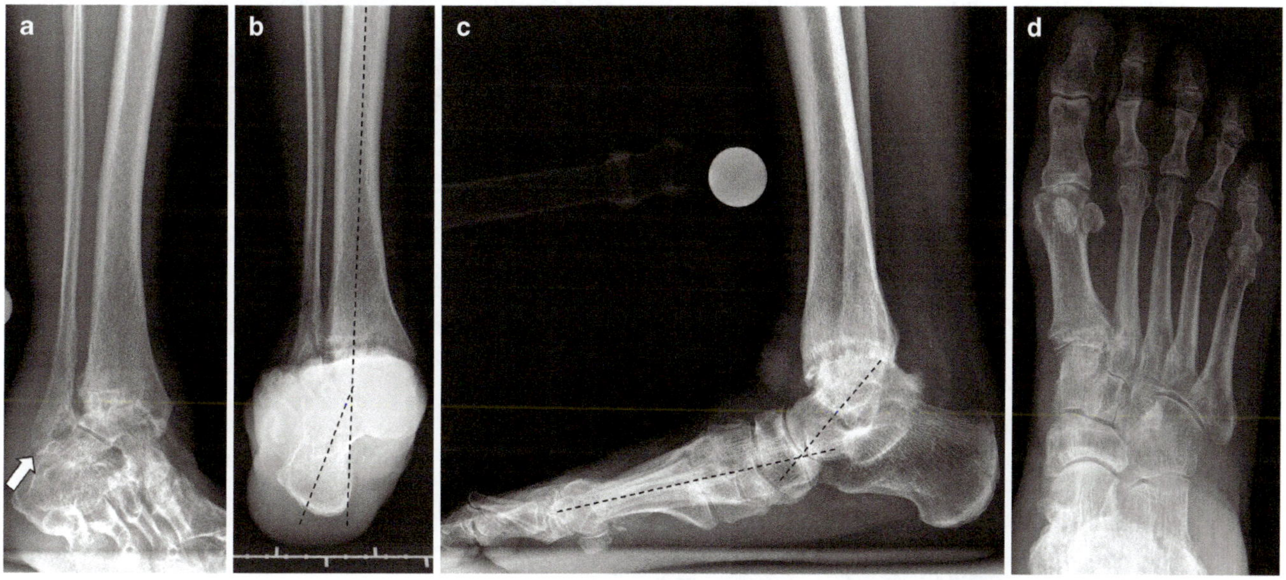

Fig. 9.12 Valgus deformity with destabilization of the foot. Ankle series of a 54-year-old female patient suffering from end-stage valgus osteoarthritis of her right ankle associated with multi-articular degeneration of the tarsometatarsal joints. (**a**) The AP view evidences a widening of distal tibiotalar joint and subfibular impingement (arrow) subsequently to the valgus collapse of the hindfoot. (**b**) The alignment view shows a significant valgus moment arm of the heel. (**c**) The lateral view shows the multisegmental breakdown of the arch with multi-articular degeneration, (**d**) whereas the alignment of the foot is preserved in the horizontal plane

guidance, a 2.0 mm K-wire is inserted to mark the planned osteotomy. The osteotomy is performed along this K-wire with a saw while paying attention to preserving the contralateral cortex. In the case of a closing wedge osteotomy (Fig. 9.14), the osteotomy is closed after removing the wedge created by a second saw cut, and plate and screw fixation is performed. In the case of an opening osteotomy (Fig. 9.15), the osteotomy is opened using a 2.5 mm K-wires-based distraction (Hintermann distractor) until the desired correction based on preoperative planning is achieved with visual confirmation from fluoroscopy. After inserting a wedged allograft into the defect, the distractor is

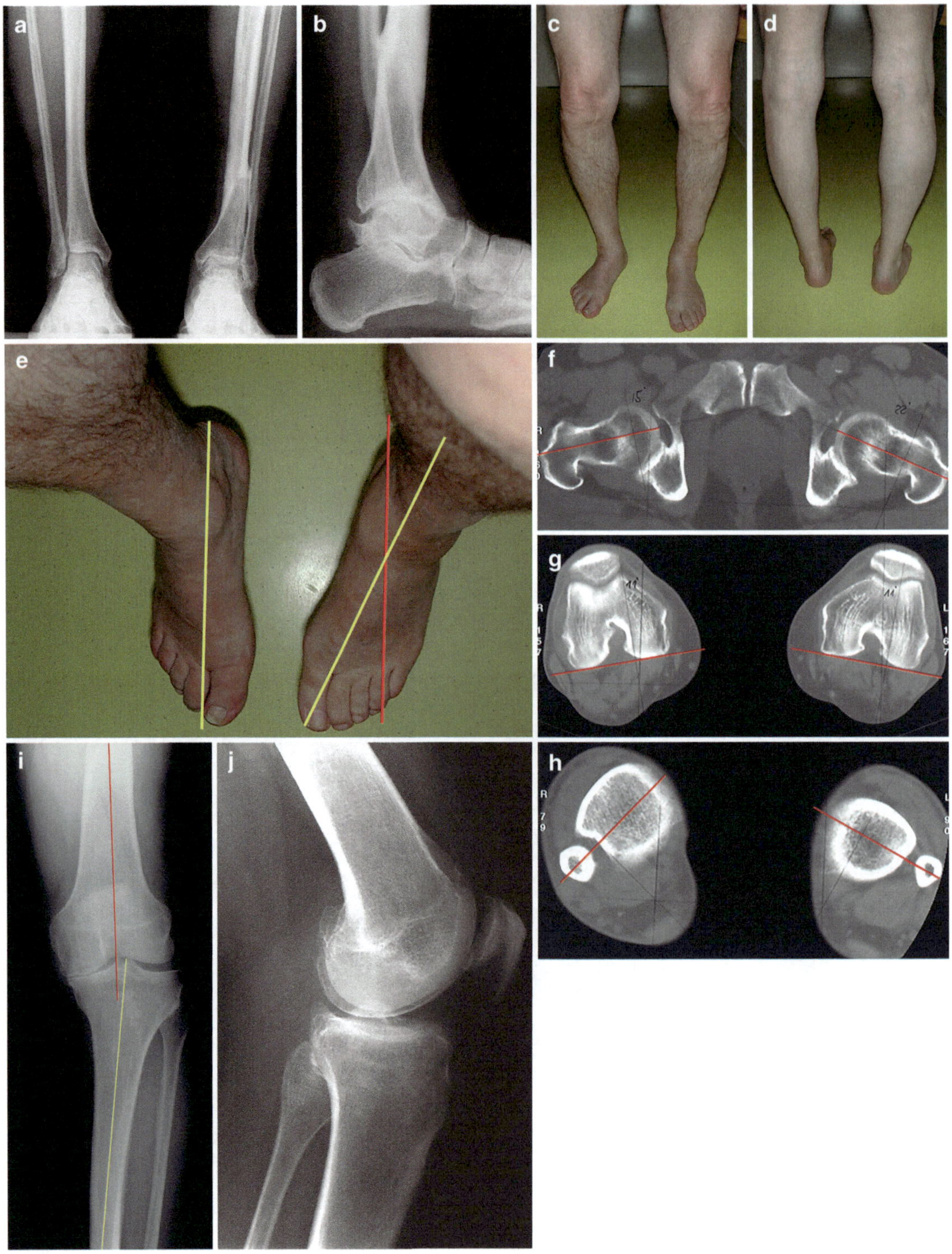

Fig. 9.13 Multiplane deformity with malrotation. A 66-year-old farmer suffering from post-traumatic ankle osteoarthritis 31 years after a conservatively treated tibial fracture. He has refused the proposed ankle fusion for 8 years. (**a–b**) The standard X-rays evidence a malunion of distal tibial diaphysis with varus and some recurvatum deformity. Besides a large osteophyte on the anterior tibia, a market osteophyte on the posterior talus indicates a rotational ankle overuse. (**c–d**) A malrotation is found clinically in a standing position and substantiated as an internal malrotation of >20° in a sitting position (**e**) and by CT scans (**f–h**). (**i** and **j**) There is also a varus deformity at the knee joint with a degenerative disease, mainly of the medial compartment. The deformity is addressed with a high tibial osteotomy because the knee function is well-preserved with only limited medial pain. (**k**) After removing a lateral wedge, the tibia is externally rotated at the osteotomy level (**l**) and fixed by a plate (**m**). The distal varus-recurvatum deformity of the tibia is addressed by correcting tibial cuts when performing the total ankle arthroplasty (**n–o**). The patient was pain-free in the knee and ankle 20 years after the one-stage surgery. (**p**) The long-standing X-rays show a correct axis of the leg, and (**q–t**) the standard ankle X-rays show a well-balanced ankle with stable components. The patient died some weeks after that of an unrelated cause to his left leg

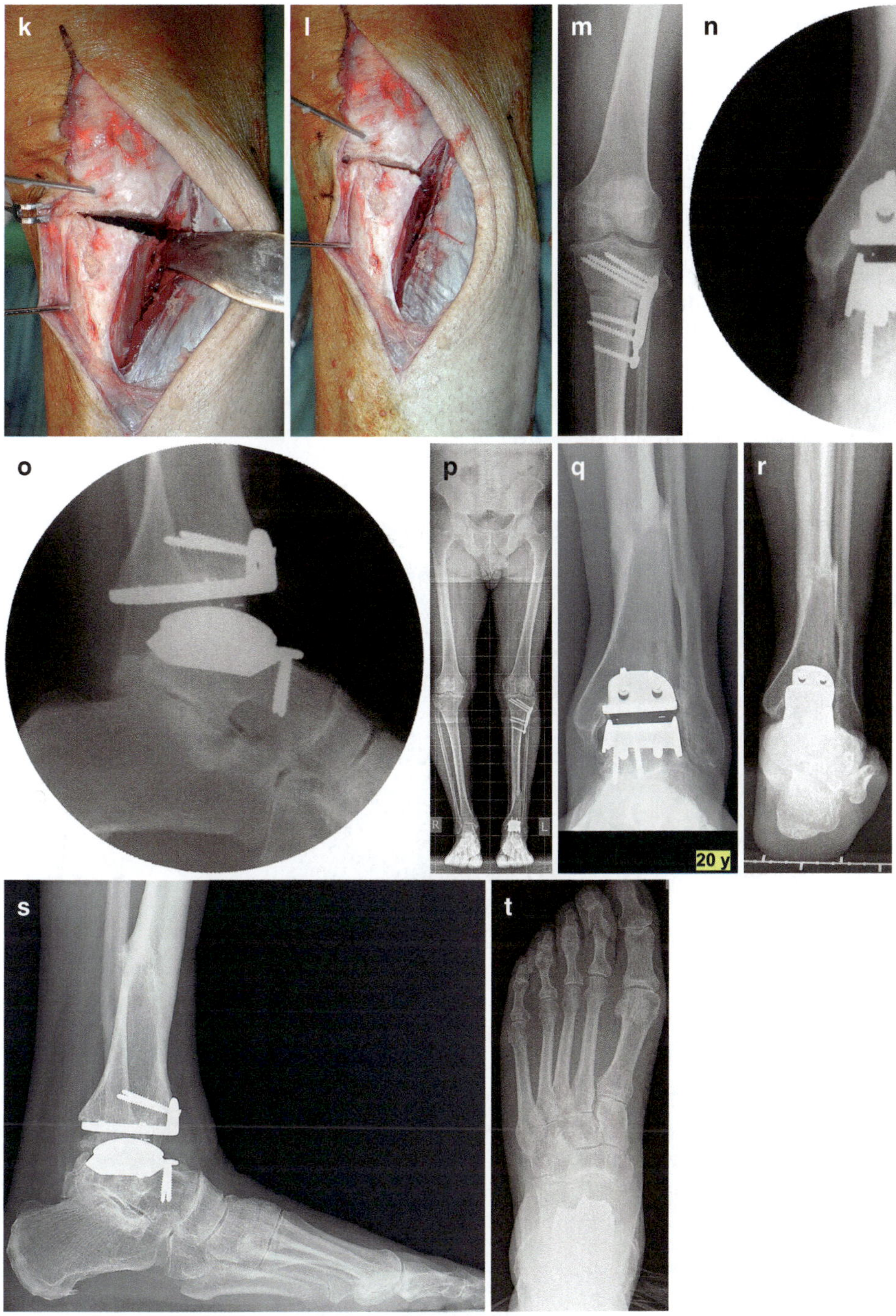

Fig. 9.13 (continued)

removed, and the osteotomy is fixed by using a plate and screws while paying attention not to conflict with subsequent total ankle arthroplasty (i.e., resection cuts and component insertion). For major correction (i.e., >6°), a dome osteotomy (Fig. 9.16) is preferred. The distal tibia is exposed through the ankle's extended anterior approach. Multiple holes with a 2.5 mm drill are performed to create a dome-shaped cut, and the osteotomy is completed with a chisel. Usually, a fibular osteotomy must be added to rotate the distal tibial bloc and fix it with one or two plates and screws.

The Authors' Approach

Following the creation of a "normal" ankle before total ankle arthroplasty, supramalleolar alignment correction is made first. The tibial bone resection will be minimized, and the final balancing of the replaced ankle will be easier and more effective.

9.1.3 Intraarticular Osteotomies

If the talus is still tilted into a varus after performing a thorough debridement of osteophytes and replacing the ankle, the underlying cause can be a too-long fibula (Fig. 9.17). The fibula is exposed through an additional lateral approach and then shortened by an oblique osteotomy. If the fibula is too short, as often seen in a valgus ankle, the fibula is lengthened instead. Another cause for a persisting varus tilt of the talus can be a medial malleolar dysplasia, subsequently to erosion often associated with soft-tissue contracture. To avoid the talus rotating internally into the spacious medial gutter, a translational and/or rotational medial malleolar osteotomy is performed (Fig. 9.18) [1, 9]. The effect of distracting an osteotomy of the medial malleolus is shown in Fig. 9.19. The main advantages of a rotational ("flip") osteotomy are a correction of the force vector of the deltoid ligament and obtaining a normal width of the medial gutter, allowing the medial malleolus to function again as a guiding structure (Fig. 9.20). Moreover, this reorientation of the medial malleolus will preserve the ankle from recurrent deltoid contracture through potential scarring.

The Authors' Approach

Creating a "normal" ankle after total ankle arthroplasty by osteotomies is most effective in avoiding the unphysiological load of ligaments and preserving ankle function and stability over time.

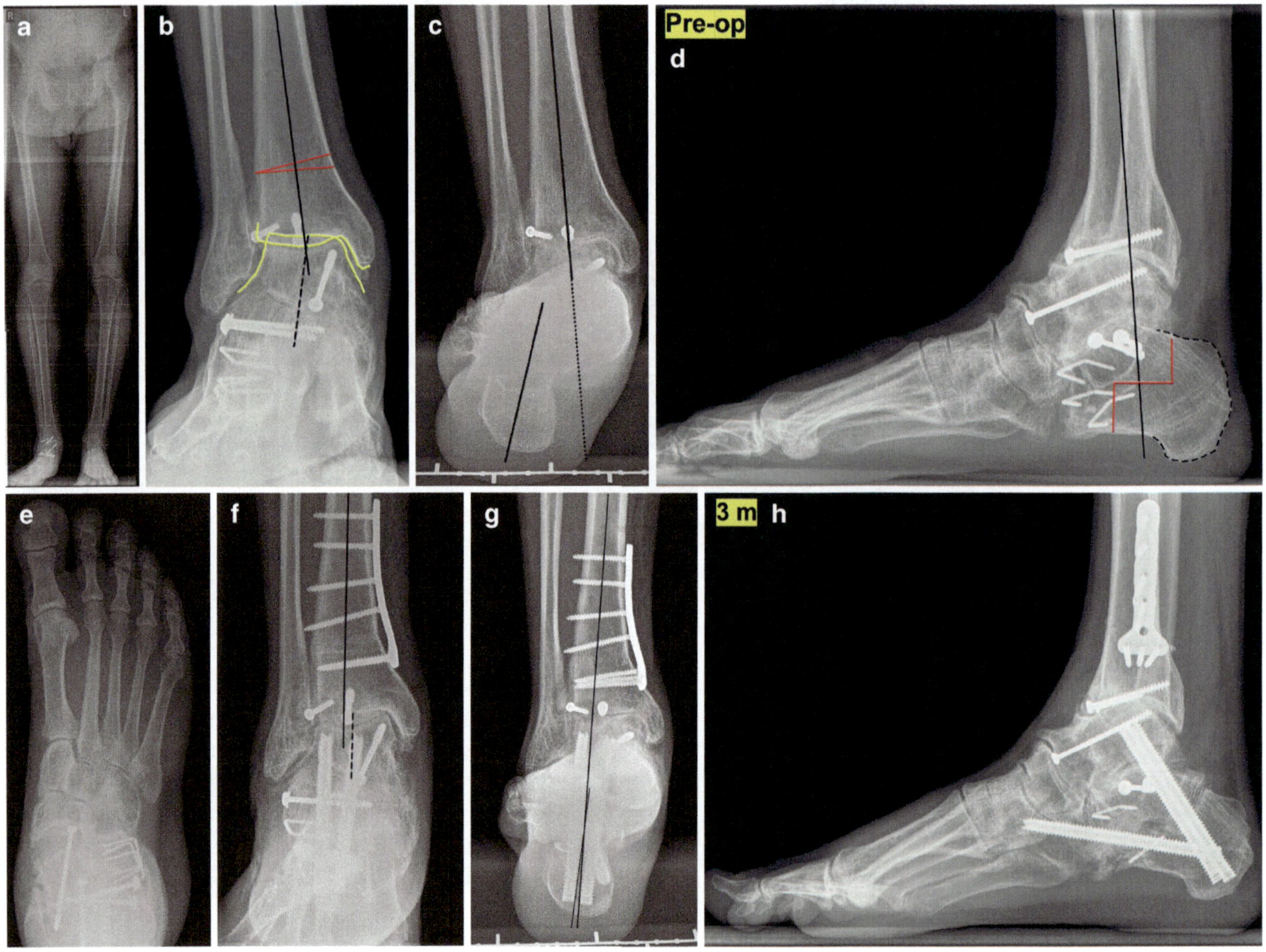

Fig. 9.14 Closing wedge osteotomy. A 41-year-old patient 5 years after a complex injury to his right hindfoot, including a talar and calcaneal fracture, suffering from progressive valgus osteoarthritis. (**a**) Long-standing radiograph shows the deformity strictly located at the ankle. (**b–e**) Preoperative radiographs showing the valgus malalignment of the tibial articular surface, the valgus position of the talus, and the calcaneus, which is also shortened. A medial closing osteotomy of the distal tibia and a Z-shaped osteotomy of calcaneus for lengthening and medial sliding, in addition to a fusion of the subtalar and calcaneocuboid joints, are done for balancing the ankle and restoring the biomechanics of the foot in the first step; the total ankle arthroplasty will be performed in a second step. (**f–i**) Result after 3 months preoperatively to the total ankle arthroplasty. (**j–m**) Radiographs at follow-up control 15 years after total ankle arthroplasty showing a well-balanced ankle with stable implants and distinct signs of asymmetric lateral polyethylene wear; the patient is delighted and is not limited in his profession as a merchant

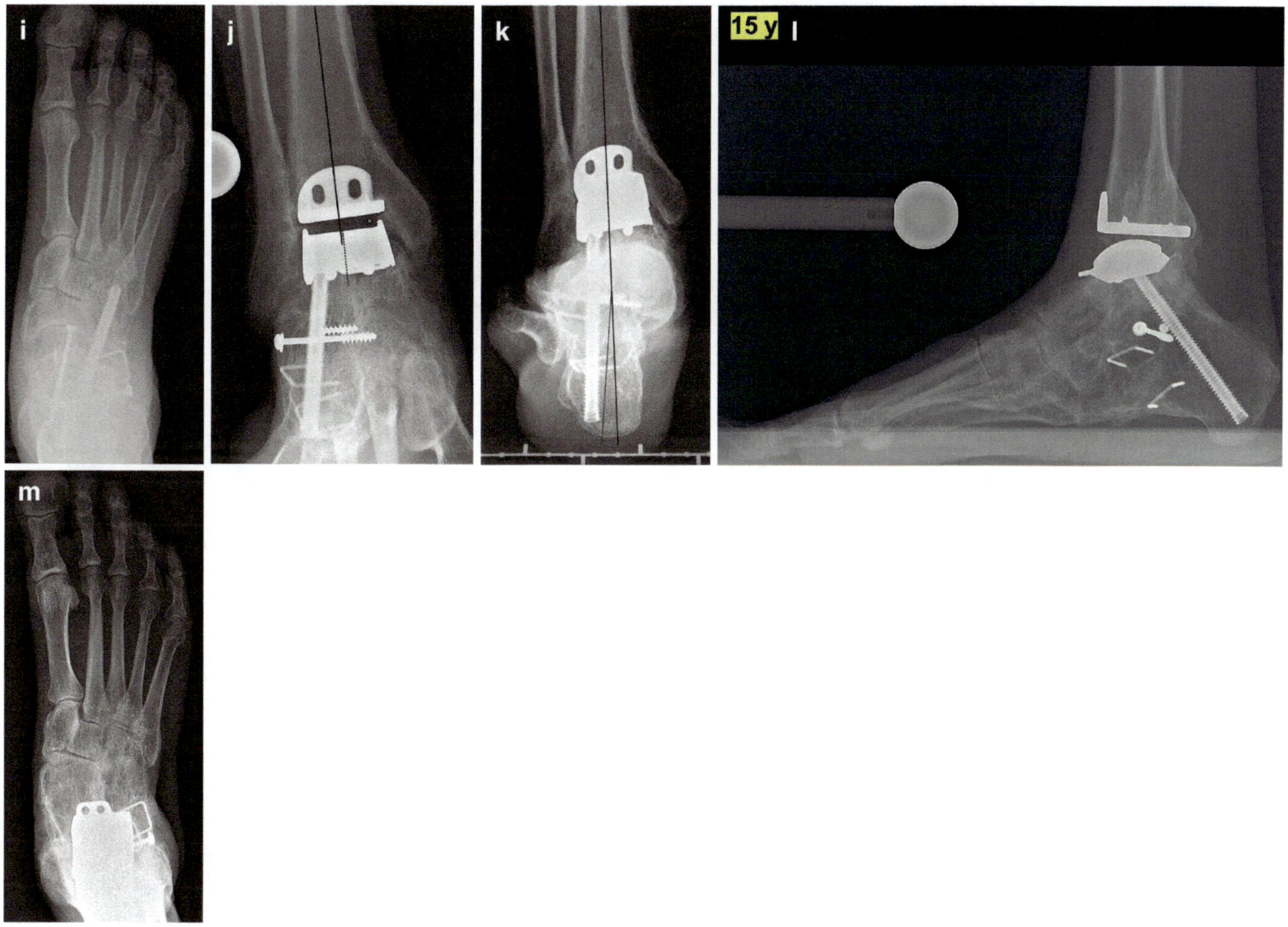

Fig. 9.14 (continued)

9.1.4 Inframalleolar Osteotomies

If the deformity is strictly localized below the ankle or if, despite the abovementioned measures, hindfoot malalignment persists, correction with a separate hindfoot procedure is required.

9.1.4.1 Varus Malalignment

In varus malalignment, a closing wedge osteotomy (Dwyer) [14] of calcaneal can be performed, but the effect is limited, and it shortens the heel. Therefore, the lateral sliding osteotomy is generally a preferred technique to correct varus deformity [15, 16]. Personally, we use a modified Italian osteotomy [17] that allows powerful correction by lateral sliding and tilting the calcaneal tuberosity into valgus (Figs. 9.21 and 9.22) [18].

9.1.4.2 Valgus Malalignment

In valgus malalignment, a medial sliding osteotomy is generally used to correct a deformity (Fig. 9.23) [19–23]. Sliding the tuber of the calcaneus medially corrects the static stability and restores a dynamic balance. If correctly aligned, the Achilles tendon pulls the hindfoot. When the distal insertion has shifted laterally, as in valgus hindfeet, the resulting vector pulling upwards creates a further eversion force to the hindfoot, contributing to the loss of medial arch stability [24]. By sliding the tuber of the calcaneus medially, this vector is neutralized, and the distal insertion of the Achilles tendon is in line with the tibiotalar and subtalar joints again.

The osteotomy is performed obliquely, approximately 10 mm posterior to the peroneal tendons (Fig. 9.24). Then, the calcaneal tuber is shifted medially as much as needed to get a well-aligned hindfoot. The effect can be increased by tilting the tuber additionally in varus. In fear that the tuber may displace cranially secondarily by the pull of the Achilles tendon, we adapted the osteotomy technique. We perform an incomplete cut, leaving the inferior cortex intact. When opening the osteotomy, the left bony bridge will fracture and form a beak anterior ward. With this adaptation, we never saw a secondary cranial displacement, although we permit full weight-bearing straight after surgery.

Occasionally, in valgus deformities associated with a flatfoot, a calcaneal lengthening osteotomy may be considered as a single measure (Fig. 9.25) [25, 26] or in addition to a medial slide [27, 28]. A calcaneal osteotomy along and parallel to the posterior facet of the subtalar joint is generally preferred.

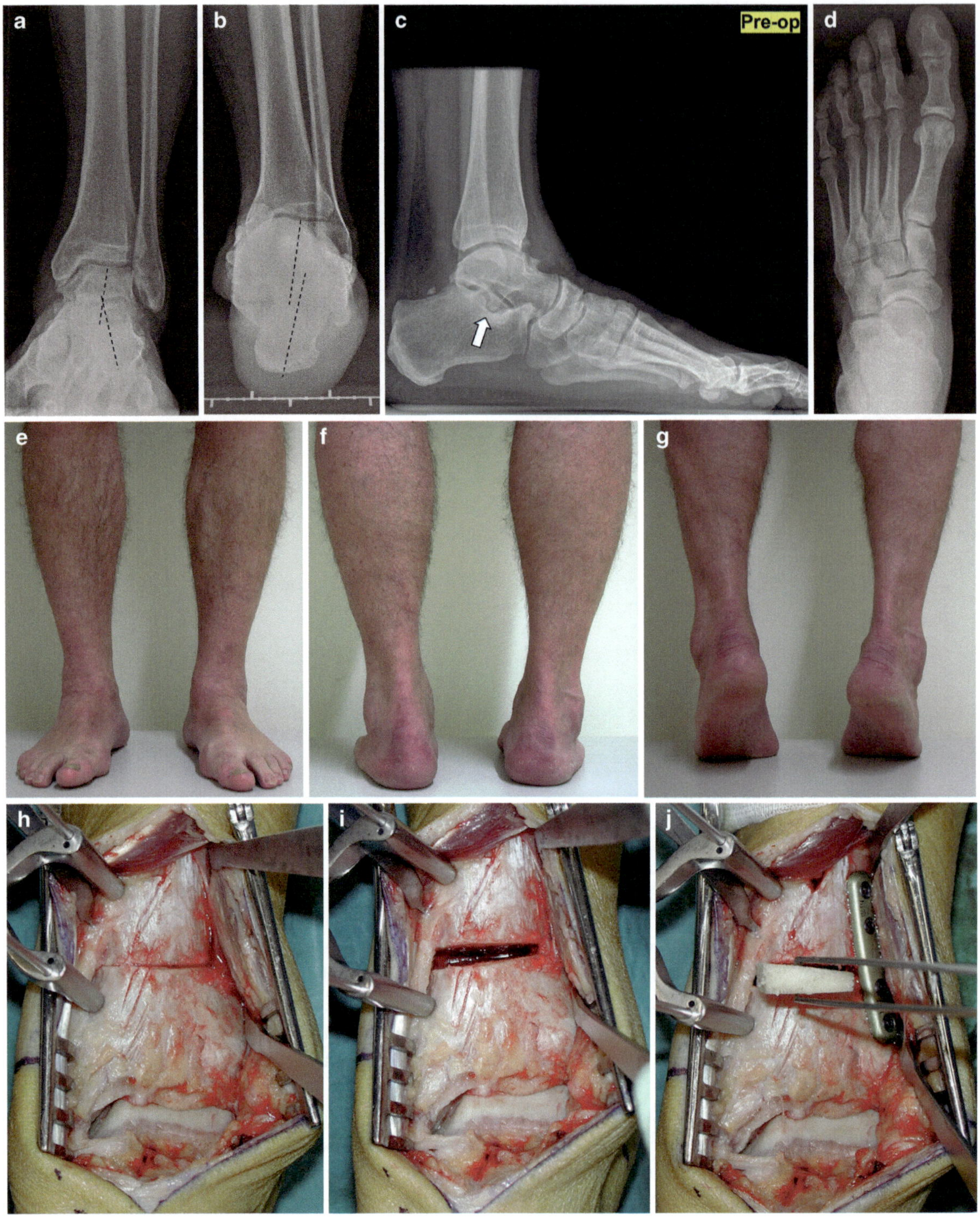

Fig. 9.15 Open wedge osteotomy. A 66-year-old passioned golfer suffering from severe ankle pain after two previous arthroscopic debridement surgeries for an osteochondral lesion at the anteromedial aspect of the talus. (**a**) Preoperative radiographs reveal a varus malalignment of 5° associated with compensatory pronation at the subtalar joint. (**b**) The heel has a slight varus. (**c**) In the lateral view, the sinus tarsi is seen to be closed due to the compensatory pronation position (arrow). (**d**) The DP view does not show any pathology. (**e–g**) The deformity is also seen clinically. (**h**) The osteotomy is made approximately 5 cm above the ankle joint. (**i**) The distractor mounted over two K-wires at the anteromedial aspect is gradually opened until the wanted correction is achieved, and an allograft wedge is prepared accordingly to the created gap (not shown). (**j**) After fixing a short plate at the anterolateral aspect of the tibia to prevent a lateral cortex fracture, the osteotomy is further open, allowing for smooth allograft insertion. (**k**) Compression is applied to the graft as the distraction is released. (**l**) An additional plate is fixed anteromedially to the tibia, paying attention not to getting into conflict with the subsequent ankle replacement. (**m**) After that, the replacement surgery is performed with the standard technique. (**n–q**) Intraoperative fluoroscopic controls showing the supramalleolar correction and the result after total ankle arthroplasty. (**r–u**) After 3 months, the osteotomy is healed, and the ankle is well-balanced. (**v–y**) Radiographs were taken at 15-year follow-up control, showing a well-balanced ankle with stable implants. (**z**) Functional result. The patient is still practicing golfing and is not limited to any activity

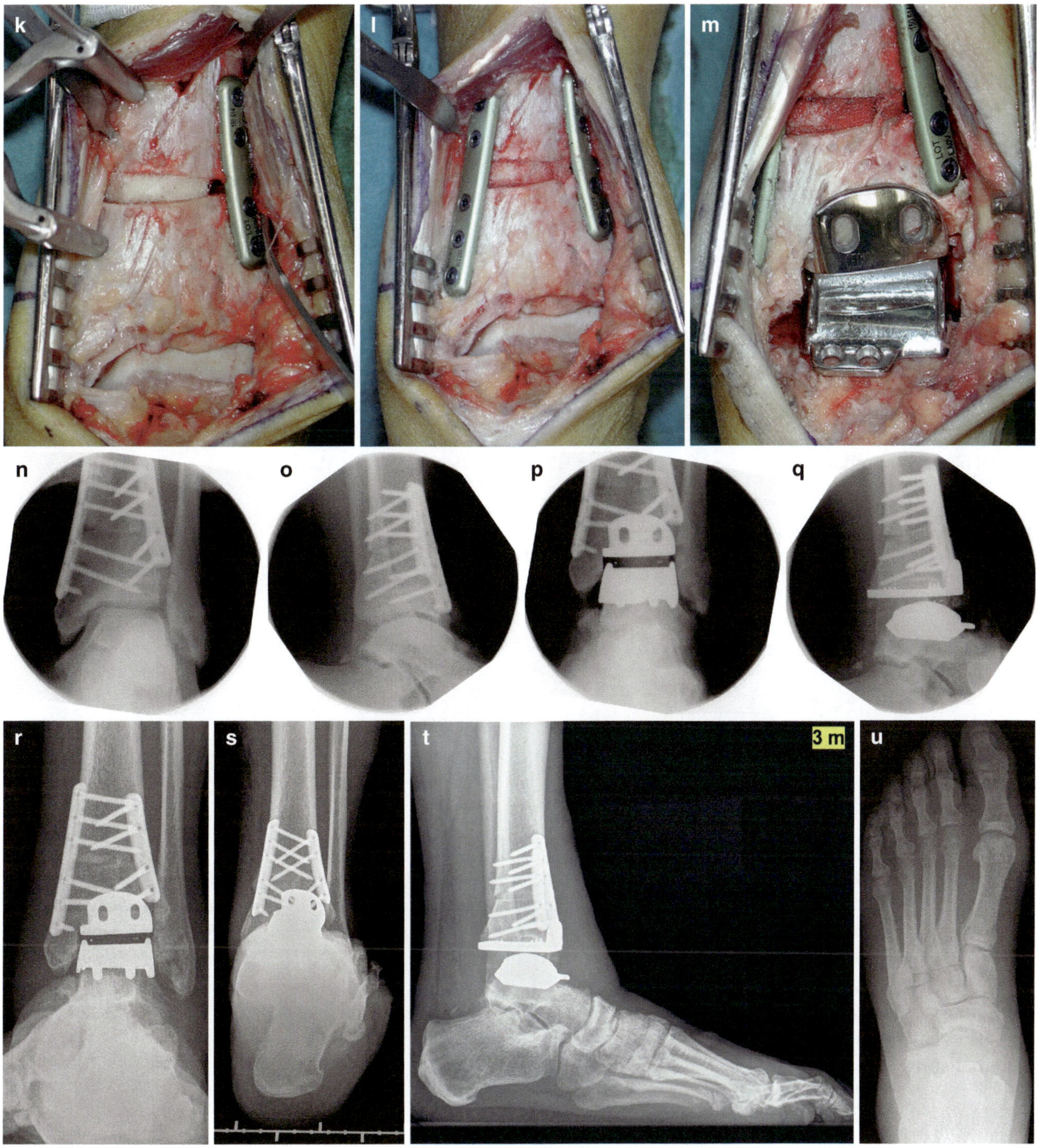

Fig. 9.15 (continued)

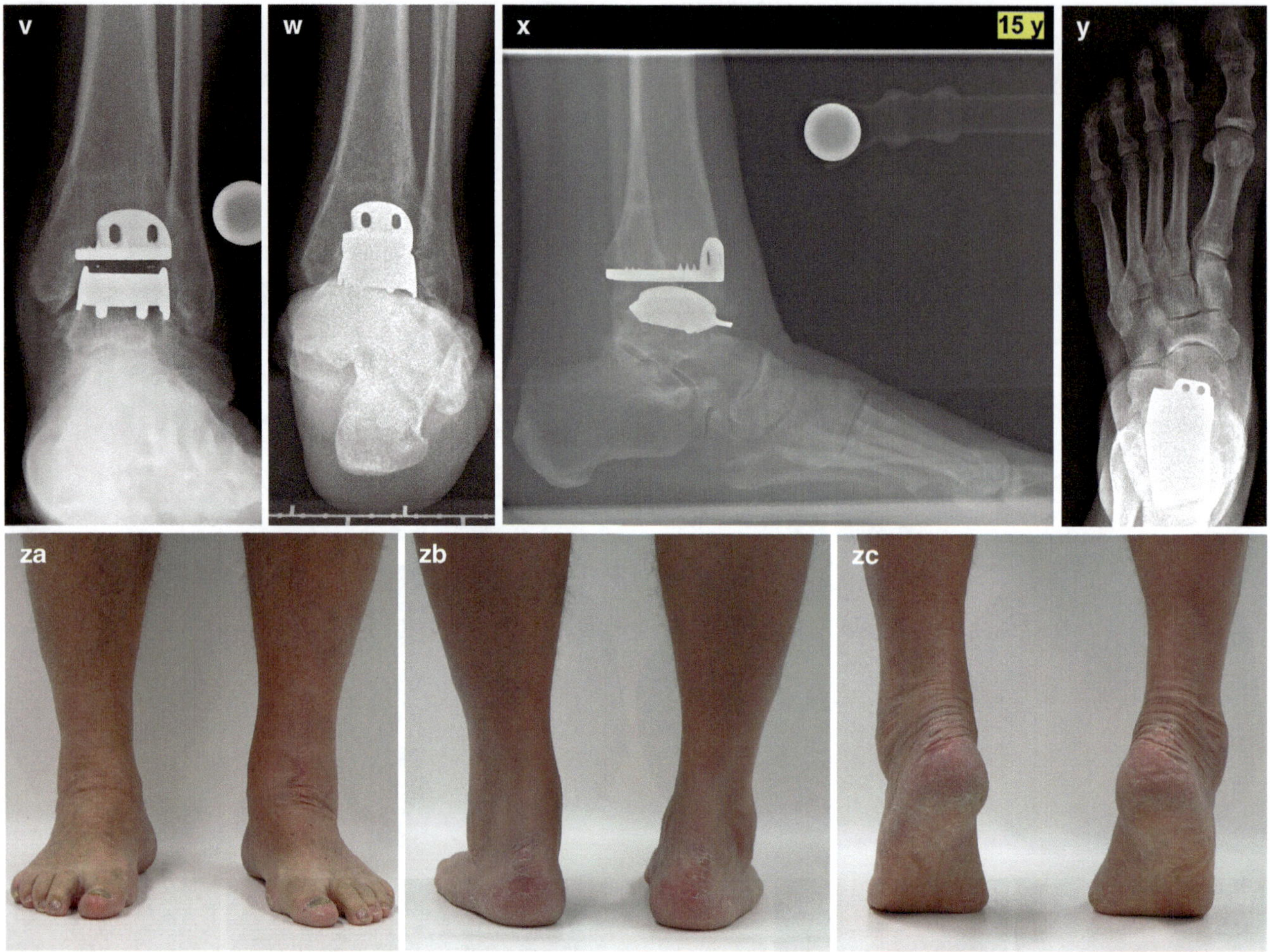

Fig. 9.15 (continued)

Since it is performed from lateral to medial, preserving the medial cortex, it is more like an opening wedge osteotomy than a lengthening osteotomy, thus being more stable [26]. As the osteotomy is widened, the pronation and abduction deformity of the foot is seen to disappear. A correctly sized allograft, or a tricortical graft from the iliac crest, is placed into the osteotomy site. A screw or a plate may protect the graft from displacing and ensure a stable osteotomy.

The Authors' Approach

Following the tightening of collapsed ligaments by the distraction of the ankle joint complex and insertion of components, the heel alignment may change. Therefore, the alignment of the heel should be carefully checked and adequately addressed at the end of replacement surgery. Remaining heel malalignment, especially in the valgus, is detrimental to the balance of the ankle prosthesis, as the asymmetric heel cord pull will continue to act as a deforming force.

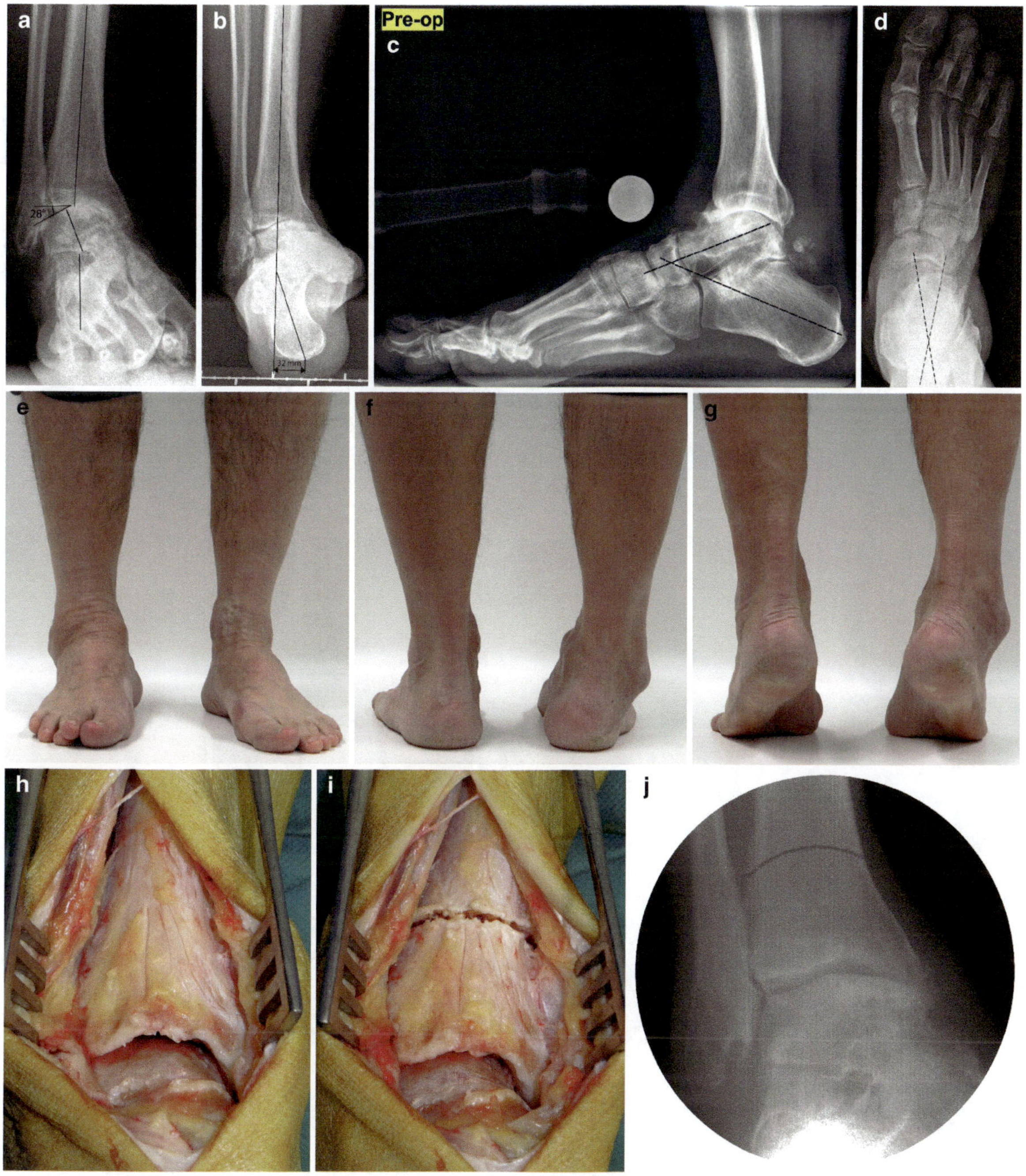

Fig. 9.16 Dome-shaped osteotomy. A 58-year-old female patient who sustained a severe ankle sprain 22 years ago. (**a**) The AP view evidences a TT angle of 28° with some articular tibial malalignment associated with a distinct compensation at the subtalar joint. (**b**) The heel varus accounts for a heel moment arm (HMA) of 32 mm. (**c**–**d**) The talocalcaneal angle has changed in both planes but more in the horizontal plane. (**e**–**g**) The marked varus deformity is also seen clinically. (**h**) After ankle exposure, the varus articular malalignment can be seen. (**i**) The dome-shaped osteotomy is made with multiple drilling and finished with a slightly curved chisel. (**j**) The osteotomy is seen by fluoroscopy. (**k**) The fibula is exposed through a short longitudinal incision, and an oblique osteotomy is performed. (**l**) This allows rotation of the whole distal tibial-fibular bloc with a distraction and a compression device mounted over K-wires on the lateral and medial sides, respectively. (**m**) A K-wire secures the position of the tibia. (**n**) The osteotomy is stabilized by two plates, such as not conflicting with subsequent total ankle arthroplasty. (**o**) A plate also fixes the fibula. (**p**–**q**) Fluoroscopies showing the achieved alignment of the tibia and the fibula; of note, the talar position has improved substantially. (**r**) The tibial resection block is mounted with reference to the tibial tuberosity, and a tibial resection cut is performed. (**s**) After having accomplished tibial and talar resection, the ankle is seen to be well-aligned before the insertion of components. (**t**) However, after insertion of the polyethylene inlay, the ankle evidences a lateral gapping due to the incompetent lateral ankle ligaments. (**u**) Therefore, the ligaments are exposed by lengthening the lateral incision and are found to be desattached entirely from the fibula. (**v**) The lateral ankle ligaments are reattached to the fibula with transosseous sutures and augmented with an internal brace. (**w**) After that, the ankle is stable. (**x**–**y**) Fluoroscopies showing the result in the coronal and sagittal planes. (**za**–**zd**) Radiographs at 5-year follow-up control show a well-aligned ankle with stable components. Notice the translational effect of the supramalleolar osteotomy and the improvement of talocalcaneal angle in the lateral and horizontal views, indicating the segmental changes of the ankle joint complex. The plate over the fibula was removed 9 months after the replacement surgery because of local irritations. (**ze**–**zh**) Clinical views show restored function and alignment

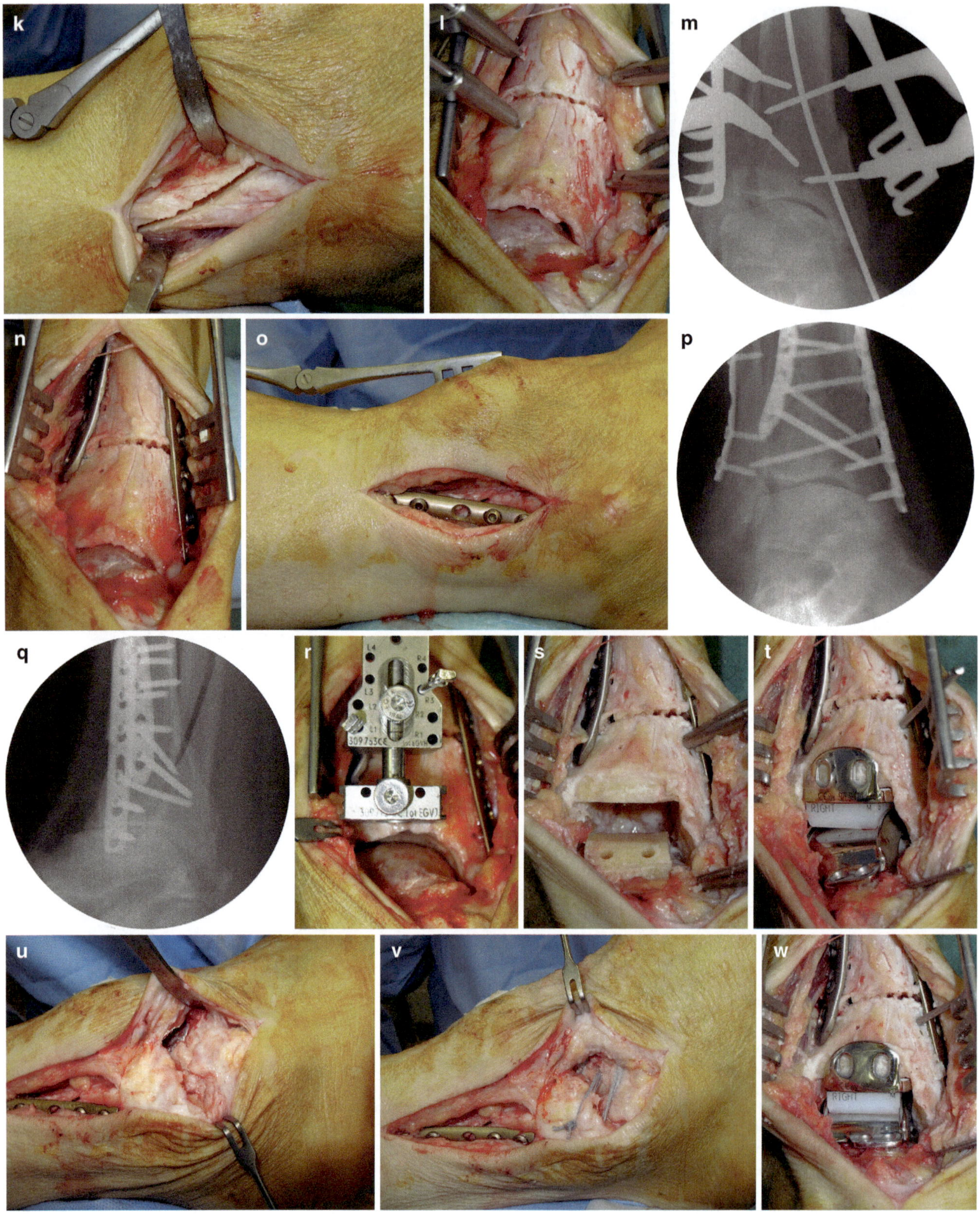

Fig. 9.16 (continued)

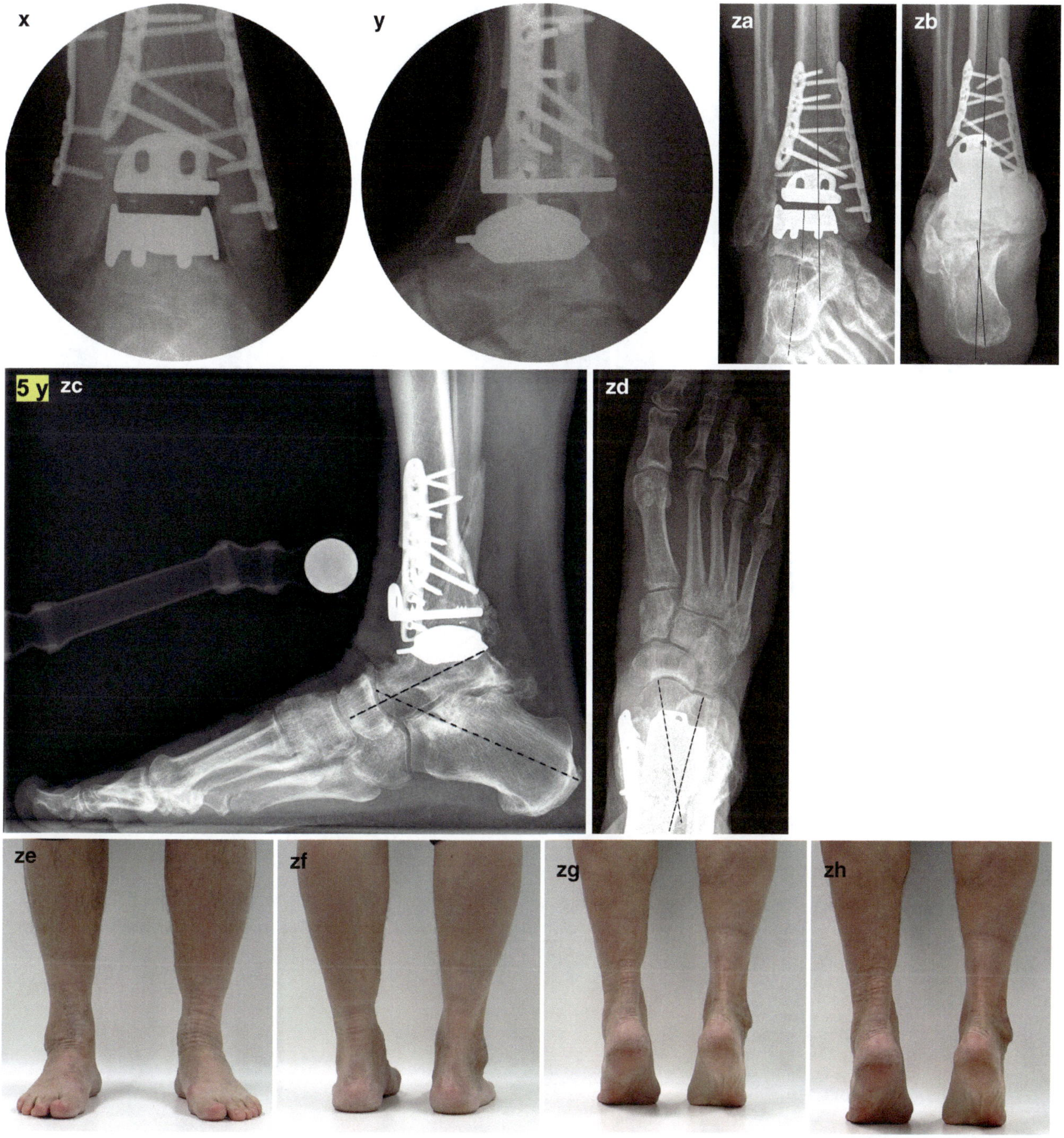

Fig. 9.16 (continued)

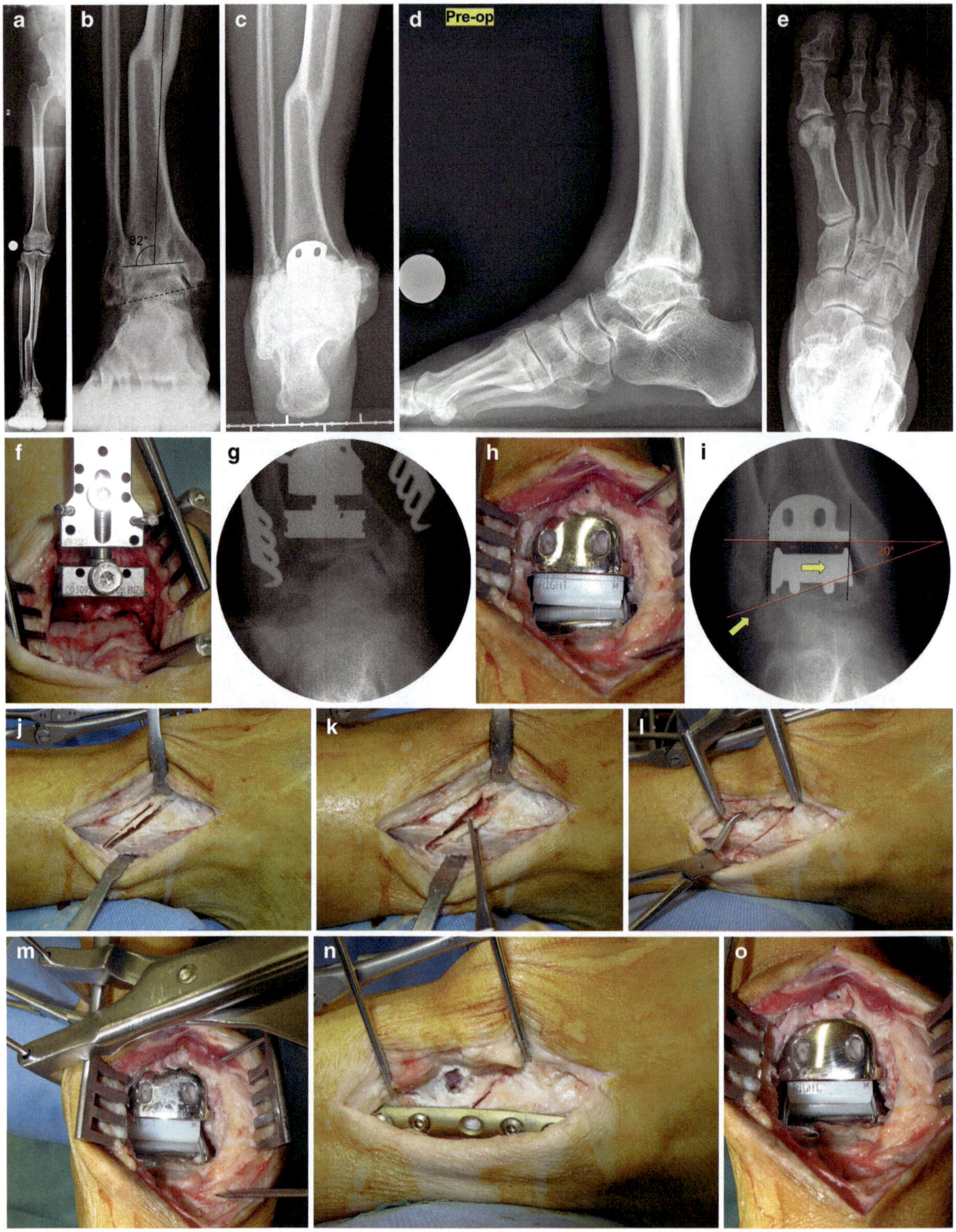

Fig. 9.17 Fibular shortening osteotomy. A 64-year-old carpenter 32 years after a tibial shaft fracture that was conservatively treated. (**a–b**) Preoperative planning on these AP views. The varus alignment is identified to be caused by a malunited tibial fracture accounting for 8° of angulation referred to as the tibial tuberosity (LDTA = 82°). (**c–e**) No deformities are detected in the other planes. (**f–g**) With the tibial resection block mounted, the attempted asymmetric tibial resection can be seen. (**h**) The ankle is not balanced after the replacement surgery because of the created overlength of the fibula, as seen by the lateral gapping. (**i**) The gapping is removed when pushing the talus toward the medial, creating space for the distal fibula (arrows). (**j**) A fibular shortening osteotomy is considered not to overstuff the ankle or to change the integrity of the medial ankle with a soft-tissue release. After exposing the fibula through a longitudinal incision, two parallel oblique osteotomies are performed, and the bone slice is removed (**k**). (**l**) A compression clamp over two K-wires shortens the fibula until the ankle is reduced (**m**). (**n**) Plate fixation is used to stabilize the osteotomy. (**o**) The ankle is now balanced and stable, as verified by fluoroscopy (**p**). Notice the medial gutter's opening and the talus' lateral translation within the mortise. (**q–t**) Standard radiographs at the 5-year follow-up show a well-balanced ankle. The plate was removed 10 months after surgery due to local discomfort

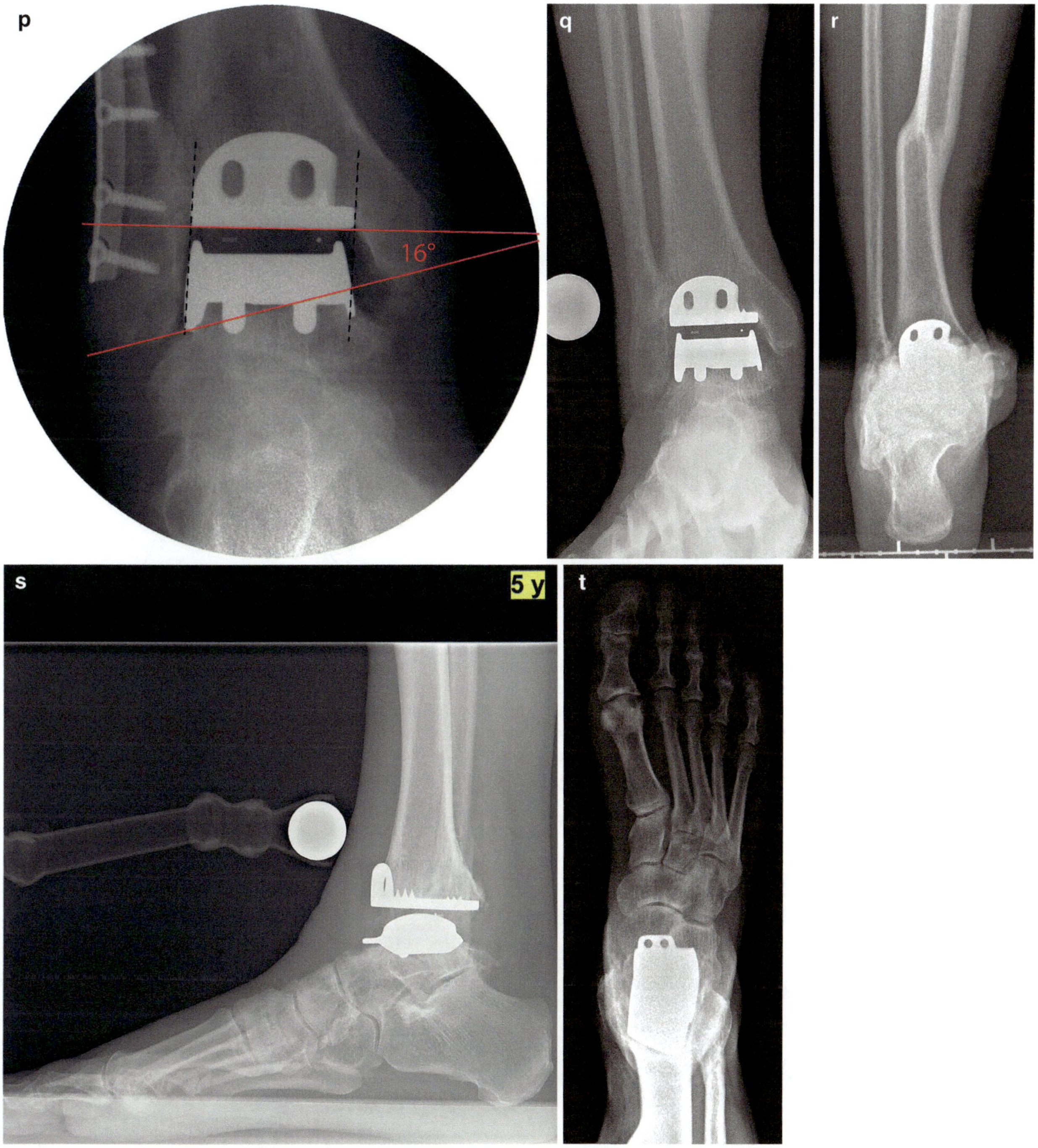

Fig. 9.17 (continued)

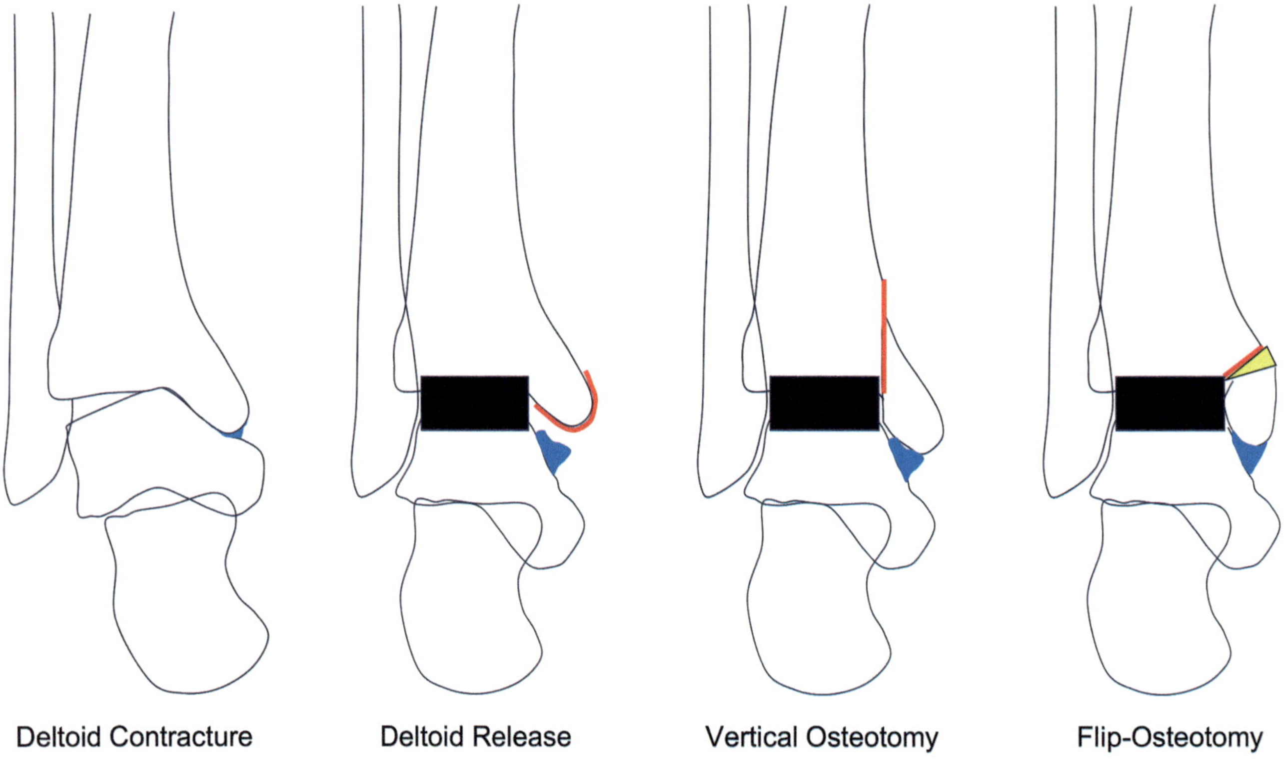

Fig. 9.18 Medial ankle release. Surgical options to address a deltoid contracture: While a deltoid release must be extended to the posteromedial aspect of the medial malleolus to be efficient, it may destabilize the medial ankle in the sagittal plane and the medial gutter remains open, giving rise to potential scarring and recurrent contracture. A vertical osteotomy permits the medial malleolus to slide distally, thus unloading the deltoid ligament. However, concerns arise with the weakening of the medial metaphysis of the distal tibia, especially after a high tibial resection. A flip osteotomy is minimally invasive and permits closure of the medial gutter, thus rotating the force vector of the deltoid toward normal. The preoperative prominence of the medial malleolus disappears without weakening the medial aspect of the distal tibia

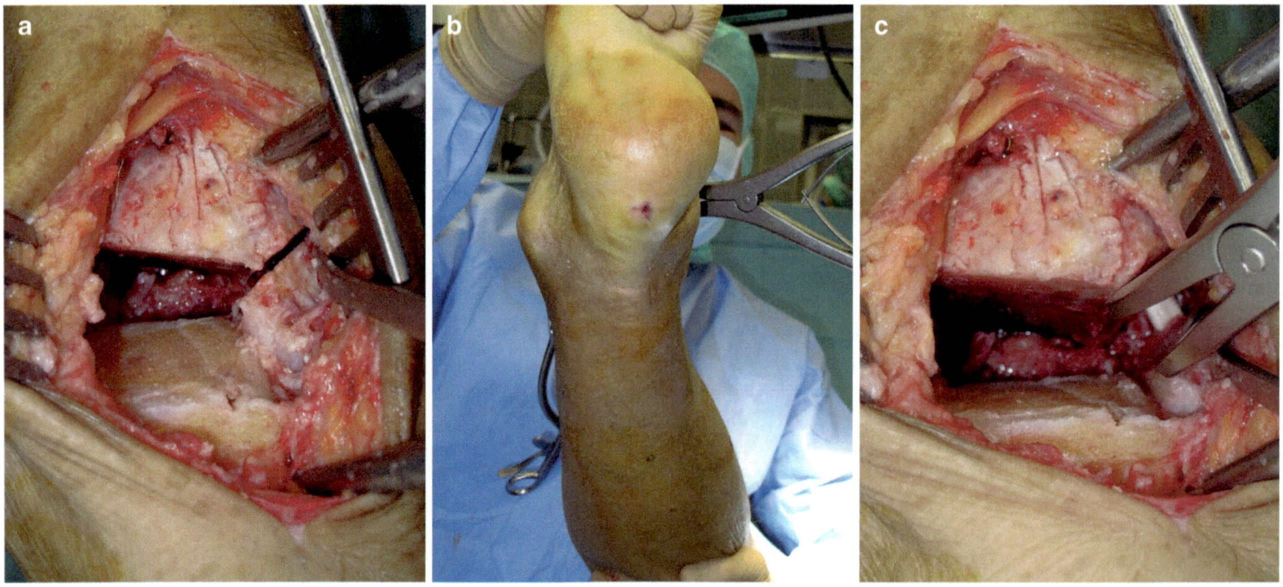

Fig. 9.19 Effect of malleolar osteotomy. (**a**) As long as no distraction to the medial malleolar osteotomy is applied, the foot is seen in varus (**b**). (**c**) With the distraction of the osteotomy, the varus deformity is seen to disappear (**d**)

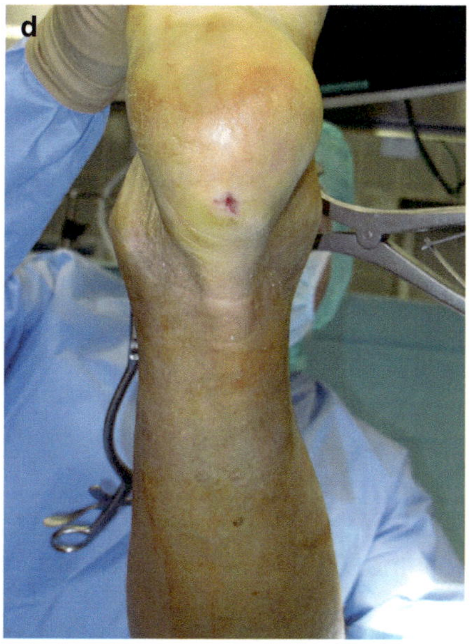

Fig. 9.19 (continued)

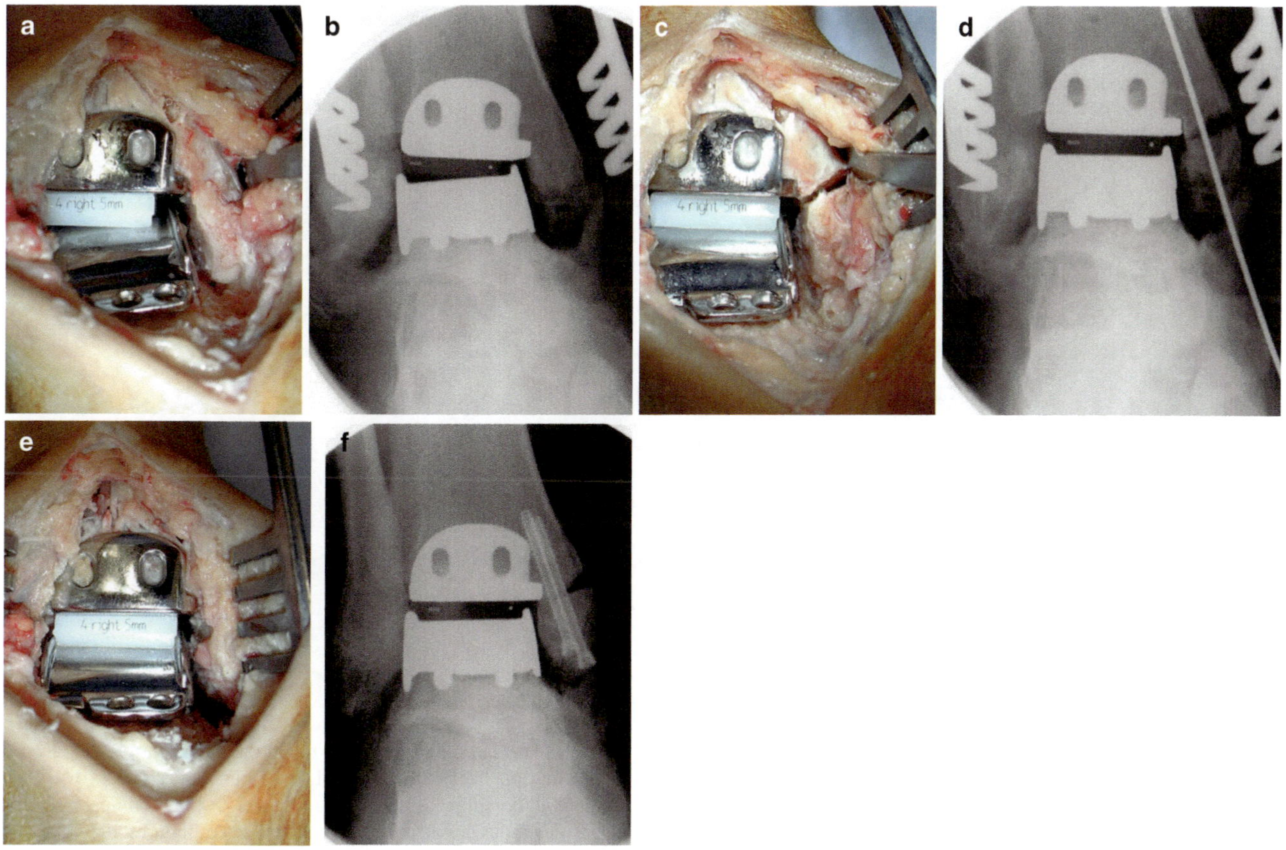

Fig. 9.20 Flip osteotomy of medial malleolus. If the ankle is not balanced at the end of the replacement surgery, as seen by a lateral gapping that will not disappear when valgus stress is applied to the heel, A bony obstacle in the lateral gutter must be excluded first. If this is not the case, it must be a medial contracture, as seen in this case visually (**a**) and with fluoroscopy (**b**). (**c**) An oblique cut in a 45° angle to the tibial component is done by a small saw and finalized with a chisel, paying attention not to damage the posterior tibial and flexor digitorum tendons. While the osteotomy is opened, the talus is seen to turn spontaneously into a normal position. (**d**) While the foot is held in a neutral position, 1 or 2 K-wires are inserted percutaneously for preliminary fixation. Additional pressure can be applied from outside the medial malleolus to close the medial gutter during this maneuver. Cannulated screws are used for final fixation. (**e**) The gap of the osteotomy is filled with bone from previous tibial resection. (**f**) Final fluoroscopic control

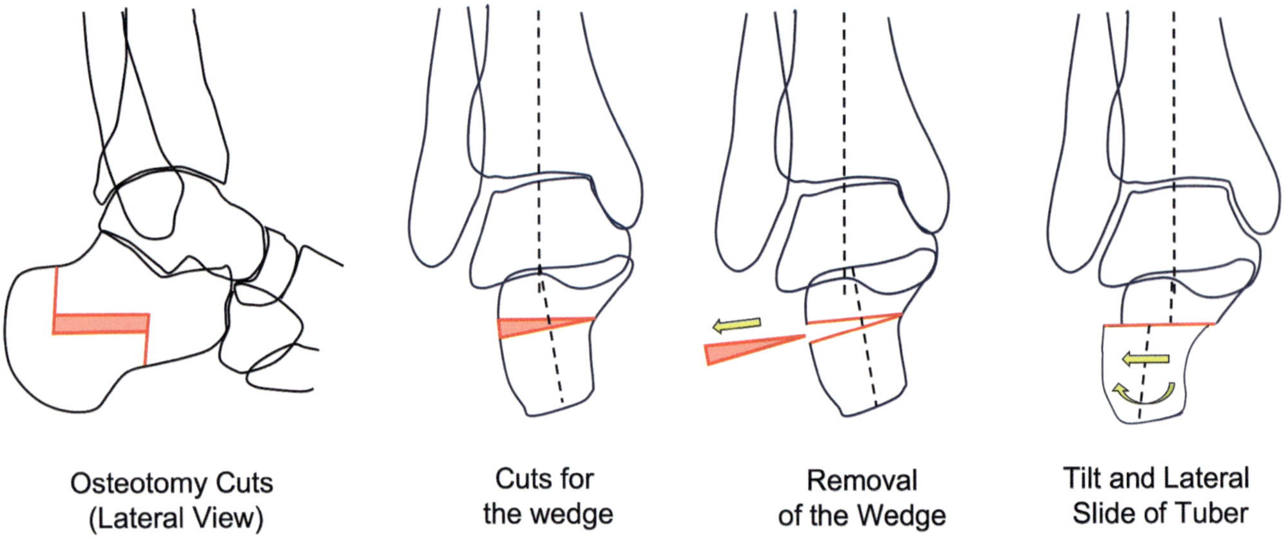

Fig. 9.21 The concept of a Z-osteotomy of calcaneus. The concept of the Z-osteotomy is to remove a wedge in the horizontal plane to tilt the calcaneal tuber into the valgus and to add a lateral sliding of the tuber fragment to increase the effect further

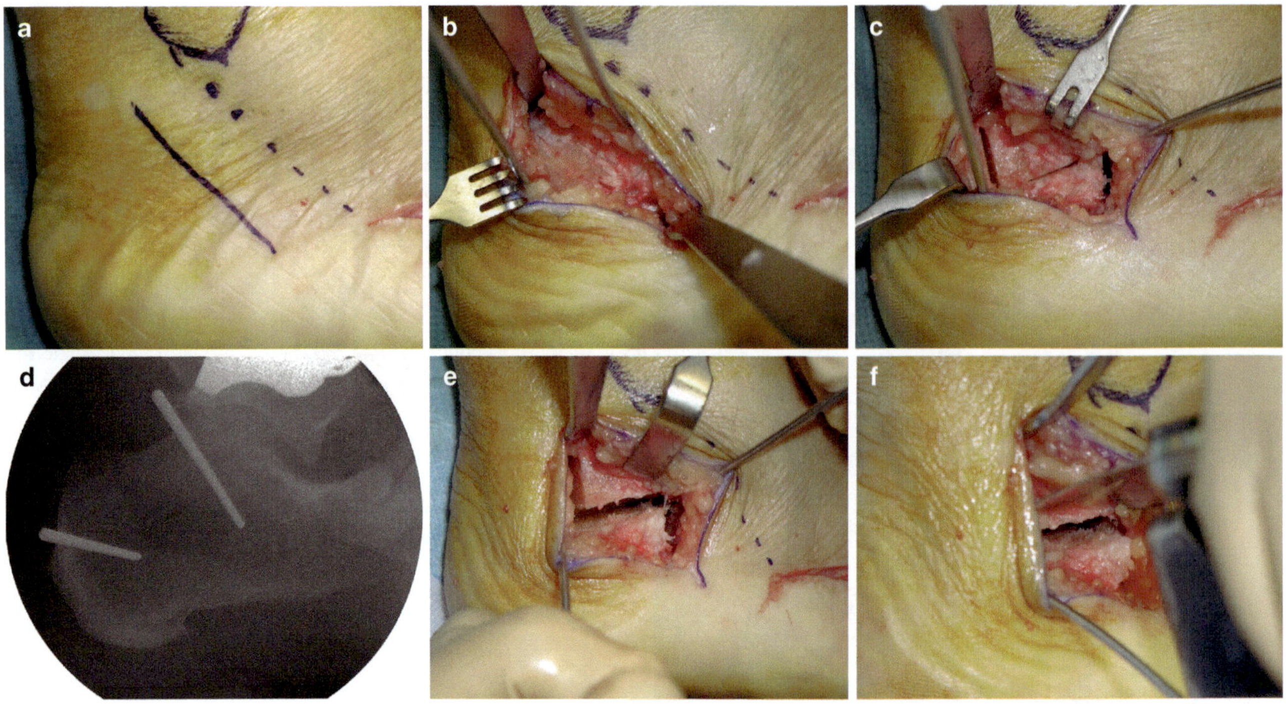

Fig. 9.22 Z-osteotomy of calcaneus. (**a**) The lateral aspect of tuber calcanei is exposed through an oblique incision. (**b–d**) A Z-shaped osteotomy, marked first by K-wires under fluoroscopy, is made with the saw. (**e**) After mobilization of the tuber fragment, a wedge-shaped osteotomy is made along the horizontal cut according to the wanted tilting into the valgus. (**f**) The bone wedge is removed. (**g**) While the foot is held in a plantarflexed position, the tuber fragment is moved lateralward by pushing the heel with one hand or a Hohmann retractor. (**h**) When the foot is dorsiflexed, the osteotomy will become compressed; the tuber undergoes valgisation movement, according to the removed wedge. (**i–j**) After preliminary fixation with K-wires, one or two cannulated screws are used for final fixation (not shown)

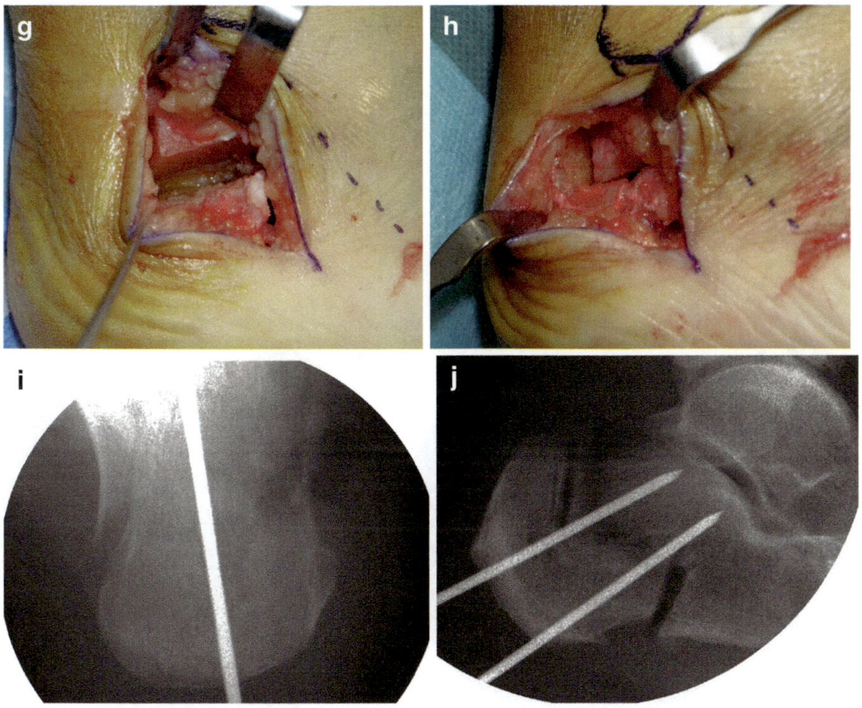

Fig. 9.22 (continued)

Fig. 9.23 The concept of a medial sliding osteotomy of calcaneus. The calcaneal tuber is moved medially as much as needed to get a neutral heel alignment

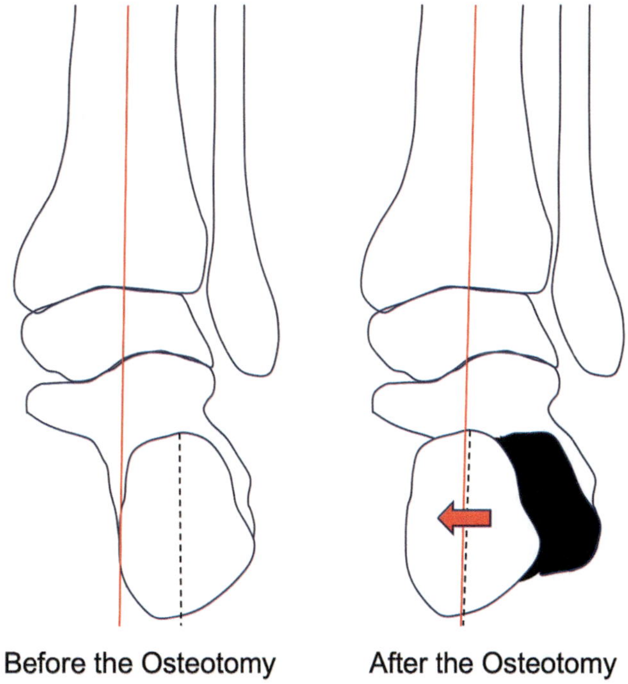

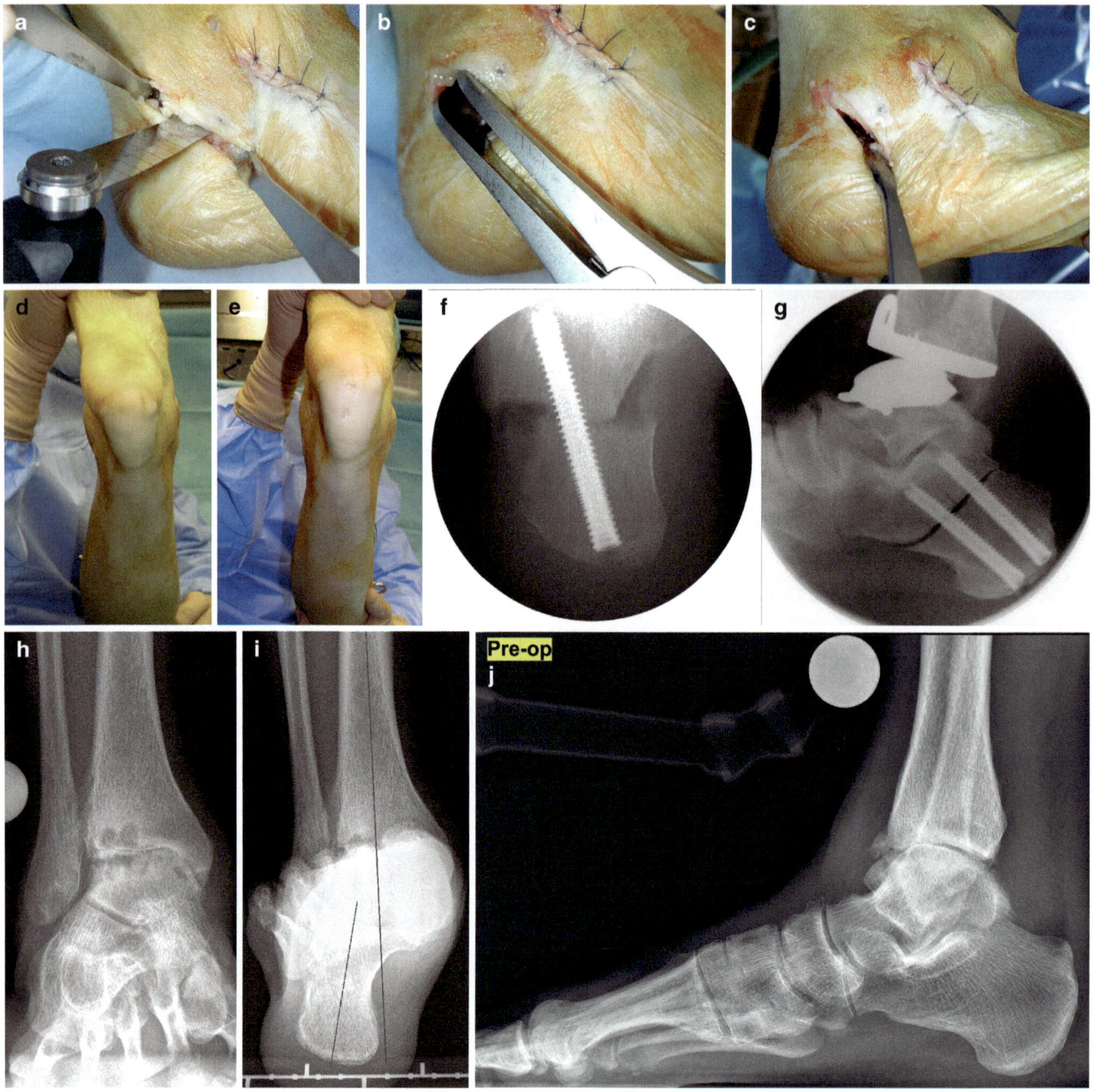

Fig. 9.24 Medial sliding osteotomy of calcaneus. (**a**) Two Hohmann retractors are inserted to protect soft tissues, and the osteotomy is made with the saw. (**b**) While the foot is held in plantarflexion, a lamina-type spreader is used to open the osteotomy and mobilize the tuber fragment. (**c**) The tuber can then be moved medially manually or with a Hohmann retractor and preliminary fixed in position by dorsiflexion of the foot as compression forces are applied to the osteotomy. The correction amount is checked clinically by leg elevation while dorsiflexion is still applied: (**d**) before and (**e**) after shifting the heel. (**f**) Once the wanted position is obtained, one or two screws are used for fixation. Depending on the amount of translation, the screws are inserted in a lateral direction to meet the calcaneal bone. (**g**) Lateral view showing the screw fixation. Notice the beak on the inferior aspect of the tuber fragment created by preserving the inferior cortex from the saw cut and subsequently fracturing it when the osteotomy was distracted. (**h**–**j**) Preoperative radiographs showing the valgus malalignment of the heel. (**k**–**m**) 6 weeks after surgery, the osteotomy is healed with the tuber in a neutral heel alignment. The correction is also seen clinically from a posterior view when comparing the heel alignment preoperatively (**n**) with postoperatively (**o**)

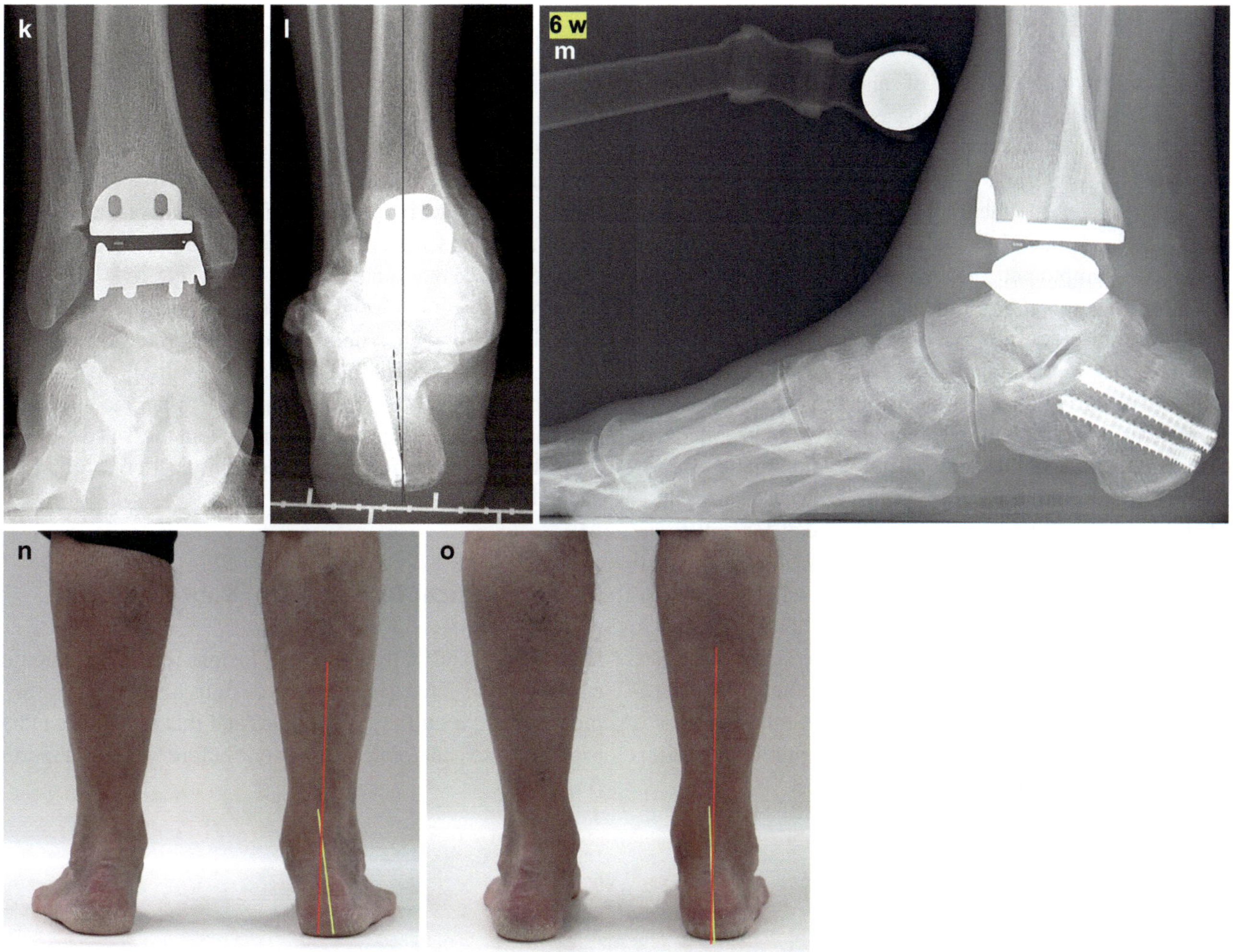

Fig. 9.24 (continued)

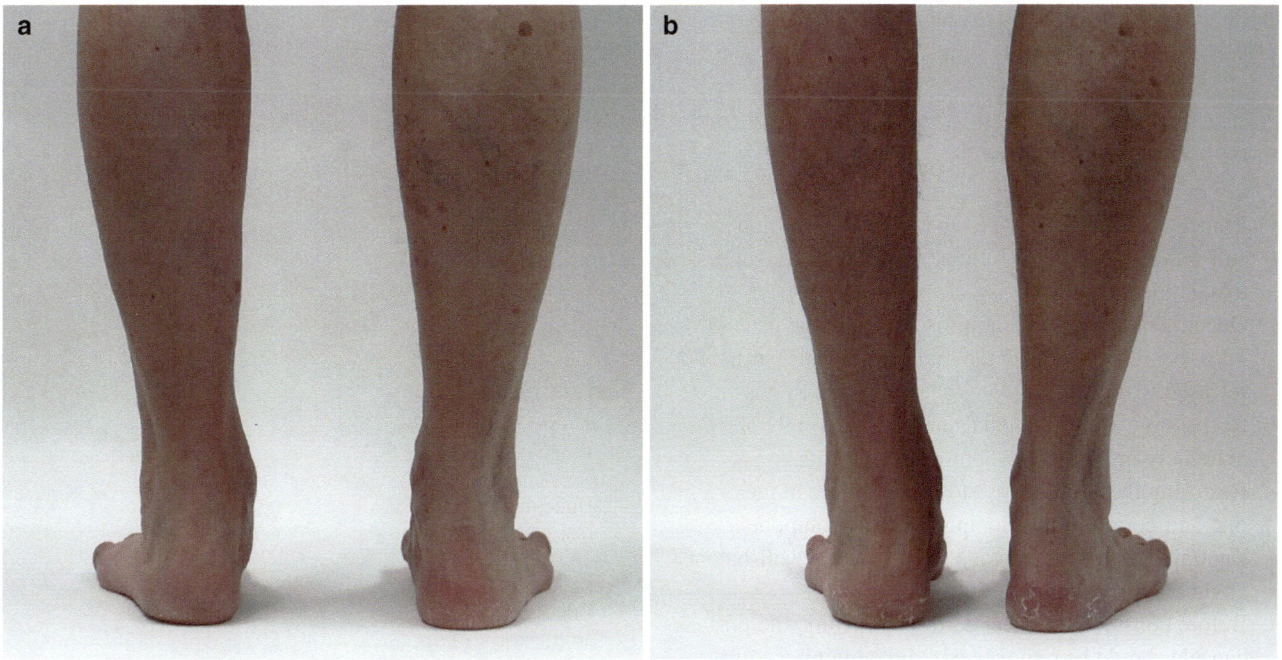

Fig. 9.25 Lateral calcaneal lengthening osteotomy. (**a**) In this 69-year-old female patient, a lateral calcaneal lengthening osteotomy was performed during total ankle arthroplasty because of chronic pain along the posterior tibial tendon associated with a forefoot abduction. (**b**) 12 months postoperatively, the deformity and the medial pain disappeared

9.2 Hindfoot Arthrodeses

Regardless of the etiology of ankle arthritis, in some instances, adjacent joint arthritis is present at the subtalar joint. It remains to be seen whether staged or simultaneous arthrodesis is preferred. The few studies demonstrated the paucity of cases in which both primary total ankle arthroplasty and ipsilateral subtalar arthrodesis are required because of symptomatic degenerative disease, and they did not show that subtalar arthrodesis in association with total ankle arthroplasty results in a decreased outcome [29].

The most common reasons for performing hindfoot arthrodeses during ankle replacement surgery are rigid (not correctable) varus deformity, progressive destabilization associated with a valgus deformity, or symptomatic osteoarthritis of one or more hindfoot joints. However, arthrodesis of the hindfoot does not eliminate the need for soft-tissue releases to correct the deformity or reconstruction to stabilize the ankle. A similar approach is taken whether performing fusions or osteotomies. To the authors' experience, remaining instability and not fully corrected deformities are the leading causes of subsequent failure of total ankle arthroplasty mid-to-long term. This is particularly true for a mobile-bearing ankle prosthesis that does provide only limited intrinsic stability to the replaced ankle.

9.2.1 Assessment and Decision-Making

Inspection of the foot while the patient is standing will allow for recognition of a deformity of the foot and ankle. Functional tests further allow us to recognize whether a deformity is correctable. Weight-bearing standard radiographs are the base for recognizing foot abnormalities and deformities, and they may also help to detect degenerative disease at adjacent joints.

In recent years, a weight-bearing CT scan has become a helpful tool for better understanding of the deformity and destabilization process in all three planes. It allows the surgeon to recognize the extent of articular wear and subchondral changes. It provides information about the 3-D deviation of the bones and the segmental instability pattern of the foot and ankle (Fig. 9.26).

9.2.2 Surgical Technique for Subtalar Fusion

Most importantly, the selected fusion technique should ensure that an extensive stripping of sinus tarsi will not compromise the vascularity of the talus and that the talus can be brought into anatomical position before screw fixation (Fig. 9.27).

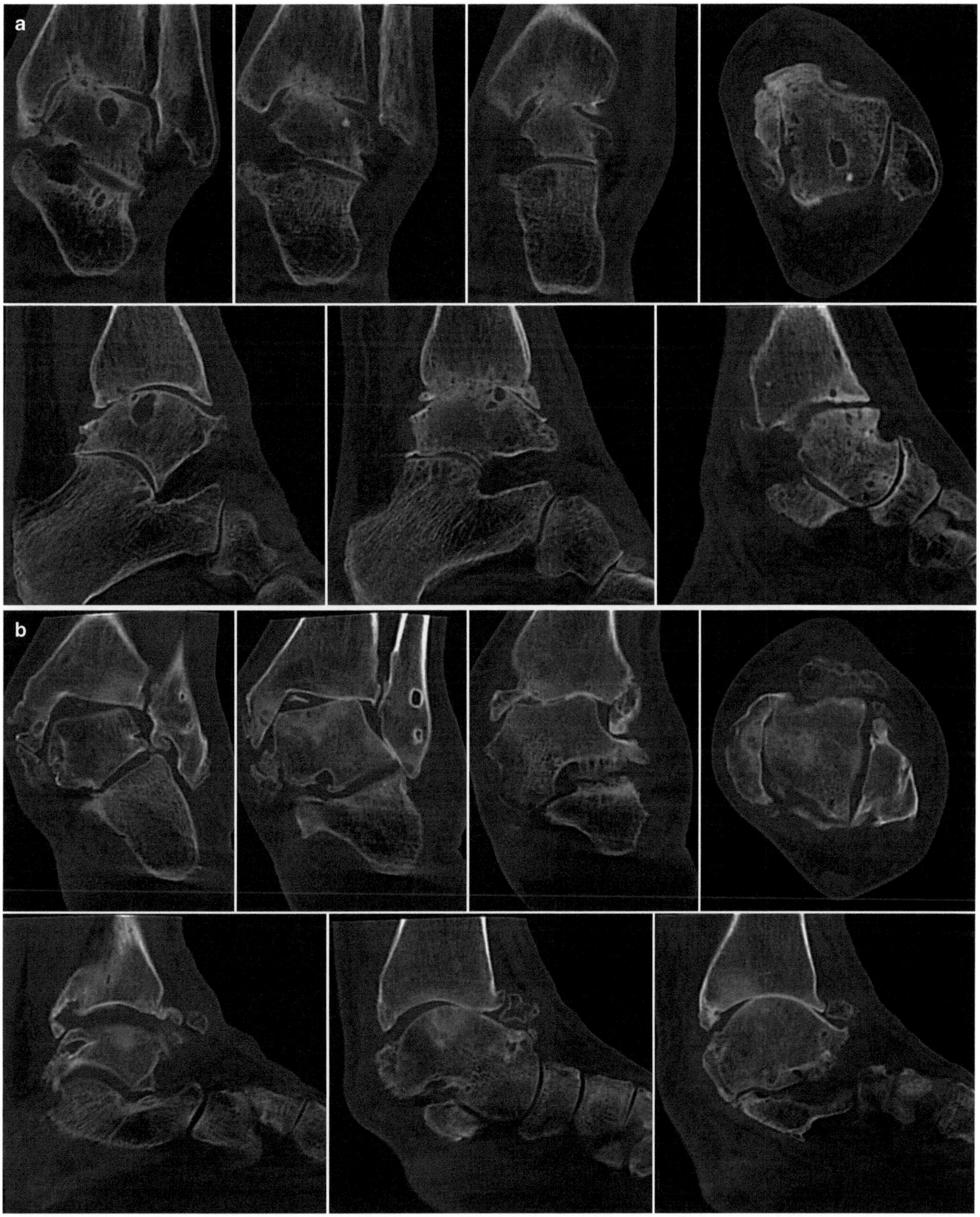

Fig. 9.26 Weight-bearing CT scan in assessing multisegmental instability. The weight-bearing CT scan shows the degenerative disease and the segmental instability in more detail; thus, it is beneficial to identify the whole pathology and make the decision-making process in planning the total ankle arthroplasty. (**a**) Varus ankle osteoarthritis and (**b**) valgus ankle osteoarthritis

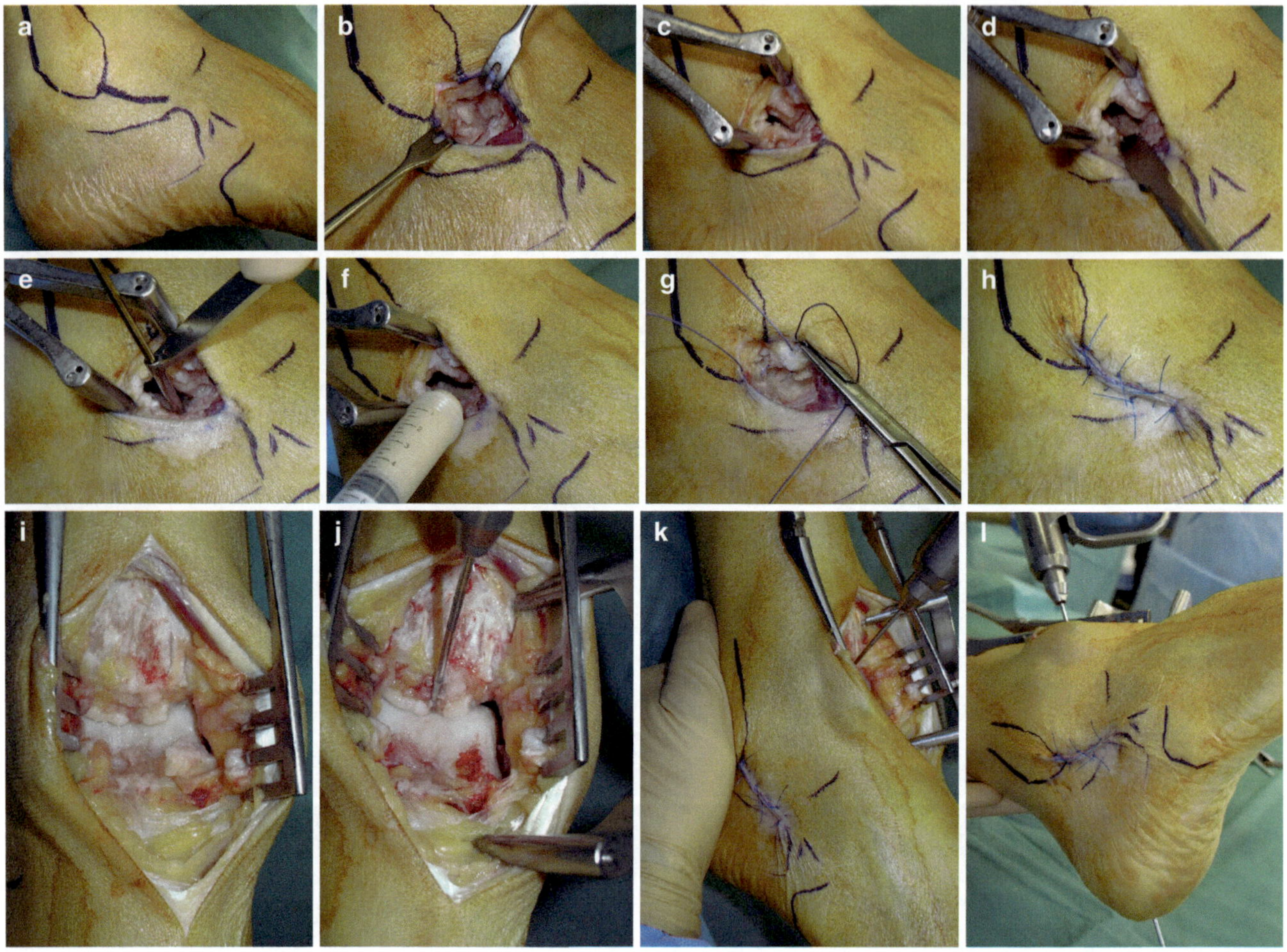

Fig. 9.27 Subtalar fusion. (**a**) The subtalar joint is exposed through a sinus tarsi approach. A 3 cm long incision starts at the anterior border of the fibula along the superior border of the peroneal tendons. (**b**) The subcutaneous layers are dissected to expose the sinus tarsi, and an arthrotomy of the subtalar joint is performed. Notice that the sinus tarsi is not stripped down to preserve the vascularity of the talus. (**c**) A 2.5 mm K-wire is inserted in the lateral process of the talus and another into the calcaneus, allowing for the mounting of the Hintermann distractor to distract the subtalar joint. (**d**) A chisel debrides the posterior facet to the subchondral bone. (**e**) After that, multiple drillings with a 2.5 mm drill are made. (**f**) Bone autograft, allograft, and bone matrix can be inserted before distraction removal. (**g**) The subcutaneous layers are closed by interrupted sutures and skin closure (**h**). (**i**) The ankle joint is exposed through a standard anterior approach. (**j**) While the ankle is sequentially distracted over two 2.5 mm K-wires on the anteromedial aspect, the collateral ligaments are tightened, and the talus is seen to take the intended position in the coronal plane. While the foot is held in a slightly plantarflexed position, the center of the talus will be exposed, allowing a guiding K-wire for the attempted cannulated screw to be inserted. (**k**) While the position of the heel is controlled by one hand, the K-wire is inserted into the direction of the heel. Attention is paid to removing the hand before the K-wire penetrates the opposite bone cortex and appears at the heel (**l**). (**m**) After having changed the power machine to the K-wire at its opposite end, it is pulled further until its end reaches the articular surface of the talus (arrow), allowing now to determine the length of the screw to be used with the aid of another K-wire and a ruler (**n**). Approximately 10 mm is deduced from the measured length to make sure that the screw will be far enough from the resection cut at the talar apex. (**o**) A cannulated screw is now inserted from the heel into the talus. If desired, a second screw can be positioned and inserted in the same way, 10 to 15 mm more posteriorly. (**p**) Finally, a guiding K-wire is brought from the talar head slightly lateralward in the anterior process of the calcaneus that will serve to insert an additional cannulated screw, providing rotational stability (**q**). Fluoroscopy is used to final check the screw position in the sagittal (**r**) and coronal (**s**) planes. Notice the central position of the screws in the talar body so there will be no fear of conflicts with the talar component. (**t**) After that, the replacement surgery uses the standard instrumentation set of the used ankle prostheses. (**u**) After the insertion of components, the ankle is well-balanced and stable. (**v–w**) Fluoroscopy for final control of the component position

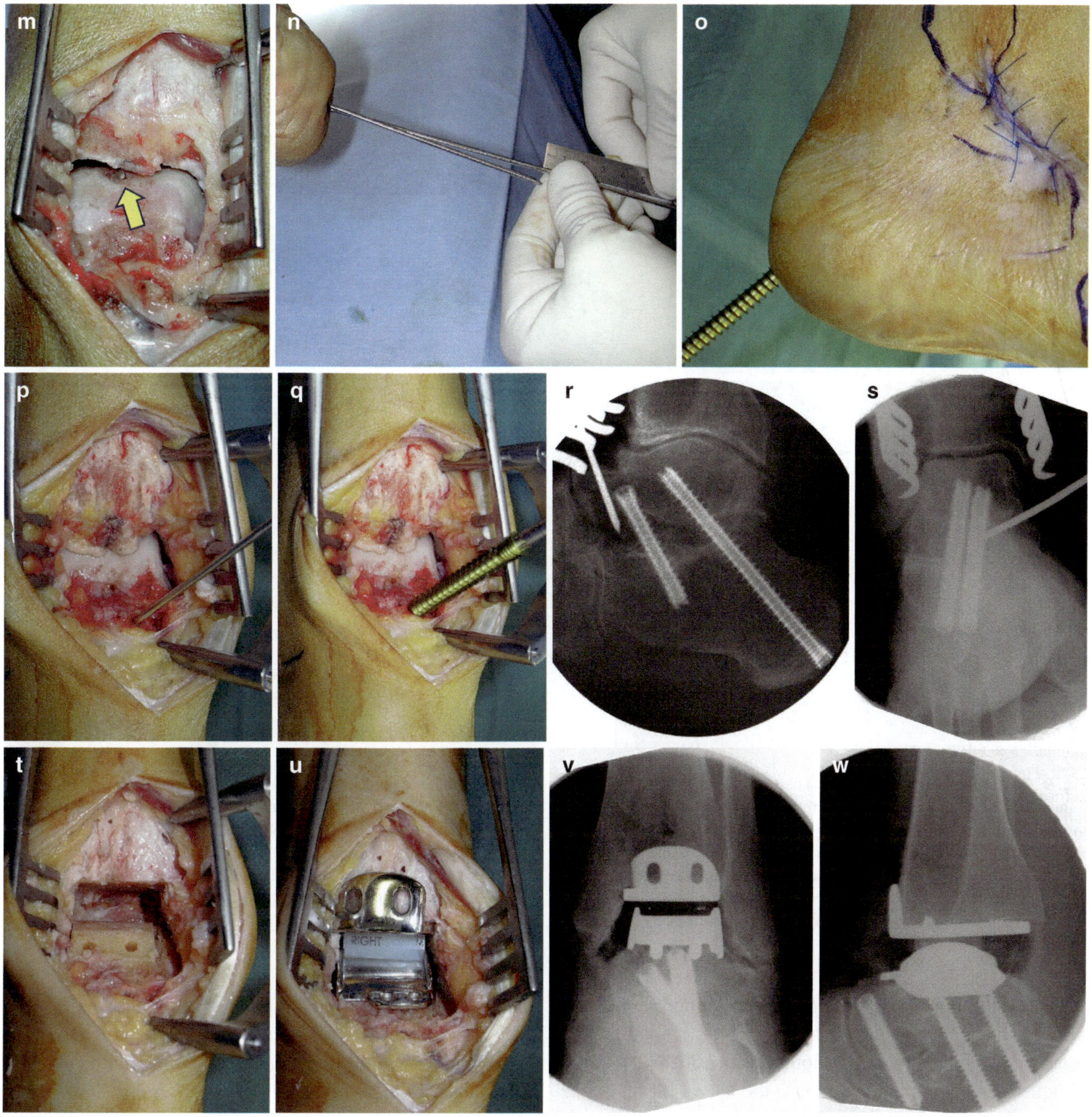

Fig. 9.27 (continued)

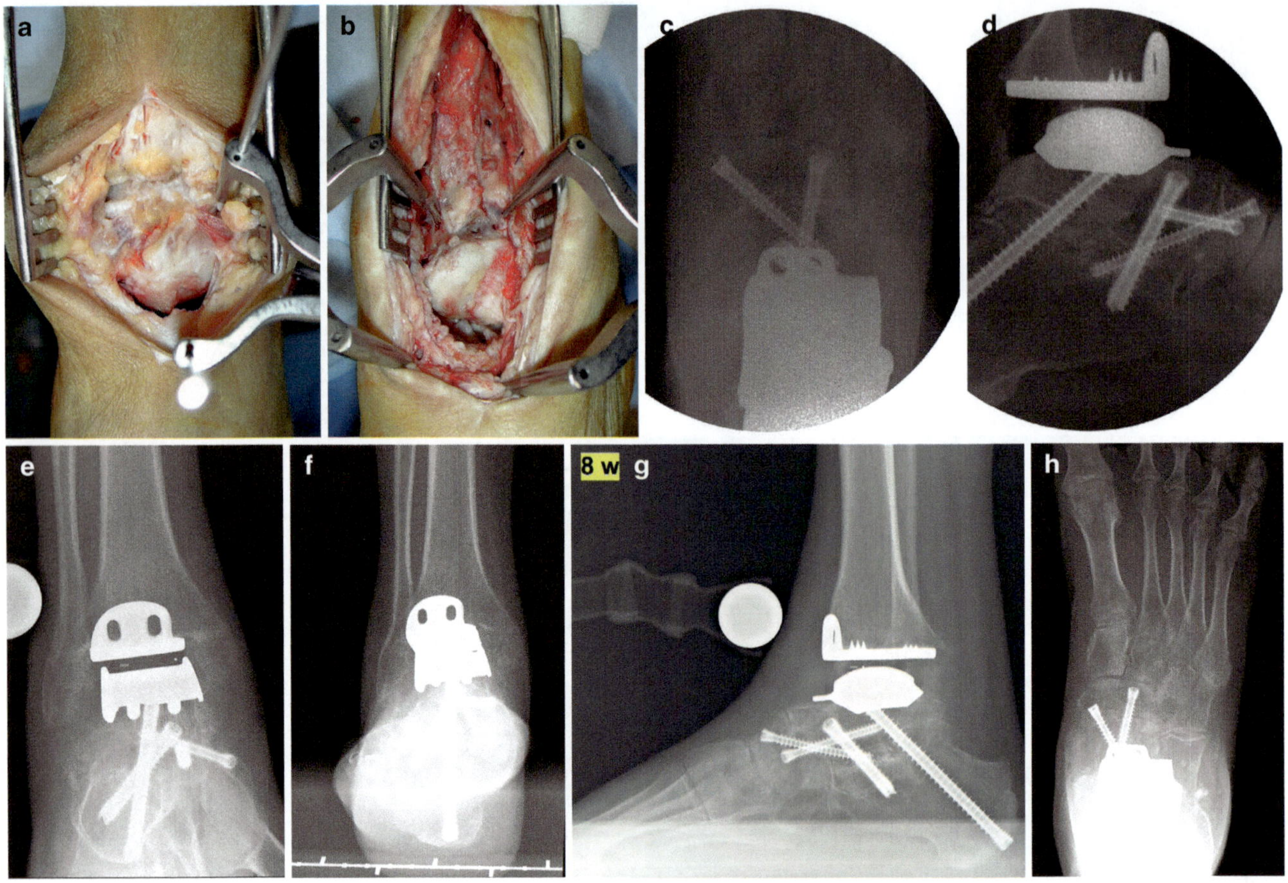

Fig. 9.28 Talonavicular fusion. (**a**) The anterior incision to the ankle joint is lengthened distally to expose the talonavicular joint. K-wires are inserted at the medial side into the talus and navicular bone, respectively, and the joint is distracted by a Hintermann distractor. (**b**) To better expose the talonavicular joint and to facilitate final correction, a second Hintermann distractor may be applied over two K-wires on the lateral aspect of these bones. The articular surfaces are debrided to the subchondral bone, and some drillings are done in the case of osteosclerosis. After that, the distraction is removed, and the foot position is corrected to neutral, paying attention to entirely correct forefoot supination and abduction. (**c**–**d**) Two to three screws are used for fixation. (**e**–**h**) Usually, the arthrodesis is seen to be united within 8 weeks while protected in a boot and permitted weight-bearing as tolerated

If the hindfoot is still in valgus after preliminary fixation of the subtalar joint with the first K-wire, a medial sliding osteotomy of the calcaneus should be considered. A short oblique incision is made to expose the lateral aspect of the calcaneal tuber. While the foot is in position, the K-wire is retracted under fluoroscopy (e.g., toward the talus) as much as needed to get it out of the intended osteotomy site. After that, the osteotomy is done with an oscillating saw, and after mobilization, the calcaneal tuber is moved toward medially as needed to get an aligned hindfoot (Fig. 9.24). Now, the K-wire is brought again anterior-ward into the tuberosity, followed by screw fixation as described above.

The Authors' Approach

Following the release of potential contractures at the subtalar joint and tightening of the ligaments by the distraction of the collapsed tibiotalar joint, anatomic talar orientation in all three planes can best be achieved when the heel is kept with one hand in a neutral position, and the foot is brought into maximal dorsiflexion with the other hand. Besides putting the subtalar joint under compression, this maneuver exercises a translational force anterior-ward to the talus. Notice that the ankle joint is distracted just as much as to get the talus in a neutral position (coronal plane); if overtightened, the talus is typically seen to tilt into the varus.

9.2.3 Surgical Technique for Talonavicular Fusion

In the case of severe degenerative changes at the talonavicular joint or in a rigid, not correctable varus deformity, a fusion of the talonavicular joint might be considered. It can be done as an isolated procedure or in addition to the subtalar joint (Fig. 9.28).

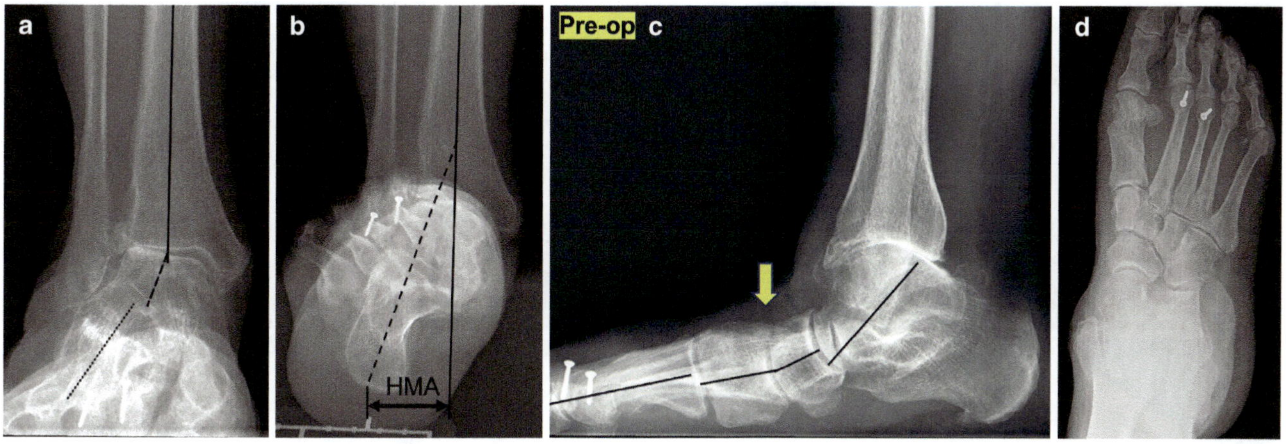

Fig. 9.29 Breakdown of medial arch. A 59-year-old female patient suffering from progressive lateral ankle pain that subsequently led to a medial arch collapse. (**a**) The AP radiograph shows a significant tilt of the talus within the widened ankle mortise, and the talus had started to tilt into the valgus. (**b**) The valgus malalignment of the heel accounts for a heel moment arm of >40 mm. (**c**) The main sag of the collapsed medial arch is located at the naviculocuneiform joints, but the talonavicular and tarsometatarsal joints are also involved. (**d**) Some talar head uncovering is also seen, but the forefoot abduction is moderate

The Authors' Approach

In the case of isolated osteoarthritis of the talonavicular joint, an isolated fusion of this joint is made. The subtalar joint should also be fused for a severe varus deformity or a peritalar instability associated with a progressive collapsing foot deformity.

9.2.4 Surgical Technique for Arthrodesis of Medial Arch

In the case of a breakdown of the medial arch (Fig. 9.29), correction and stabilization arthrodesis might be considered at naviculocuneiform (Fig. 9.30) and/or tarsometatarsal (Fig. 9.31) joints, in most instances in addition to a subtalar fusion. If so, the subtalar fusion is made first.

In the case of a breakdown at the tarsometatarsal joint, the incision is made more distally, and the first tarsometatarsal joint is exposed, distracted, and debrided to the subchondral bone. The same technique is used to apply compression at the attempted fusion site, and stable fixation is achieved by one to two screws and a plate (Fig. 9.31).

The Authors' Experience

Achieving a stable foot in the neutral position in total ankle arthroplasty is a vital portion of the operative procedure, and its effectiveness directly influences the quality of the replacement. This is particularly true for the collapsed foot, typically associated with peritalar destabilization and breakdown of the medial arch. The main working horse is the subtalar joint fusion; however, an additional fusion of talonavicular or naviculocuneiform joints is often necessary to achieve this goal. If hindfoot misalignment persists despite these measures, a medial sliding osteotomy should be performed to obtain a neutral ankle joint load. Though fusion procedures are most effective for proper reorientation and stabilizing the ankle, there is, in some instances, a need for additional soft-tissue procedures.

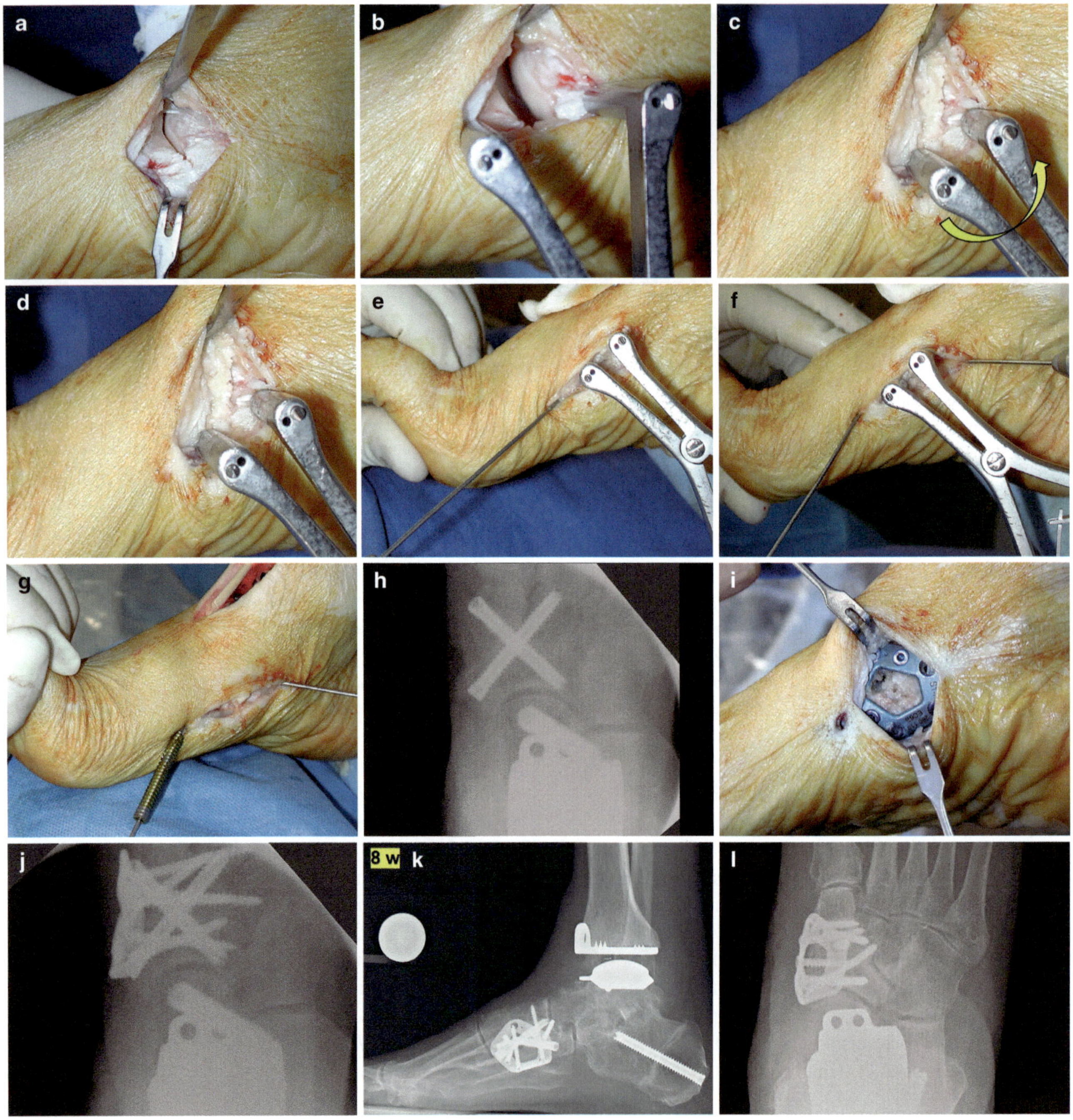

Fig. 9.30 Naviculocuneiform fusion. (**a**) The naviculocuneiform joints are exposed through a 3–4 cm incision at the medial aspect of the foot. (**b**) Distraction is applied over two K-wires to expose the three joints. After that, the naviculocuneiform joints I–III are debrided to the subchondral bone, carefully resecting as minimal bone as possible and preserving the joints' original rounded shape. Some subchondral drilling may be added. (**c**) The distractor is then replaced by a compression device using the same K-wires, and compression is applied. During this maneuver, most importantly, the compression device is swayed until the forefoot is seen to be in the neutral position, e.g., the forefoot supination has disappeared (**d**). Enforced dorsiflexion of the great toe may assist in achieving an appropriate plantarflexed position of the first ray and additional compression at the fusion site. (**e**) First, a guiding K-wire is inserted from the distal aspect of cuneiform I into the lateral navicular and (**f**) then a second one from the tuberosity of the navicular into the cuneiform II. (**g**) A 5-mm-full-treated screw is inserted over each guiding wire, and the final position is checked by fluoroscopy (**h**). (**i**) A medioplantar tension bending plate is used to enhance stability. (**j–l**) The final check by fluoroscopy shows an appropriate realignment at the talonavicular joint. Postoperatively, the foot is protected by a walking boot, and weight-bearing as tolerated was permitted. After 8 weeks, the fusion is seen to be united

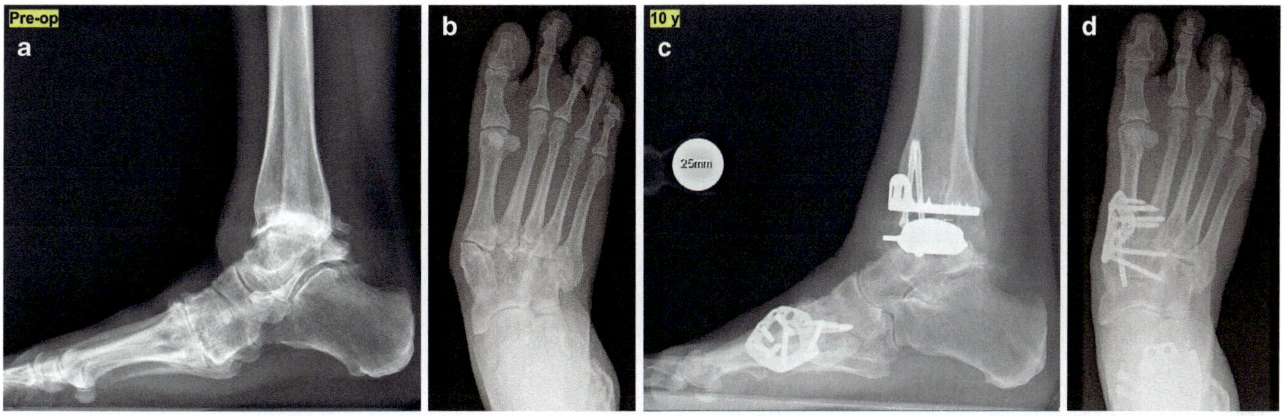

Fig. 9.31 Tarsometatarsal fusion. See text. In this 56-year-old former high-level runner, the preoperative radiographs show the sag clearly at tarsometatarsal joints in the sagittal (**a**) and horizontal (**b**) plane. (**c–d**) 10 years after tarsometatarsal I and II fusion and replacement surgery, the foot is stable, with a well-balanced ankle

9.3 Ligament Reconstructions

Proper soft-tissue balancing during total ankle arthroplasty is paramount to ensure long-term success postoperatively. Even minimal coronal plane deformity may necessitate some degree of soft-tissue release for balancing. Suppose the talus tends to invert, lateral ligament reconstruction is inadequate to reposition the talus, and further bone resection, a medial release of soft tissues, or osteotomy of medial malleolus should be performed. Addressing the challenge of coronal plane deformities by various ancillary procedures simultaneously with total ankle arthroplasty has shown comparable outcomes in ankles with moderate-to-severe deformity [30–32]. Instability after primary total ankle arthroplasty, in contrast, has been reported as one of the major factors for early revision and poor outcomes [33].

If the ankle sits in a neutral position at rest but demonstrates significant instability with an inversion stress test (lateral joint opens), then lateral ligament reconstruction should be performed.

9.3.1 Assessment and Indication

Medial or lateral instability of the ankle joint complex and a destabilization of the medial arch can best be seen when the patient is asked to load the foot [34]. The anterior drawer test may indicate instability while sitting. However, its reliability could have been better, likely because the average amount of clinically meaningful talocrural laxity is small and varies considerably, making it difficult to perceive with a manual test [35]. Recently, the weight-bearing CT scan has evolved to be a helpful tool for better understanding the deformity and destabilization process in all three planes (Fig. 9.32). It allows the surgeon to recognize the extent of articular wear and subchondral changes. It provides information about the 3-D deviation of the bones and the segmental instability pattern of the foot and ankle. Stress-testing the ankle under fluoroscopy in the coronal (Fig. 9.33) and sagittal (Fig. 9.34) plane provides additional information on what the surgeon must expect during surgery. While varus tilt of the talus increases under varus stress, it may indicate incompetence of lateral ligaments. If the valgus test does not reduce talar tilt, a medial soft-tissue contracture or bony obstacle in the lateral gutter may hinder the talus from moving back against neutral. In a valgus ankle, varus stress may detect lateral ankle instability, whereas valgus stress associated with foot abduction may evidence syndesmotic incompetence. Anterior and posterior drawer tests may provide further information about the instability pattern.

9.3.2 Lateral Ligament Reconstruction

In most instances, a primary Broström-type reconstruction of lateral ligaments is possible [34, 36, 37]. If there is an anterolateral instability with only distinct lateral gapping when applying varus stress, a ligament repair through the anterior incision can be considered (Fig. 9.35). In major lateral ankle instability, the lateral ligaments are exposed through a slightly curved 3- to 4-cm-long incision (Fig. 9.36). After bone removal and re-shaping of the fibula to normal contour, ligaments can be re-attached using transosseous sutures or bony anchors. If the remaining ligamentous tissue is incompetent, augmentation by an internal brace or tendon graft may support the reconstruction [34, 38] (Fig. 9.37). However, isometric reconstruction of the ligaments is mandatory to ensure free motion and stability (Fig. 9.38).

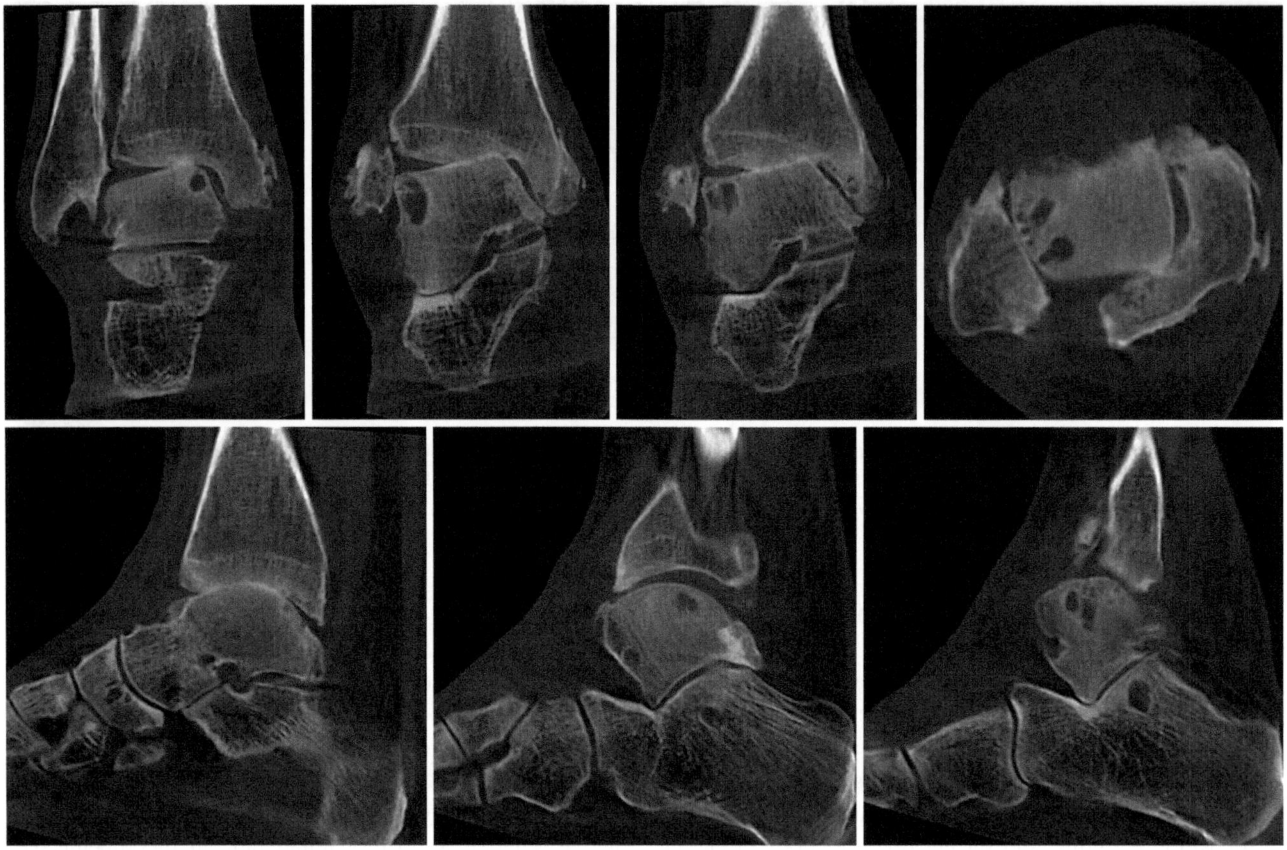

Fig. 9.32 Weight-bearing CT scan in assessing segmental instability. The weight-bearing CT scan shows the degenerative disease and the segmental instability in all three planes; in particular, it shows the position of the subtalar joint as opposed to the ankle joint and the malrotation of the talus within the ankle mortise

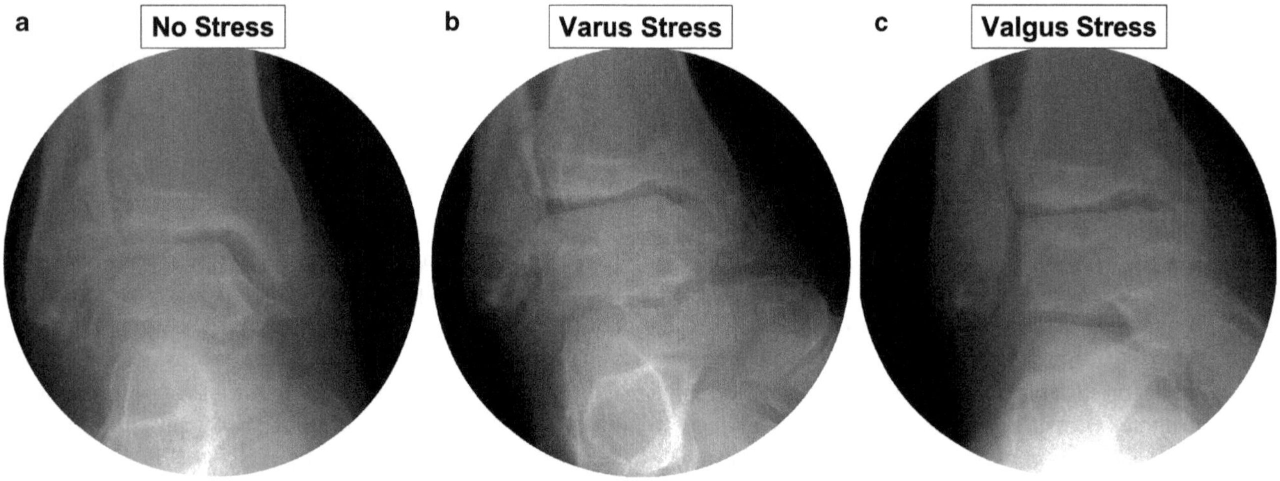

Fig. 9.33 Assessment of coronal plane instability. (**a**) No stress, (**b**) varus stress, and (**c**) valgus stress (see text)

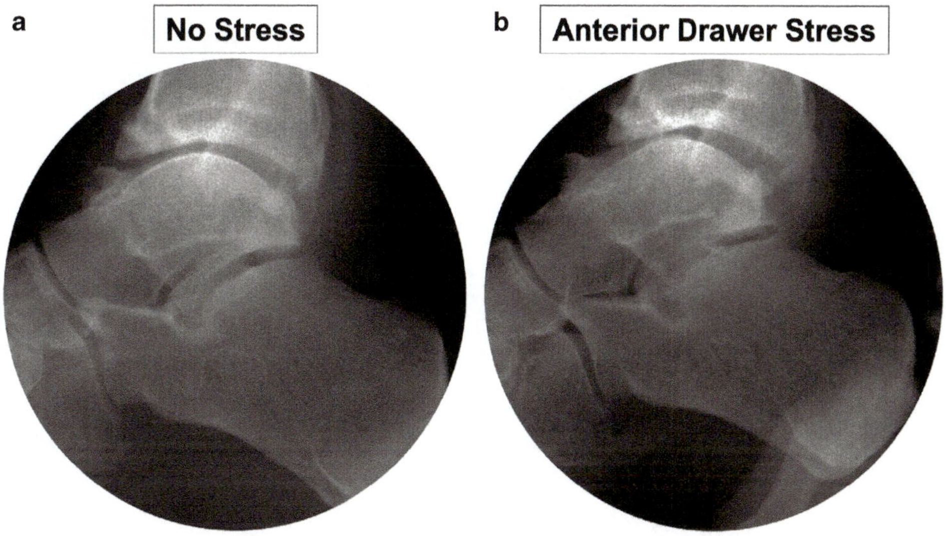

Fig. 9.34 Assessment of sagittal plane instability. (**a**) No stress and (**b**) anterior drawer stress (see text)

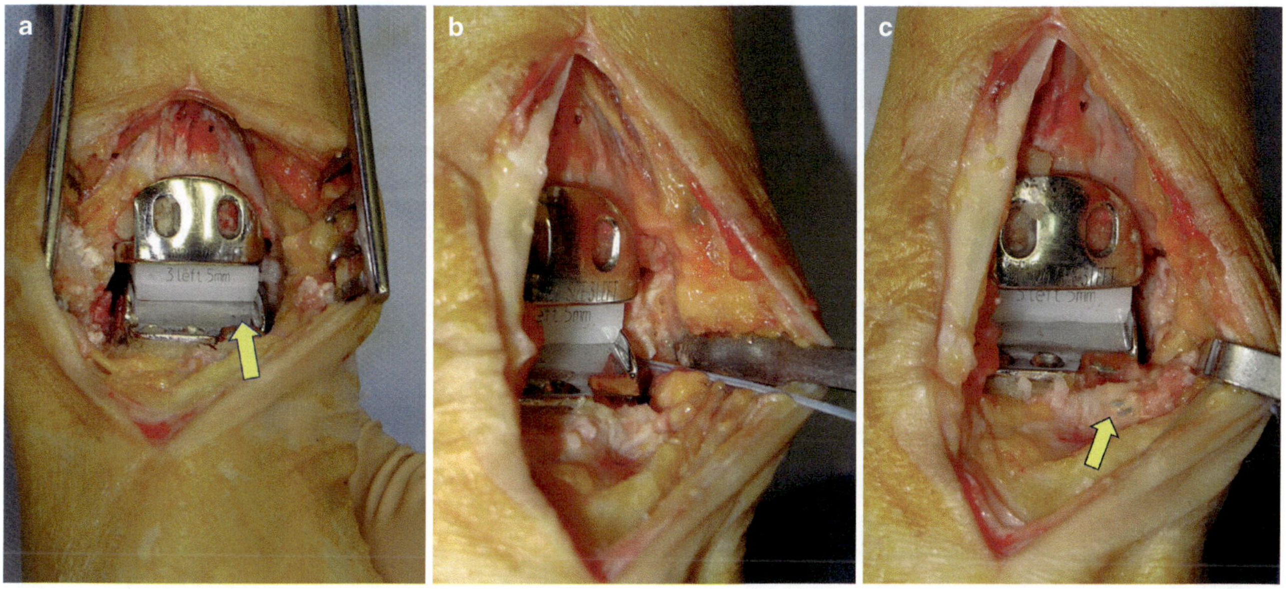

Fig. 9.35 Repair anterior talofibular ligament. (**a**) A distinct lateral gapping (arrow) can be seen in this left ankle when varus stress is applied to the foot. (**b**) The lateral malleolus is exposed through the anterior approach, and a bone anchor is placed as distally as possible. (**c**) The desattached ligament is caught with the suture and tightened. The arrow shows the knot close to the insertion of the anterior talofibular ligament to the talar neck

9.3.3 Medial Ligament Reconstruction

Deltoid ligament insufficiency is the most challenging issue to address adequately during ankle replacement surgery. Many methods of repair and reconstruction of the deltoid ligament have been described, but no single method has demonstrated superior results thus far [34, 39–44].

In distinct instability caused by an incompetent superficial deltoid ligament, a repair can be considered through the anterior approach analogously to the lateral side (Fig. 9.39). The incompetence of the deep deltoid ligament is typically associated with a talar tilt within the ankle mortise. If medial talar tilt does not exceed 10° or half of the length of the medial malleolus, a medially stable ankle can be achieved

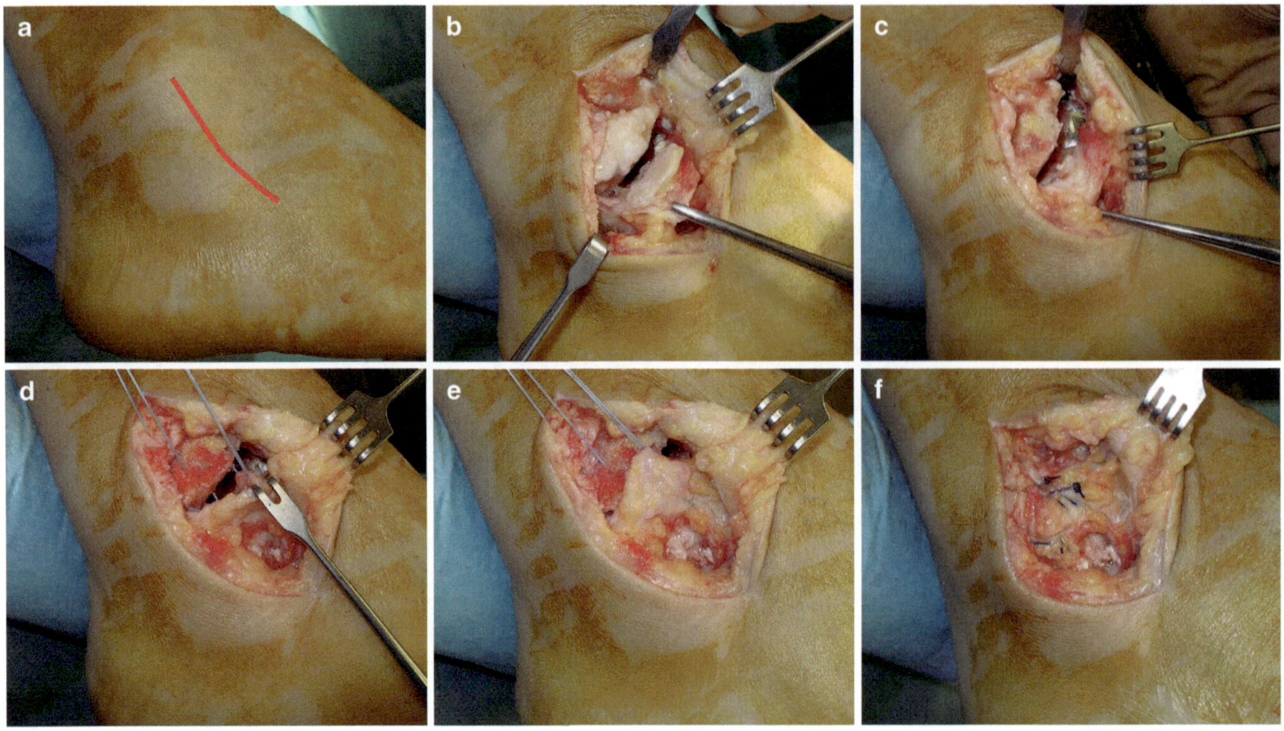

Fig. 9.36 Broström-type reconstruction lateral ankle ligaments. (**a**) A 3- to 4-cm-long incision starts over the distal fibula and ends close to the sinus tarsi. (**b**) An old bony avulsion is attached to well-preserved ligaments in this case. (**c**) The fragment is removed, and the fibula is debrided. (**d**) The ligaments are cached with strong sutures, and a transosseous fixation is prepared. (**e**) While the sutures are tightened, the ankle ligaments are seen to get restored as a fan-shaped anatomical construct. (**f**) Final sutures are used to get a strong ligament construct

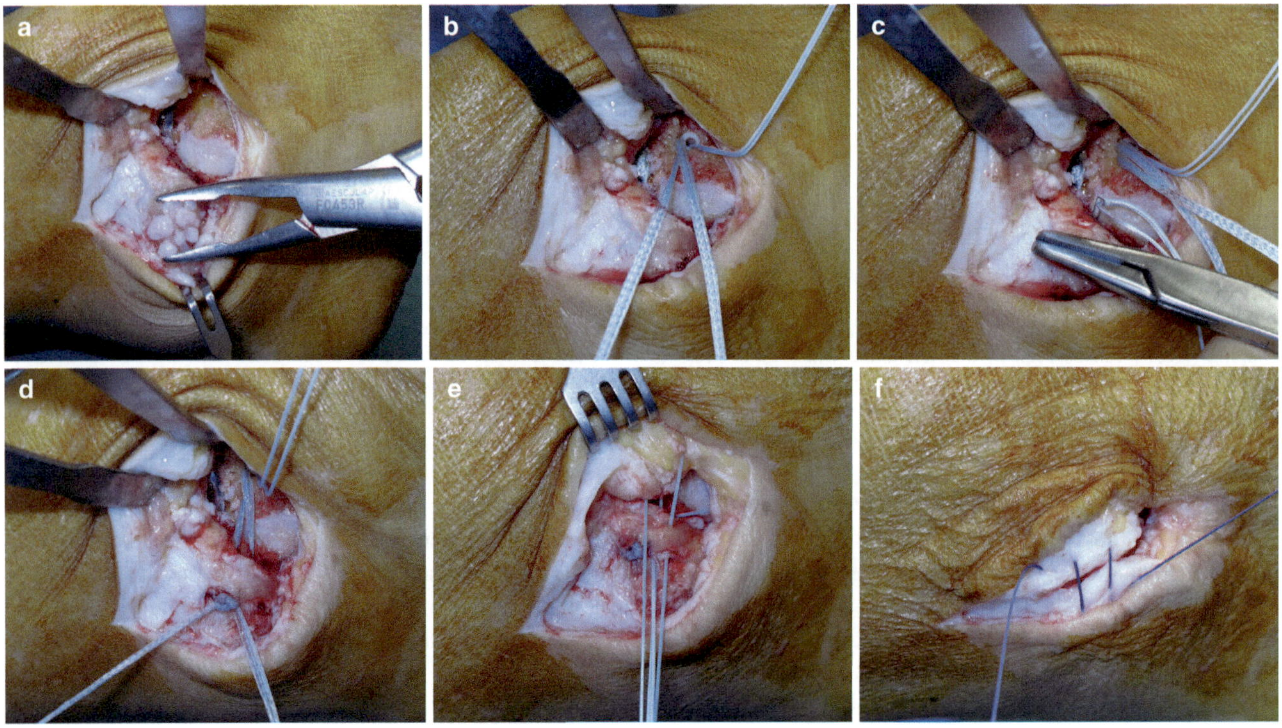

Fig. 9.37 Reconstruction of lateral ankle ligaments with internal brace. (**a**) In this case, insufficient ligament material is preserved for appropriate reconstruction. The insertion area of the fibula and the talar neck is debrided. (**b**) The internal brace is fixed to the talar neck. (**c**). Transosseous fixation is prepared at the fibula site. (**d**) The internal brace is tightened, and a knot is made. (**e**) The second fiber wire caches the remaining scarred ligament tissue. (**f**) Final side-to-side repair of the scarred superficial layers

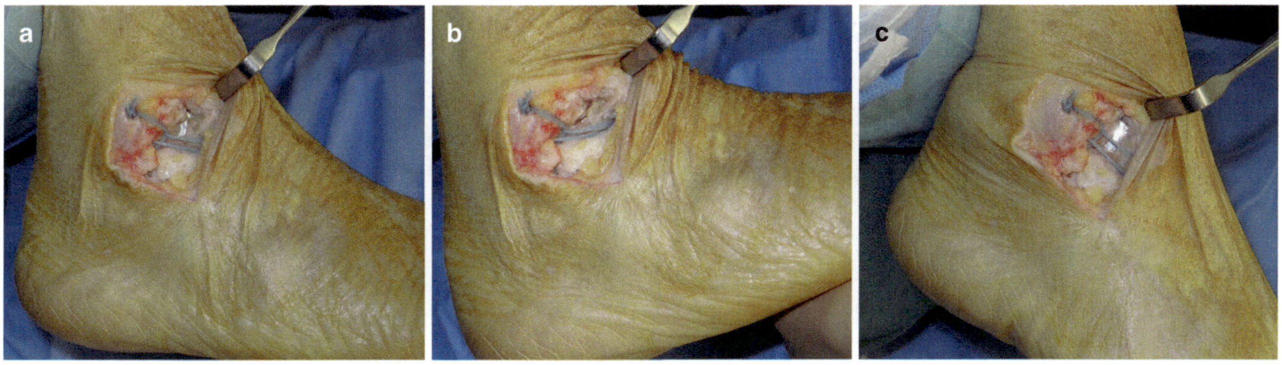

Fig. 9.38 Testing of isometric position. In this patient, a reconstruction of the lateral ankle ligaments was done with an internal brace, including a second loop to the calcaneus (calcaneofibular ligament). The isometric of the reconstructed ligaments can be tested when the foot I brought from neutral (**a**) into a dorsiflexed (**b**) and plantarflexed (**c**) position

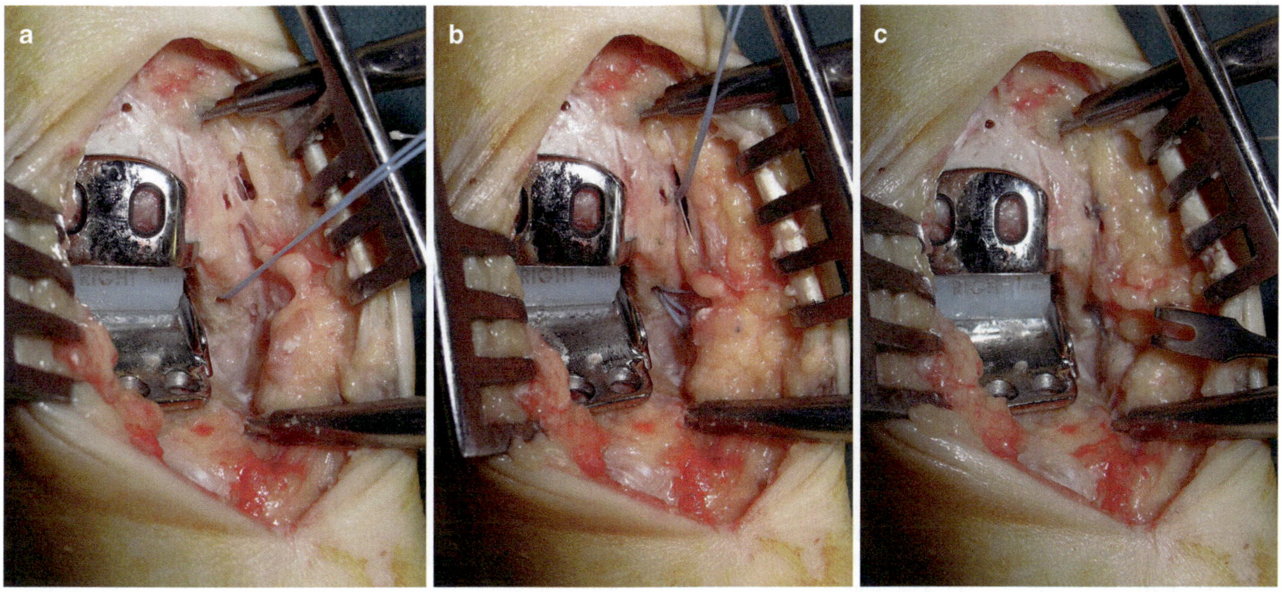

Fig. 9.39 Repair of superficial deltoid ligament. The incompetence of the superficial deltoid ligament can be recognized in an anteromedial rotational instability of the talus within the mortise as provoked by the anterior drawer test. (**a**) The medial malleolus is roughened with a rongeur, and a suture anchor is inserted at the anterior aspect of the anterior colliculus. (**b**) The superficial deltoid complex is then reefed and repaired to the medial malleolus using the suture anchor. (**c**) Final result

with the use of the prosthesis as a spacer (Fig. 9.40). In this case, minimal bone resection is attempted on the tibial side, and a thicker polyethylene insert may be used to tension the medial ankle ligaments properly. If the valgus is >10° and the deltoid ligament is grossly incompetent, a two-stage procedure with first a ligament reconstruction and, if necessary, additional fusions or an ankle fusion are considered.

Some techniques for reconstructing incompetent medial ankle ligaments have been proposed in the literature, but they have yet to prove long-term success. Most proposed techniques use non-anatomic deltoid ligament reconstruction by tendon grafts or internal braces, including tibionavicular tenodesis [39, 45, 46]. The authors prefer an anatomic reconstruction using a free plantaris tendon graft, with or without internal brace augmentation [34]. However, there is consent that deltoid ligament incompetence resulting in a talar tilt of >10° is a relative contraindication for a total ankle arthroplasty.

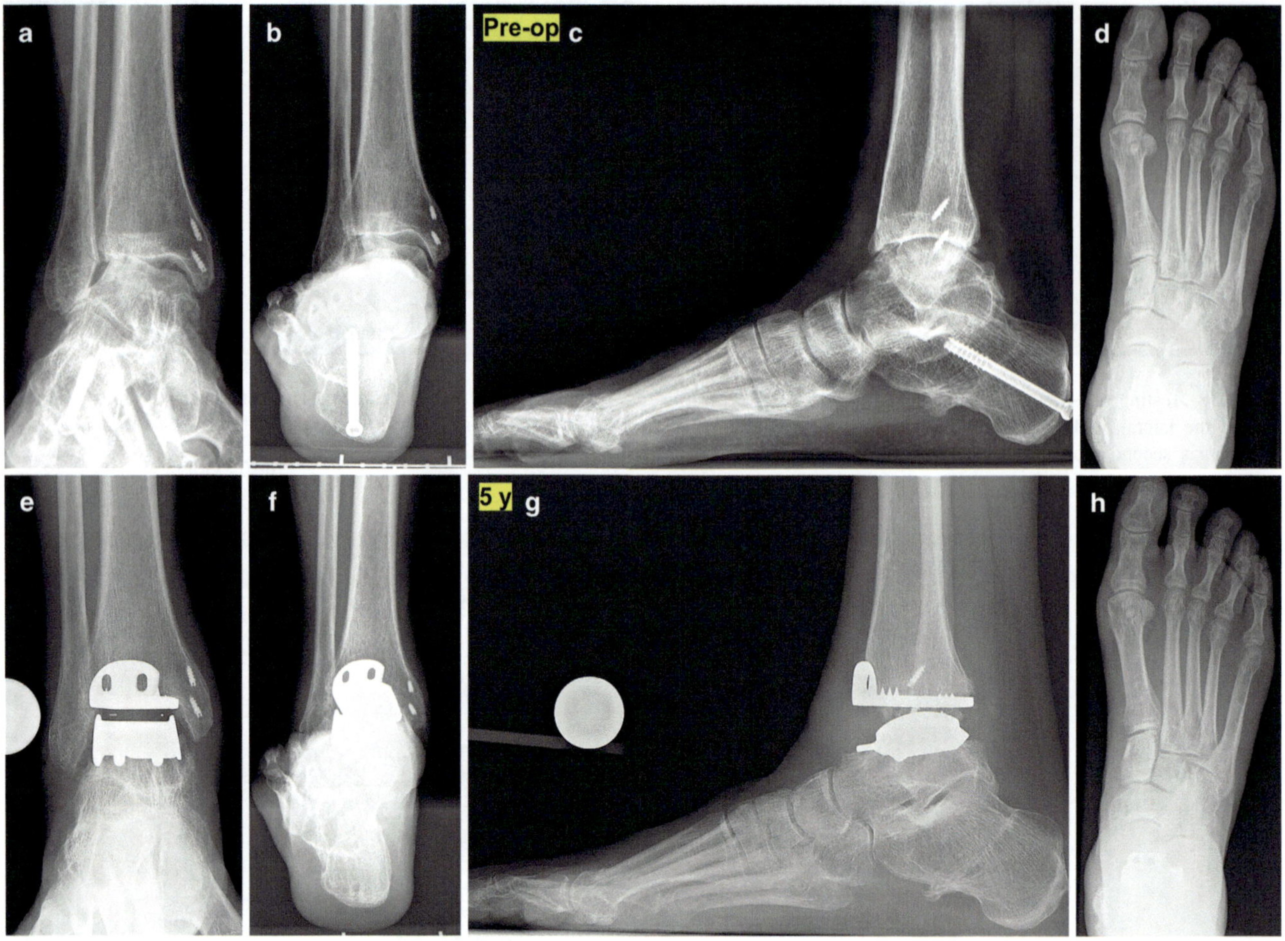

Fig. 9.40 Tightening of the deltoid ligament by the prosthesis ("spacer effect"). This 67-year-old retired gardener underwent previous deltoid reconstruction combined with a medial sliding osteotomy of the calcaneus. (**a**) He presents with a recurrent talar valgus corresponding to 50% of the height of the medial malleolus. (**b**) The hindfoot is in valgus malalignment. (**c**) The lateral view shows the talus in pronation position with closed sinus tarsi. (**d**) In contrast, the DP view of the foot does not show much deformity. (**e**) 5 years after the isolated ankle replacement surgery without any ancillary measure, the ankle is well aligned and balanced. (**f**) The heel is also well-aligned. (**g**) The effect of tightening the deltoid ligament complex is best seen in the lateral view; the talus is again regularly positioned on the top of the calcaneus, and the sinus tarsi impingement has disappeared. (**h**) No position changes are seen in the DP view of the foot

9.3.4 Syndesmotic Instability

Syndesmotic instability in total ankle arthroplasty is more common than generally believed [47]. First, as most osteoarthritic ankles that qualify for total ankle arthroplasty are post-traumatic, the previous trauma may have left some instability (Fig. 9.41). Second, when resecting the tibia, the syndesmosis may be weakened; this is particularly true when using components that need higher tibial resection (Fig. 9.42). Another issue is that, in some ankles, the syndesmotic ligaments are seen to be stable at ankle replacement surgery, but they will become incompetent over time due to chronic overload [47]. This may be especially true for ankles with incompetent deltoid ligament, post-traumatic origin, or after extended deltoid release at total ankle arthroplasty.

Syndesmotic instability can be seen in the coronal, sagittal, or both planes. Testing the syndesmotic ligaments specifically after component insertion is thus mandatory. The Hintermann distractor, fixed on the anteromedial aspect of the tibia and talus over two K-wires, can push the talus lateralward and anterior-posterior (Fig. 9.43). If the syndesmosis is seen to open or demonstrate anteroposterior instability, specific measures are necessary for stabilization.

Theoretically, in a strict coronal plane instability, a TightRope (Fig. 9.44) or position screw (Fig. 9.45) may be appropriate to stabilize the ankle mortise. However, this is seldom the case, and most instabilities are also seen in the sagittal plane. Therefore, a syndesmotic fusion is advised in most cases of syndesmotic instability (Fig. 9.46).

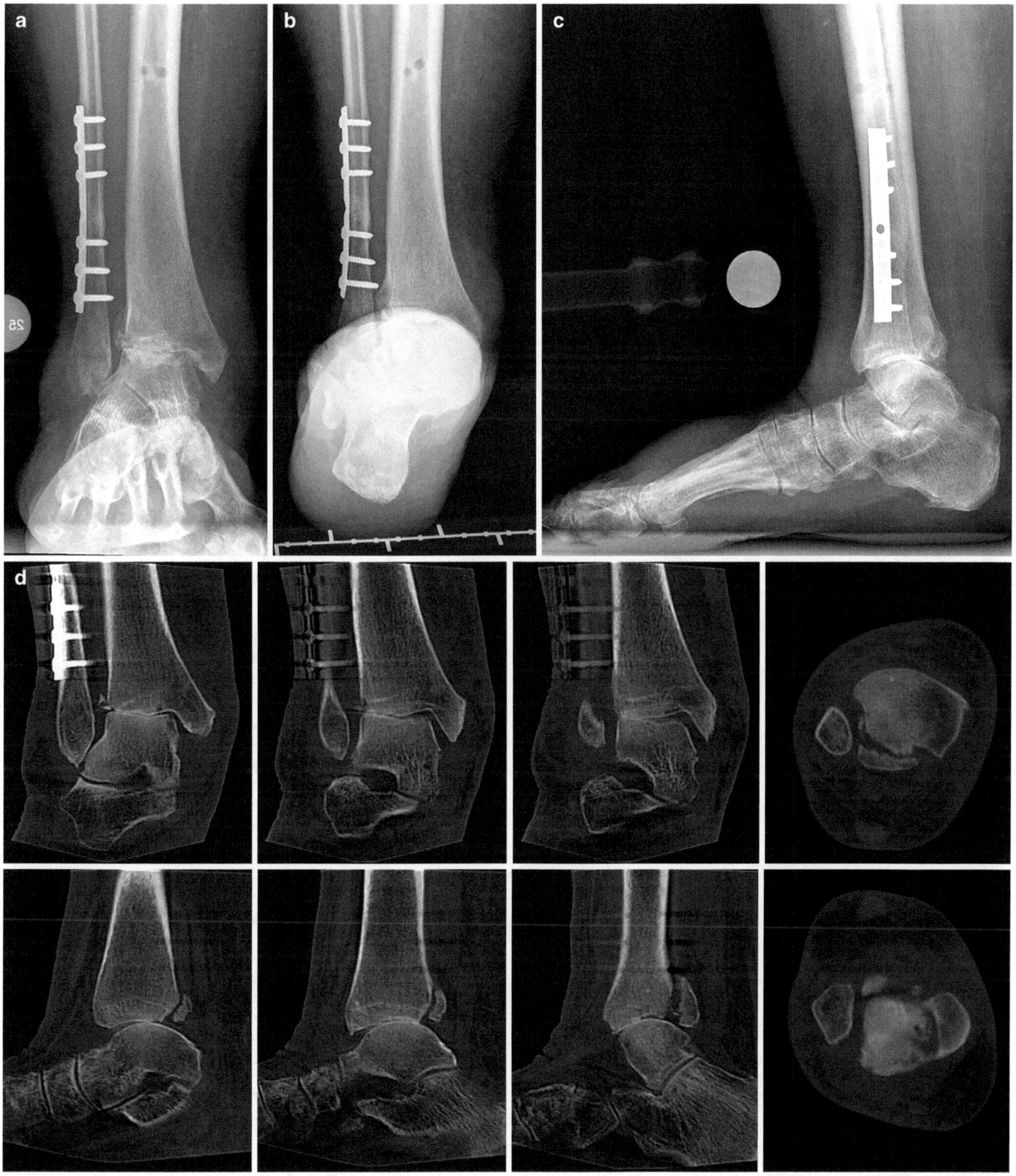

Fig. 9.41 Post-traumatic syndesmotic instability. This 66-year-old female patient presents with a progressive hindfoot valgus deformity associated with lateral ankle pain 18 months after an ankle fracture. (**a**) An apparent widening of the distal tibiofibular joint and the ankle mortise, resulting in a valgus tilt of the talus. (**b**) The valgus malalignment of the hindfoot is also seen in the alignment view. (**c**) A posterior shift of the talus is seen in the lateral view, and a too-anterior position of the fibula indicates a sagittal plane instability of the syndesmosis. (**d**) A non-united posterior malleolar fragment can be detected in the weight-bearing CT scan, explaining the posterior destabilization of the ankle joint and the syndesmotic instability

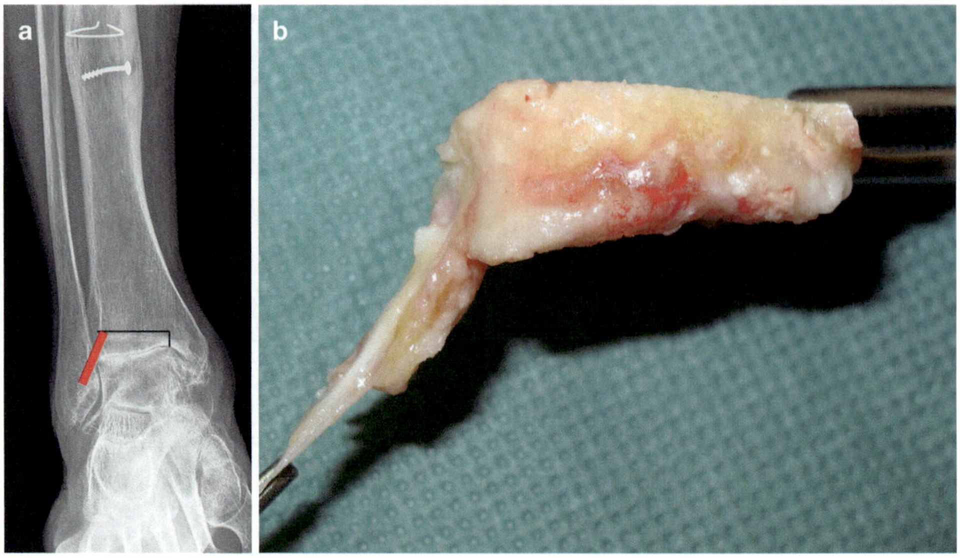

Fig. 9.42 Incompetent syndesmosis after high tibial resection. This 62-year-old retired navy officer sustained a tibial shaft fracture 28 years ago, resulting in a varus malunion with some internal malrotation. (**a**) A high-correcting tibial cut is performed to address the varus malunion, thus putting the syndesmotic ligaments at risk to be dissected. (**b**) The resected distal tibial fragment shows the resected syndesmotic ligaments that might have substantially weakened the distal tibiofibular joint

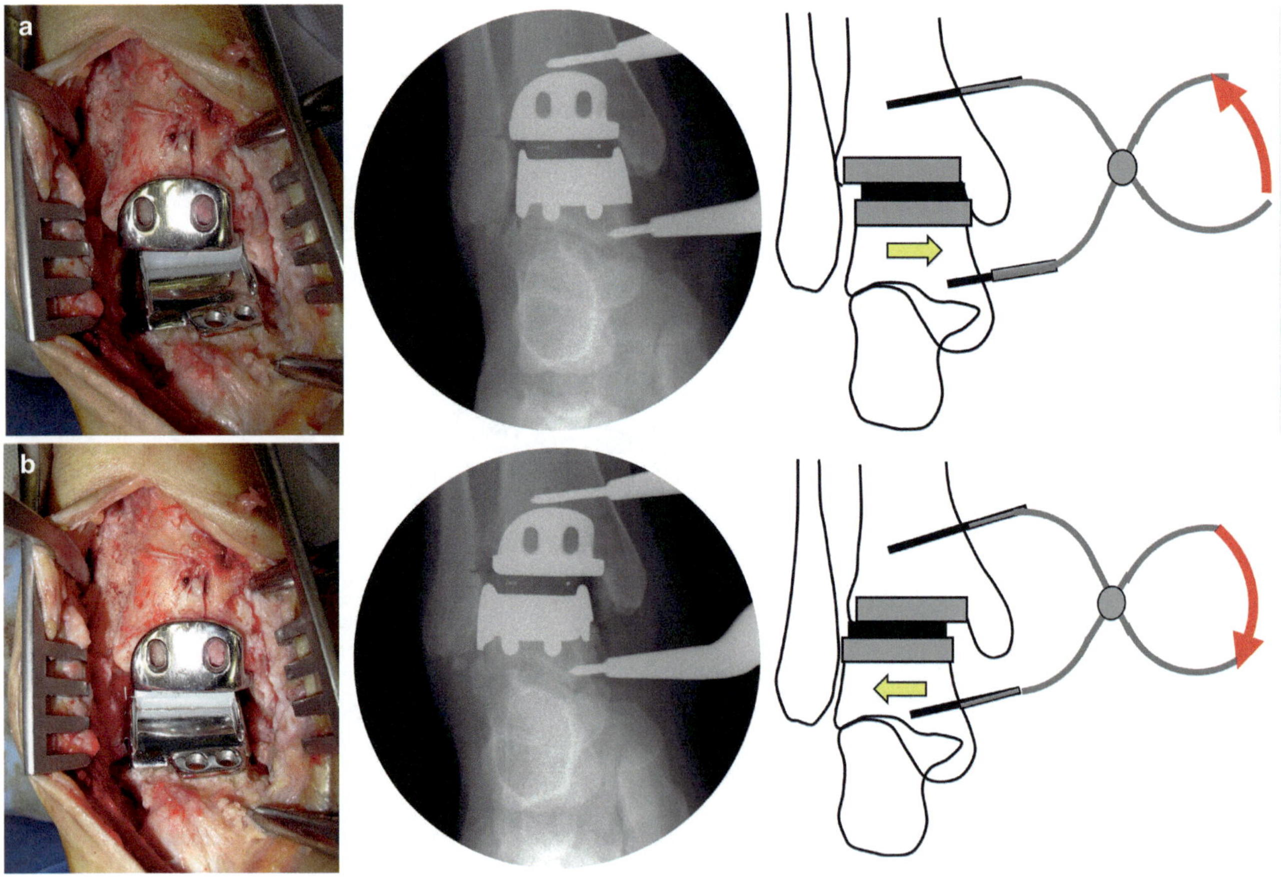

Fig. 9.43 Intraoperative testing of syndesmotic stability. The Hintermann distractor mounted over two K-wires in the anteromedial tibia and talus, respectively, is used to sway it upwards, thereby pushing the talus against the medial malleolus (**a**) and then downwards, thereby pushing the talus against the fibula (**b**). The amount of resulting translational movement of the talus and widening of syndesmotic clear space can best be quantified under fluoroscopy

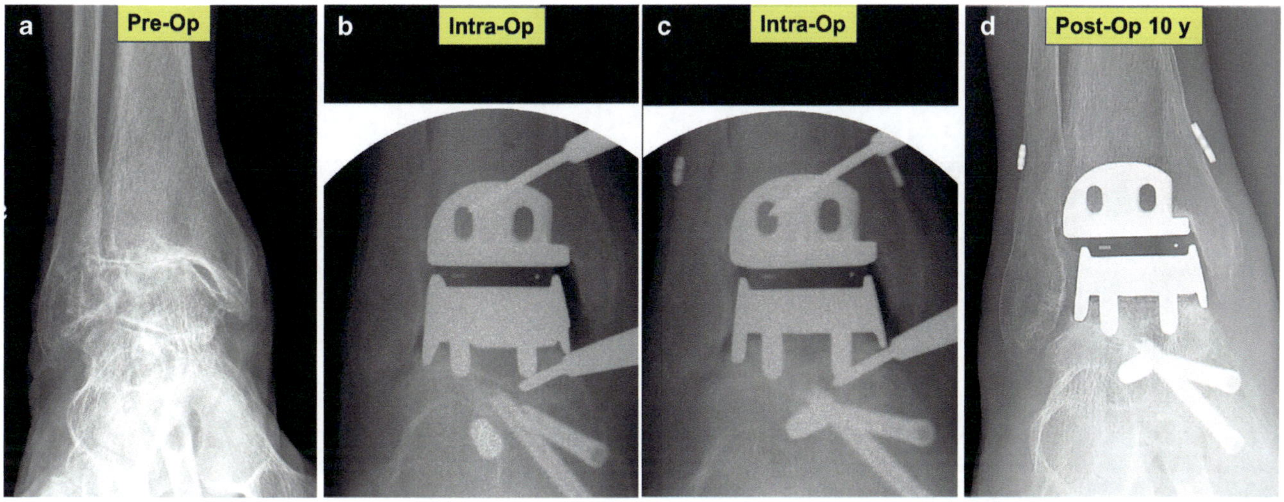

Fig. 9.44 Syndesmosis stabilization with a TightRope. (**a**) A distinct lateral shift of talus with the widening of the medial clear space is seen in this 58-year-old female patient with post-traumatic ankle osteoarthritis after a severe ankle sprain. (**b–c**) Intraoperative testing substantiated the coronal plane instability. Therefore, a TightRope was used to enhance the syndesmotic stability. (**d**) At 10-year-control, the ankle was well-aligned and stable

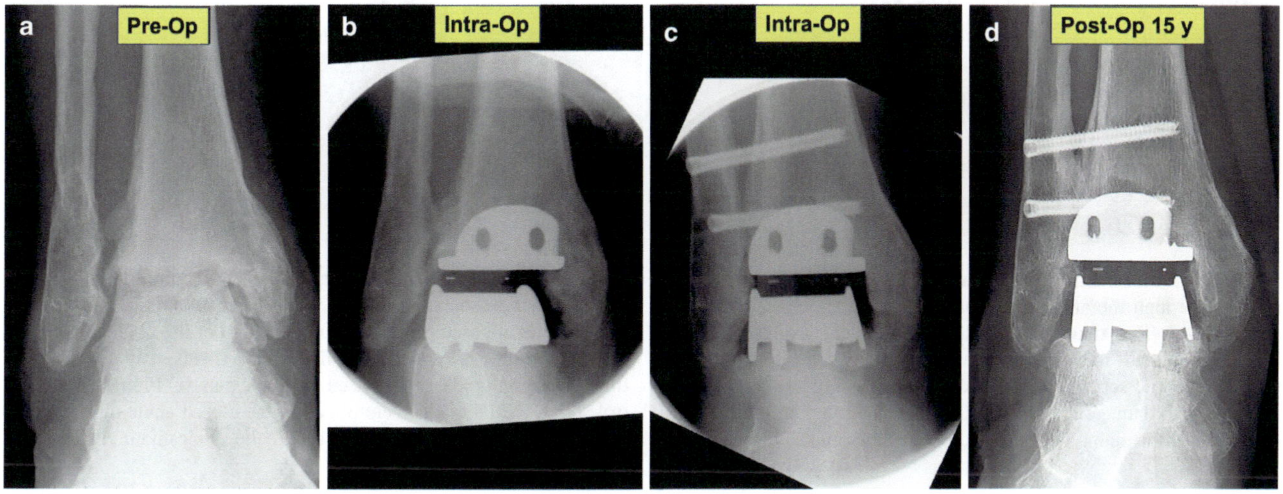

Fig. 9.45 Syndesmosis stabilization with positioning screws. (**a**) An increased tibiofibular clear space is seen in this osteoarthritic ankle with the tibial articular surface's erosion and subsequent talus impaction into the tibia and overlength of malleoli. (**b**) After the replacement surgery, as a result of ligament tensioning, the talus is seen to follow the talus, while the medial clear space is widened. (**c**) Two position screws were inserted to stabilize the distal tibiofibular joint. (**d**) At 15-year control, the syndesmosis was found to be fused, the ankle being stable and pain-free

The Authors' Experience

Mediolateral ligament balancing is crucial for the long-term success of total ankle arthroplasty. Thus, besides medial release, lateral ligament reconstruction is advised if lateral gapping of the replaced ankle is seen at the end of total ankle arthroplasty. Deltoid ligament reconstruction, in contrast, is critical to achieve. Distal tibiofibular instability following not addressed syndesmotic instability or chronic stress on the syndesmosis creates instability of the total ankle arthroplasty, which may lead to early failure. A distal tibiofibular fusion is the best option to restore the stability of ankle mortise.

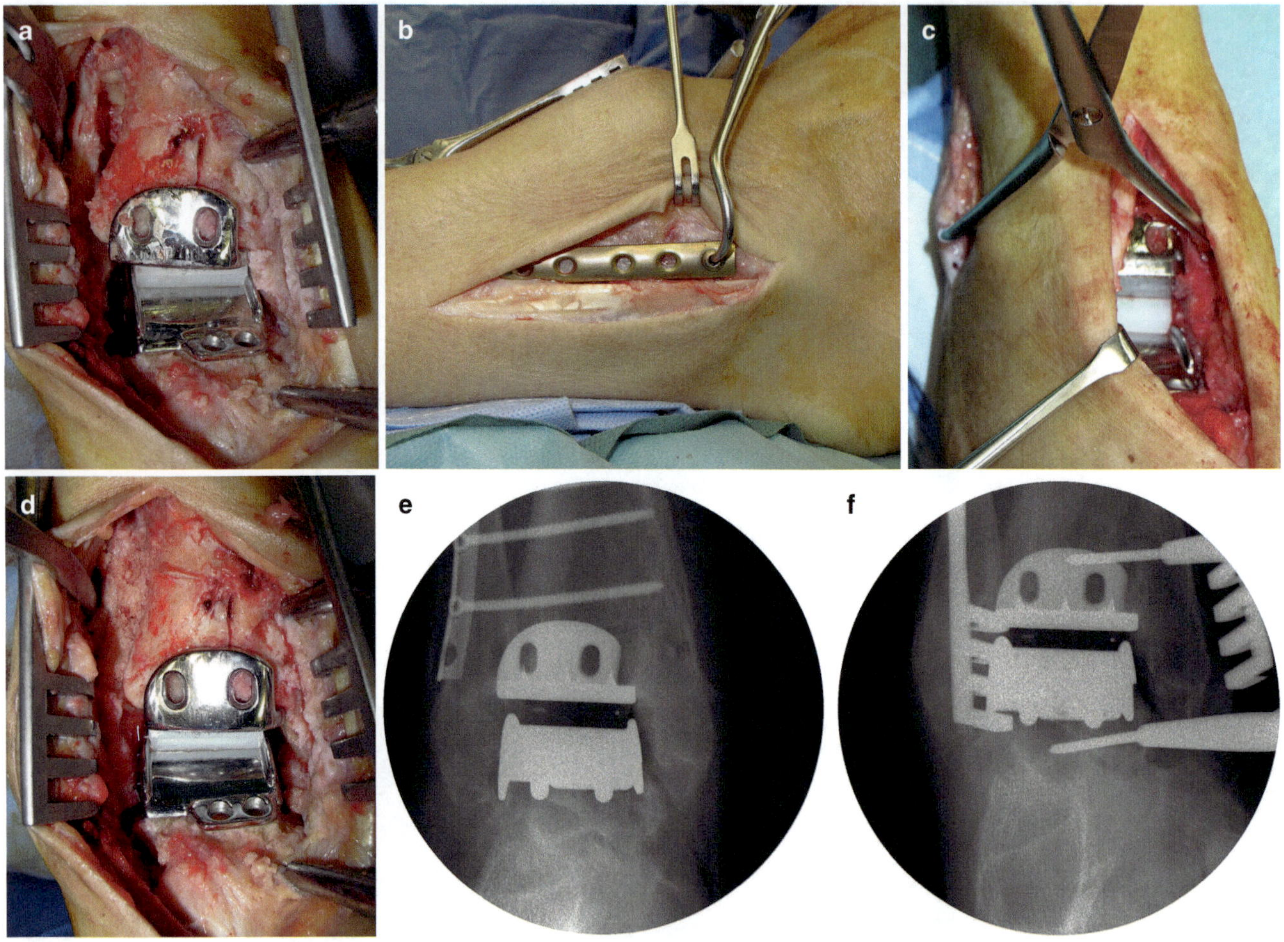

Fig. 9.46 Syndesmotic fusion. (**a**) The distal tibiofibular joint is exposed through the anterior approach and cleaned with a chisel and rongeur. (**b**) The fibula is exposed through an additional lateral approach, and a 4- to 5-hole plate is preliminarily fixed distally with a short screw. The screw imbue is taken by one arm of the compression clamp (not to damage the fibula when applying compression). (**c**) The other arm of the clamp is positioned on the anteromedial aspect of the distal tibia, where the bone is usually solid. While the foot is held in a neutral position, maximal compression force is applied, and two to three screws are used for four-cortical fixation of the fibula to the tibia. (**d**) If the tibiofibular space is not firmly closed, a bone from a previous tibial resection or allograft is used to fill the gap. (**e**) Fluoroscopic control shows the talus well centralized in the closed ankle mortise compared to the translational freedom before the syndesmotic fusion (**f**)

9.4 Tendon Transfers

The relative weakness of the peroneus brevis and tibialis anterior muscles compared with the posterior tibial and peroneus longus muscles is often associated with a cavovarus deformity. The peroneus brevis tendon may also be dysfunctional due to partial or complete rupture.

9.4.1 Peroneus Longus to Peroneus Brevis Tendon Transfer

A peroneus longus to peroneus brevis tendon transfer may be considered when eversion power is grade 3/5 or less (Fig. 9.47) [9]. The concept is to convert the peroneus longus to a foot abductor and evertor; thus, an attachment to the base of the fifth metatarsal bone associated with a side-to-side suture to the distal peroneus brevis tendon is performed (Fig. 9.48). Simple tendon reconstruction is no longer feasible if both the peroneus brevis and peroneus longus tendons are dysfunctional and incompetent. If muscular force is preserved, a tendon allograft may be considered (Fig. 9.49).

9.4.2 Tibialis Posterior Tendon Transfer

If both the peroneus brevis and peroneus longus tendons are dysfunctional and/or incompetent, and/or if muscular power is significantly reduced or lost, a posterior tibial tendon transfer may be considered (Fig. 9.50). The harvested tendon is brought behind the tibia into the peroneal tendon sheath and rerouted distally toward the base

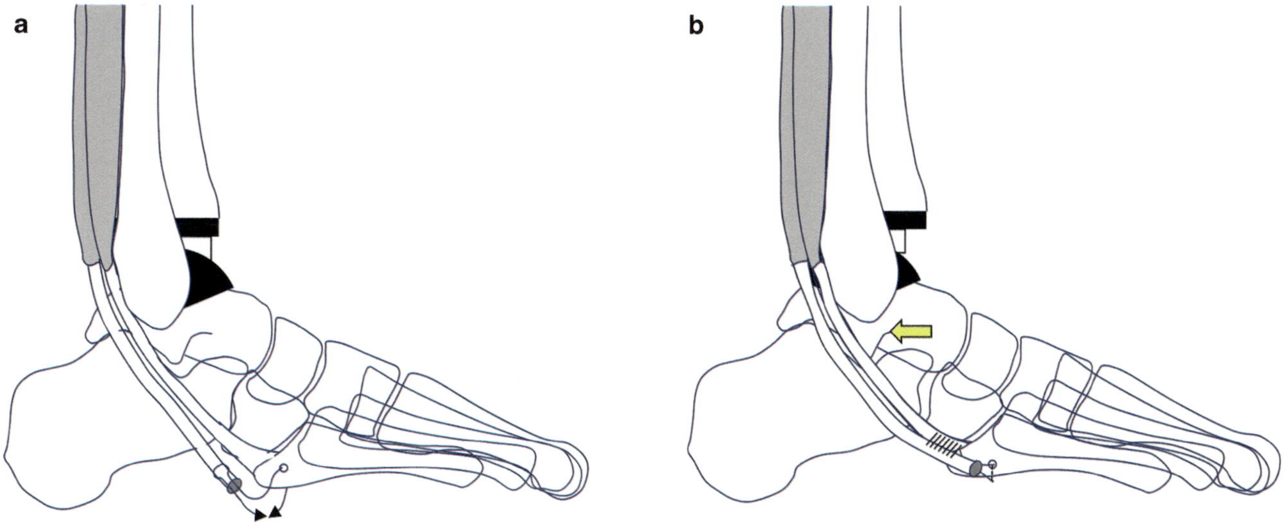

Fig. 9.47 Ratio and concept of peroneus longus to peroneus brevis tendon transfer. A long-standing varus-supination deformity is often associated with an anterolateral extrusion of talus out of the mortise, thus exposing the peroneus brevis tendon to a higher load with subsequent incompetence. As the peroneus longus tendon acts with its insertion at the base of the first metatarsal as plantarflector of the first ray, it increases the varus-supination deformity of the foot. The idea of this tendon transfer is, therefore, to convert the peroneus longus to an everter-abductor of the foot, thus supporting the incompetent peroneus brevis on one side, and to remove its plantarflector force to the first metatarsal on the other side. (**a**) The dissected peroneus longus tendon is prepared for attachment to the base of the fifth metatarsal. (**b**) After the fixation, an additional side-to-side suture to the peroneus brevis tendon is performed. As a result, the talus will be actively stabilized within the ankle mortise against anterolateral translation, seen as a change of distal fibula position

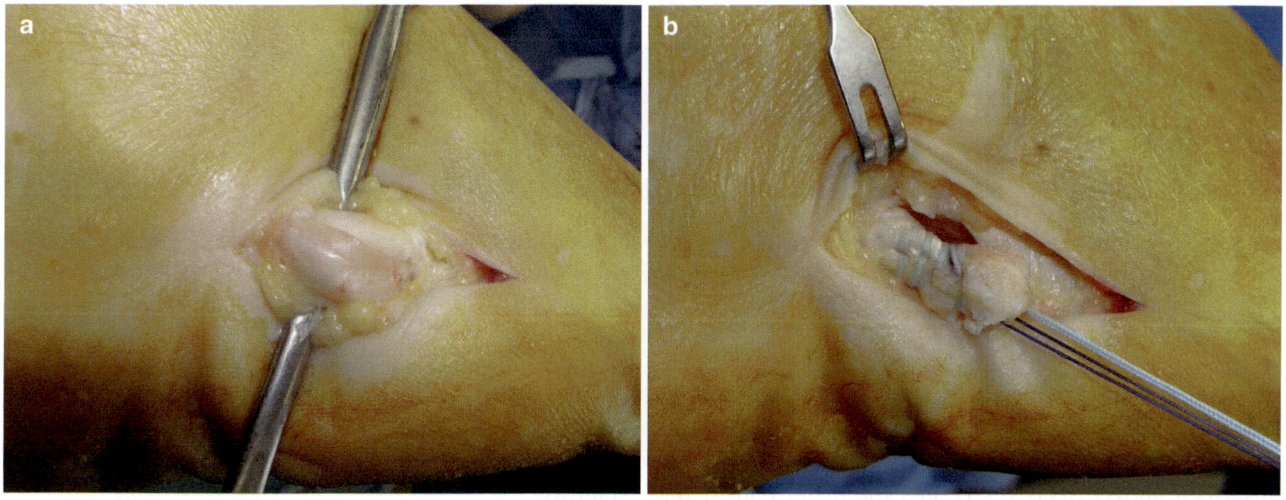

Fig. 9.48 Peroneus longus to peroneus brevis tendon transfer. (**a**) A 2- to 3-cm-long lateral incision is made to expose the base of the fifth metatarsal and the distal insertion area of the peroneus brevis tendon. The peroneus longus tendon that runs behind the peroneus brevis tendon is identified and dissected at its most distal portion, with the ankle in full plantarflexion and eversion. (**b**) A fiber wire mounted to the stump is used for transosseous fixation to the base of the fifth metatarsal. Alternatively, a suture anchor is inserted at the base of the fifth metatarsal, just plantar and lateral, to insert the peroneus brevis tendon. The peroneus longus tendon is secured to the base of the fifth metatarsal with the foot in a slightly plantarflexed and everted position. (**c**) The peroneus longus tendon is attached by a side-to-side suture to the brevis tendon for additional fixation. (**d**) Then, the wound is closed by interrupted sutures

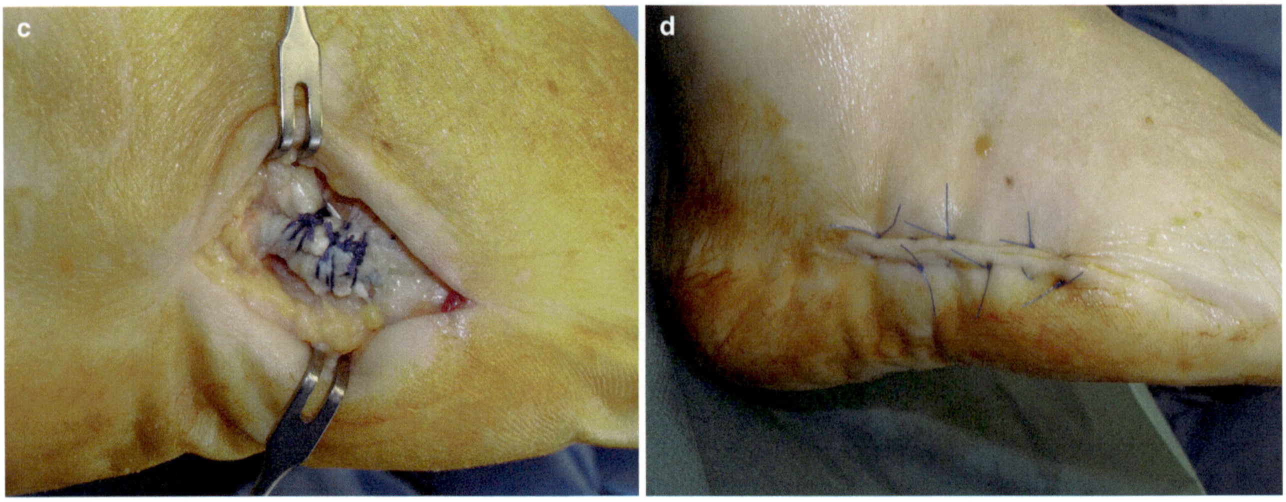

Fig. 9.48 (continued)

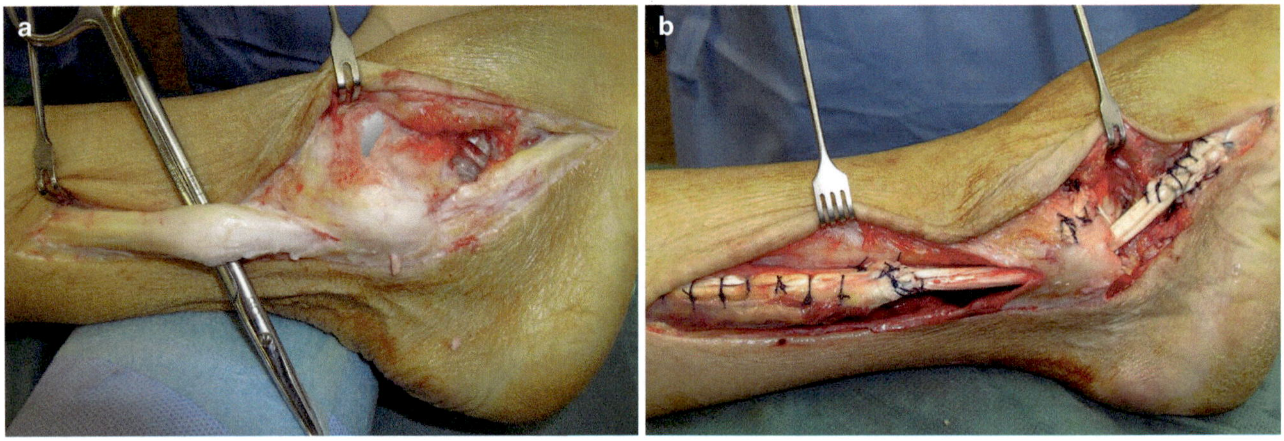

Fig. 9.49 Tendon allograft. (**a**) In this patient, the peroneus brevis tendon is dysfunctional with chronic tendinosis and degeneration. (**b**) Thus, it is resected and replaced with a tendon allograft. Notice that the peroneus longus tendon is transferred to the base of the fifth metatarsal and side-to-side fixed to the distal stump of the peroneus brevis tendon

of the fifth metatarsal. Usually, it needs to be longer to reach the fifth metatarsal. Therefore, the peroneus longus tendon is transferred to the base of the fifth metatarsal (as described above, Sect. 9.3.3), and the distal end of the posterior tibial tendon is sutured to the peroneus longus tendon. Side-to-side sutures to the distal stump of the peroneus brevis tendon may enhance the primary stability.

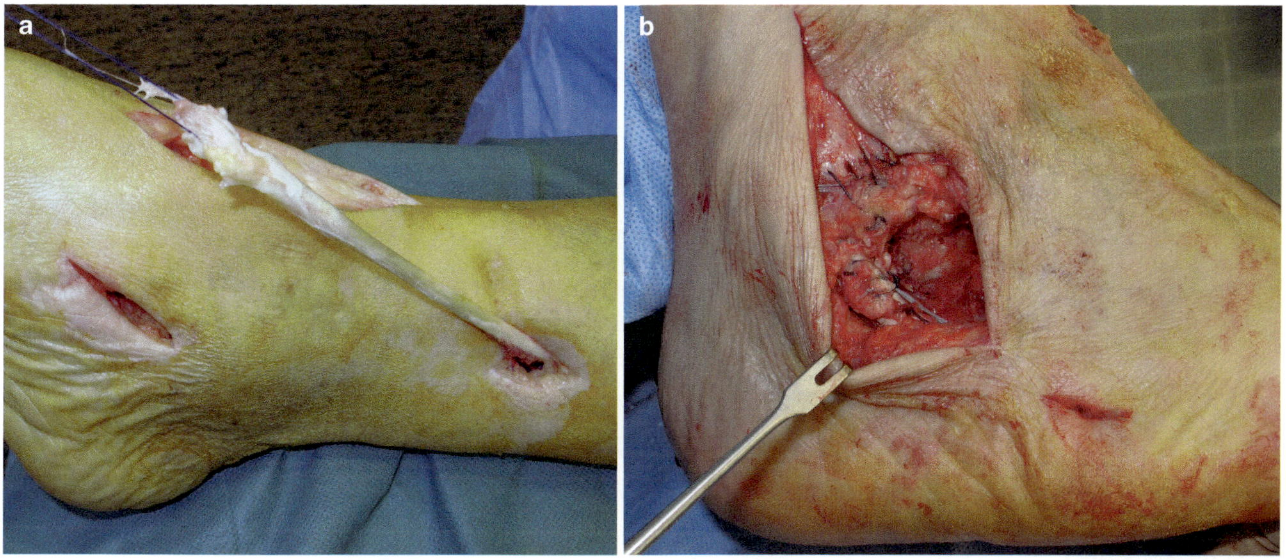

Fig. 9.50 Posterior tibial tendon transfer. (**a**) The posterior tibial tendon is exposed at its insertion to the navicular tuberosity and dissected sharply to the bone. A second incision is made 10–15 cm cranial to the ankle joint. After having identified the tendon, it is pulled out. (**b**) The suture mounted to the end of the tendon is crabbed with a long-curved clamp inserted from the lateral incision behind the fibula and the tibia and brought to the lateral side to pull out the tendon. While the foot is held in maximal eversion, the transferred tendon is fixed to the peroneus brevis tendon or, in this case, to the peroneus longus tendon that was transferred before to the peroneus brevis tendon

9.5 Posterior Soft-Tissue Release

Besides obtaining functional alignment of a total ankle arthroplasty, physiologic sagittal plane range of motion is paramount for a successful outcome. If the foot cannot be moved into a minimal 10° of dorsiflexion at the end of the reconstruction surgery, a posterior release of soft tissues should be considered. Soft-tissue ankle equinus correction with either Achilles tendon lengthening or gastrocnemius recession and posterior ankle capsule release and, in more significant contractures, medial and lateral collateral ligament complex release after osseous joint resection has been described [3, 48–51].

9.5.1 Periarticular Posterior Soft-Tissue Release

Of note, dorsiflexion is primarily controlled and restricted not by a single structure but by the interaction between most ankle ligaments. The periarticular soft-tissue release starts with the posterior ankle capsule, which should be excised until the posterior tibial and flexor digitorum longus tendons are visualized medially, the flexor hallucis longus muscle and tendon centrally, and the peroneal tendons laterally (Fig. 9.51). The adipose tissue within the retro Achilles area can be removed to expose the deep crural fascia, which can be released with a narrow-curved osteotomy to reduce posterior soft-tissue constraint further. The final step would be to perform the release of the posterior deep deltoid ligament and then, if needed, the talofibular ankle ligament, as these ligaments provide dorsiflexion restraint. The release is complete medially when the posterior tibial tendon can be visualized adjacent to the central portion of the medial malleolus. The release laterally is complete once the peroneal tendons can be visualized adjacent to the central portion of the lateral malleolus. Following the abovementioned procedures, the ankle should be able to achieve full dorsiflexion and plantarflexion with no frontal plane instability tested manually.

9.5.2 Achilles Tendon Lengthening Versus Gastrocnemius Recession

If, after periarticular posterior soft-tissue release, the foot with the extended knee can passively not bring to 10° of dorsiflexion (Fig. 9.52), Achilles tendon lengthening and gastrocnemius recession are both commonly used to increase dorsiflexion during total ankle arthroplasty procedures. Theoretically, a gastrocnemius recession is performed when Silfverskiöld's test determines an isolated gastrocnemius contracture. Achilles tendon lengthening is indicated when both the gastrocnemius and soleus are contracted. However, though it has been demonstrated that gastrocnemius recession does increase dorsiflexion while preserving nearly normal plantarflexion strength, Achilles tendon lengthening procedures are not without fear of the potential shortcomings, including loss of plantarflexion strength, push-off

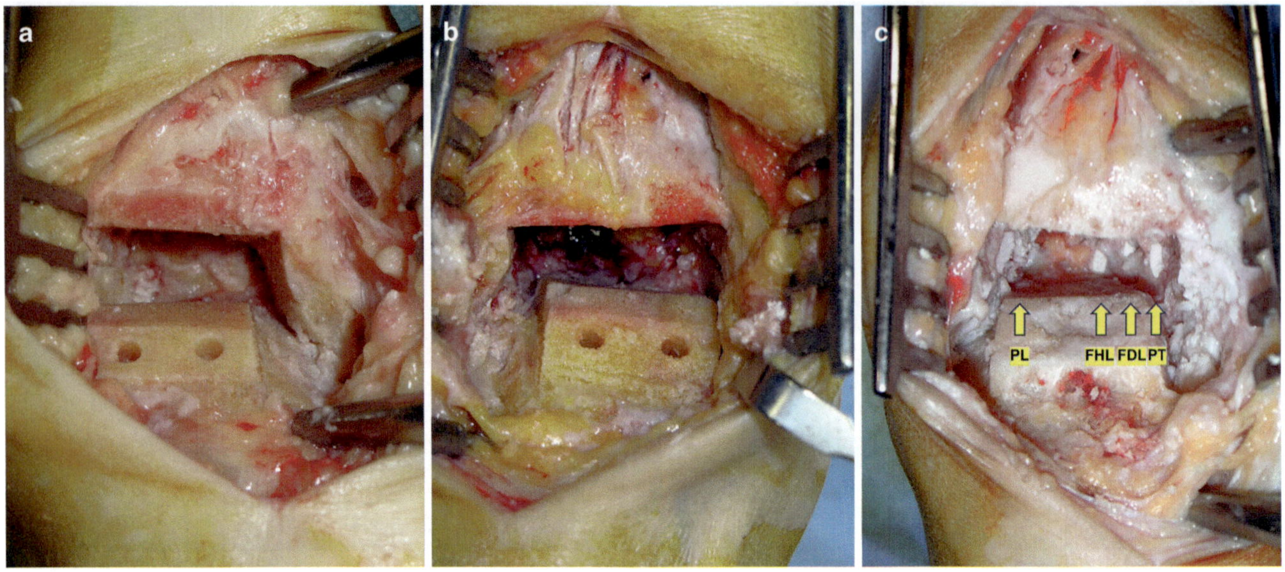

Fig. 9.51 Periarticular posterior soft-tissue release. The posterior capsule is excised completely, including the posteromedial (**a**) and posterolateral (**b**) corners. (**c**) The deep flexor and peroneal tendons can be seen after complete capsular resection: PL = peroneus longus, FHL = flexor hallucis longus, FDL = flexor digitorum longus, and PT = posterior tibial

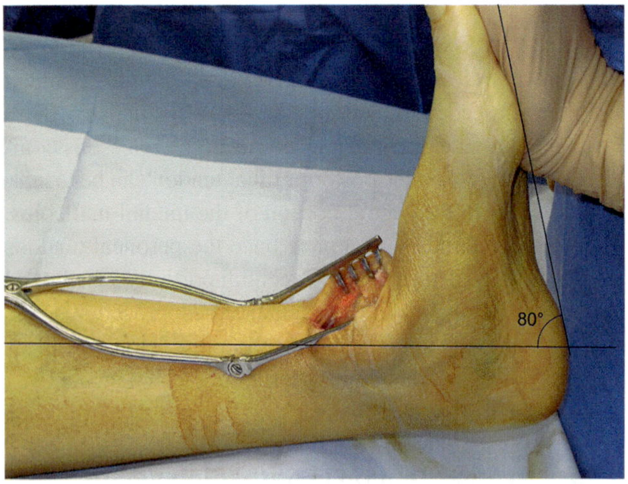

Fig. 9.52 Dorsiflexion after posterior soft-tissue release. In this ankle, 10° of dorsiflexion can be achieved by forced passive dorsiflexion, making an additional lengthening of the heel cord unnecessary

weakness during gait, loss of terminal plantarflexion, and risk of overlengthening [52–54]. By measuring the range of motion on lateral dorsiflexion-plantarflexion radiographs using reference lines on the surface of the implants, Jeng et al. [55] found an increased tibiotalar dorsiflexion following arthroplasty in those patients who underwent Achilles tendon lengthening and gastrocnemius recession. However, Achilles tendon lengthening had the unexpected effect of significantly decreasing plantarflexion, which was not found after gastrocnemius recession. They concluded that gastrocnemius recession might be a better choice when faced with a tight ankle replacement because it increases dorsiflexion without a compensatory loss of plantarflexion.

For Achilles tendon lengthening (Fig. 9.53a), an initial percutaneous stab incision is performed longitudinal at the center of the Achilles tendon 2 cm proximal to its insertion onto the calcaneus [48, 56]. The blade should advance only through the Achilles tendon properly. The blade is turned medially to transect the medial half of the tendon. A second longitudinal stab incision is made 3 cm proximal to the first, with the blade turned laterally to incise the lateral half of the Achilles tendon. Then, a third stab incision is made 3 cm proximal to the second for transection of the medial half of the tendon. The foot is moved at the ankle into controlled dorsiflexion to achieve between 5 and 10° of passive ankle dorsiflexion with the knee fully extended.

For gastrocnemius recession (Fig. 9.53b), a posteromedial incision is made on or just below the posterior knee crease [57]. The crural fascia is divided, and the proximal insertion of the medial gastrocnemius is identified. Performing the "hook maneuver" with a curved dissector is helpful at this step. Only the white fibers are sectioned to allow for a lengthening of the muscular fibers completed with forceful ankle dorsiflexion. After proper hemostasis has been achieved, the subcutaneous layer and skin are closed, leaving the fascia open. Alternatively, gastrocnemius recession can also be made more distally, following the techniques of Strayer [58, 59], Vulpius [60], or Baumann [61].

The effect of heel cord lengthening is demonstrated in Fig. 9.54.

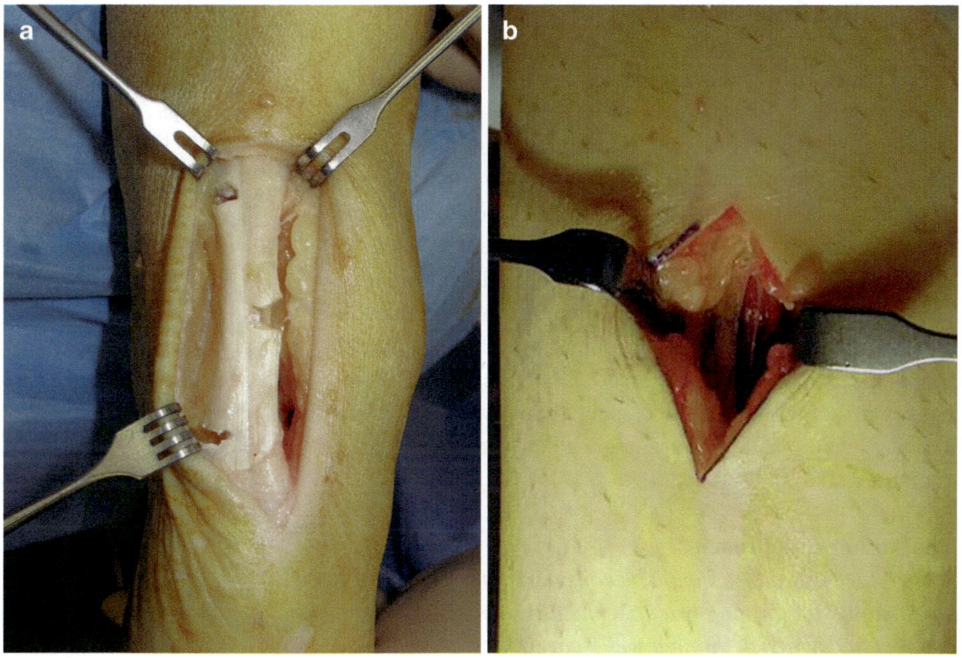

Fig. 9.53 Heel cord lengthening. (**a**) Achilles tendon lengthening by the triple-hemi-section technique is shown as an open procedure; usually, this procedure is done as percutaneous surgery. (**b**) Gastrocnemius recession can occur at various levels (see text)

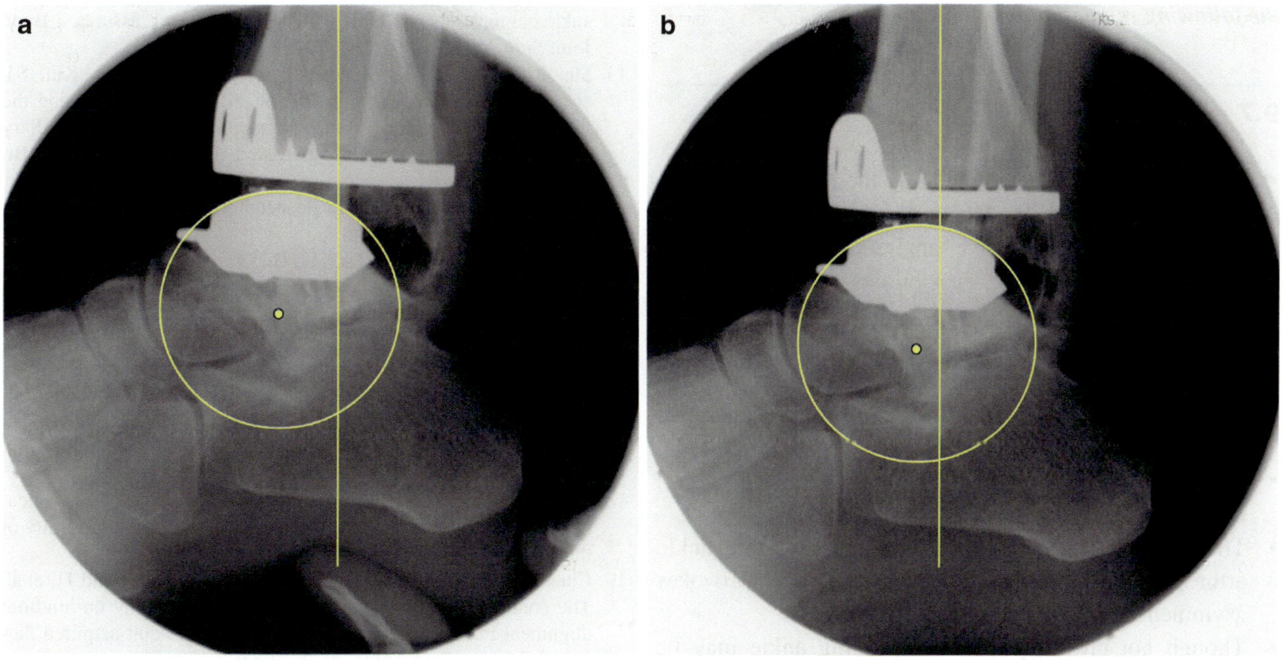

Fig. 9.54 Effect of heel cord lengthening. (**a**) A tight heel cord results in an anterior translational force to the talus, as shown with a mobile-bearing prosthesis. (**b**) After a percutaneous lengthening of the Achilles tendon, the talus is seen to have moved back

The Authors' Approach

If, at the end of the replacement surgery, the foot cannot be rotated at the ankle into 10° of dorsiflexion even after completed periarticular soft-tissue release, we consider an Achilles tendon lengthening to achieve minimally 10° of dorsiflexion. Before, a contracture of posterior tibial and deep flexor tendons should be excluded and, if present, released first.

9.6 The Role of Staging

There are no firm rules regarding whether staged procedures may be necessary to safely perform a total ankle arthroplasty. However, approaching these procedures and total ankle arthroplasty should be done cautiously because they may add considerable time under a tourniquet and increase the risk of vascular embarrassment caused by multiple incision placement, dissection, and manipulation of all vasculatures. The counterargument to this caveat is that achieving neutral foot alignment may be easier with the ankle appropriately reduced after the arthroplasty. However, surgeons should respect their own limitations about speed and experience when making these decisions.

The Authors' Approach

A one-stage procedure should be considered if the surgeon is comfortable performing brief, technically reproducible procedures and low risk through well-spaced incisions. In general, it facilitates achieving a stable foot in a neutral position in total ankle arthroplasty, and it may be advantageous for the following rehabilitation program.

9.7 Conclusions

- Balancing and properly stabilizing the replaced ankle is the key to success in the long term.
- A meticulous preoperative analysis is mandatory to understand deformities, instabilities, and deforming forces.
- Ultimately, deformities must also be addressed at their origin by correcting osteotomies or arthrodeses below the ankle, especially for peritalar instability or degenerative disease as the origin.
- Proper surgical technique is imperative to achieve an optimal outcome.
- The heel should never be left in the valgus after total ankle arthroplasty; it alters the mechanics of the joint, provokes asymmetric wear, and may also progress.
- Though not proven yet, a fixed-bearing ankle may be more forgiving in balancing and stabilizing than a mobile-bearing ankle, but with the fear of generating rotational torque or translational forces as the geometry of the prosthesis attempts to seek congruency.

References

1. Hintermann B, Ruiz R. Total replacement of varus ankle: three-component prosthesis design. Foot Ankle Clin. 2019;24(2):305–24.
2. Brunner S, Knupp M, Hintermann B. Total ankle replacement for the valgus unstable osteoarthritic ankle. Foot Ankle Tech. 2010;9:174–9.
3. Hintermann B. Total ankle arthroplasty—historical overview, current concepts and future perspectives. Wien-New York: Springer; 2004. p. 195.
4. Scheidegger P, Horn Lang T, Schweizer C, Zwicky L, Hintermann B. A flexion osteotomy for correction of a distal tibial recurvatum deformity. Bone Joint J. 2019;101-B(6):682–90.
5. Franz AC, Krahenbuhl N, Ruiz R, Susdorf R, Horn-Lang T, Barg A, et al. Hindfoot balancing in total ankle replacement: the role of supramalleolar osteotomies. Int Orthop. 2020;44(9):1859–67.
6. Hintermann B, Knupp M, Barg A. Supramalleolar osteotomies for the treatment of ankle arthritis. J Am Acad Orthop Surg. 2016;24(7):424–32.
7. Hintermann B. What the orthopaedic foot and ankle surgeon wants to know from MR imaging. Semin Musculoskelet Radiol. 2005;9(3):260–71.
8. Gauvain TT, Hames MA, McGarvey WC. Malalignment correction of the lower limb before, during, and after total ankle arthroplasty. Foot Ankle Clin. 2017;22(2):311–39.
9. Dodd A, Daniels TR. Total ankle replacement in the presence of Talar Varus or valgus deformities. Foot Ankle Clin. 2017;22(2):277–300.
10. Tarr RR, Resnick CT, Wagner KS, Sarmiento A. Changes in tibiotalar joint contact areas following experimentally induced tibial angular deformities. Clin Orthop Relat Res. 1985;199:72–80.
11. Ting AJ, Tarr RR, Sarmiento A, Wagner K, Resnick C. The role of subtalar motion and ankle contact pressure changes from angular deformities of the tibia. Foot Ankle. 1987;7(5):290–9.
12. Espinosa N, Walti M, Favre P, Snedeker JG. Misalignment of total ankle components can induce high joint contact pressures. J Bone Joint Surg Am. 2010;92(5):1179–87.
13. Sun XT, Easwar TR, Manesh S, Ryu JH, Song SH, Kim SJ, et al. Complications and outcome of tibial lengthening using the Ilizarov method with or without a supplementary intramedullary nail: a case-matched comparative study. J Bone Joint Surg Br. 2011;93(6):782–7.
14. Dwyer FC. Osteotomy of the calcaneum for pes cavus. J Bone Joint Surg Br. 1959;41-B(1):80–6.
15. Schmid T, Zurbriggen S, Zderic I, Gueorguiev B, Weber M, Krause FG. Ankle joint pressure changes in a pes cavovarus model: supramalleolar valgus osteotomy versus lateralizing calcaneal osteotomy. Foot Ankle Int. 2013;34(9):1190–7.
16. Krause FG, Sutter D, Waehnert D, Windolf M, Schwieger K, Weber M. Ankle joint pressure changes in a pes cavovarus model after lateralizing calcaneal osteotomies. Foot Ankle Int. 2010;31(9):741–6.
17. Malerba F, De Marchi F. Calcaneal osteotomies. Foot Ankle Clin. 2005;10(3):523–40. vii
18. Knupp M, Horisberger M, Hintermann B. A new Z-shaped calcaneal osteotomy for 3-plane correction of severe varus deformity of the Hindfoot. Tech Foot Ankle Surg. 2008;7(2):90–5.
19. Chan JY, Williams BR, Nair P, Young E, Sofka C, Deland JT, et al. The contribution of medializing calcaneal osteotomy on hindfoot alignment in the reconstruction of the stage II adult acquired flatfoot deformity. Foot Ankle Int. 2013;34(2):159–66.
20. Greenfield S, Cohen B. Calcaneal osteotomies: pearls and pitfalls. Foot Ankle Clin. 2017;22(3):563–71.
21. Nyska M, Parks BG, Chu IT, Myerson MS. The contribution of the medial calcaneal osteotomy to the correction of flatfoot deformities. Foot Ankle Int. 2001;22(4):278–82.
22. Stufkens SA, Knupp M, Hintermann B. Medial displacement calcaneal osteotomy. Tech Foot Ankle Surg. 2009;8(2):85–90.
23. Weinfeld SB. Medial slide calcaneal osteotomy. Technique, patient selection, and results. Foot Ankle Clin. 2001;6(1):89–94. vii
24. Trnka HJ, Easley ME, Myerson MS. The role of calcaneal osteotomies for correction of adult flatfoot. Clin Orthop Relat Res. 1999;365:50–64.
25. Evans D. Calcaneo-valgus deformity. J Bone Joint Surg Br. 1975;57(3):270–8.

26. Hintermann B, Valderrabano V, Kundert HP. Lengthening of the lateral column and reconstruction of the medial soft tissue for treatment of acquired flatfoot deformity associated with insufficiency of the posterior tibial tendon. Foot Ankle Int. 1999;20(10):622–9.
27. Aly AS, Abdel Rahman AF, Mahmoud S. Double calcaneal osteotomy in treatment of flexible planovalgus foot deformity in ambulatory cerebral palsy. A case series study. Foot Ankle Surg. 2019;25(5):640–5.
28. Didomenico LA, Haro AA 3rd, Cross DJ. Double calcaneal osteotomy using single, dual-function screw fixation technique. J Foot Ankle Surg. 2011;50(6):773–5.
29. Kim BS, Knupp M, Zwicky L, Lee JW, Hintermann B. Total ankle replacement in association with hindfoot fusion: outcome and complications. J Bone Joint Surg Br. 2010;92(11):1540–7.
30. Kim BS, Choi WJ, Kim YS, Lee JW. Total ankle replacement in moderate to severe varus deformity of the ankle. J Bone Joint Surg Br. 2009;91(9):1183–90.
31. Kim BS, Lee JW. Total ankle replacement for the varus unstable. Foot Ankle Tech. 2010;9:157–67.
32. Choi WJ, Kim BS, Lee JW. Preoperative planning and surgical technique: how do I balance my ankle? Foot Ankle Int. 2012;33(3):244–9.
33. Richter D, Krahenbuhl N, Susdorf R, Barg A, Ruiz R, Hintermann B. What are the indications for implant revision in three-component total ankle arthroplasty? Clin Orthop Relat Res. 2021;479(3): 601–9.
34. Hintermann B, Ruiz R. Foot and ankle instability—a clinical guide to diagnosis and surgical management. 1st ed. Springer International Publishing; 2021.
35. Fujii T, Luo ZP, Kitaoka HB, An KN. The manual stress test may not be sufficient to differentiate ankle ligament injuries. Clin Biomech (Bristol, Avon). 2000;15(8):619–23.
36. Brostrom L. Sprained ankles. VI. Surgical treatment of "chronic" ligament ruptures. Acta Chir Scand. 1966;132(5):551–65.
37. Coetzee JC. Surgical strategies: lateral ligament reconstruction as part of the management of varus ankle deformity with ankle replacement. Foot Ankle Int. 2010;31(3):267–74.
38. Comfort SM, Marchetti DC, Duncan PP, Dornan GJ, Haytmanek CT, Clanton TO. Brostrom repair with and without augmentation: comparison of outcomes at median follow-up of 5 years. Foot Ankle Int. 2023;44:691–701.
39. Deland JT, de Asla RJ, Segal A. Reconstruction of the chronically failed deltoid ligament: a new technique. Foot Ankle Int. 2004;25(11):795–9.
40. Haddad SL, Dedhia S, Ren Y, Rotstein J, Zhang LQ. Deltoid ligament reconstruction: a novel technique with biomechanical analysis. Foot Ankle Int. 2010;31(7):639–51.
41. Hintermann B, Valderrabano V, Boss A, Trouillier HH, Dick W. Medial ankle instability: an exploratory, prospective study of fifty-two cases. Am J Sports Med. 2004;32(1):183–90.
42. Hintermann B. Medial ankle instability. Foot Ankle Clin. 2003;8(4):723–38.
43. Jeng CL, Bluman EM, Myerson MS. Minimally invasive deltoid ligament reconstruction for stage IV flatfoot deformity. Foot Ankle Int. 2011;32(1):21–30.
44. Kim J, Mizher R, Sofka CM, Ellis SJ, Deland JT. Medium- to long-term results of nonanatomic spring ligament reconstruction using an allograft tendon in progressive collapsing foot deformity with severe abduction deformity. Foot Ankle Int. 2023;44(4):363–74.
45. Ellis SJ, Williams BR, Wagshul AD, Pavlov H, Deland JT. Deltoid ligament reconstruction with peroneus longus autograft in flatfoot deformity. Foot Ankle Int. 2010;31(9):781–9.
46. Kim DH, Berkowitz MJ, Pressman DN. Avulsion fractures of the medial tubercle of the posterior process of the talus. Foot Ankle Int. 2003;24(2):172–5.
47. Ruiz R, Susdorf R, Krahenbuhl N, Barg A, Hintermann B. Syndesmotic overload in 3-component total ankle replacement. Foot Ankle Int. 2020;41(3):275–85.
48. Roukis TS, Simonson DC. Management of osseous and soft-tissue ankle equinus during total ankle replacement. Clin Podiatr Med Surg. 2015;32(4):543–50.
49. DeOrio JK, Lewis JS Jr. Silfverskiold's test in total ankle replacement with gastrocnemius recession. Foot Ankle Int. 2014;35(2): 116–22.
50. Queen RM, Grier AJ, Butler RJ, Nunley JA, Easley ME, Adams SB Jr, et al. The influence of concomitant triceps surae lengthening at the time of total ankle arthroplasty on postoperative outcomes. Foot Ankle Int. 2014;35(9):863–70.
51. Gerard R, Unno-Veith F, Fasel J, Stern R, Assal M. The effect of collateral ligament release on ankle dorsiflexion: an anatomical study. Foot Ankle Surg. 2011;17(3):193–6.
52. Chimera NJ, Castro M, Manal K. Function and strength following gastrocnemius recession for isolated gastrocnemius contracture. Foot Ankle Int. 2010;31(5):377–84.
53. Delp SL, Statler K, Carroll NC. Preserving plantar flexion strength after surgical treatment for contracture of the triceps surae: a computer simulation study. J Orthop Res. 1995;13(1):96–104.
54. Sammarco GJ, Bagwe MR, Sammarco VJ, Magur EG. The effects of unilateral gastrocsoleus recession. Foot Ankle Int. 2006;27(7):508–11.
55. Jeng CL, Campbell JT, Maloney PJ, Schon LC, Cerrato RA. Effect of achilles tendon lengthening and gastrocnemius recession on radiographic tibiotalar motion following total ankle replacement. Foot Ankle Int. 2021;42(4):476–81.
56. Hatt RN, Lamphier TA. Triple hemisection: a simplified procedure for lengthening the achilles tendon. N Engl J Med. 1947;236(5):166–9.
57. Gamba C, Alvarez Gomez C, Martinez Zaragoza J, Leal Alexandre C, Bianco Adames D, Gines-Cespedosa A. Proximal medial gastrocnemius release: surgical technique. JBJS Essent Surg Tech. 2022;12(1).
58. Pinney SJ, Sangeorzan BJ, Hansen ST Jr. Surgical anatomy of the gastrocnemius recession (Strayer procedure). Foot Ankle Int. 2004;25(4):247–50.
59. Strayer LM Jr. Recession of the gastrocnemius; an operation to relieve spastic contracture of the calf muscles. J Bone Joint Surg Am. 1950;32-A(3):671–6.
60. Tinney A, Khot A, Eizenberg N, Wolfe R, Graham HK. Gastrocsoleus recession techniques: an anatomical and biomechanical study in human cadavers. Bone Joint J. 2014;96-B(6):778–82.
61. Herzenberg JE, Lamm BM, Corwin C, Sekel J. Isolated recession of the gastrocnemius muscle: the Baumann procedure. Foot Ankle Int. 2007;28(11):1154–9.

10 Algorithms for the Treatment of Complex Deformities

A conflicting problem for the surgeon to replace the ankle is that, subsequently, due to structural changes, the mechanics of the osteoarthritic ankle may have critically changed, thus making it unrealistic to determine exactly the axis of rotation of the ankle. Instability, coronal plane, and hindfoot deformity may have also caused axial malrotation of the talus, resulting in a three-dimensional deformity. At the time of surgery, it remains unclear to which extent osteophyte removal, osteotomies, and release or reconstruction of soft tissues can normalize the talar position within the ankle mortise and to which extent a mismatch will persist after the final insertion of the implants. Theoretically, an intraarticular deformity can be addressed intraoperatively with correcting cuts. Still, obvious limitations exist, and often, additional measures are necessary to obtain a balanced ankle. Extraarticular deformities, in contrast, may need periarticular osteotomies. If not addressed, concomitant instabilities may progress and disbalance the replaced ankle. This section presents solutions and algorithms for balancing and stabilizing a replaced ankle.

10.1 Total Ankle Arthroplasty in a Varus Osteoarthritic Ankle

The ankle prosthesis for the varus malaligned and varus unstable ankle can only be successfully done if the surgeon can adequately balance and stabilize the ankle. A primary challenge to address is the deforming forces. While standing, the center of force transmission is medialized. The forces within the joint are amplified by activating the triceps surae, and the Achilles tendon may become an invertor, thereby acting as an additional deforming force on the hindfoot.

10.1.1 Preoperative Assessment and Planning

Besides thorough clinical investigation (Fig. 10.1), diagnostic imaging under weight-bearing conditions is essential in the preoperative workup of the varus osteoarthritic ankle (Fig. 10.2). Differentiating between symmetrical and asymmetrical deformities is paramount, as asymmetrical deformities indicate a loss of ligamentous support, resulting in a disbalanced ankle, whereas, in symmetrical deformities, the ankle remains somehow balanced [1–5]. While symmetrical coronal plane deformities can be addressed by supramalleolar and inframalleolar correcting osteotomies alone [4, 6], asymmetrical deformities may need additional ligament reconstruction and tendon transfers [7–10]. For the surgeon, it is essential to understand whether an asymmetrical deformity is correctable (Fig. 10.3).

A varus-tilted talus can be associated with a calcaneus in varus ("varus-varus" deformity), as typically seen in a cavovarus deformity (Fig. 10.2). However, it can be associated with a calcaneus in the valgus, resulting in a "varus-valgus" deformity that indicates a peritalar instability with the collapse of the ankle joint complex (Figs. 9.7 and 9.11). The underlying cause is chronic lateral ankle instability that has led to multidirectional ankle instability associated with a destabilization of peritalar joints. As the pre-existing hindfoot varus orientation is associated with compensatory eversion to maintain a plantigrade foot, the calcaneus rotates into a relative valgus position, resulting in a "zig-zag" deformity. The talar tilt into varus and the rotation of calcaneus into valgus is further increased by loading the foot and the pull of the Achilles tendon during push-off, with subsequent stress overload to the anteromedial aspect of the ankle joint with the gradual erosion of medial tibial plafond and medial malleolus. It is challenging to appreciate this deformity on clinical examination because the hindfoot may appear to be in a neutral position.

10.1.2 Algorithm for Surgical Treatment of a Varus-Varus Ankle

The authors' proposed step-by-step algorithm for a "varus-varus" ankle is as follows (Fig. 10.4):

B. Hintermann, R. Ruiz, *Total Ankle Replacement*, https://doi.org/10.1007/978-3-031-56810-7_10

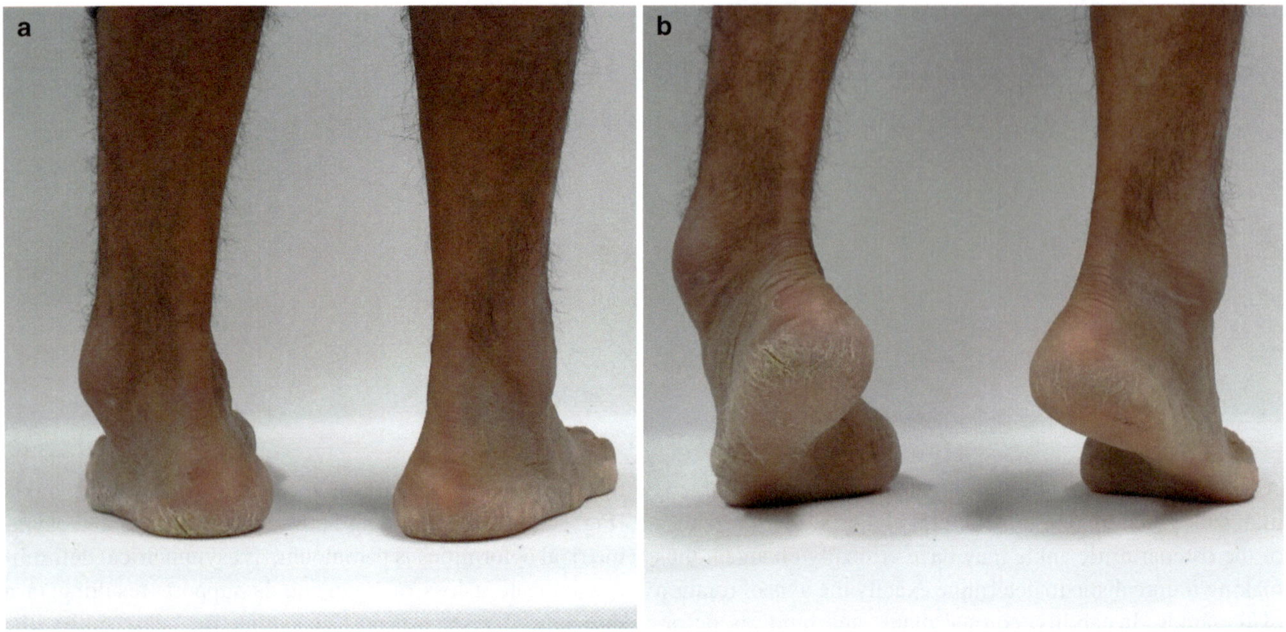

Fig. 10.1 Clinical investigation of varus deformity. The posterior view shows a complex varus deformity when standing (**a**) that increases in tiptoe position due to a fixed forefoot pronation (**b**)

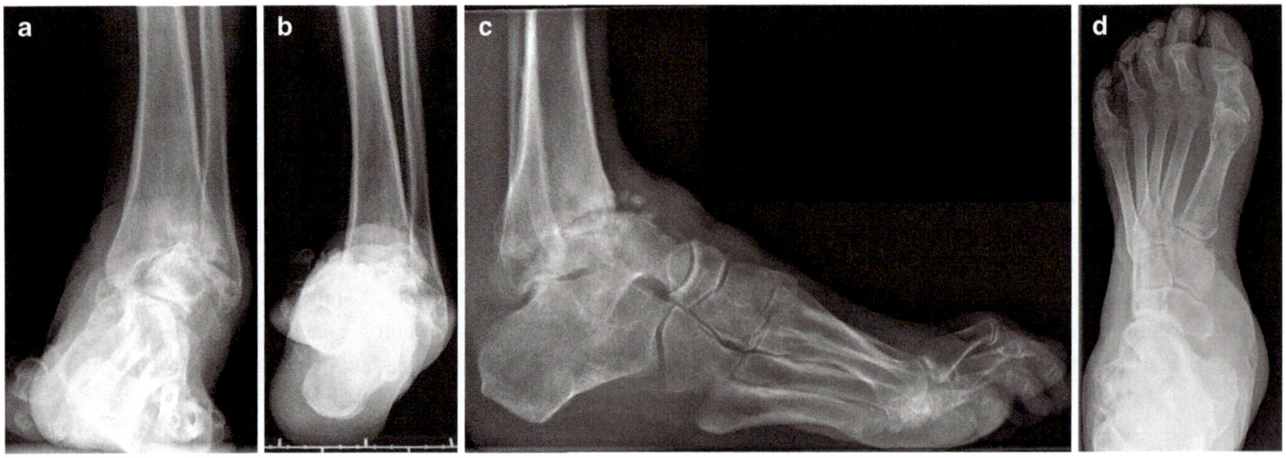

Fig. 10.2 Radiographic assessment of varus deformity. The standard radiographs permit us to understand the 3-D deformity in more detail. In this case, an anterolateral extrusion of the talus is associated with significant erosion of the anterior tibia. In contrast, the foot is in a supination position, suggesting a medial soft-tissue contracture, including the deltoid ligament and posterior tibial tendon, and incompetence of lateral soft tissues, including the lateral ankle ligaments and the peroneus brevis tendon. (**a**) AP view, (**b**) alignment view, (**c**) lateral view, and (**d**) DP view (same patient as Fig. 10.1)

10.1.2.1 Supramalleolar Correction

A minor varus deformity can be addressed by correcting the cut of the distal tibia; however, an LDTA angle <85° usually necessitates a supramalleolar osteotomy (Figs. 9.14–9.15).

10.1.2.2 Total Ankle Arthroplasty

Total ankle arthroplasty is now performed using the standard technique. Final correction of the distal tibia is achieved with the tibial resection cut.

10.1.2.3 Medial Ankle Release

A deltoid release is done in a mild medial contracture (Fig. 9.18). This can be done at the beginning of total ankle arthroplasty while the medial ankle is distracted over two K-wires with the Hintermann distractor. However, in the case of medial malleolus dysplasia, as it typically results in an offset position of the medial malleolus, our preferred technique is a flip osteotomy of the medial malleolus (Figs. 9.19 and 9.20) [7]. The same measure is considered if, after the polyethyl-

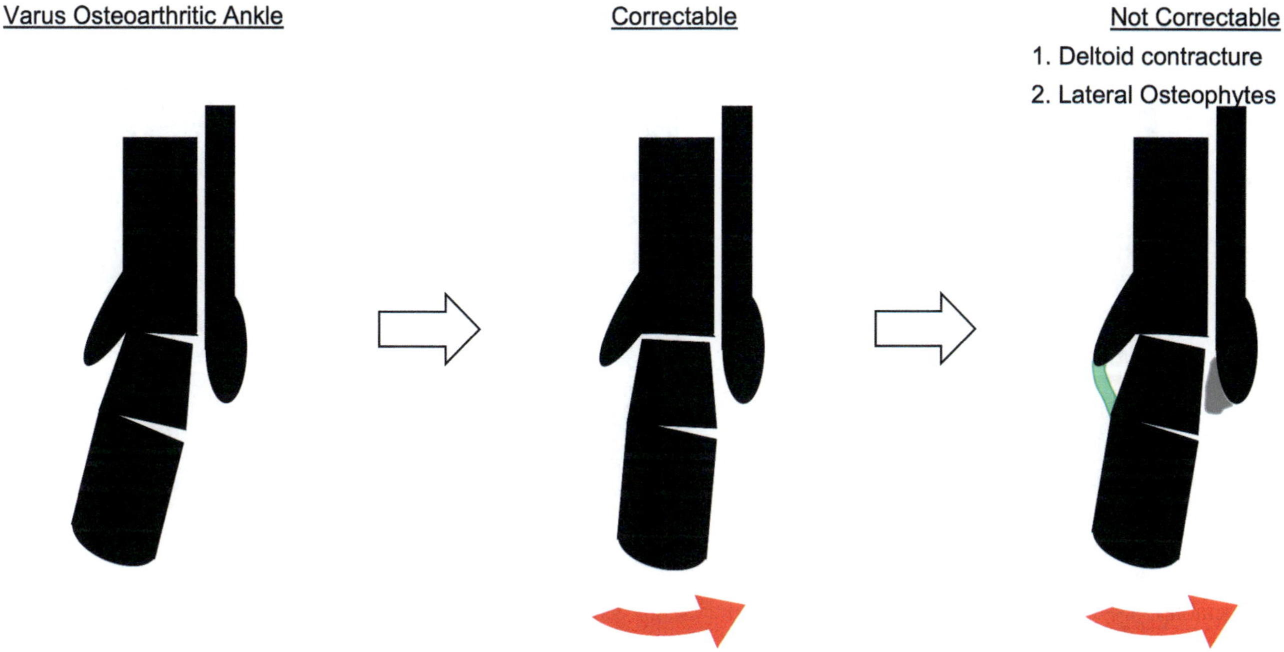

Fig. 10.3 Manual testing. The surgeon can recognize whether the varus deformity is correctable by applying valgus stress to the heel. The underlying cause for an uncorrectable deformity can be a deltoid ligament contracture, osteophytes in the lateral gutter, or both

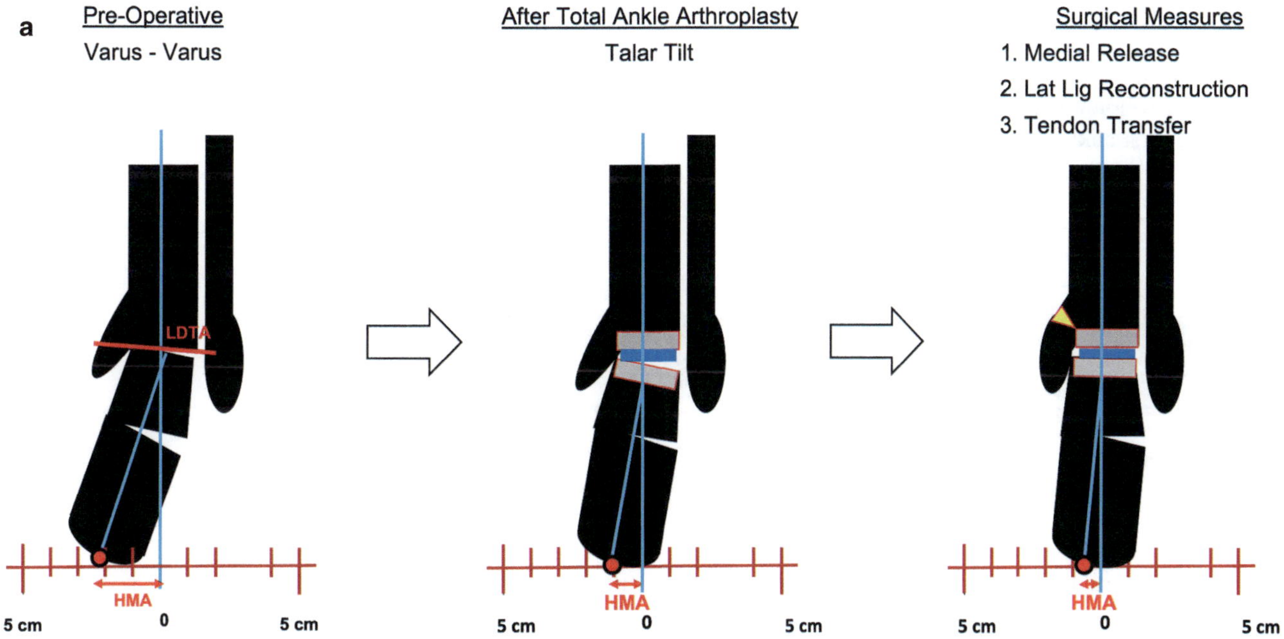

Fig. 10.4 Algorithm for surgical measures of a varus-varus deformity. (**a**) If the talus remains tilted into the varus after the total ankle arthroplasty, a medial release is done first, followed by a lateral ligament reconstruction. If necessary, a peroneal longus to brevis transfer is added. (**b**) A calcaneal osteotomy is performed if the heel remains in a varus malaligned position. In severe deformities, especially when the subtalar joint is irreducible, a correcting subtalar fusion might be considered, with or without including the talonavicular joint. (**c**) In the case of fixed forefoot pronation, a dorsiflexion osteotomy is performed to elevate the first ray

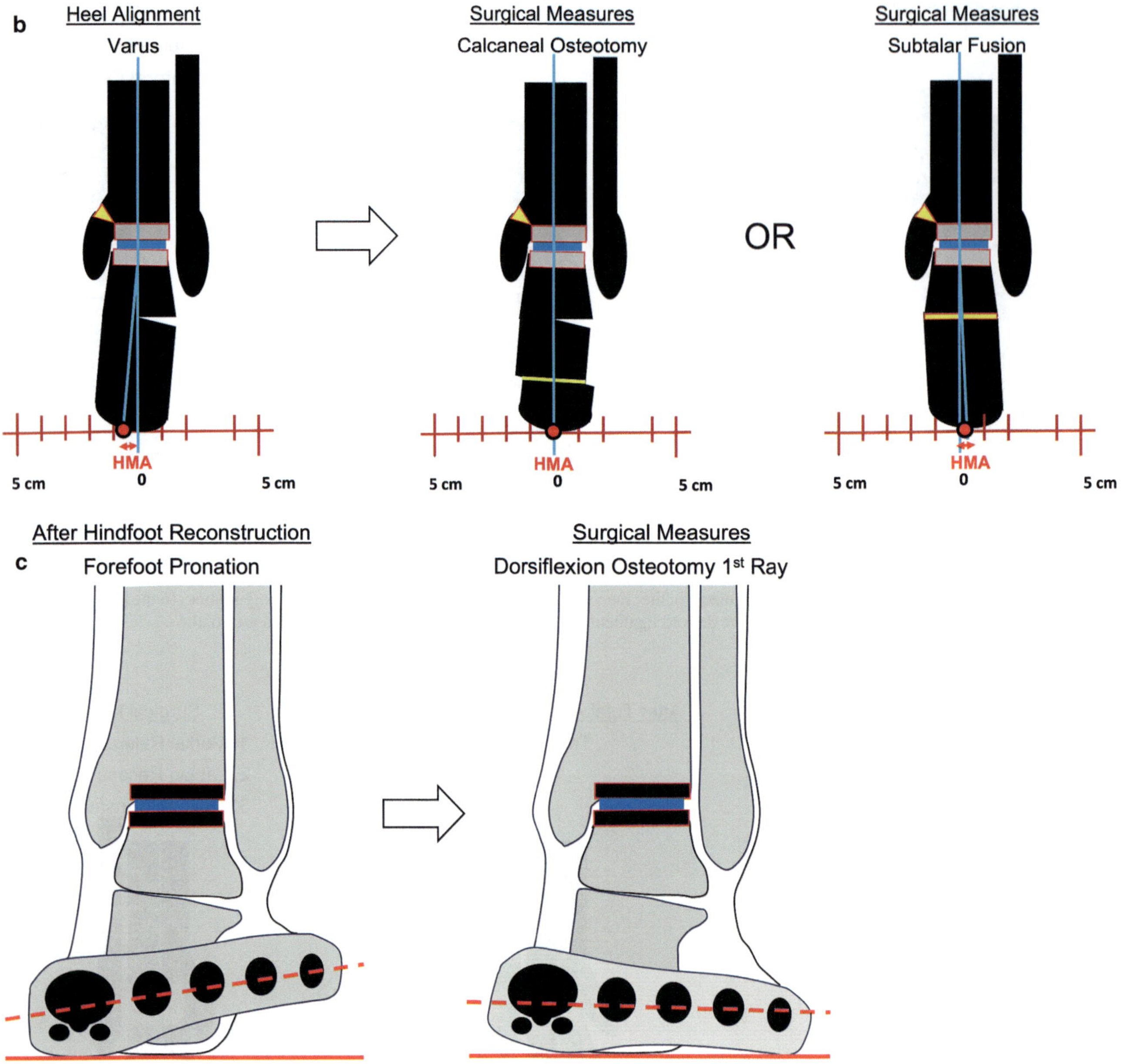

Fig. 10.4 (continued)

ene inlay is inserted, a lateral gapping of the joint is seen as a consequence of remaining medial contracture. This rotational osteotomy results in a correction of the force vector of the deltoid ligament, and a regular width of the medial gutter will be obtained, allowing the medial malleolus to function again as a guiding structure. Moreover, this reorientation of the medial malleolus will preserve the ankle from recurrent deltoid contracture through potential scarring.

10.1.2.4 Release of Posterior Tibial Tendon

Diagnosing a posterior tibial tendon contracture is often not easy to make, as it may be or is not associated with pain over the tendon. Typically, the foot presents in a supination-adduction position that cannot be manually corrected, and often, it is in an equinus position (Fig. 10.5a). The most reliable finding is a decrease of talocalcaneal angle in the DP view of the foot associated with a tilt of the navicular toward medially (Fig. 10.5b). After having exposed the tendon sheath, the posterior tibial tendon is debrided and mobilized. If, with this, the foot cannot be turned to neutral, the tendon can be lengthened by a Z-shaped dissection. However, if the posterior tibial tendon, after being mobilized, does not evidence any excursion indicating a loss of elasticity of its muscle, it is resected (Fig. 10.6).

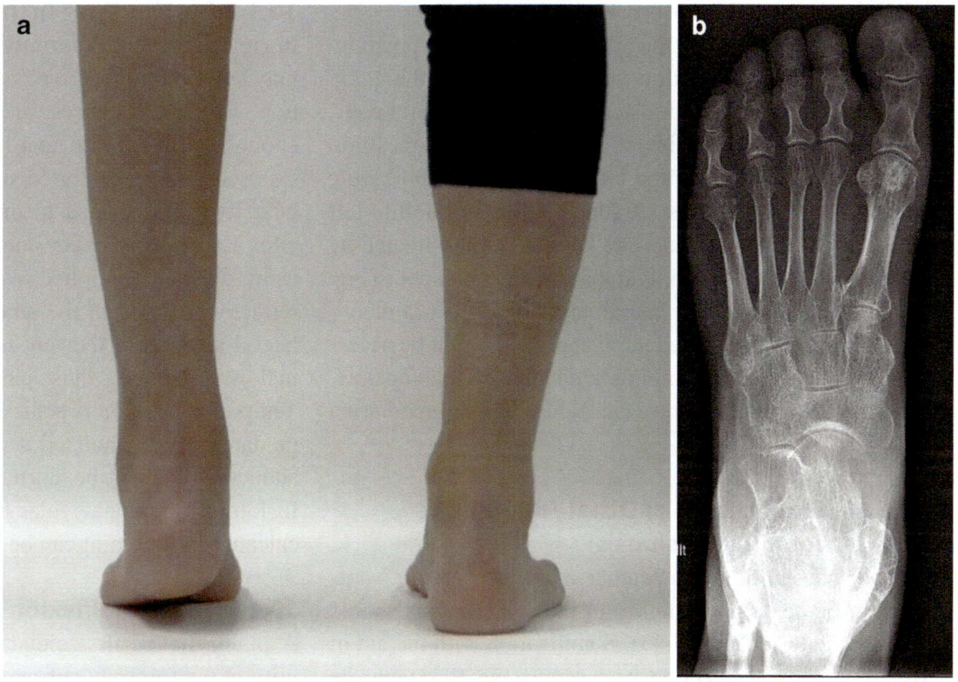

Fig. 10.5 Appearance of posterior tibial tendon contracture. (**a**) This 46-year-old female patient suffers from end-stage ankle osteoarthritis after a severe soft-tissue trauma 6 years ago. The foot is seen in a fixed equinus of 12°. (**b**) Though there is no supination deformity and only a distinct tilt of the navicular seen in the X-rays, a contract posterior tibial tendon was suspected because of severe pain along the tight tendon

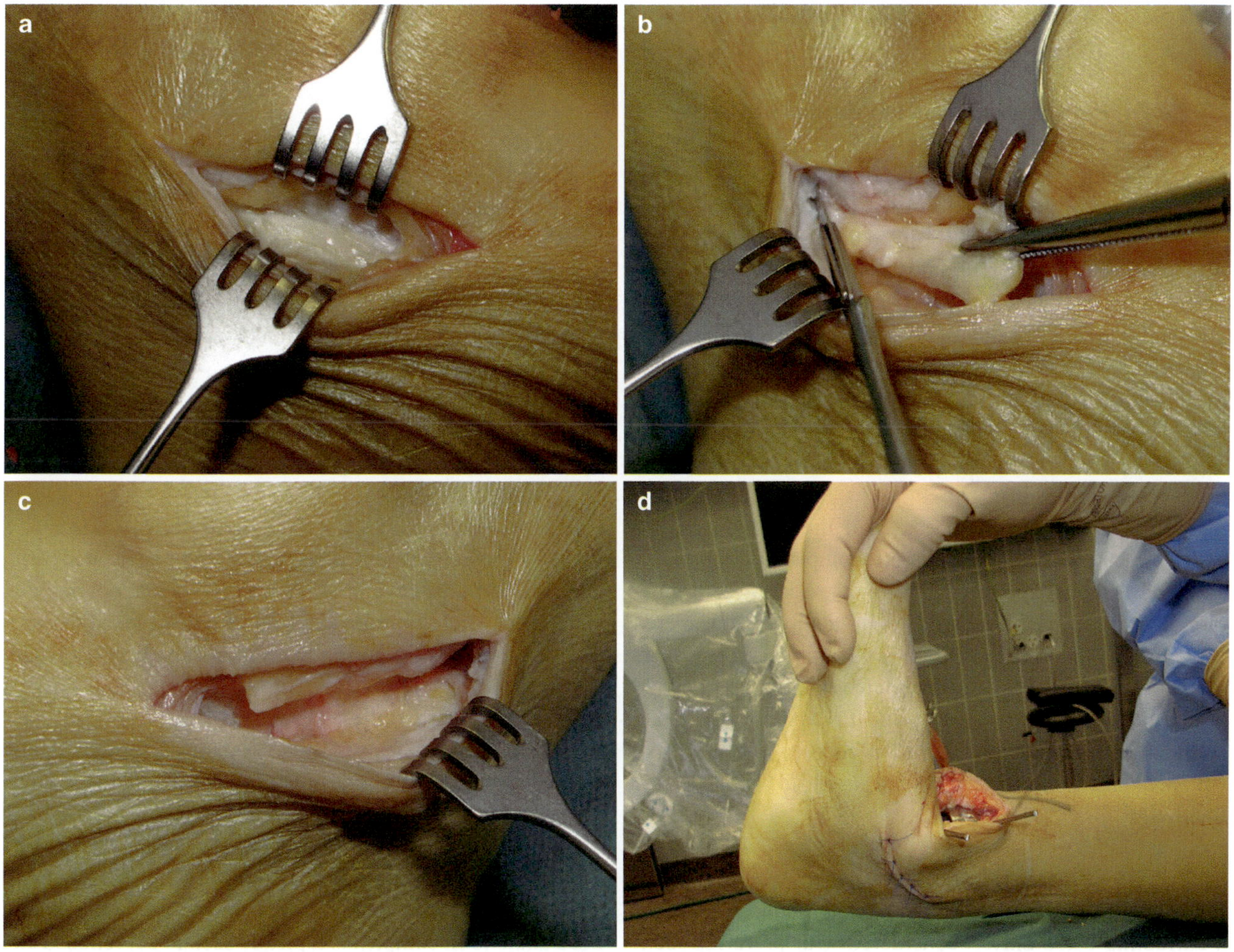

Fig. 10.6 Release of posterior tibial tendon. (**a**) Surgical exploration evidences a scarred posterior tibial tendon. (**b**) After dissection and surgical mobilization of the tendon, no excursion can be obtained, indicating that its muscle has lost its elasticity. (**c**) Therefore, the tendon is resected. (**d**) Thereafter, the foot can be forced into a dorsiflexed position without the additional release of the heel cord (same patient as Fig. 10.5)

10.1.2.5 Lateral Ligament Reconstruction

It is essential to ensure that the talus sits in a neutral position. Suppose an adequate position of the talus within the ankle mortise cannot be achieved, osteophytes in the lateral compartment or a too-long fibula can hinder the reposition (Fig. 10.3). If so, cleaning the lateral gutter and shortening the fibula must be done first. A supple lateral instability left after insertion of the implants can be successfully treated by reattachment of the scarred ligament by a bone anchor (Fig. 9.35); in the case of major lateral ankle instability, a reconstruction through a separate lateral approach might be necessary (Fig. 9.36). If the remaining ligaments are incompetent, a tendon graft or internal brace can be used for augmentation (Fig. 9.37).

10.1.2.6 Stabilization of Distal Tibiofibular Joint (Syndesmosis)

Though syndesmotic incompetence is rarely seen in a varus osteoarthritic ankle, the stability of the syndesmosis should constantly be tested (Fig. 9.43). Stabilization with the aid of a TightRope (Fig. 9.44) or position screw (Fig. 9.45) may be considered for minor instability, whereas, for gross instability, a fusion of the distal tibiofibular joint might be considered (Fig. 9.46).

10.1.2.7 Peroneus Longus to Peroneus Brevis Tendon Transfer

A long-standing varus deformity is often associated with the incompetence of the peroneus brevis tendon, resulting in an anterolateral extrusion of the talus out of the ankle mortise. As the peroneus longus has its attachment at the plantar aspect of first metatarsal, it acts as a plantar flexor of first ray, thus supporting supination and adduction of the foot. The effect of converting the peroneus longus tendon to an evertor by dissecting it at its entrance into the tunnel and transferring it to the base of the fifth metatarsal is therefore bifold, as its supination force is eliminated, and its action converted to a foot evertor (Fig. 9.48).

A tendon allograft may be used if the peroneus brevis and peroneus longus tendons are incompetent (Fig. 9.49). However, suppose the muscles do not work correctly anymore, a transfer of the posterior tibial tendon is considered (Fig. 9.50). The posterior tibial tendon is dissected at its insertion to the navicular and rerouted behind the tibia and fibula into peroneal tendon sheath. It is fixed to the distal stump of the peroneus brevis tendon. Side-to-side sutures to the peroneus longus tendon are used to enhance the fixation.

10.1.2.8 Calcaneal Osteotomy

If the calcaneus evidences persistent varus malalignment, a correcting osteotomy is considered. Our preferred technique is a Z-shaped osteotomy, allowing us to tilt the tuber calcanei into the valgus and slide it lateralward (Figs. 9.21 and 9.22).

10.1.2.9 Hindfoot Arthrodesis

In rigid or severe deformity, the above-described measures may not be sufficient to obtain a stable foot in a neutral position. In most instances, an isolated subtalar arthrodesis is enough to obtain this goal (Fig. 9.27). The subtalar joint is exposed through a limited sinus tarsi approach, and the subtalar joint is debrided to the subchondral bone. While the talus is forced to rotate internally on top of the calcaneus using distraction applied over two K-wires and a Hohmann retractor inserted in the sinus tarsi and pressed against the lateral talar neck, the foot is additionally forced into maximal dorsiflexion, thus pushing the talus anterior-ward. Temporary fixation is achieved by two K-wires that serve as guidance for cannulated screws. If, with this, the forefoot adduction cannot be corrected sufficiently, an additional fusion of the talonavicular joint (Fig. 9.28) and even of the calcaneocuboid joint can be considered.

10.1.2.10 Dorsiflexion Osteotomy of First Ray

A plantarflexed first metatarsal causes a pronation deformity of the forefoot, subsequently acting as a hindfoot supinator (Fig. 10.4c). A correcting osteotomy aims to elevate the first ray, which can be achieved by a closing wedge osteotomy at the medial cuneiform or base of first metatarsal (Fig. 10.7).

10.1.2.11 Heel Cord Lengthening

At the very end of the surgery, the foot is moved into maximal dorsiflexion. If <10° of dorsiflexion can be achieved, a lengthening of the Achilles tendon or a gastrocnemius recession is considered (Fig. 9.53b). If maximal dorsiflexion remains <10°, lengthening the heel cord is mandatory to restore a satisfactory foot function (Fig. 9.53a).

10.1.3 Algorithm for Surgical Treatment of a Varus-Valgus Ankle

Compared with an ankle with a varus-varus deformity, a varus-valgus deformity is typically not associated with medial soft-tissue contracture, a posterior ankle contracture, and a fixed forefoot pronation due to a plantarflexed first ray. The treatment algorithm is adapted accordingly (Fig. 10.8):

10.1.3.1 Supramalleolar Osteotomy

An LDTA angle <85° usually necessitates a supramalleolar osteotomy (Figs. 9.14–9.16).

10.1.3.2 Total Ankle Arthroplasty

Total ankle arthroplasty is performed using the standard technique. With the insertion of the prosthesis, the destabilized ankle joint complex is typically seen to get reduced and stabilized, and the varus-valgus deformity will disappear. Sometimes, a bigger polyethylene insert is necessary to achieve this goal.

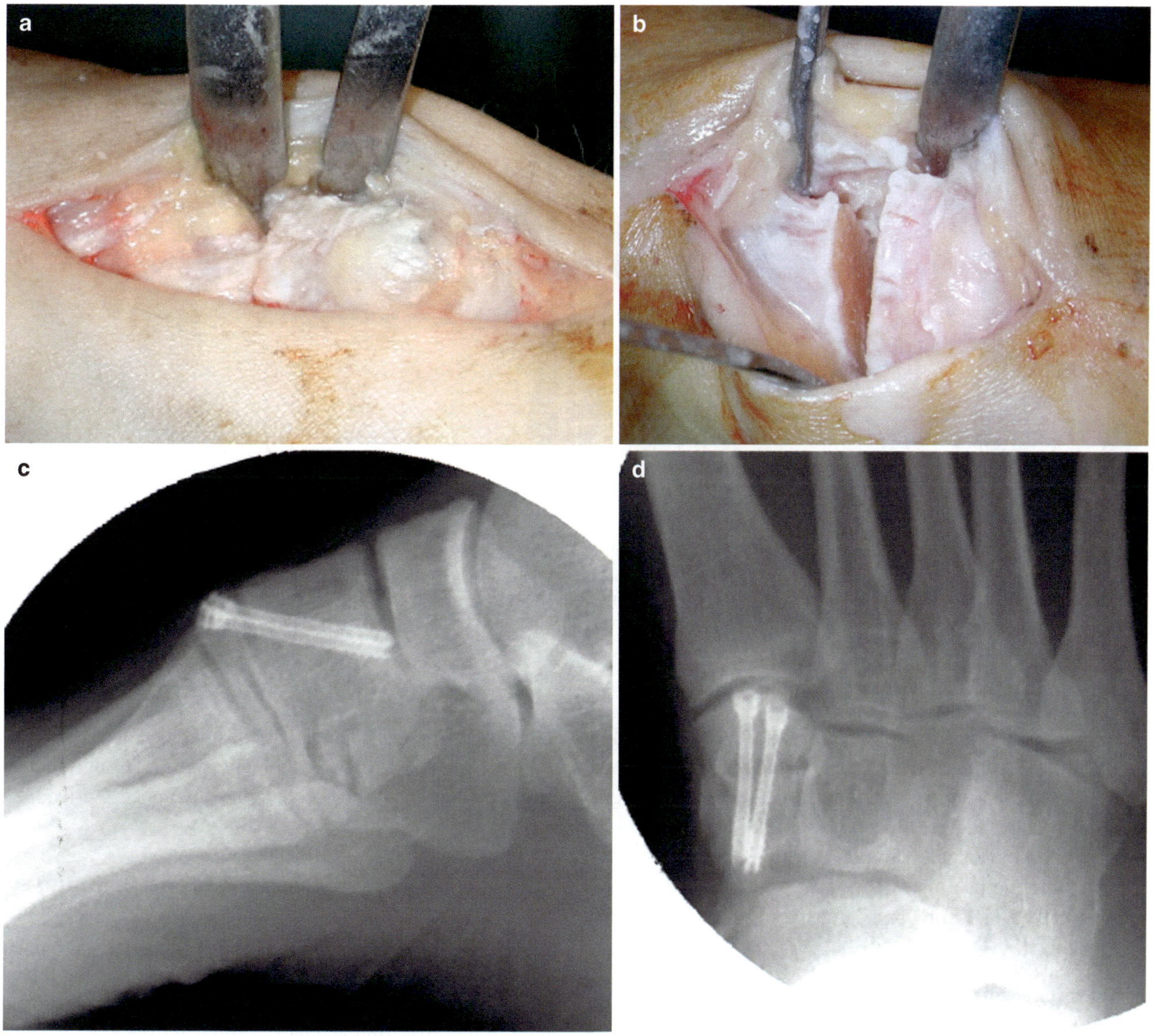

Fig. 10.7 Dorsiflexion osteotomy of first ray. (**a**) The medial cuneiform is exposed through a short longitudinal incision. (**b**) A double osteotomy is performed, and the wedge is removed. Attention is paid to preserving the plantar cortex. (**c**) Lateral view and (**d**) DP view showing the osteotomy after closure and fixation by two screws

10.1.3.3 Lateral Ligament Reconstruction

A supple lateral instability left after insertion of the implants can be successfully treated by reattachment of the scarred ligament by a bone anchor (Fig. 9.35); in the case of major lateral ankle instability, a reconstruction through a separate lateral approach might be necessary (Fig. 9.36). If the remaining ligaments are incompetent, a tendon graft or internal brace can be used for augmentation (Fig. 9.37).

10.1.3.4 Calcaneal Osteotomy

Supramalleolar and intraarticular correction of varus deformity may result in a valgus malalignment of the heel (Fig. 10.8). If not addressed, the eccentric lateral pull of the Achilles tendon would exert a medialization force on the talus, which may result in a painful medial impingement of the replaced ankle. Therefore, a medial sliding osteotomy should be performed to get a neutral heel position (Fig. 9.23).

10.1.4 Conclusions

Addressing all underlying components of the varus deformity meticulously is mandatory to obtain a well-balanced and stable ankle. In a cavovarus ("varus-varus") deformity, medial soft-tissue contractures and deforming forces must be eliminated to ensure a successful total ankle arthroplasty in the long term. In a "varus-valgus" deformity, in contrast,

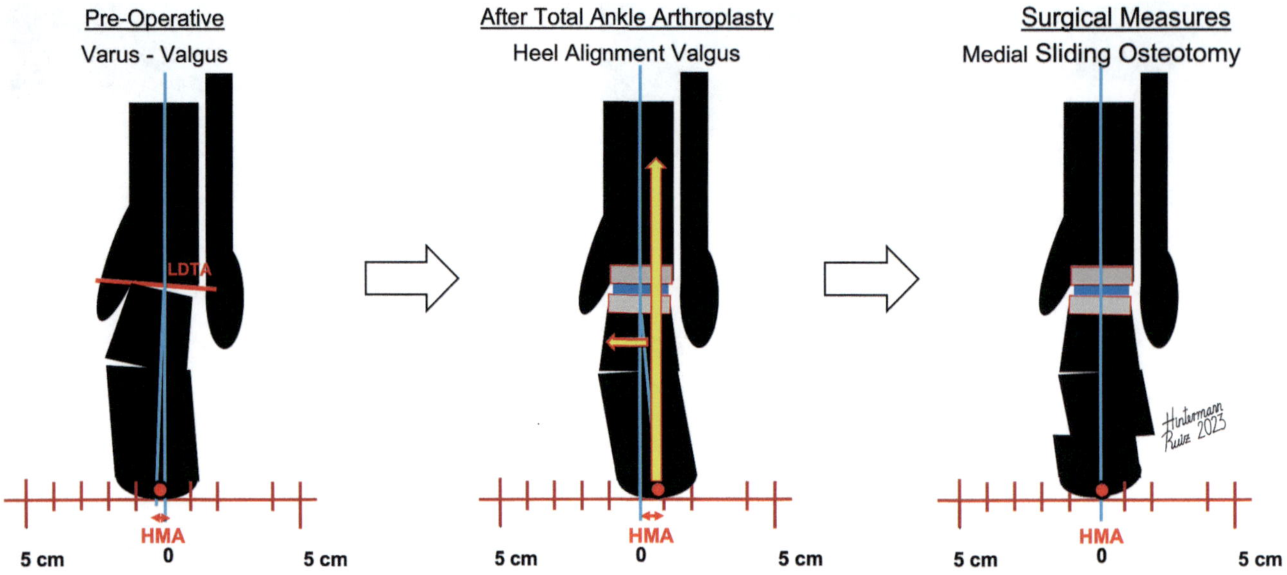

Fig. 10.8 Algorithm for surgical measure of a varus-valgus deformity. After the total ankle arthroplasty, the hindfoot is typically well-aligned due to the tightening of the ligaments. However, in the case of a major correction, especially in the presence of a subtalar joint contracture, the heel may become overcorrected into a valgus position, necessitating a medial sliding osteotomy to align the heel properly. If the heel valgus remains unresolved, an asymmetric pull of the heel cord will be created that exercises a translational force to the talus toward medially (arrow), which may result in a painful medial impingement

tightening and, if necessary, reconstruction of lateral ankle ligaments is essential for getting a stable and well-aligned ankle. Of note, an over-correction of the heel into a valgus position must be addressed by a medial sliding osteotomy to avoid painful medial ankle impingement, especially with the use of a mobile-bearing ankle where the second interface allows the talus for free translational and rotatory movement.

10.2 Total Ankle Arthroplasty in a Valgus Osteoarthritic Ankle

Total ankle arthroplasty is only successful when the replaced ankle is stable and the implants are well-positioned. This is particularly challenging in ankles, where the talus has tilted into valgus within the ankle mortise because of medial soft-tissue incompetence and a valgus malalignment of the heel associated with a breakdown of the medial arch, respectively. While standing, the center of force transmission is lateralized. The forces within the joint are amplified by activation of the triceps surae, and the Achilles tendon may become an evertor, thereby acting as an additional deforming force on the hindfoot.

In contrast to a varus deformity, a valgus deformity is usually associated with a significant destabilization of the foot that progresses over time. Therefore, as a rule, appropriate realignment of the bony structures is mandatory for success. If osteotomies cannot achieve this alone, arthrodesis procedures at the inframalleolar side must be considered. Contrary to general belief, the heel cord is seldom too short in a valgus deformity, thus making a heel cord lengthening unnecessarily.

10.2.1 Preoperative Assessment and Planning

Besides thorough clinical investigation (Fig. 10.9), diagnostic imaging under weight-bearing conditions is essential in the preoperative workup of the valgus osteoarthritic arthritic ankle. Weight-bearing standard X-rays are the base for recognizing foot abnormalities and deformities; primarily, they serve to assess the talar position within the ankle mortise in all three planes, which also provides information about segmental instability of the ankle joint complex (Fig. 10.10). The weight-bearing CT scan has evolved to be a helpful tool for better understanding the deformity and destabilization process in all three planes (Fig. 10.11). It allows the surgeon to recognize the extent of articular wear and subchondral changes. It provides information about the 3-D deviation of the bones and the segmental instability pattern of the foot and ankle.

A valgus-tilted talus can be associated with a calcaneus in valgus ("valgus-valgus" deformity), as typically seen in a valgus deformity and flatfoot deformity (Figs. 9.12 and 10.10). However, it can be associated with a calcaneus in varus, resulting in a "valgus-varus" deformity that indicates a peritalar instability with the collapse of the ankle joint complex (Fig. 9.26).

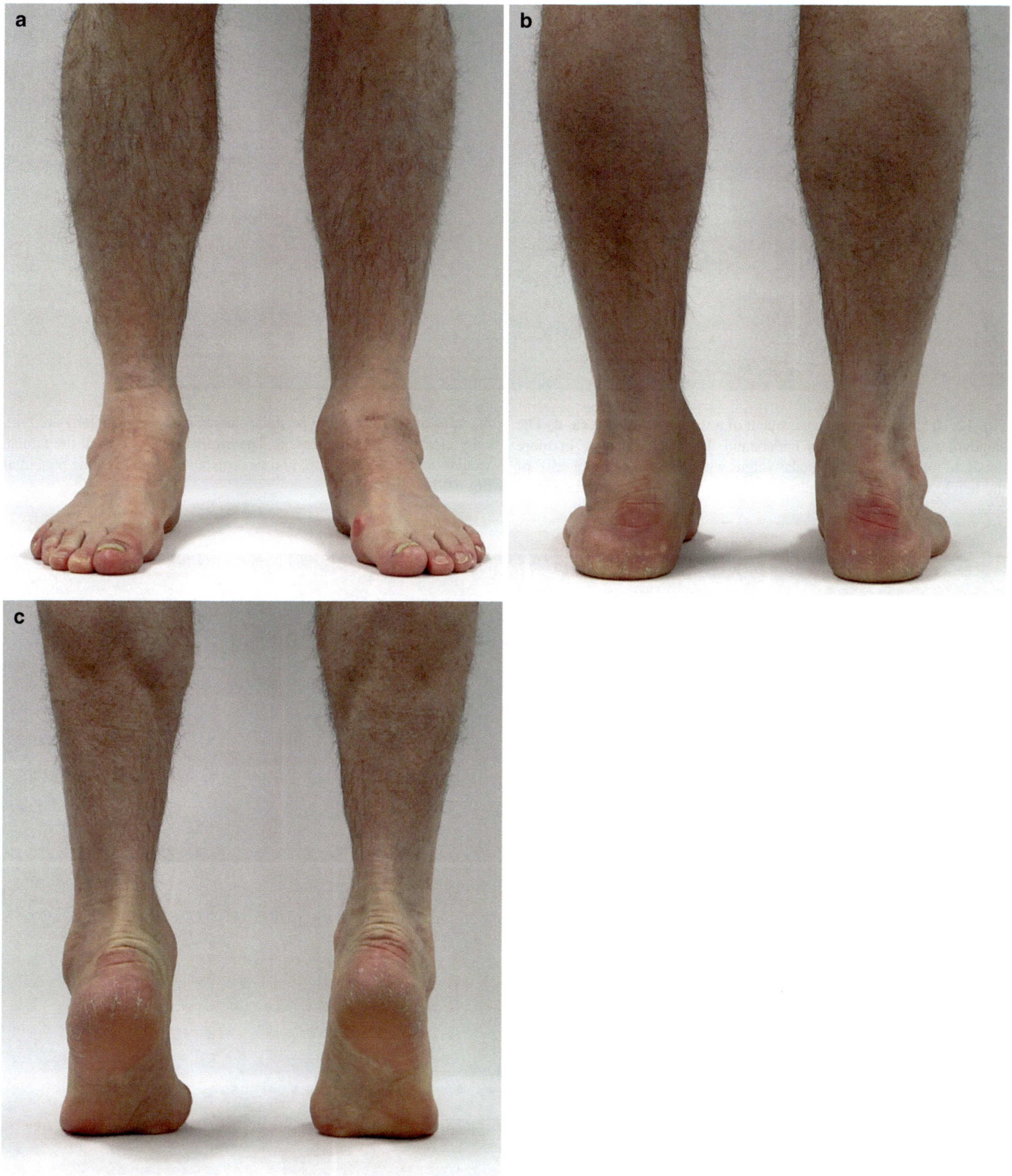

Fig. 10.9 Clinical investigation of a valgus deformity. The anterior (**a**) and posterior (**b**) view shows a complex valgus deformity when standing that is corrected in the tiptoe position due to the activation of the posterior tibial tendon, also meaning that the deformity is correctable (**c**)

Theoretically, the malalignment can be treated with correcting cuts. Still, there are apparent limits to getting a balanced ankle. Thus, additional measures are necessary, namely, osteotomies, arthrodesis, and ligament reconstructions, with the specific aims of (1) to realign the hindfoot, (2) to stabilize the foot and ankle joint complex, (3) to transfer the ankle joint under the weight-bearing axis, and (4) to normalize the direction of the force vector of the triceps surae. Suppose the sub-

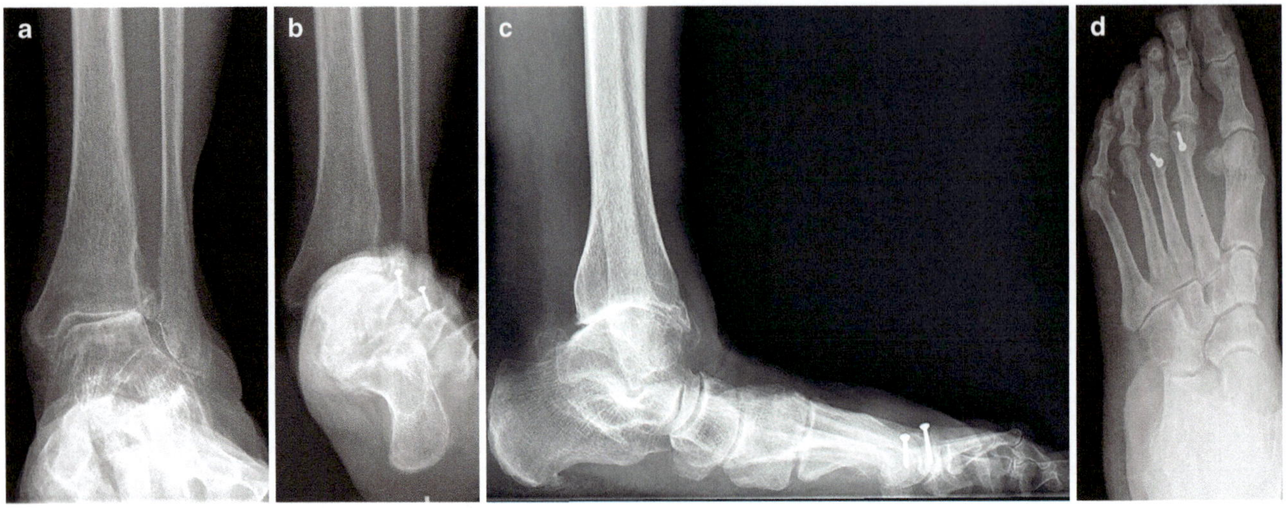

Fig. 10.10 Radiographic assessment of a valgus deformity. (**a–d**) The standard radiographs let us understand the 3-D deformity in more detail. In this case, there is a talar valgus with a medial gapping <50° of the height of the medial malleolus associated with a plantarflexion of the talus as a cause of the peritalar instability. The sinus tarsi are typically closed with impingement. The arc is broken down at the talonavicular, naviculocuneiform, and tarsometatarsal joints (same patient as Fig. 10.10)

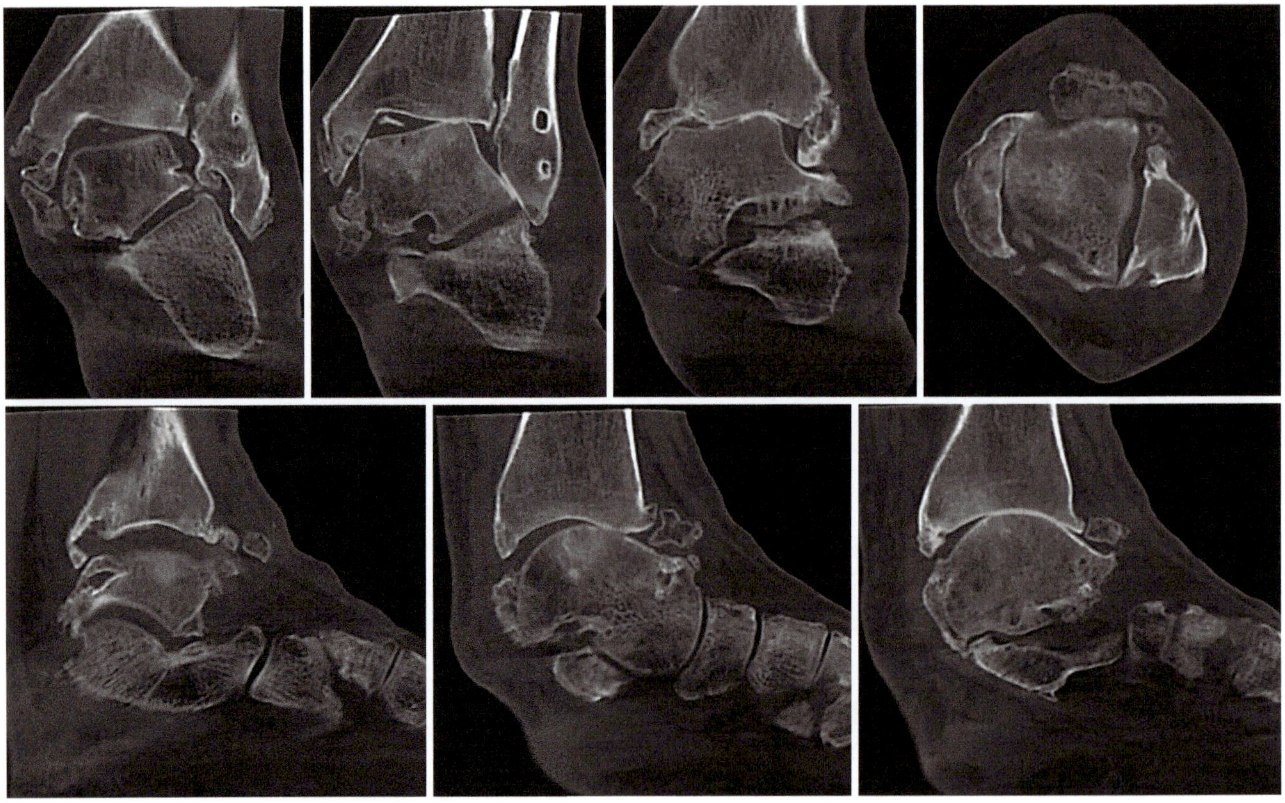

Fig. 10.11 Weight-bearing CT scan in a valgus deformity. The weight-bearing CT scan shows the degenerative disease and the segmental instability in all three planes; in particular, it evidences an old bony avulsion of the deltoid ligament and the severe talus tilt resulting in subfibular impingement. The peritalar instability pattern can also be understood in more detail (same patient as Fig. 10.10)

talar joint is highly unstable, thus allowing the talus to glide toward the medial and anterior on the calcaneus. In that case, a subtalar fusion is essential to get a stable hindfoot and avoid a deformity progression. Similarly, if the subtalar joint is not reducible or in an advanced stage of degenerative disease, a subtalar fusion will also be necessary (Fig. 10.12).

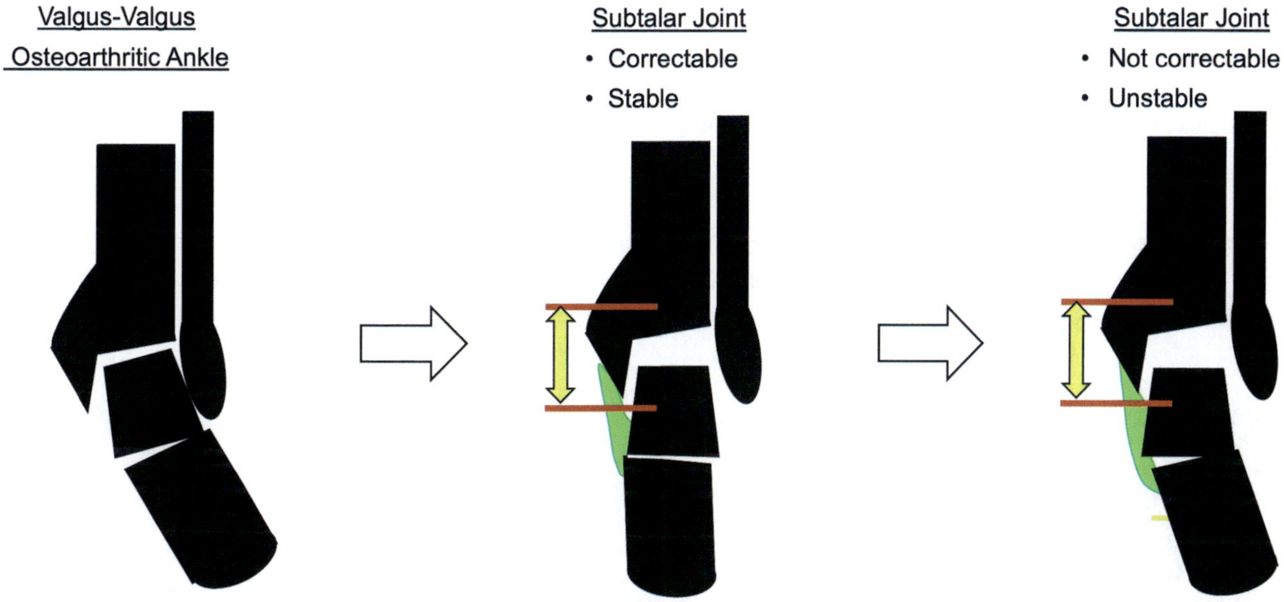

Fig. 10.12 Testing the subtalar joint by distraction. The surgeon can recognize whether the subtalar joint is contract or highly unstable by distracting the ankle joint. If so, a subtalar joint will be necessary

10.2.2 Algorithm for Surgical Treatment of a Valgus-Valgus Ankle

A "valgus-valgus" deformity is typically seen in a flatfoot deformity with a progressive breakdown of the medial arch, thus making additional measures necessary to restore the incompetent medial arch. As a rule, it will need less bone resection on the tibial side; as the inserted ankle prosthesis will work as a spacer, the ligaments will be tensioned, and the ankle joint will be realigned. However, in the great majority, an additional medial sliding osteotomy (Fig. 9.24) or subtalar fusion (Fig. 9.27) will be mandatory to obtain a stable and well-aligned ankle joint complex. Bony procedures along the medial foot are often also necessary to obtain a stable foot.

The authors' proposed step-by-step algorithm for a "valgus-valgus" ankle is as follows (Fig. 10.13):

10.2.2.1 Supramalleolar Correction

A minor valgus deformity can be addressed by correcting the cut of the distal tibia; however, an LDTA angle >5° usually necessitates a supramalleolar osteotomy (Fig. 9.14).

10.2.2.2 Subtalar Fusion

A subtalar fusion is done before the replacement surgery in significant medial destabilization of peritalar joints or rigid valgus deformities (Fig. 9.27). Appropriate repositioning of the talus on top of the calcaneus is essential to stabilize it and protect it against the progression of the deformity.

10.2.2.3 Total Ankle Arthroplasty

Total ankle arthroplasty is now performed using the standard technique. The prosthesis is a spacer to tension the worn-out ligaments (Fig. 10.14). The tibial resection cut is done more distally to preserve as much bone as possible and avoid using an oversized polyethylene insert. It might be favorable to leave the trial insert in place and wait to select and insert the final polyethylene insert until additional measures achieve alignment and stabilization of the ankle joint complex.

10.2.2.4 Intraarticular Correcting Osteotomy

A fibular osteotomy may be considered for malunion after ankle fracture with shortening and external malrotation of the distal fibula. Another indication for a distal fibular osteotomy may be a lateral malleolus dysplasia caused by the long-standing valgus position of the talus and subsequent erosion of the lateral malleolus. To close the created capacious lateral gutter, a transverse opening wedge osteotomy is performed to close the gutter to the appropriate width.

10.2.2.5 Calcaneal Osteotomy

If the hindfoot is still in valgus after the ankle replacement surgery, a medial sliding osteotomy of the calcaneus should be considered (Fig. 9.24). The goal is to obtain a neutral or slightly varus-aligned hindfoot.

10.2.2.6 Medial Ligament Reconstruction

In mild medial ligament incompetence, e.g., if the lateral tibiotalar gapping is <50% of the height of the medial malleolus, medial ligament reconstruction may be considered (Fig. 9.39). This is particularly true for an old bony avulsion injury to the superficial deltoid. After having debrided the colliculus anterius of the medial malleolus, the trial insert is removed, and reattachment of the deltoid to the medial malleolus is achieved with the aid of an anchor or transosseous sutures. The trial insert is inserted again, thereby tightening the reconstructed ligaments. Once the appropriate size of the insert is determined, the final polyethylene inlay is inserted.

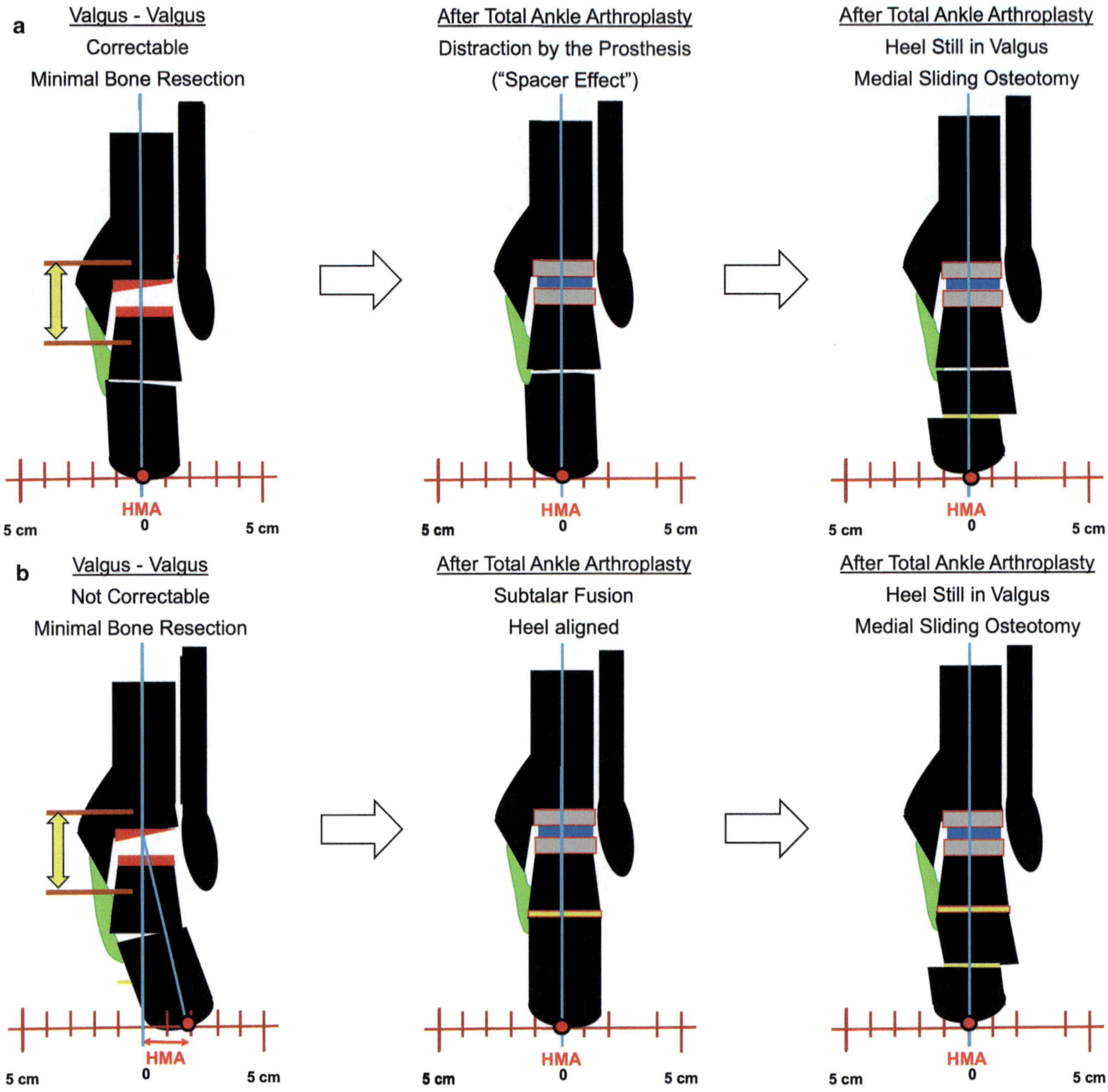

Fig. 10.13 Algorithm for surgical measures of a valgus-valgus ankle. After ankle exposure, the joint is distracted with a distraction device mounted over two K-wires at the medial side. (**a**) If the subtalar joint is seen to be reduced and stable, minimal bone is resected on the tibial side, and talar resection cuts are performed to replace the ankle. The inserted implants preserve the joint distraction when the distraction device is removed. If the heel is still in valgus, an osteotomy of the calcaneal tuber slides the tuber fragment medial-ward until a neutral alignment is achieved. (**b**) If the subtalar joint is contract or highly unstable, a subtalar joint is performed. If, with this, the heel remains in a valgus position, a medial sliding osteotomy is added to get the heel in a neutral position. (**c**) If lateral ankle instability occurs, lateral ligament reconstruction is performed. If the syndesmotic ligaments are incompetent, as seen by manual stress testing, a fusion of the distal tibiofibular joint is performed. At this stage, a stable hindfoot is achieved. (**d**) If there is evidence of an incompetent medial arch, as seen by a minor correctable forefoot supination deformity, a plantarflexion osteotomy of the first cuneiform or metatarsal bone is added. In a significant forefoot supination deformity, mainly when fixed, a fusion at the level of the primary deformity is performed to achieve a neutral and stable forefoot position

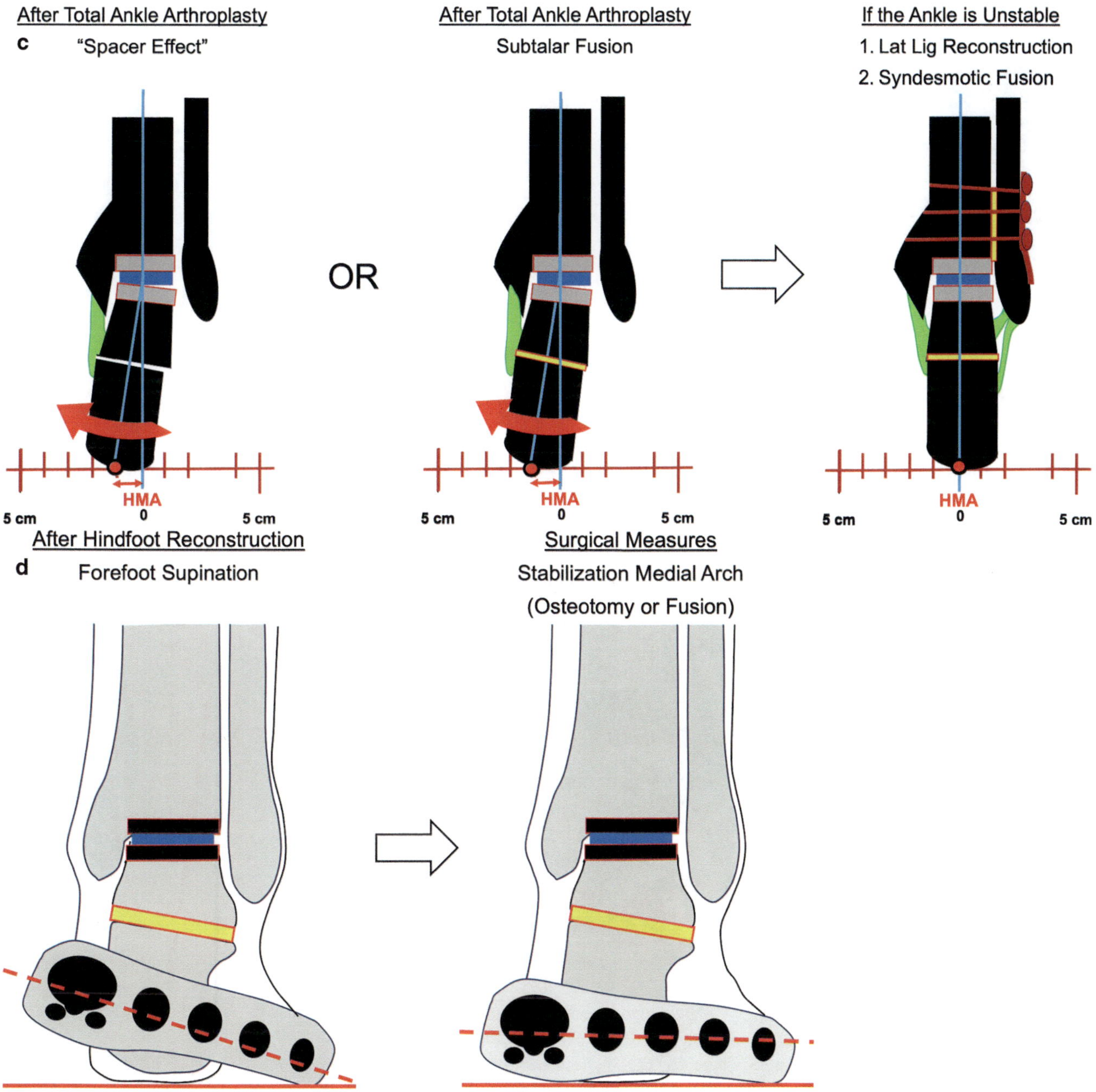

Fig. 10.13 (continued)

10.2.2.7 Lateral Ligament Reconstruction

In valgus ankle osteoarthritis, a lateral ligament insufficiency due to previous injuries can often be found in addition to deltoid incompetence. Another reason can be that the valgus position of the calcaneus leads to calcaneofibular impingement, and the lateral ankle ligaments can be ground off the lateral malleolus. Not addressing the lateral instability is especially critical if the lax medial ankle ligaments are tightened with a too-big polyethylene insert, which may result in lateral gapping of the inserted prosthesis (Fig. 10.13c). A lateral ankle ligament reconstruction is made through a separate lateral approach with transosseous reattachment of the ligaments to the fibula or using a tendon graft or internal brace (Figs. 9.35–9.37).

10.2.2.8 Syndesmotic Stabilization

In valgus ankle or hindfoot deformities, chronic stress on the syndesmotic ligaments may result in distal tibiofibular instability (Fig. 9.43). Such instability may occur in the coronal, sagittal, or both planes. If not addressed, this can create instability of the replaced ankle, which may lead to early failure. Suppose gapping and sagittal plane instability of the

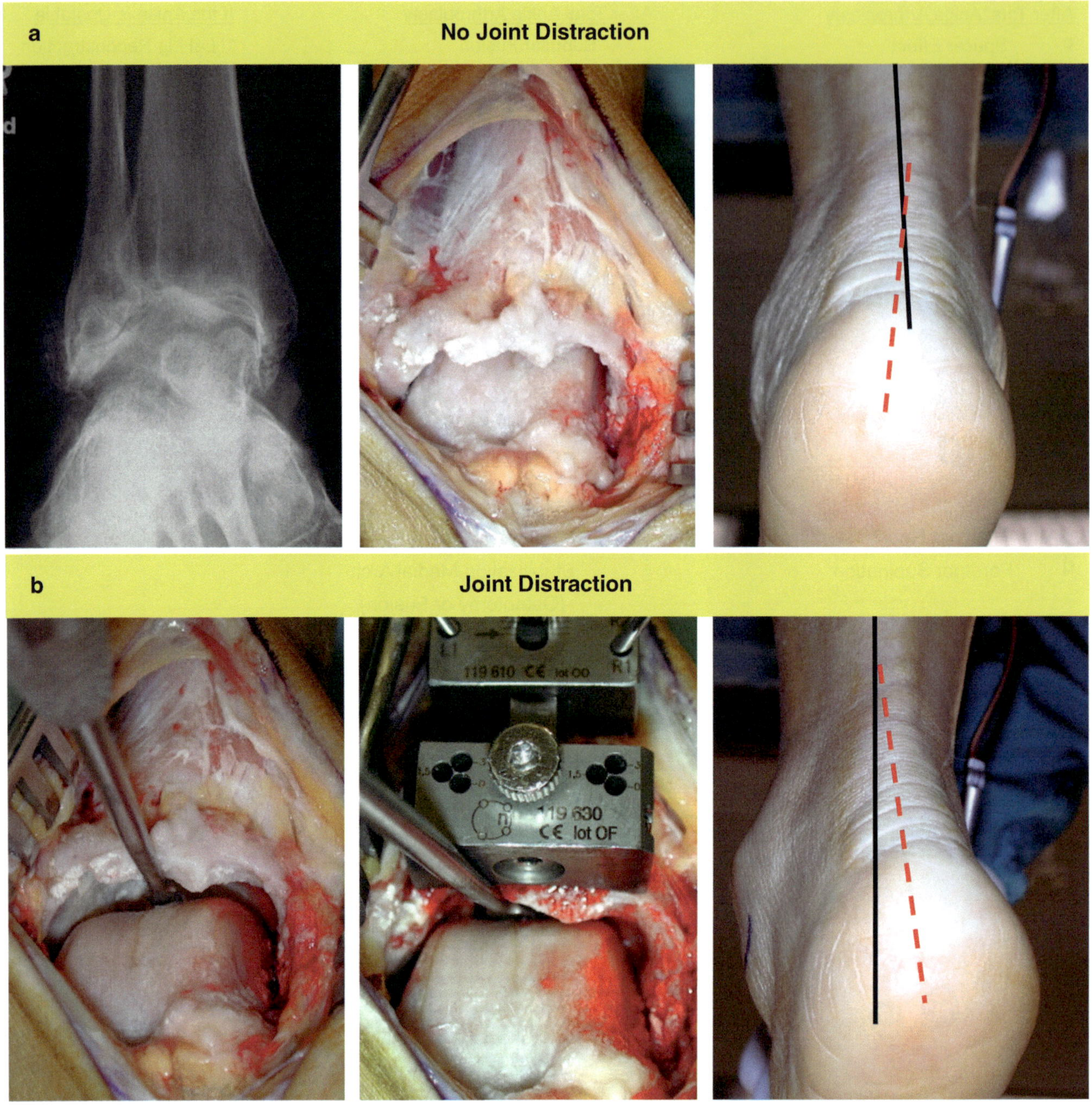

Fig. 10.14 Total ankle arthroplasty in a valgus-valgus deformity. A 57-year-old wife of a farmer suffering from severe valgus osteoarthritis of her right ankle. (**a**) Without distraction, the whole ankle joint complex is in a valgus position. (**b**) When the ankle joint is distracted, as shown with a raspatorium inserted, the ankle joint complex is seen to be realigned. This signalizes the surgeon that minimal bone resection will be necessary for the prosthesis to act as a spacer, thus being capable of tensioning the ligaments and realigning the hindfoot

fibula is found by manual testing, debridement of the distal tibiofibular joint, and stabilization, performing a fusion with the aid of a plate and two to three screws is recommended (Figs. 9.44–9.46, and 10.13c).

10.2.2.9 Reconstruction of Medial Arch

In the case of a progressive breakdown of the medial arch with a sag at the talonavicular, naviculocuneiform, or tarsometatarsal joint, a plantarflexing osteotomy or a fusion at the affected joint level is considered (Fig. 9.29). In our experience, in most instances, the breakdown is located at naviculocuneiform level (Fig. 9.31). After a subtalar fusion, a fusion at the affected level is performed to restore the arch, address the associated peritalar instability, and correctly reposition the talus on top of the calcaneus. In a consecutive series of 32 patients, subtalar and naviculocuneiform fusion was very effective, providing excellent stability over time [11].

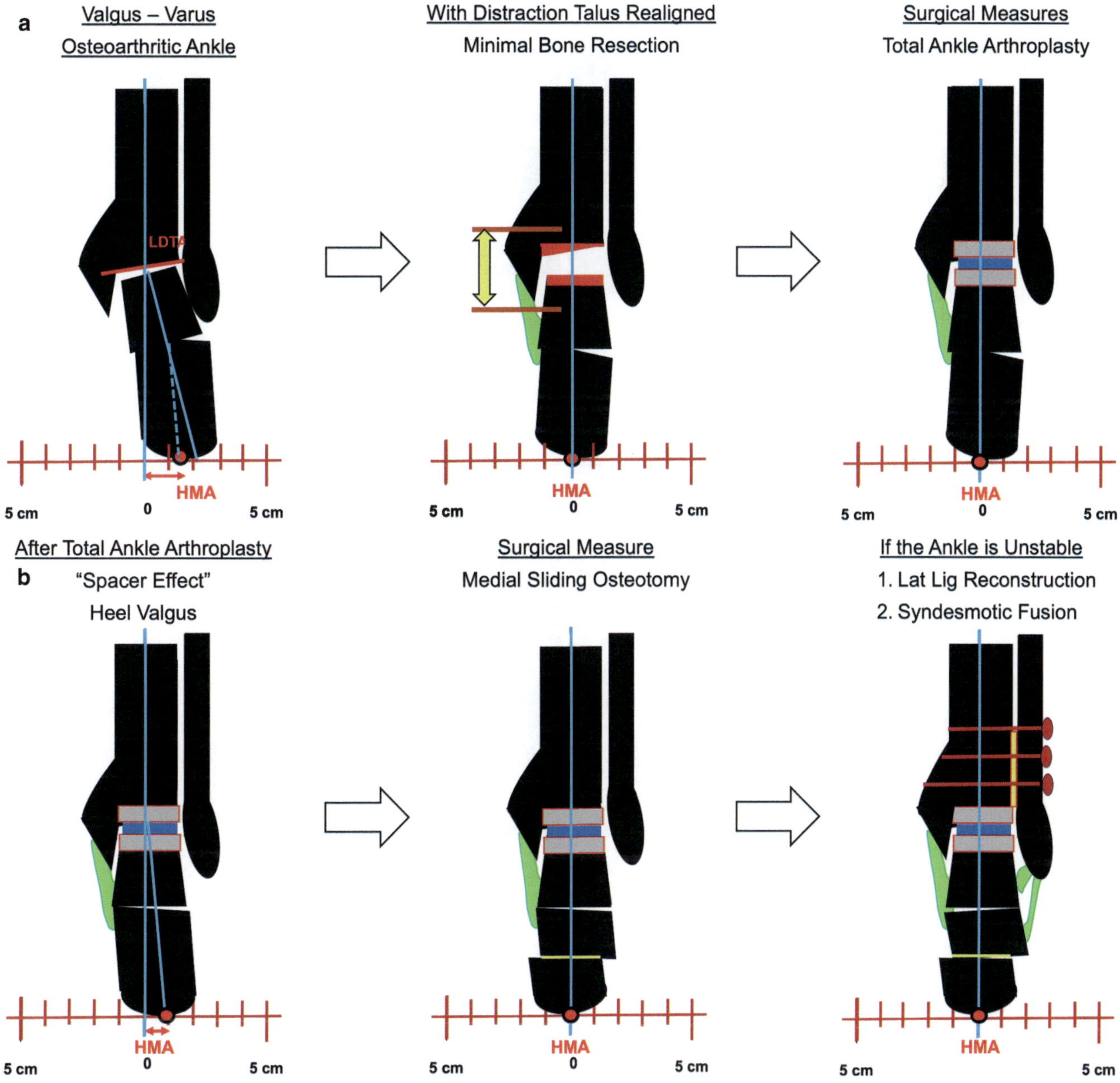

Fig. 10.15 Algorithm for surgical measures of a valgus-varus ankle. (**a**) After ankle exposure, the joint is distracted over two K-wires at the medial side as much as the hindfoot is seen to get into a neutral position. The resection cuts are done by the instrumentation set of the selected ankle prosthesis, and the components are inserted. (**b**) If a valgus position of the hindfoot persists, an additional medial sliding osteotomy may be considered. Finally, if needed, reconstruction of medial and lateral ligaments is performed. An unstable syndesmosis, often more pronounced in the sagittal than the coronal plane, might be considered a fusion of the distal tibiofibular joint

10.2.3 Algorithm for Surgical Treatment of a Valgus-Varus Ankle

Compared with an ankle with a valgus-valgus deformity, a valgus-varus deformity is typically not associated with a progressive flatfoot deformity with a breakdown of the arch. The subtalar joint may show degenerative changes but does not evidence instability with medial subluxation of the talus on top of the calcaneus. The treatment algorithm is adapted accordingly (Fig. 10.15):

10.2.3.1 Supramalleolar Osteotomy

An LDTA angle >5° usually necessitates a supramalleolar osteotomy (Fig. 9.14).

10.2.3.2 Total Ankle Arthroplasty

Total ankle arthroplasty is performed using the standard technique. With the distraction of the exposed tibiotalar joint, the destabilized ankle joint complex is typically seen to get reduced and stabilized, and the valgus-varus deformity will disappear (Fig. 10.15a). The same effect is seen after

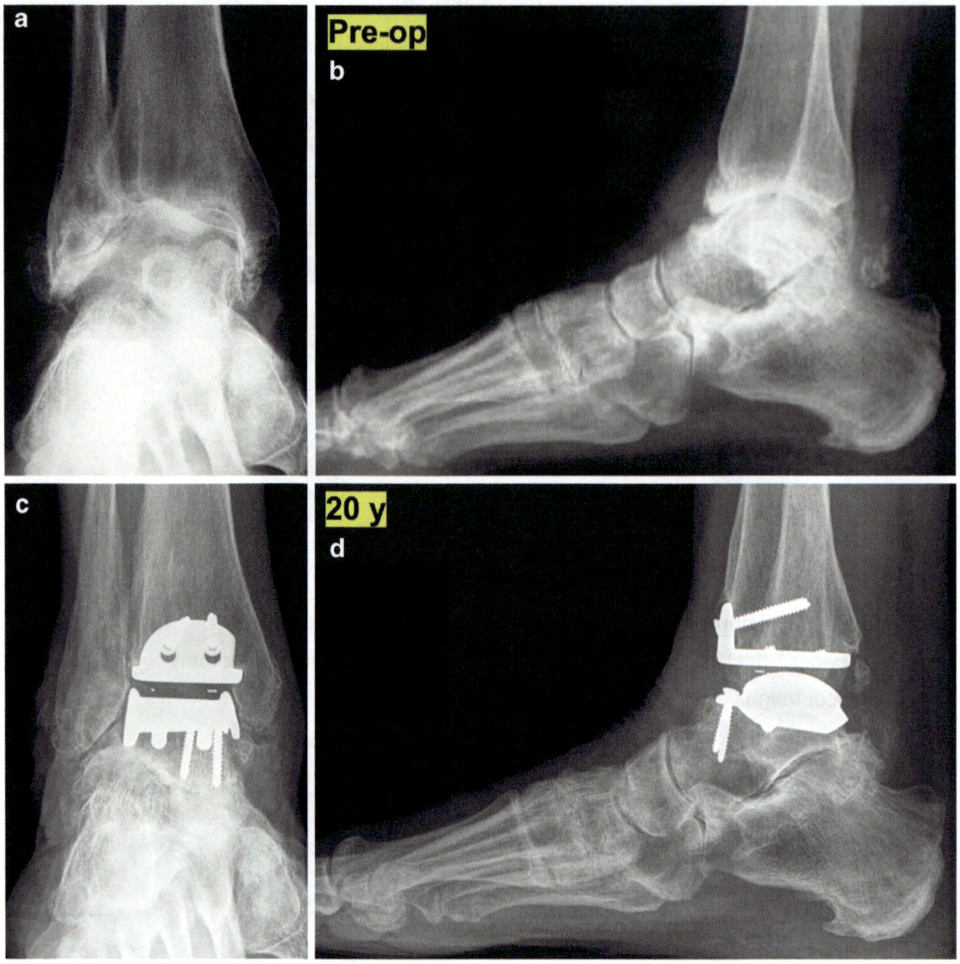

Fig. 10.16 Effect of distraction by the prosthesis. (**a–b**) This 61-year-old patient who presented with a significant valgus deformity was treated solely with an ankle replacement surgery. (**c–d**) 20 years later, the hindfoot was still well-aligned, without evidence of the incompetence of the medial arch. Notice the improved position of the subtalar joint with well-preserved articular surfaces

prosthesis insertion (Fig. 10.16). Sometimes, a thicker polyethylene insert is necessary to achieve this goal.

10.2.3.3 Intraarticular Correcting Osteotomy

A fibular osteotomy may be considered in the case of malunion after ankle fracture with shortening and external malrotation of the distal fibula or if the lateral malleolus shows a dysplasia caused by erosion of lateral malleolus subsequently to the valgus position of the talus. To close the created capacious lateral gutter, a transverse opening wedge osteotomy is performed to close the gutter to the appropriate width.

10.2.3.4 Lateral Ligament Reconstruction

A supple lateral instability left after the insertion of the implants can be successfully treated by reconstruction through a separate lateral approach (Fig. 9.36). If the remaining ligaments are incompetent, a tendon graft or internal brace can be used for augmentation (Fig. 9.37).

10.2.3.5 Syndesmotic Stabilization

Analogously to a valgus-valgus deformity, chronic stress on the syndesmotic ligaments may result in distal tibiofibular instability, necessitating a syndesmotic fusion to stabilize the replaced ankle properly and to prevent early failure (Fig. 9.46).

10.2.3.6 Calcaneal Osteotomy

Supramalleolar and intraarticular correction of valgus deformity may not sufficiently correct the valgus malalignment of the heel. If this is the case, a medial sliding osteotomy should be performed to get a neutral or slightly varus heel position (Fig. 9.24).

10.2.3.7 Conclusions

As a valgus deformity usually progresses, addressing all underlying components is mandatory to obtain a well-balanced and stable ankle. This is, in particular, true for the "valgus-valgus" deformity, which is typically associated with a progressive flatfoot deformity and breakdown of the arch, where obtaining a stable foot and ankle in a neutral position is essential for the success of total ankle arthroplasty in the long term. In a "valgus-varus" deformity, in contrast, tightening of medial and lateral ankle ligaments by insertion of the ankle prosthesis is often sufficient for getting a well-aligned ankle.

In any case of valgus deformity, an unstable distal tibiofibular joint may be present due to chronic overload, and if so, it must be addressed by a stabilization procedure. At the end of the surgery, the heel should never be left in a valgus malaligned position, as this might result in early failure.

10.3 Total Ankle Arthroplasty in Sagittal Plane Deformities

Sagittal plane deformities include recurvatum and procurvatum deformities.

10.3.1 Recurvatum Deformity

A recurvatum deformity is typically associated with a stiff ankle with limited dorsiflexion, leading to anterior plafond wear due to the talus being repetitively driven into the anterior tibia. It can also result from avascular necrosis or defect at the anterior tibia with the subsequent intrusion of the talar body into the tibial plafond. The resulting anterior escape of the talus may cause or result from a tight posterior capsule and Achilles tendon contracture.

10.3.1.1 Preoperative Assessment and Planning

Differentiating between intraarticular and extraarticular deformities is of utmost importance, as extraarticular deformities involve an anterior translation with loss of leverage of the Achilles tendon about the ankle joint axis, whereas, in intraarticular deformities, the ankle itself remains somehow balanced. In any case, the deviation of the center of rotation of the ankle, as indicated by the center of a circle given by the talus' articular surface, to the tibia's mechanical axis should be calculated and compared to the contralateral non-affected ankle. Particular attention should be paid to a malunited fibula that can be the underlying cause of anterior extrusion of the talus with subsequent erosion of the distal tibia. The talus will remain fixed in the anterior position if not addressed, resulting in non-balanced total ankle arthroplasty.

10.3.1.2 Surgical Technique

Theoretically, an intraarticular recurvatum can be addressed through the joint by performing appropriate resection for the arthroplasty at the level of the anterior ledge of cortical tibial bone (Fig. 10.17a). However, this procedure may leave an extensive resection of the posterior bone of the tibia that can be challenging to remove and result in significant bone loss at the distal tibia. Alternatively, an open wedge osteotomy of the distal tibia performed before the tibial resection cut is made will prevent unnecessary bone loss and, in addition, move the mechanical axis of the tibia anterior ward (Fig. 10.17b). An extraarticular recurvatum deformity, in contrast, always requires an open wedge osteotomy of the distal tibia about the CORA (Fig. 10.17c). Besides a complete posterior release, aggressive debridement of medial and lateral gutters is often necessary to allow the talus to translate posterior wards.

The Authors' Approach

*With an increased ADTA angle of > 5° compared to the contralateral ankle, a correcting osteotomy is indicated to avoid unnecessary bone loss and to balance the replaced ankle. An osteotomy is also considered for fear of overstuffing the ankle instead of getting it balanced in the sagittal plane. The same strategy may be used for avascular necrosis of the anterior tibial plafond (*Fig. 10.18*).*

10.3.2 Procurvatum Deformity

A procurvatum deformity is the least common of the deformities seen at the osteoarthritic ankle joint. An intraarticular deformity usually results from posterior bony wear, allowing posterior escape and some proximal migration, often due to global instability of the foot associated with a plantarflexed talus in the presence of a breakdown of the arch. In contrast to a recurvatum deformity, an extraarticular deformity is rarely seen.

10.3.2.1 Preoperative Assessment and Planning

A thorough imaging workup of the foot and ankle is necessary to fully understand the deformity and identify the underlying causes, especially to substantiate a potential posterior position of the fibula due to syndesmotic instability or malunion after a fracture.

10.3.2.2 Surgical Technique

A procurvatum deformity is generally corrected through the joint with a tibial resection based on the posterior ledge of the tibial cortical bone at its lowest level. In the case of distal tibiofibular instability or a fibular malunion, a syndesmotic fusion or a correcting fibula osteotomy should be performed before ankle replacement surgery.

The Authors' Approach

To counteract the translation forces toward the posterior, we aim to achieve a slightly increased ADTA angle (posterior tilt) with the resection cut of the tibia.

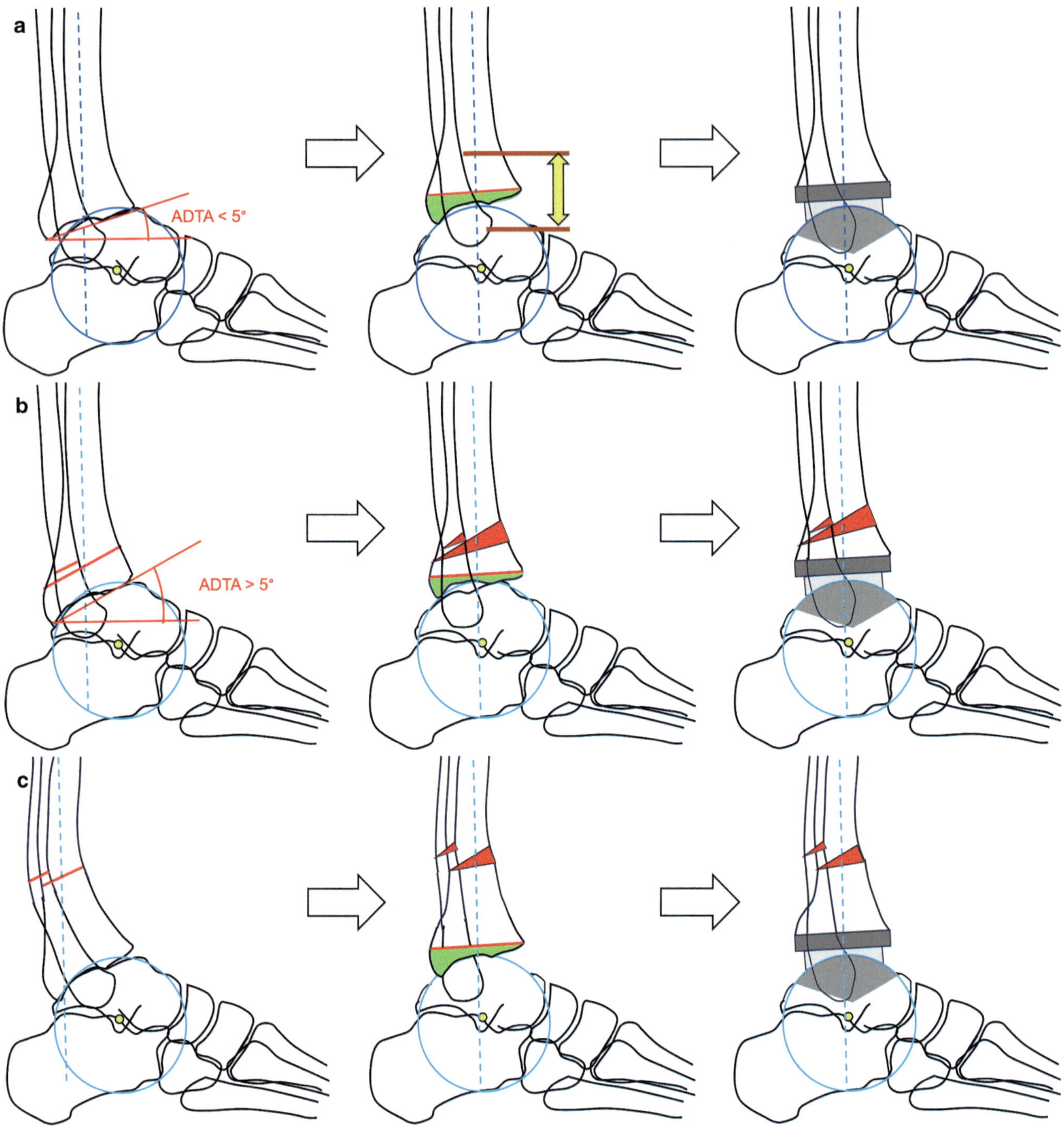

Fig. 10.17 Algorithm for addressing the recurvatum deformity. (**a**) If, in an intraarticular recurvatum deformity, the anterior ledge of the tibia is well-preserved and the ADTA angle increased by <5°, a correcting tibial cut is made, paying attention to preserving the anterior cortex of the tibia. When the joint is distracted, the tibial alignment should be restored; if not, there might be a posterior contracture, a fibular malunion, or both that must be addressed first. (**b**) If the ADTA angle is increased by >5° or the erosion process has weakened the anterior cortex, a correcting osteotomy of the distal tibia should be done before the tibial resection. This allows the preservation of bone and efficiently realigns the ankle in the sagittal plane. (**c**) If there is an extraarticular recurvatum deformity, a correcting osteotomy must always be done first

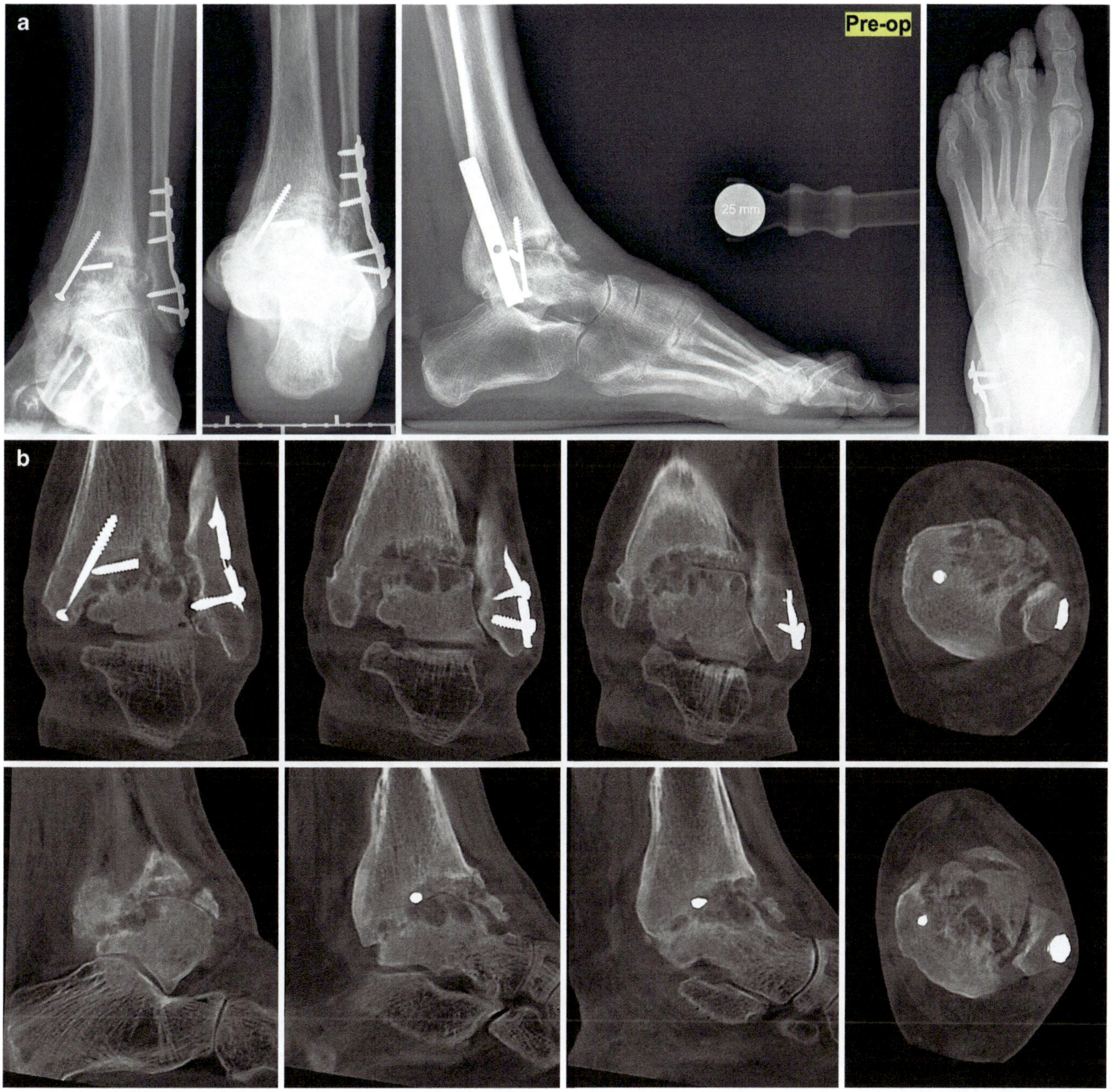

Fig. 10.18 Anterior opening wedge osteotomy. A 54-year-old female patient 14 months after an ankle fracture that was treated operatively. (**a**) The standard radiographs show the extended bone loss of the anterior part of the tibial plafond. (**b**) The weight-bearing CT scan evidences the extent of bone loss in more detail. (**c**) The extent of bone loss is also seen after ankle distraction. Thus, an osteotomy is aimed to recentralize the ankle and preserve the bone. The K-wire is inserted for planning the osteotomy with a CORA close to the joint. (**d**) The osteotomy is open step by step until the wanted correction is achieved, as checked by fluoroscopy. (**e**) An allograft is inserted, and the distraction is removed. (**f**) A plate is used for stabilization, paying attention to not getting into conflict with the subsequent total ankle arthroplasty (**g**–**h**). (**i**) Radiographs at 5-year follow-up control show a well-balanced ankle joint and stable components. Notice the load transmission, which is slightly posterior to the mechanical axis of the tibia

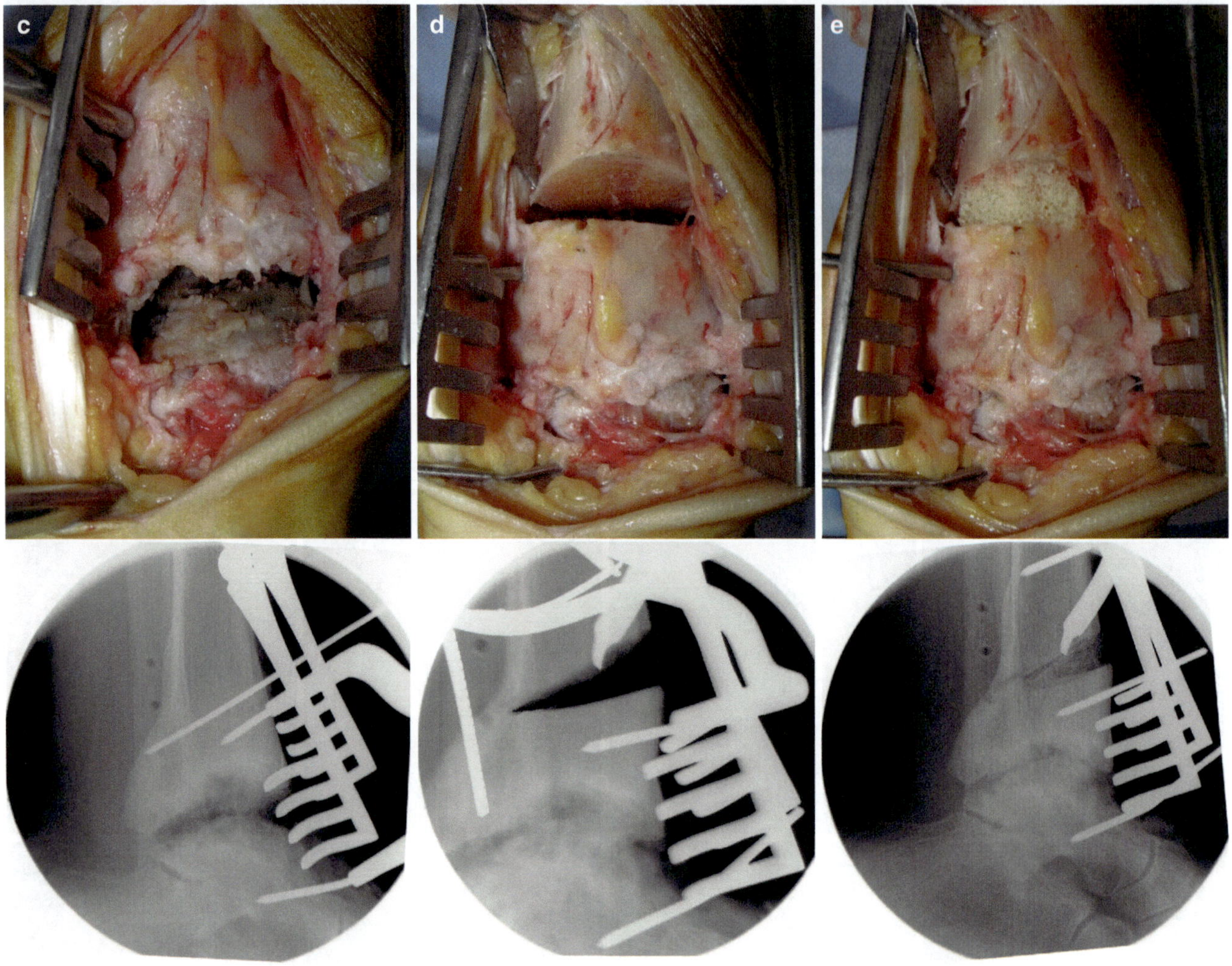

Fig. 10.18 (continued)

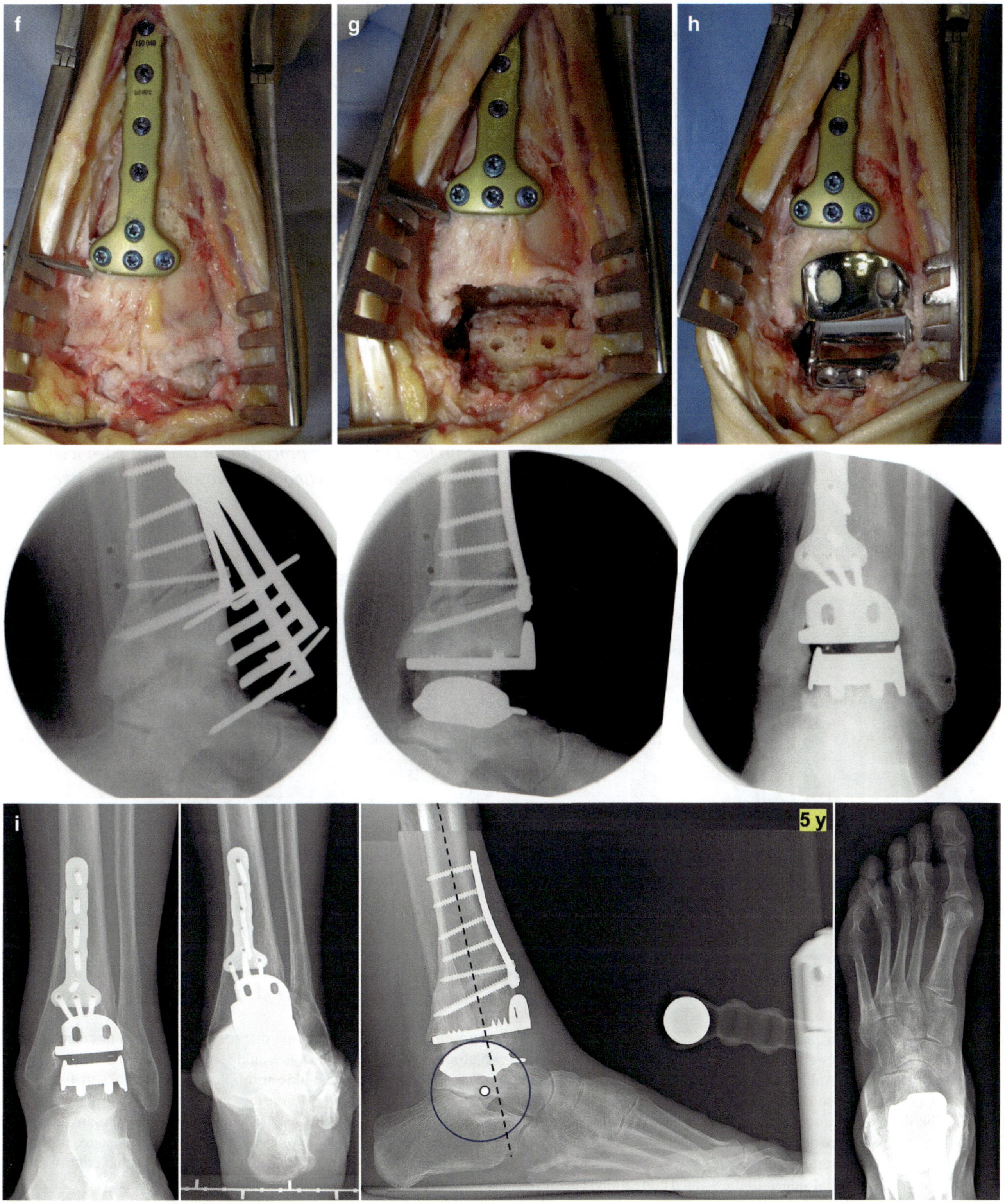

Fig. 10.18 (continued)

10.4 Total Ankle Arthroplasty in Multiplanar Deformities

Multiplanar deformities usually occur due to prior trauma but may also be present due to congenital deformity, previous infection, or metabolic bone disorder. These deformities should be addressed before undertaking resection cuts for the prosthesis to avoid postoperative deformity.

10.4.1 Preoperative Assessment and Planning

All facets of deformity must be considered and factored into the planning, including alterations in length, angulation, rotation, translation, and joint posture or position. Soft tissues are also included in the deformity and must be considered when contemplating a correction method.

10.4.2 Surgical Technique

Treatment options include traditional osteotomy at the apex of the deformity or multilevel osteotomies (Figs. 10.19 and 10.20). Besides fewer and smaller incisions, osteoplasty with external fixation has the advantage of gradual correction and adjusting the deformity correction based on progression to make it as accurate as possible and not lose length or bone stock. The disadvantages are the length of time in the frame, the pin tract problem, and delayed union or nonunion.

The Authors' Approach

Except for a significant length discrepancy to be corrected, we prefer osteotomy-adapted techniques, allowing us triplane and rotational correction in the first stage. As, after that, patients may recover some ankle function and report pain relief, total ankle arthroplasty can be postponed. However, we prefer a one-stage procedure in cases of advanced-stage ankle osteoarthritis without the prospect of any recovery.

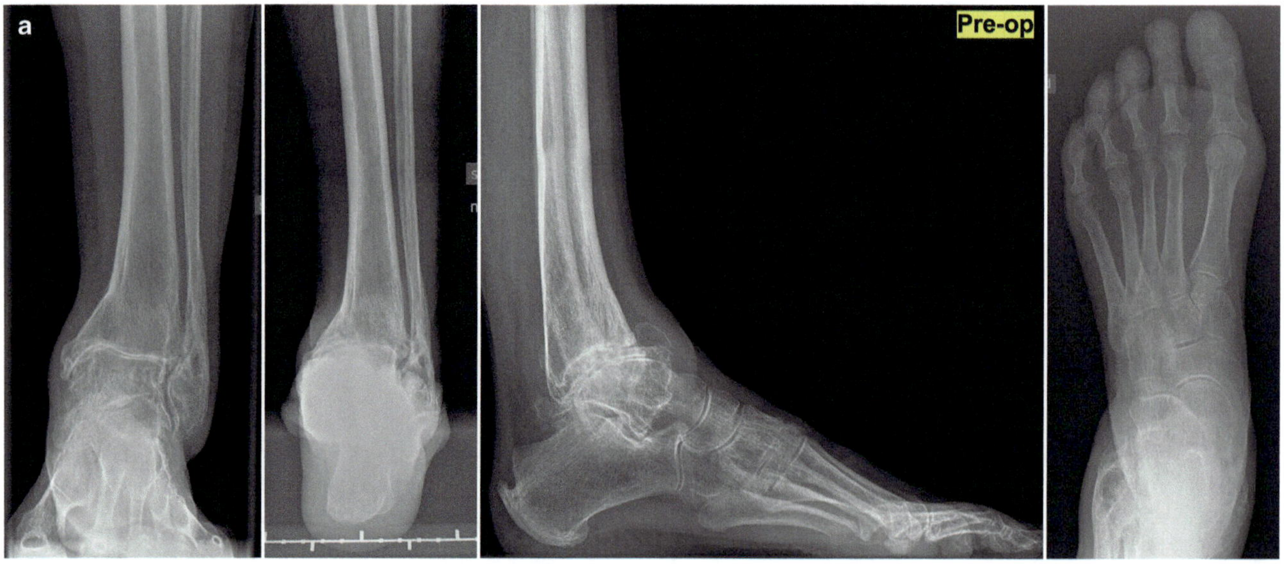

Fig. 10.19 Multilevel triplane correcting osteotomies. A 54-year-old former ski racer 29 years after a complex injury to her left ankle that stopped her career. (**a**) Ankle series showing the complex three-plane deformity, the apex for both the coronal and sagittal plane extraarticular. (**b**) The deformity can also be seen clinically. (**c**) After ankle and distal tibia exposure, an osteotomy is made in the horizontal plane (arrow). (**d**) After osteotomy of the fibula (not shown), a distraction is applied at the anteromedial side until the wanted correction is achieved. (**e**) A wedged allograft is inserted, and the distraction is removed. (**f**) Fixation with two plates is performed at the tibial side and with another plate at the fibular side (not shown). Notice the persisting intraarticular deformity in the coronal plane due to the erosion of the medial tibial plafond. (**g**) The tibia and the ankle are well-aligned in the sagittal plane. (**h**) After the total ankle arthroplasty, the medial soft-tissue contracture is addressed by a flip osteotomy of the medial malleolus (not shown). (**i**) Fluoroscopic views showing a well-aligned ankle in both planes. (**j**) A dorsal closing wedge osteotomy is finally added to address the hyperflexed first ray. (**k**) Postoperative radiographic control and (**l**) clinical results after 4 months. (**m**) 15 years after the surgery, the patient is very pleased with her ankle and is particularly happy that skiing and golfing are possible without limitations. The radiographs show a well-balanced ankle and stable components

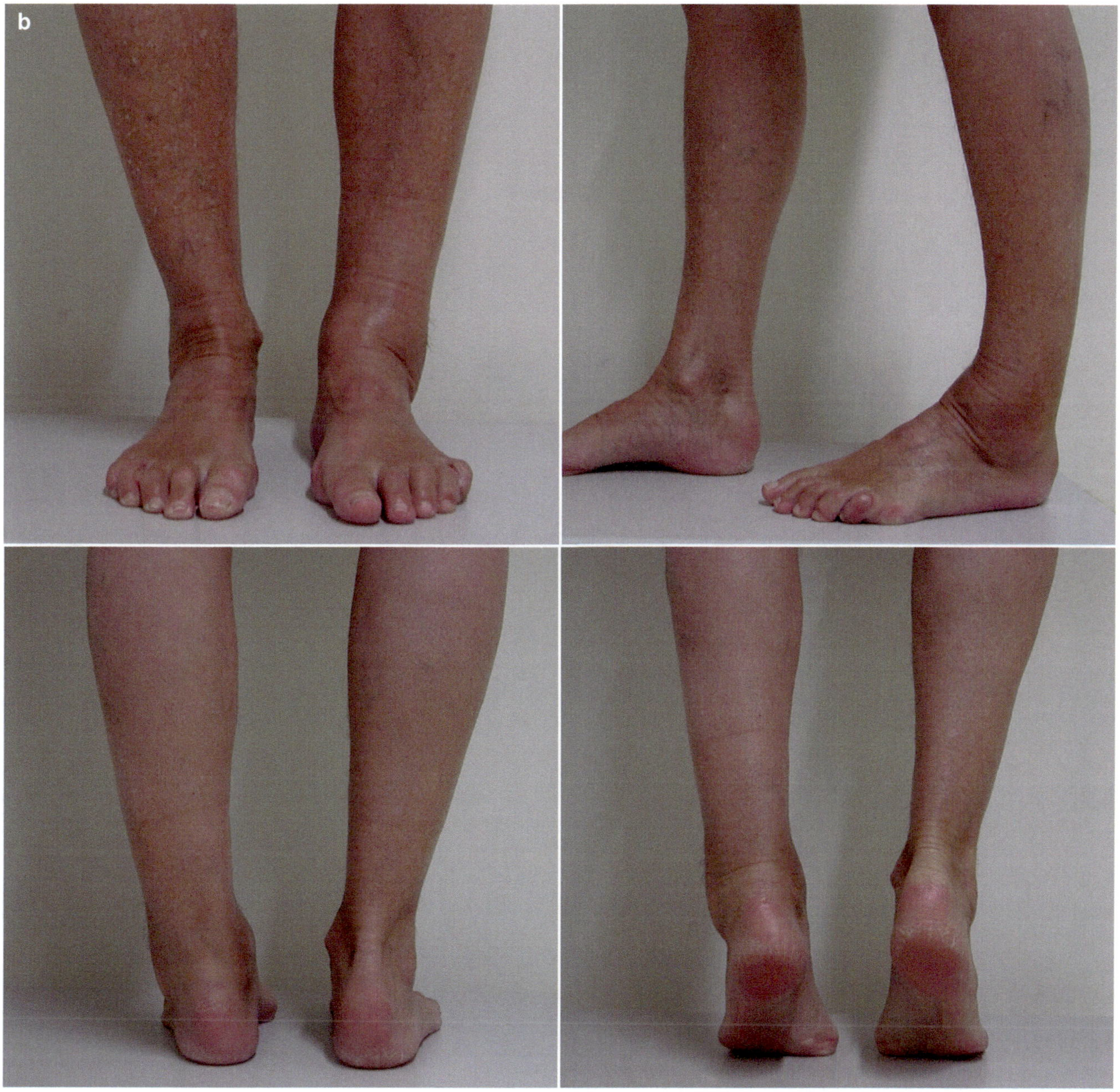

Fig. 10.19 (continued)

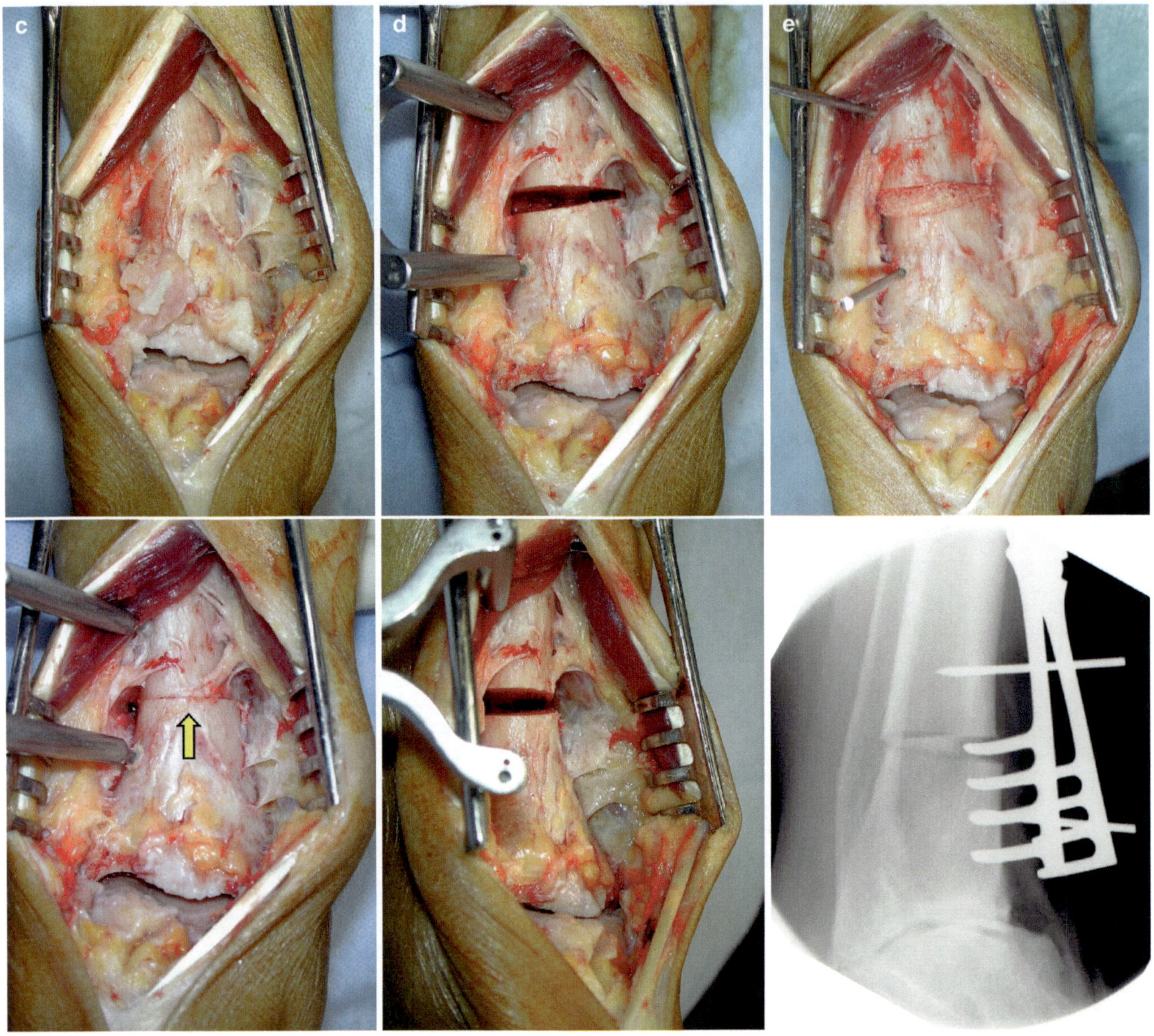

Fig. 10.19 (continued)

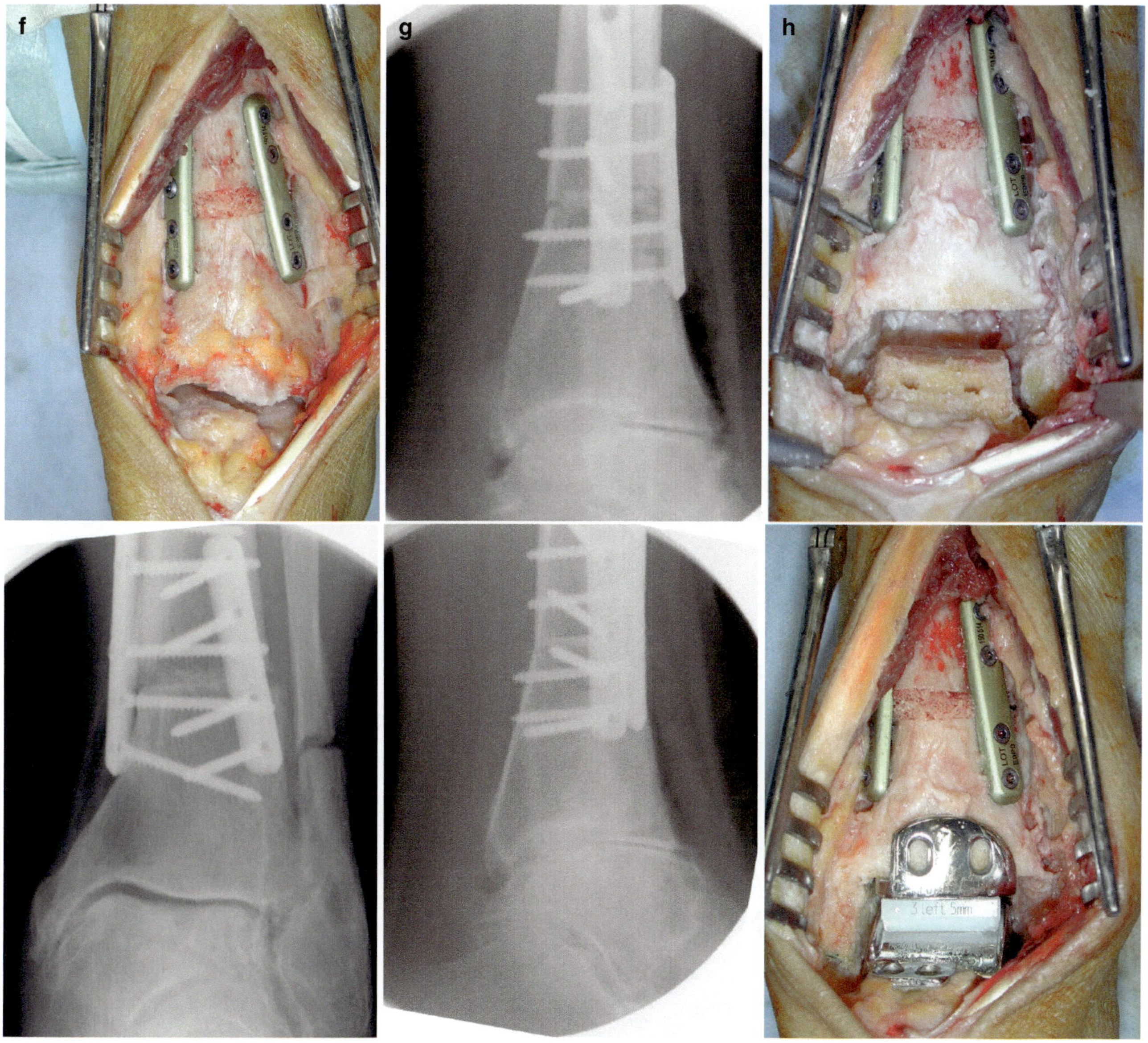

Fig. 10.19 (continued)

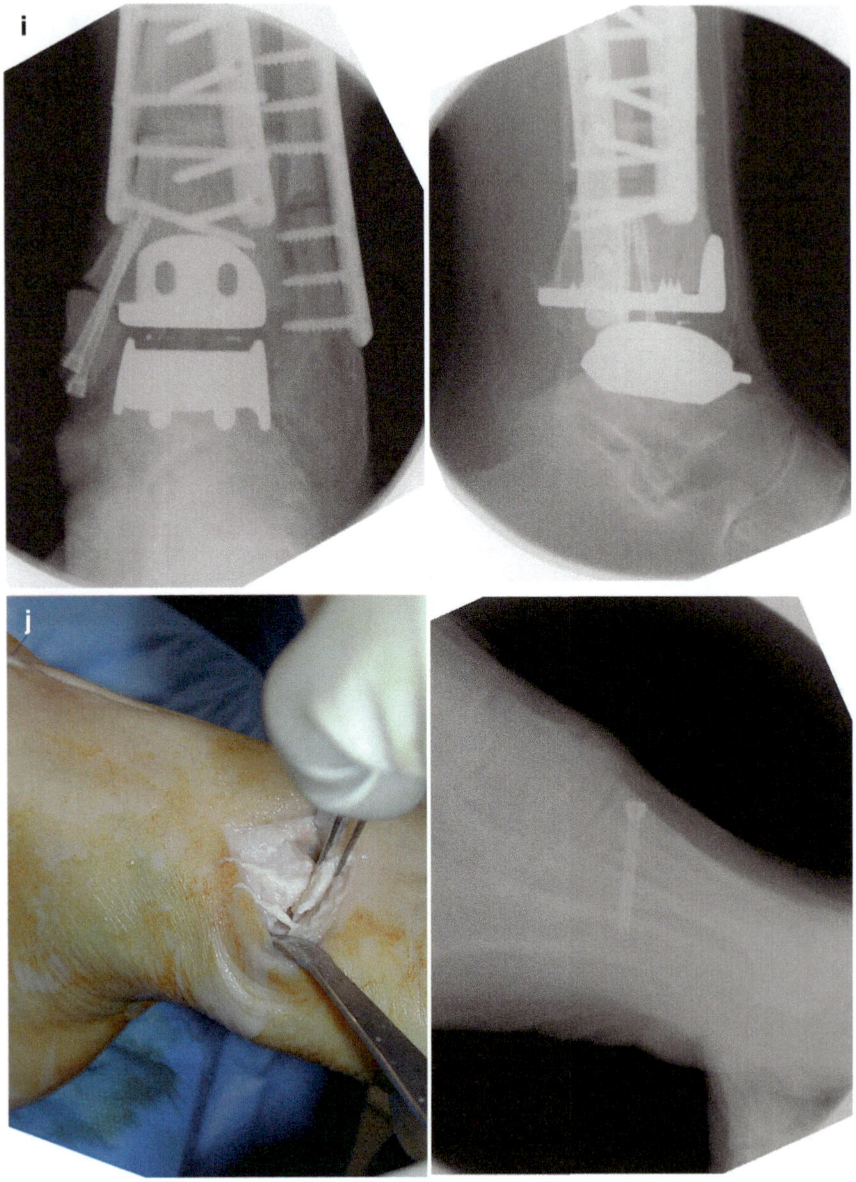

Fig. 10.19 (continued)

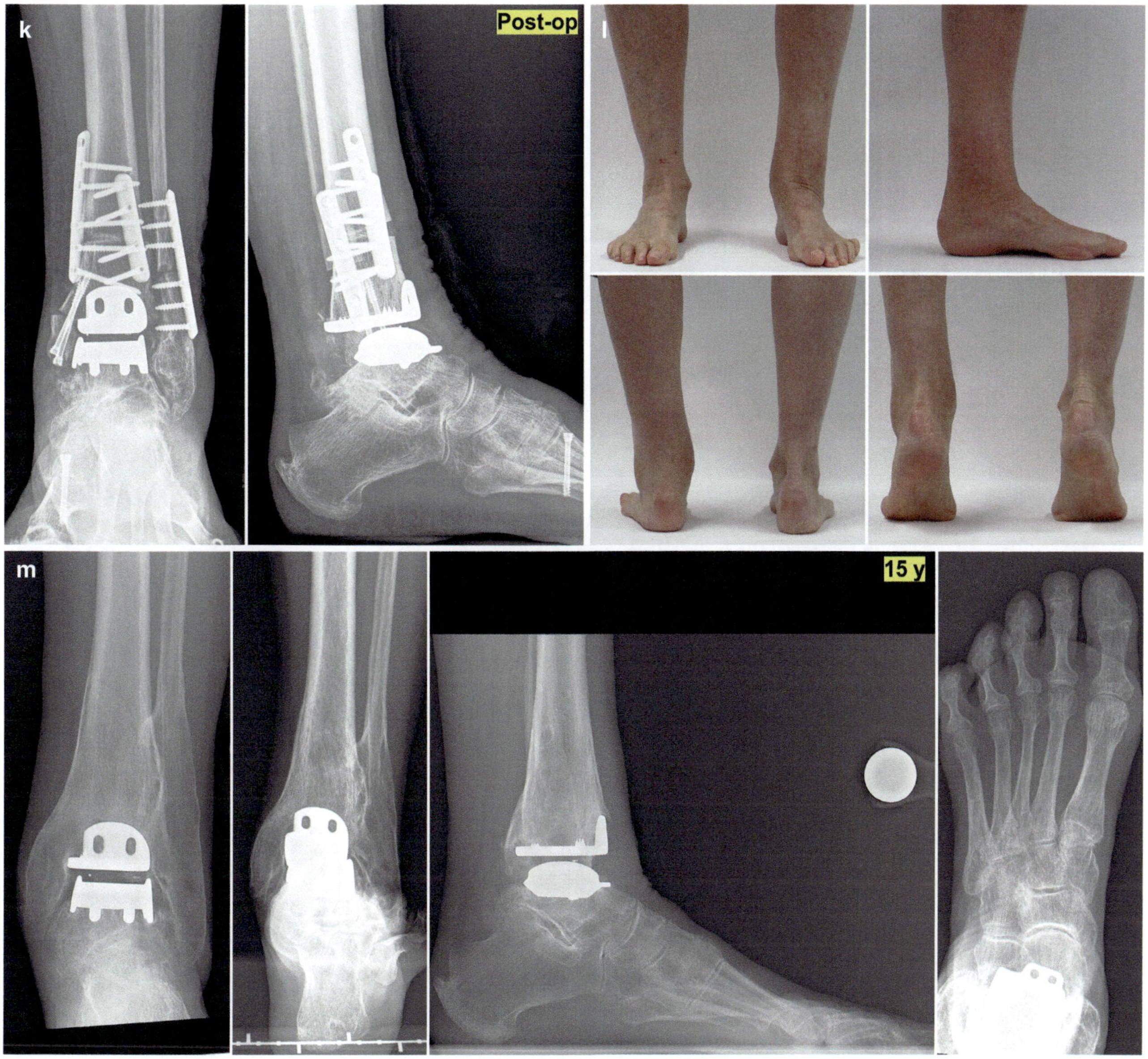

Fig. 10.19 (continued)

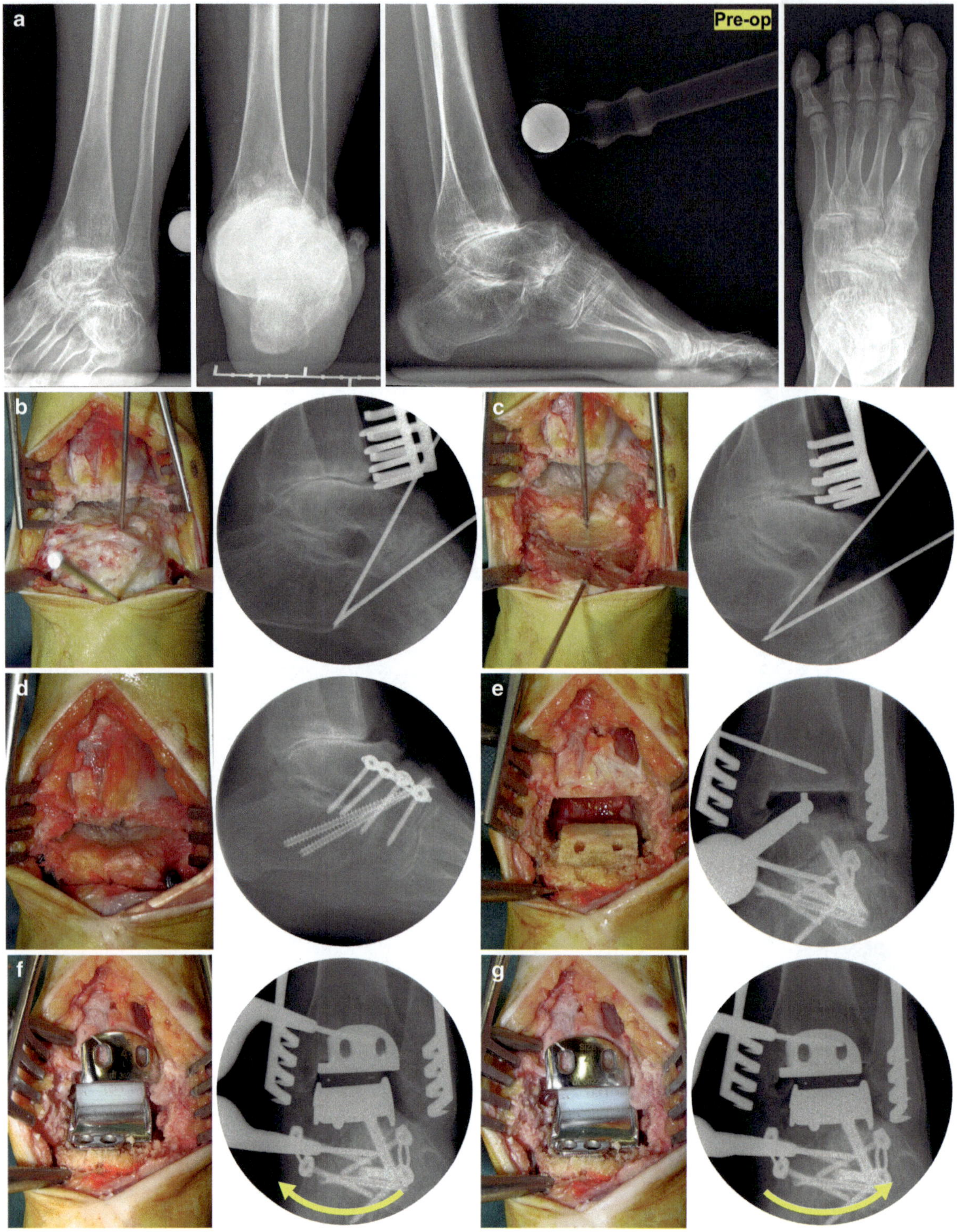

Fig. 10.20 Inframalleolar triplane correction. A 43-year-old patient who sustained a complex injury to his left foot in a motorcycling accident. (**a**) The main deformity is located at peritalar joints, with a dorsiflexed and externally rotated talus associated with a retro dislocation of the tibia and a mild intraarticular recurvatum deformity. (**b**) After exposure of the ankle joint, the planned osteotomy is marked by two K-wires. (**c**) After a first cut proximally, the second cut is done in an angulation of approximately 20° toward laterally (to address the supination component of the deformity), and the wedge is removed. (**d**) The osteotomy is closed and fixed with a plate dorsolaterally and additional screws. (**e**) After that, the replacement surgery is performed with the aid of the instrumentation in a standard way. (**f**) While applying a rotational force to the distractor, the talus is seen to move slightly medially. In contrast, by changing the rotational force in the opposite direction, the talus moves markedly lateralward, while the syndesmosis is widened (**g**). (**h**) Therefore, the distal tibiofibular joint is debrided, and a compression force is applied with a clamp while the foot is held in a neutral position. (**i**) Anterior view of this maneuver and a fluoroscopic check after fixation of the distal tibiofibular joint with screws. (**j**) Through fixation of the syndesmosis, the talus is still found to be not sufficiently stabilized against anterolateral rotation forces; therefore, the lateral ankle ligaments are reconstructed. (**k**) Radiographs at 2-year follow-up control show a well-aligned ankle and the foot in a plantigrade position

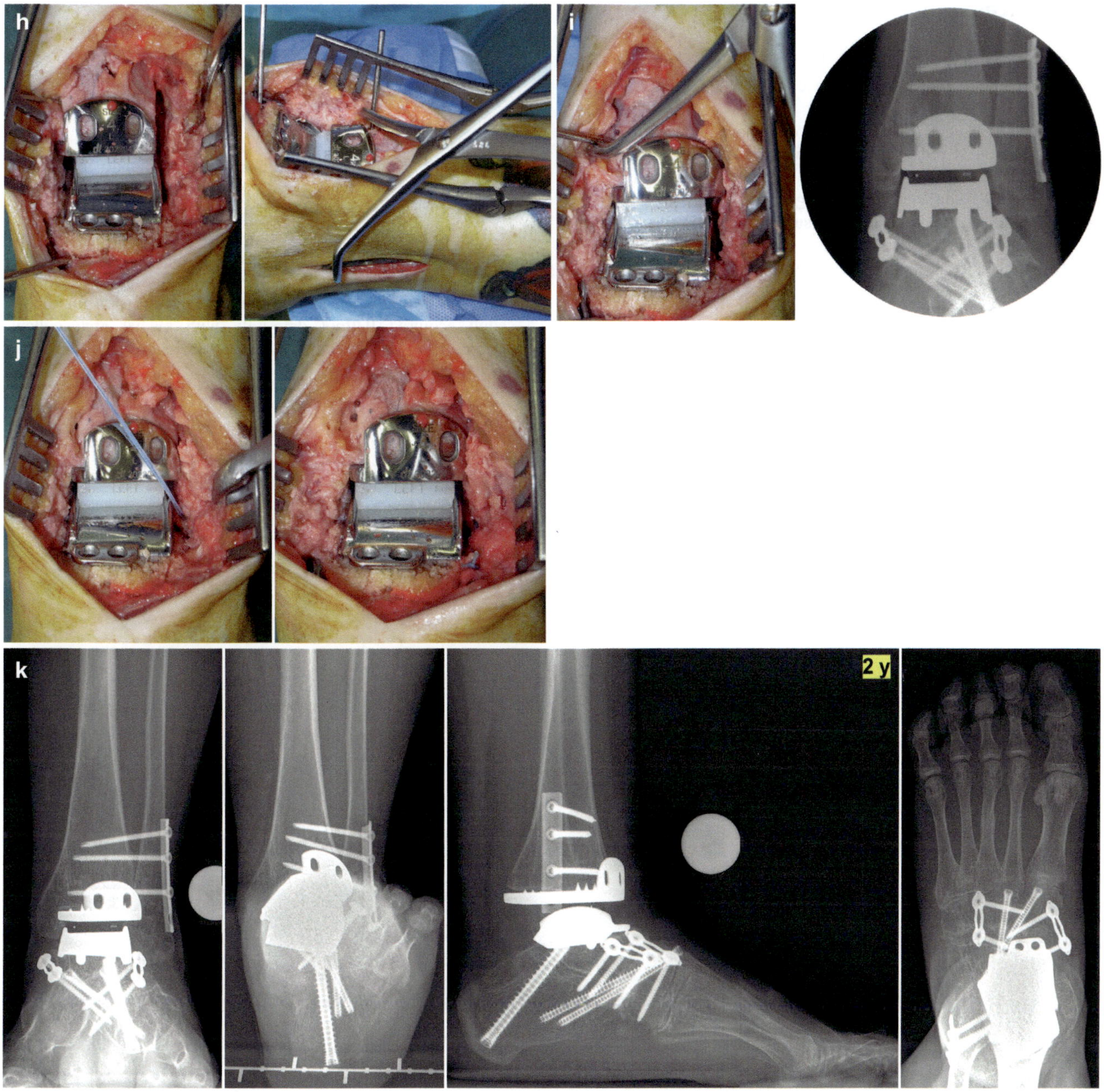

Fig. 10.20 (continued)

10.5 Conclusions

- Careful radiographic assessment of the talar position in all three planes is mandatory to successfully replace an end-stage osteoarthritic ankle joint associated with a concomitant major deformity.
- Correcting resection cuts for the prosthesis may not be able to restore proper position of the talus within the ankle mortise and provide overall stability of the ankle.
- Additional osteotomies above or below the ankle or selective fusions may be necessary to obtain a well-balanced ankle and hindfoot joint complex.
- The key to success is to use all treatment modalities necessary to restore appropriate alignment and stability of the hindfoot complex.
- The use of established algorithms may be helpful and lead to an improved outcome.

References

1. Choi WJ, Kim BS, Lee JW. Preoperative planning and surgical technique: how do I balance my ankle? Foot Ankle Int. 2012;33(3):244–9.
2. Haskell A, Mann RA. Perioperative complication rate of total ankle replacement is reduced by surgeon experience. Foot Ankle Int. 2004;25(5):283–9.
3. Knupp M, Stufkens SA, Bolliger L, Barg A, Hintermann B. Classification and treatment of supramalleolar deformities. Foot Ankle Int. 2011;32(11):1023–31.
4. Hintermann B, Knupp M, Barg A. Supramalleolar osteotomies for the treatment of ankle arthritis. J Am Acad Orthop Surg. 2016;24(7):424–32.
5. Hintermann B, Ruiz R. Joint preservation strategies for managing varus ankle deformities. Foot Ankle Clin. 2022;27(1):37–56.
6. Knupp M, Horisberger M, Hintermann B. A new Z-shaped calcaneal osteotomy for 3-plane correction of severe Varus deformity of the Hindfoot. Tech Foot Ankle Surg. 2008;7(2):90–5.
7. Hintermann B, Ruiz R. Total replacement of varus ankle: three-component prosthesis design. Foot Ankle Clin. 2019;24(2):305–24.
8. Kim BS, Lee JW. Total ankle replacement for the varus unstable. Foot Ankle Tech. 2010;9:157–67.
9. Brunner S, Knupp M, Hintermann B. Total ankle replacement for the valgus unstable osteoarthritic ankle. Foot Ankle Tech. 2010;9:174–9.
10. Kilger R, Knupp M, Hintermann B. Peroneus longus to peroneus brevis tendon transfer. Tech Foot Ankle Surg. 2009;8(3):146–9.
11. Steiner CS, Gilgen A, Zwicky L, Schweizer C, Ruiz R, Hintermann B. Combined subtalar and naviculocuneiform fusion for treating adult acquired flatfoot deformity with medial arch collapse at the level of the naviculocuneiform joint. Foot Ankle Int. 2019;40(1):42–7.

Part III

Outcomes, Complications and Complex Scenarios

Possibilities and Limitations of Total Ankle Arthroplasty

11

Over the past decade, there has been a vast change in the treatment approach for managing ankle osteoarthritis. Not only has the surgical treatment armamentarium expanded, but the viable options are now more numerous, and total ankle arthroplasty is emerging as an alternative to ankle arthrodesis. It is apparent that there are several arthroplasty designs to choose from, and each has its staunch advocates. The complications experienced by total ankle arthroplasty patients in the early days of the procedure remain a concern, but one which fortunately seems to be overcome by gaining a more thorough understanding of the prostheses, the literature, and the execution of the surgery. As the available knowledge of total ankle arthroplasty increases, more interest is given to how far total ankle arthroplasty can go and what is feasible. This section summarizes some of the authors' experiences with the possibilities and limitations of total ankle arthroplasty based on a case-based series. The goal is to demonstrate the potential benefit of using total ankle arthroplasty as a part of the hindfoot reconstruction and its limits.

11.1 The Varus Ankle

A varus deformity associated with end-stage ankle osteoarthritis is generally a complex three-dimensional deformity with the talus tilted into a varus and rotated internally, combined with an anterior extrusion out of the mortise. While, for the surgeon, the progressive incompetence of lateral ankle ligaments is apparent, the deforming forces behind the deformation process often remain unpredictable (Figs. 11.1, 11.2, and 11.3).

The Authors' Experience

A severe varus deformity, mainly when associated with a cavus and supinatus deformity, should be investigated preoperatively for a neurologic disorder. Even if not confirmed, it is wise to release the posterior tibial tendon and use it to enhance the eversion force. Further, a flip osteotomy of the medial malleolus effectively releases the medial contracture, as it closes the medial gutter and normalizes the direction of the deltoid ligament. A fixed-bearing ankle might be superior to a mobile-bearing ankle in treating a severe varus osteoarthritic ankle as it provides additional intrinsic stability in all planes but at the expense of increased forces at bone-implant interfaces associated with a higher risk of implant failure.

B. Hintermann, R. Ruiz, *Total Ankle Replacement*, https://doi.org/10.1007/978-3-031-56810-7_11

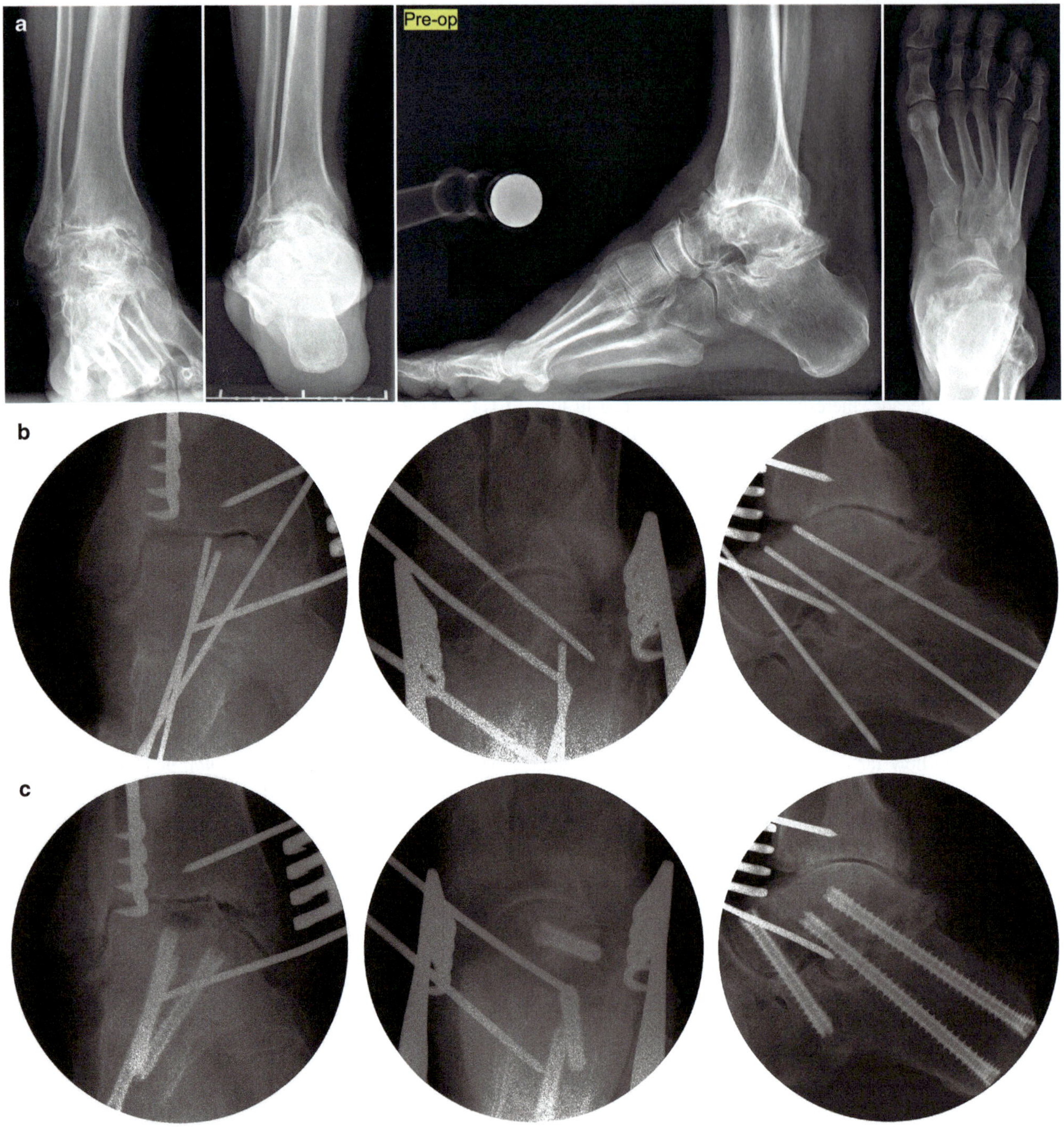

Fig. 11.1 Varus ankle managed with a mobile-bearing ankle. A 67-year-old retired captain presents with end-stage varus ankle osteoarthritis after a talar fracture 22 years ago. He observed an increase in varus deformity in the last years. (**a**) Preoperative series showing the varus tilt of the talus and the advanced stage of osteoarthritis of the ankle and the subtalar joint. Notice the supination deformity of the foot with the medial tilt of the navicular in the DP view. (**b**) First, the subtalar joint is debrided to subchondral bone. After that, the talus is moved to a neutral position on top of the calcaneus, and K-wires are used for preliminary fixation, including transfixation of the talonavicular joint. (**c**) Cannulated screws are then inserted using the K-wires as a guide. With this, a stable foot in a plantigrade position is obtained. (**d**) The replacement surgery is now performed, followed by the fusion of the distal tibiofibular joint. (**e**) Radiographs taken at 5-year control show a well-aligned and balanced ankle, and the former supination deformity of the foot is fully corrected. The patient is delighted with his forgotten ankle, allowing him an everyday life

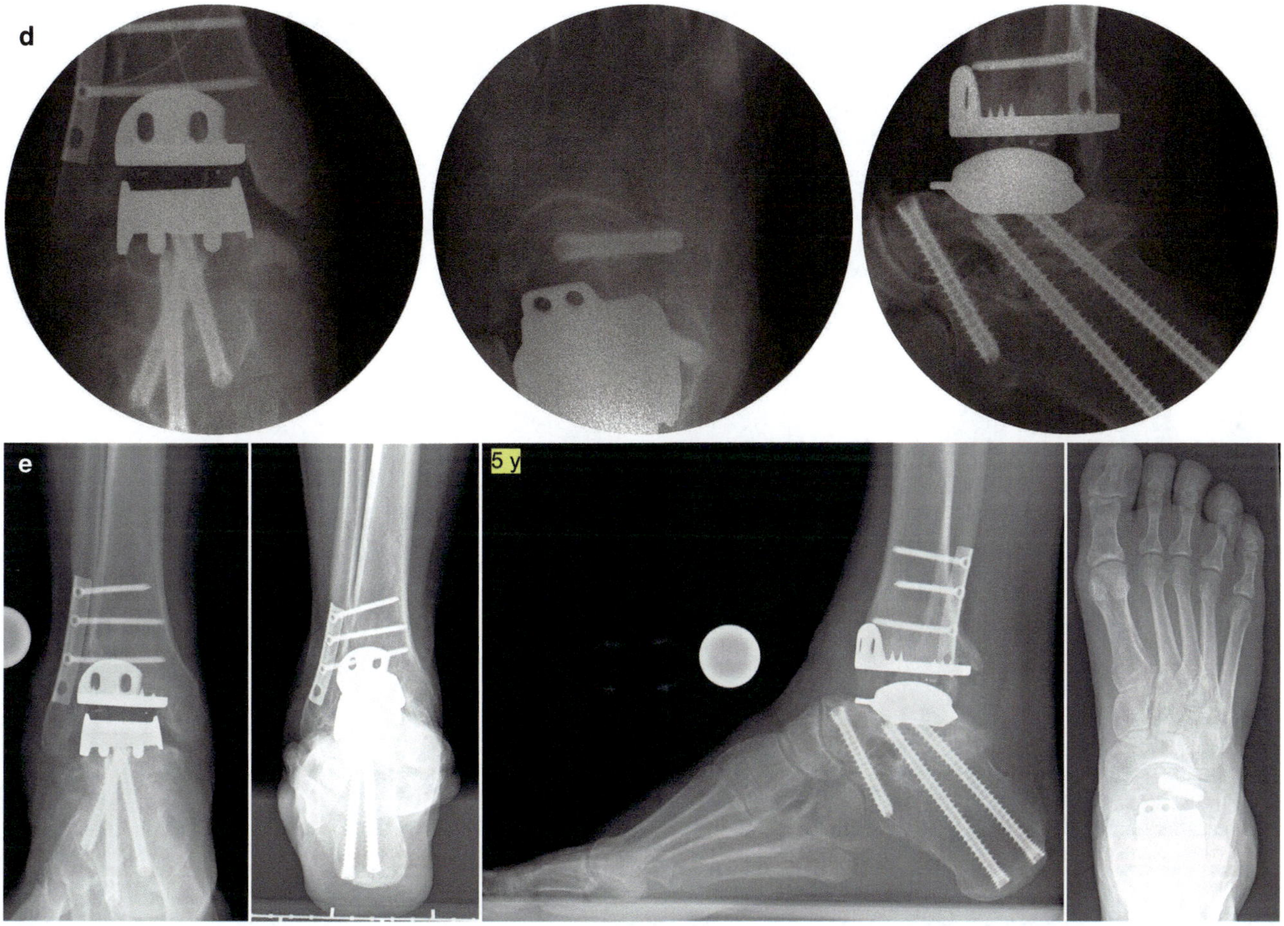

Fig. 11.1 (continued)

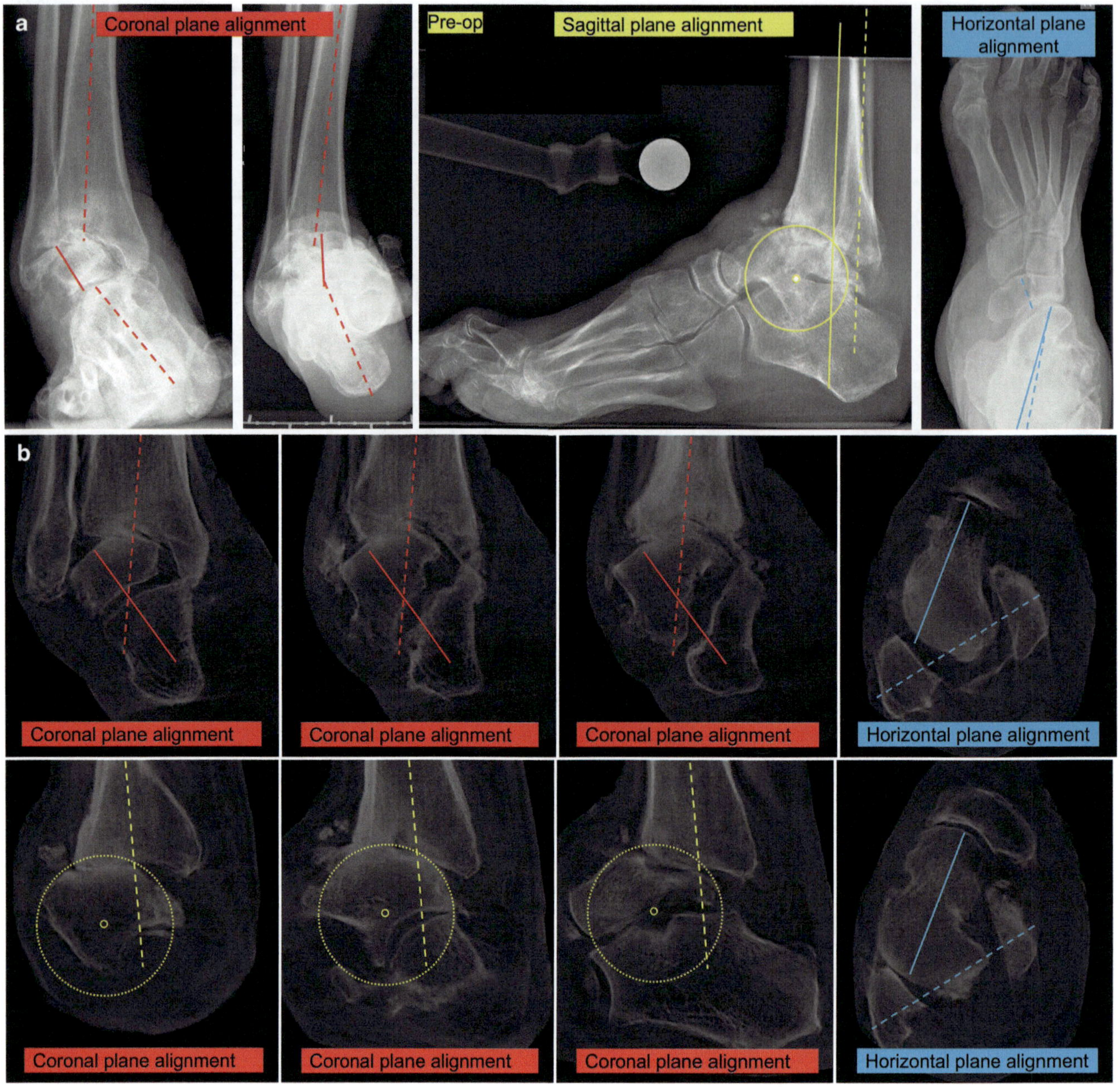

Fig. 11.2 Extreme varus ankle managed with a fixed-bearing ankle. A 69-year-old retired teacher and former soccer player presents with end-stage varus ankle osteoarthritis. (**a**) Standard radiographs showing the complex varus and supination deformity with anterior extrusion of the talus in the three planes. (**b**) Weight-bearing CT scans showing the deformity in more detail: the varus tilt with impaction of the talus into the tibial plafond, the anterior extrusion of the talus, and the internal rotation of the extruded talus. (**c**) Compared with the preoperative condition, standard radiographs at 5-year follow-up control show the correction achieved by replacing the ankle with a fixed-bearing prosthesis. Surgical technique: (**d**) The defect in the medial tibial plafond is visible after ankle exposure. (**e**) Minimal bone resection is attempted to preserve as much bone as possible. (**f**) The posterior tibial tendon is dissected at its insertion to the tuberosity of the navicular bone and retracted through a medial incision proximal to the ankle joint. (**g**) Despite this, after resectioning the tibia and the talus, the distraction sees a lateral gapping of the ankle on the medial side, indicating significant lateral instability. (**h**) The posterior tibial tendon is rerouted behind the tibia into the peroneal tendon sheath and fixed to the peroneal longus tendon, which is transferred to the base of the 5th metatarsal. In addition, lateral ligament reconstruction is performed, augmented by an internal brace. (**i**) Despite this extended soft tissue balancing, the ankle still has a distinct tendency for lateral gapping (arrow), so a flip osteotomy of the medial malleolus is added (not shown)

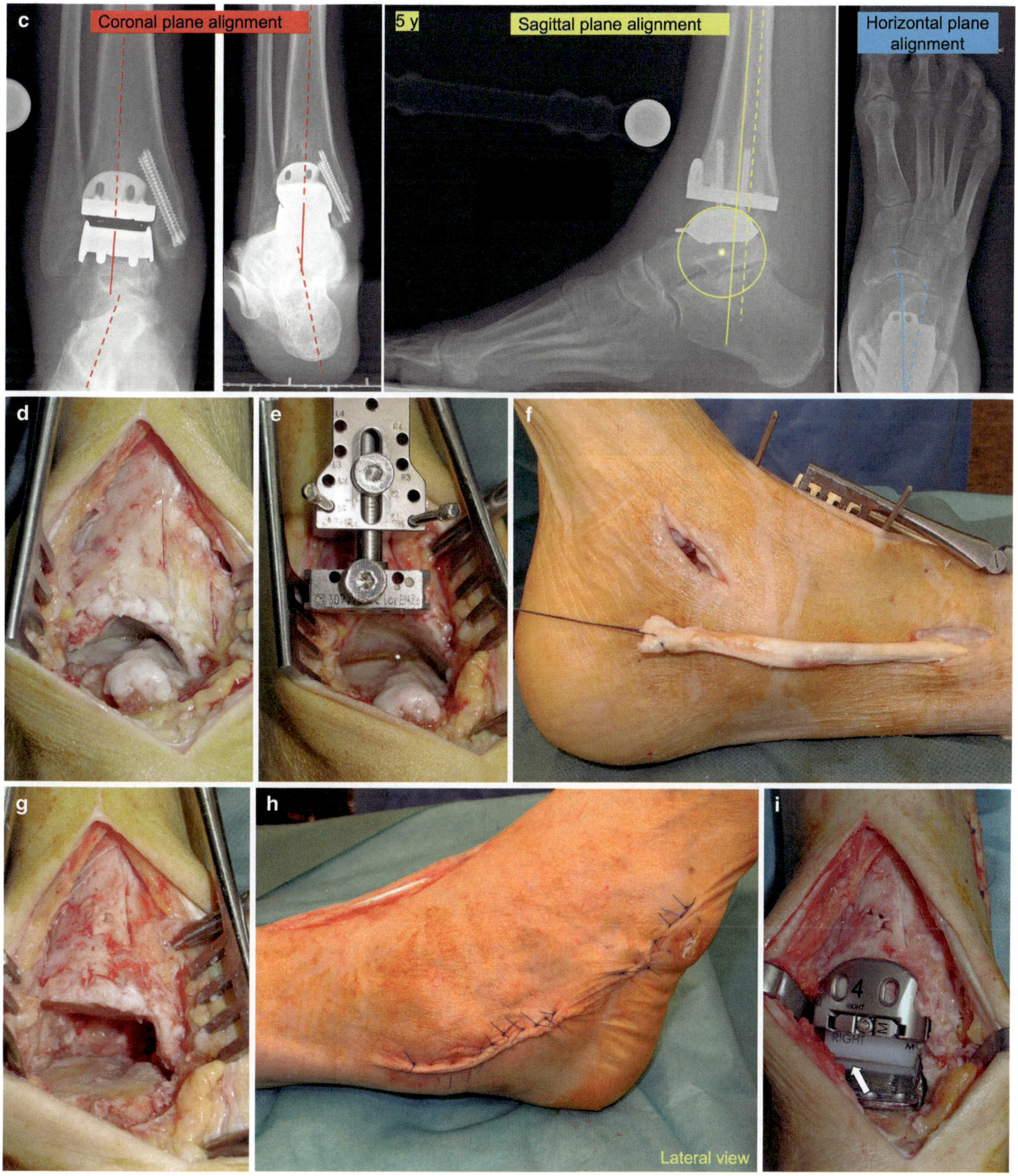

Fig. 11.2 (continued)

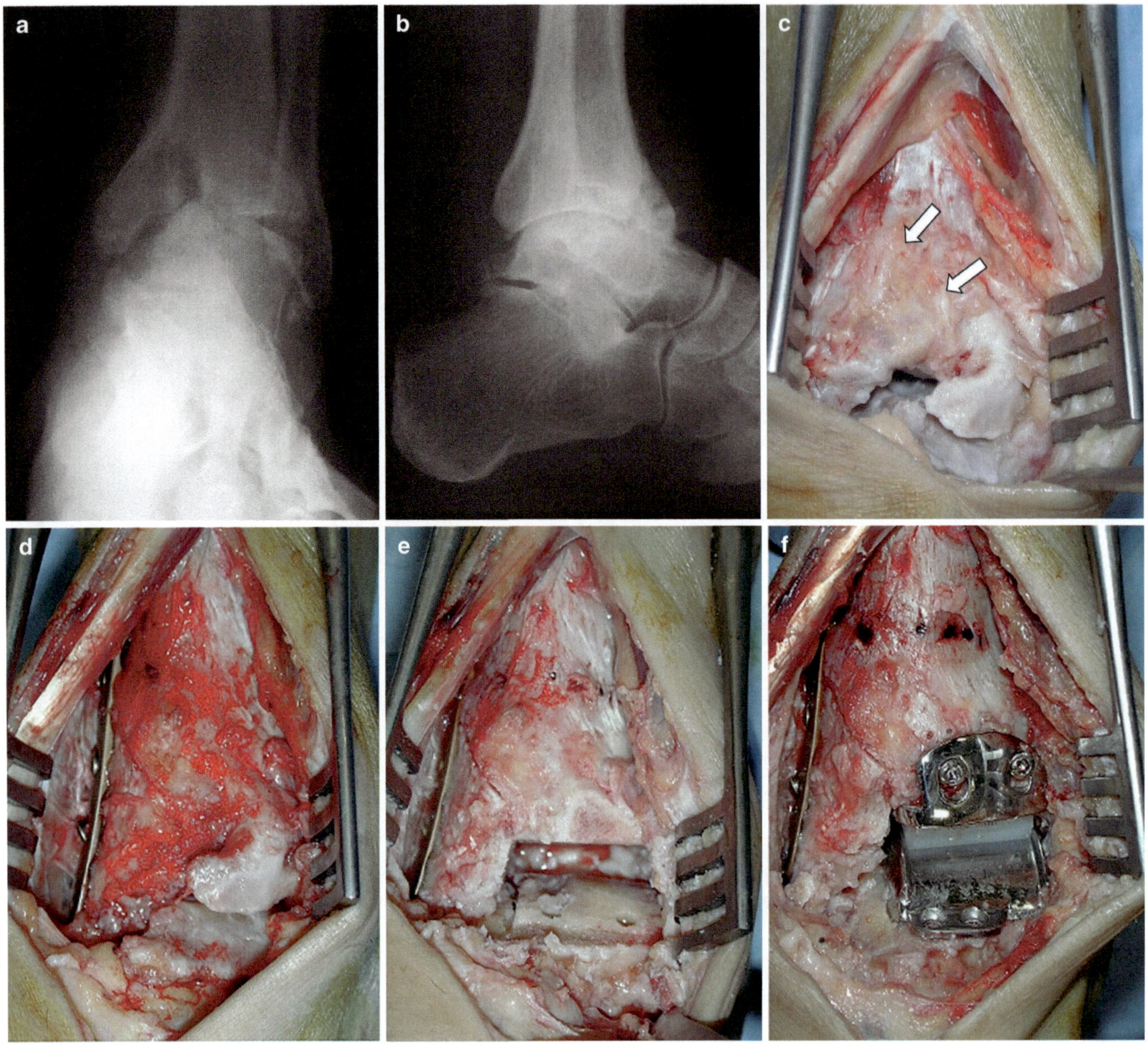

Fig. 11.3 Not manageable varus forces with pathologic fracture of medial tibial pilon. A 49-year-old supervisor with a primarily sedentary job presents with a pathologic fracture of the medial tibial pilon associated with a progressive varus deformity. No smoking, no alcohol, no diabetes. (**a**) AP view; (**b**) lateral view of the ankle. (**c**) After ankle exposure, the fracture line is almost not visible (arrows). (**d**) A buttress plate is mounted. (**e**) Ten, the resection cuts for the ankle implants are made. An area of avascular bone is seen at the medial talar apex. (**f**) Final situation after the total ankle arthroplasty. A calcaneal osteotomy is also performed to address the heel varus. (**g**) The AP view after 2 months shows stable implants, and the fracture healed, but a distinct internal rotation of the talus. (**h**) Stable implants are also seen on lateral view. (**i, j**) At 4-month follow-up control, the talus is found to have tilted again into a varus, with asymmetric subsidence of the tibial component into the tibial pilon. There is also a fracture of the medial malleolus. (**k**) The plate and the tibial component are removed. (**l**) Minimal bone is resected on the tibial side for a new implant. (**m**) A fibular osteotomy is added to shorten it. (**n**) Final situation in the lateral view. (**o, p**) The ankle looks aligned 2 months after the revision surgery, and the implants are stable. (**q**) 1.5 months later, the patient returned because he felt a crack in his medial ankle. The X-ray shows a fracture of the medial malleolus and, in addition, a fibular fracture (arrow) in the CT scan (**r**). (**s, t**) Plate fixation of the medial malleolus and the fibula is performed. (**u, v**) After 2 months, the ankle was well-aligned with stable implants. (**w–y**) While the components remain stable over the next 8 years, progressive lateralization of the talus with some tilting into varus subsequently to asymmetric polyethylene wear is seen. As the patient has no pain, the following control is planned after one year. (**z**) Series of the contralateral ankle where a dome osteotomy was performed to correct the varus deformity in combination with a calcaneal sliding osteotomy. Sixteen months later, a fracture of the medial tibial plafond occurred, in combination with a varus tilt of the talus due to the impaction into the tibia. After bolstering the medial malleolus with a strong plate and a replacement of the ankle, a loosening with asymmetric subsidence of the tibial component is associated with a plate fracture

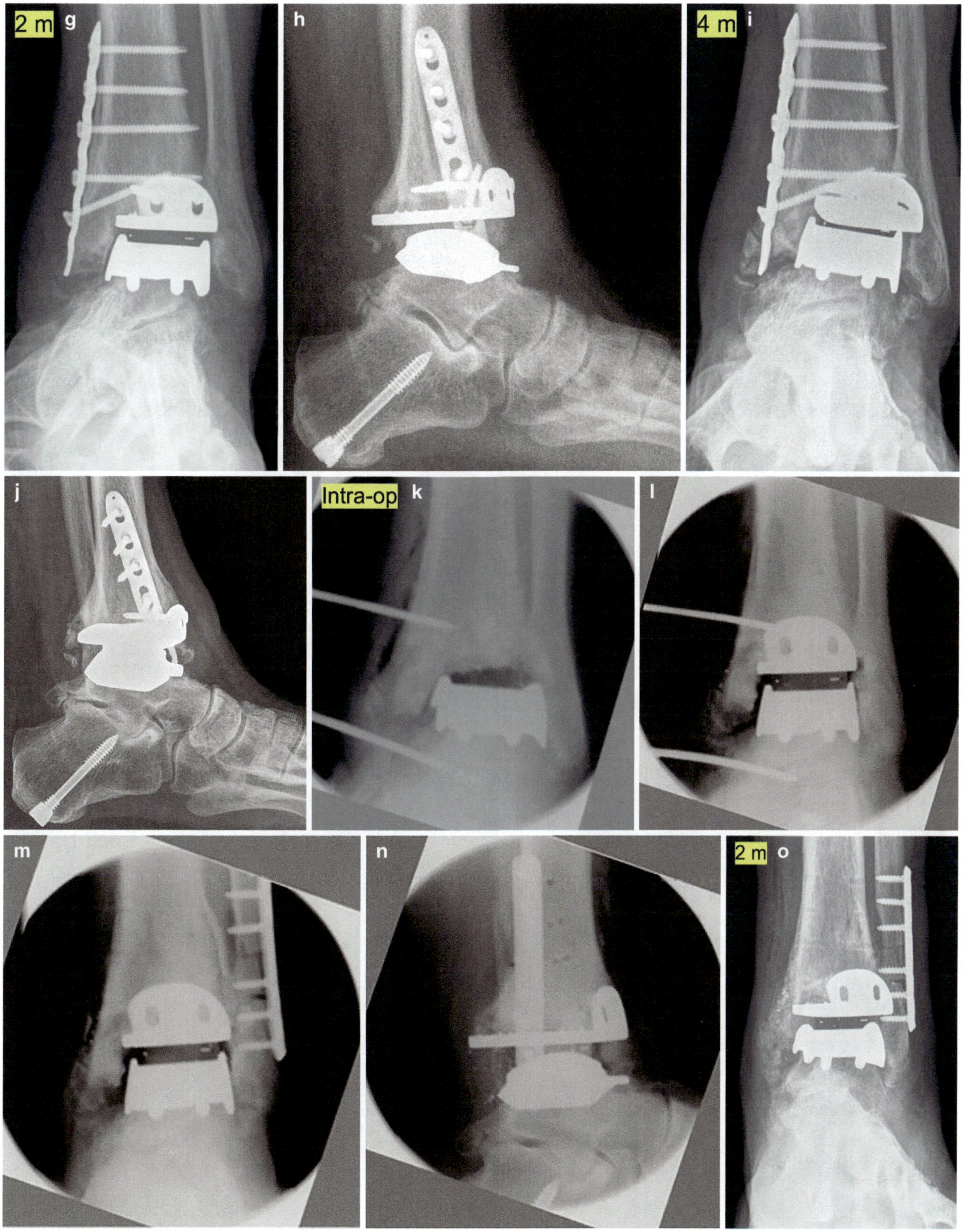

Fig. 11.3 (continued)

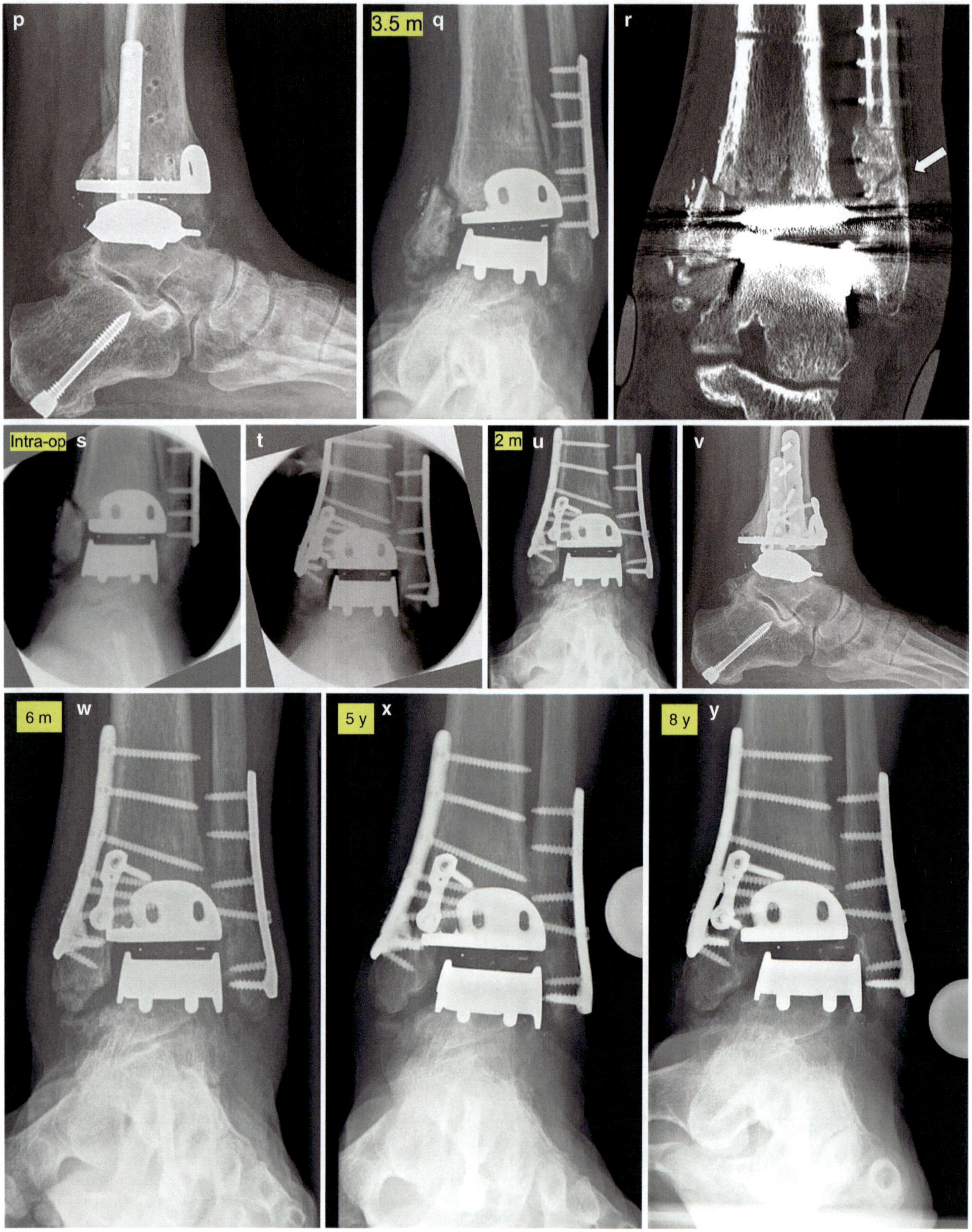

Fig. 11.3 (continued)

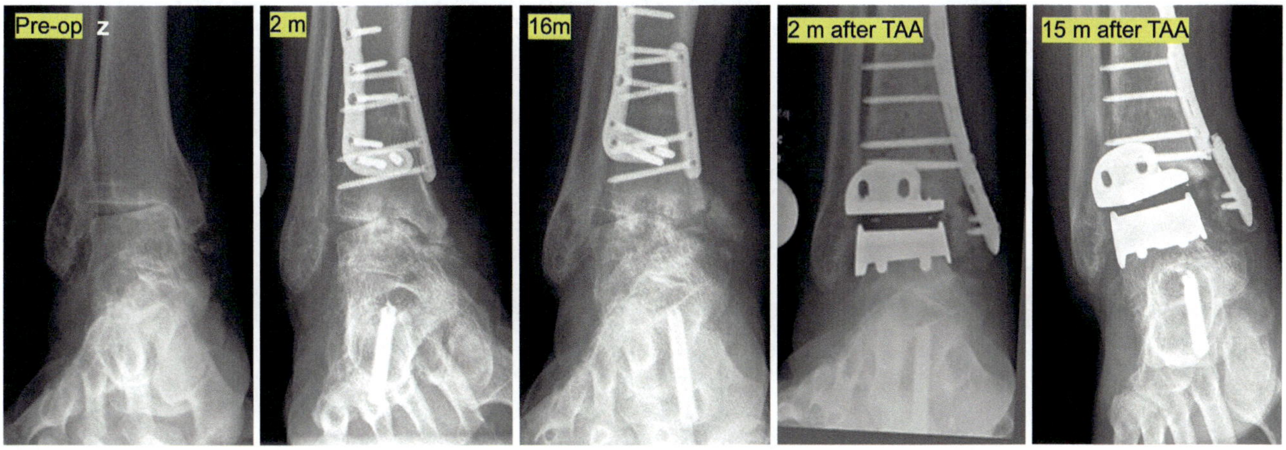

Fig. 11.3 (continued)

11.2 The Valgus Ankle

A valgus deformity associated with end-stage ankle osteoarthritis is generally associated with a progressive destabilization process of the foot, resulting in a flatfoot deformity. As the heel moves laterally, the heel cord becomes an evertor, thus increasing the pronation forces to the foot and destabilizing the midfoot, which also results in an abduction and supination deformity of the forefoot. With the increase of the valgus tilt of the talus, the syndesmotic ligaments become under stress and subsequently incompetent. The better the surgeon can address the unidirectional deforming and destabilization process, the more likely the replacement surgery will succeed (Figs. 11.4 and 11.5).

The Authors' Experience

A valgus deformity and destabilization of the foot is always a unidirectional process that will increase over time. Total ankle arthroplasty can only be successful in the long-term if the destabilization process is stopped and the deformity is corrected before the ankle replacement. The best option for treating peritalar instability is a subtalar fusion. The heel should be corrected to neutral or better to slightly varus. A challenging problem is the breakdown of the medial arch. If not appropriately addressed, the replaced ankle will be exposed to enormous valgus forces when moving from the stance phase to push-off with progressive incompetence of the deltoid ligament complex. In general, less bone should be resected at the tibial side. With this, the loosened ligaments will be tightened by moving the articulating joint line more distally. A fixed-bearing ankle might be superior to a mobile-bearing ankle in treating a severe varus osteoarthritic ankle as it provides additional intrinsic stability in all planes but at the expense of increased forces at bone-implant interfaces associated with a higher risk of implant failure.

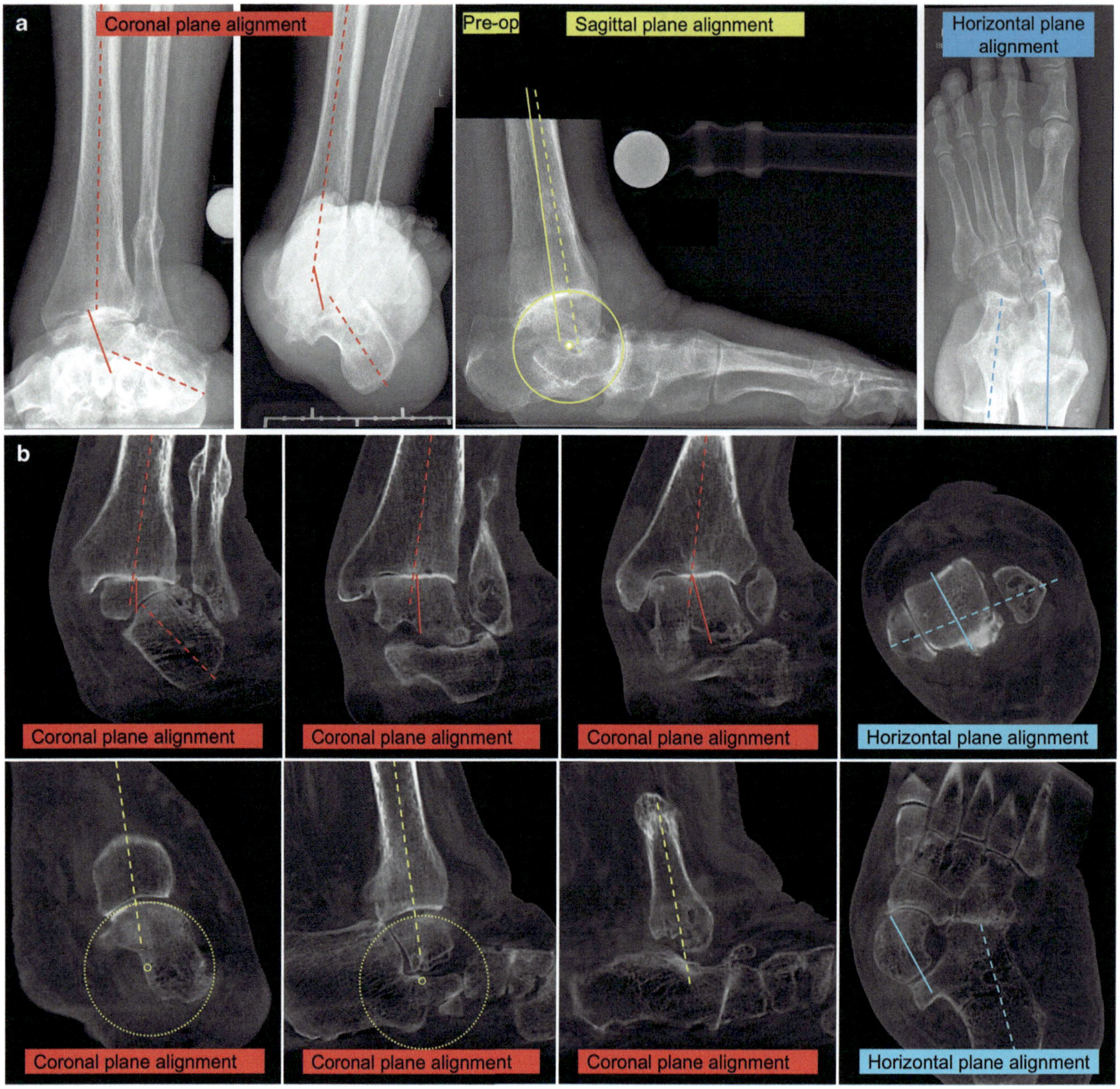

Fig. 11.4 Extreme valgus malaligned flatfoot managed with a fixed-bearing ankle. A 55-year-old female patient presents with end-stage valgus ankle osteoarthritis and flatfoot deformity of her left foot and, less progressed, of her right foot. BMI 48, no smoking, no diabetes. (**a**) Standard radiographs showing the complex valgus and flatfoot deformity with peritalar subluxation, former stress fracture of the fibula, and a severe hindfoot valgus. (**b**) Weight-bearing CT scans showing the deformity in more detail: moderate valgus tilt of the talus, indicating that the deltoid ligaments are competent, severe peritalar instability with the medial slide of the talus, sinus tarsi, and subfibular impingement, widening of distal tibiofibular joint (incompetence of the syndesmosis), and the status after fibular stress fracture. (**c**) Compared with the preoperative condition, standard radiographs at 5-year follow-up control show the correction achieved by a diple fusion, syndesmotic fusion, medial sliding osteotomy, and replacing the ankle with a fixed-bearing prosthesis. Surgical technique: (**d**) After ankle exposure, the talonavicular joint is distracted with a Hintermann spreader on its medial and lateral sides, allowing the debride of the talonavicular and subtalar joint to the subchondral bone. (**e**) After changing the distraction to the medial aspect of the ankle and holding the foot in a plantigrade position, the diple fusion is preliminarily fixed by K-wires. (**f**) After that, the heel is seen as well-aligned. (**g**) Fluoroscopies after screw fixation showing a correct talus position on top of the calcaneus. Notice the laxity in the tibiotalar joint and the gapping of the calcaneocuboid joint. (**h**) Final situation after the total ankle arthroplasty with a fixed-bearing ankle. (**i**) Final AP view under fluoroscopy after having added a syndesmotic fusion. Notice the minimal bone resection on the distal tibia and the distalization of the joint line to tension the collateral ligaments, thereby obtaining a stable ankle. (**j**) Lateral view showing the corrected position of the talus. Because the hindfoot showed a recurrent valgus alignment of the heel as a result of asymmetric physiologic subsidence of the tibial component and probably of some recurrent pronation at the fused subtalar site during the healing process, a medial sliding osteotomy is performed 6 months after the replacement surgery

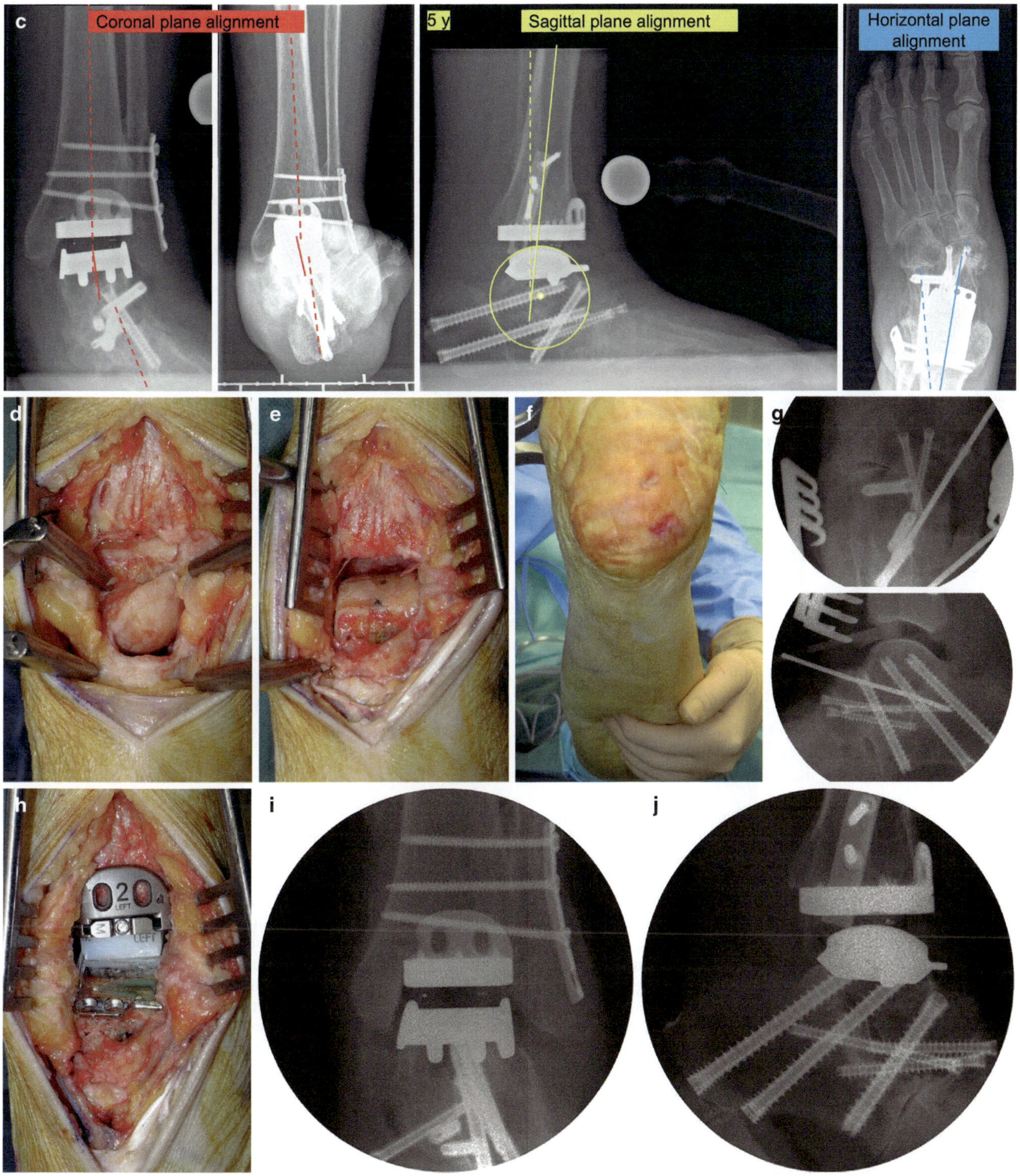

Fig. 11.4 (continued)

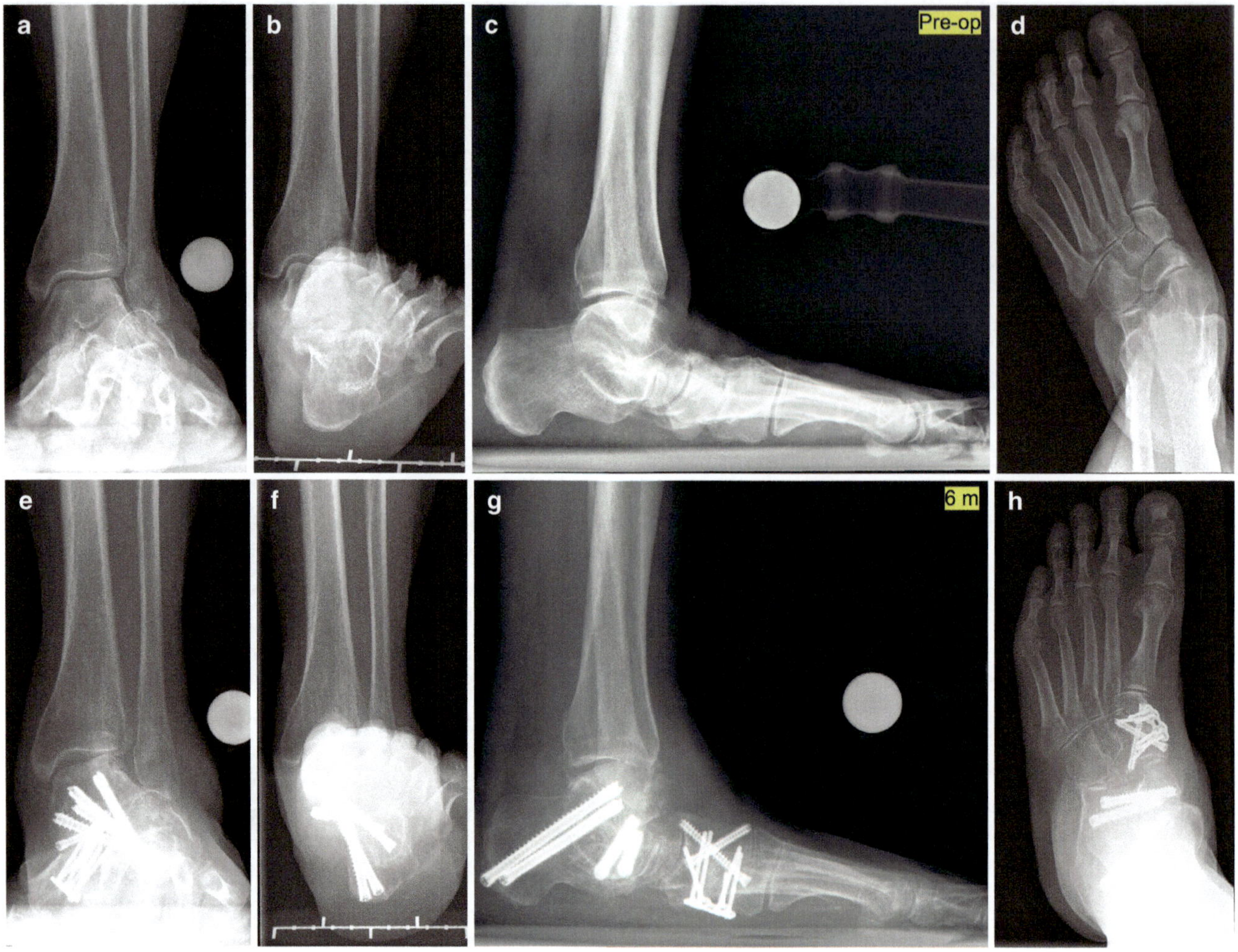

Fig. 11.5 Failed total ankle after failed hindfoot fusion in an extreme flatfoot and abductus deformity. A 65-year-old retired nurse with a flatfoot and abductus deformity complains about severe lateral ankle pain. Immunosuppression because of an unspecific autoimmune illness, no smoking, no alcohol, no diabetes. (**a**) AP view shows a significant lateral deviation of the calcaneus; (**b**) the hindfoot alignment view, in contrast, shows a neutral alignment. (**c**) The lateral view shows a multi-level breakdown of the medial arch and a peritalar subluxation with sinus tarsi impingement. (**d**) The DP view evidences a severe forefoot abduction. (**e**) Six months after a subtalar and naviculocuneiform fusion, the ankle is seen to have tilted into a valgus, causing a subfibular impingement and a diastasis stress to the syndesmosis. (**f**) The valgus tilt of the fused hindfoot can also be seen in the alignment view. (**g**) The lateral view shows the recurrent breakdown of the medial arch, more pronounced at the talonavicular and the tarsometatarsal joints after fusion of the naviculocuneiform joint. (**h**) The DP view shows the significant correction of the previous abduction deformity. (**i–l**) Postoperative views after total ankle replacement and correcting talonavicular fusion. The fracture of the medial malleolus is also fixed, as it fractured the day before surgery. (**m**) Eight weeks postoperatively, the patient complained again of lateral pain beneath the fibula. On the AP view, an asymmetric subsidence of the tibial component explains the recurrent valgus deformity. (**n**) In this situation, a revision to a tibiotalocalcaneal fusion is indicated. The alignment is correct 8 weeks postoperatively, with the fresh-frozen femoral head allograft in place. (**o**) Because of delayed healing at the fusion site, the position screws are removed for dynamization 7 months after the surgery. However, fusion does not occur 20 months after the salvage procedure. (**p**) The nail is thus removed and replaced by a plate and screw fixation, using the fibula as a vascularized lateral autograft. This resulted in a stable and pain-free fusion 9 months later. *TAA* total ankle arthroplasty, *TTC* tibiotalocalcaneal

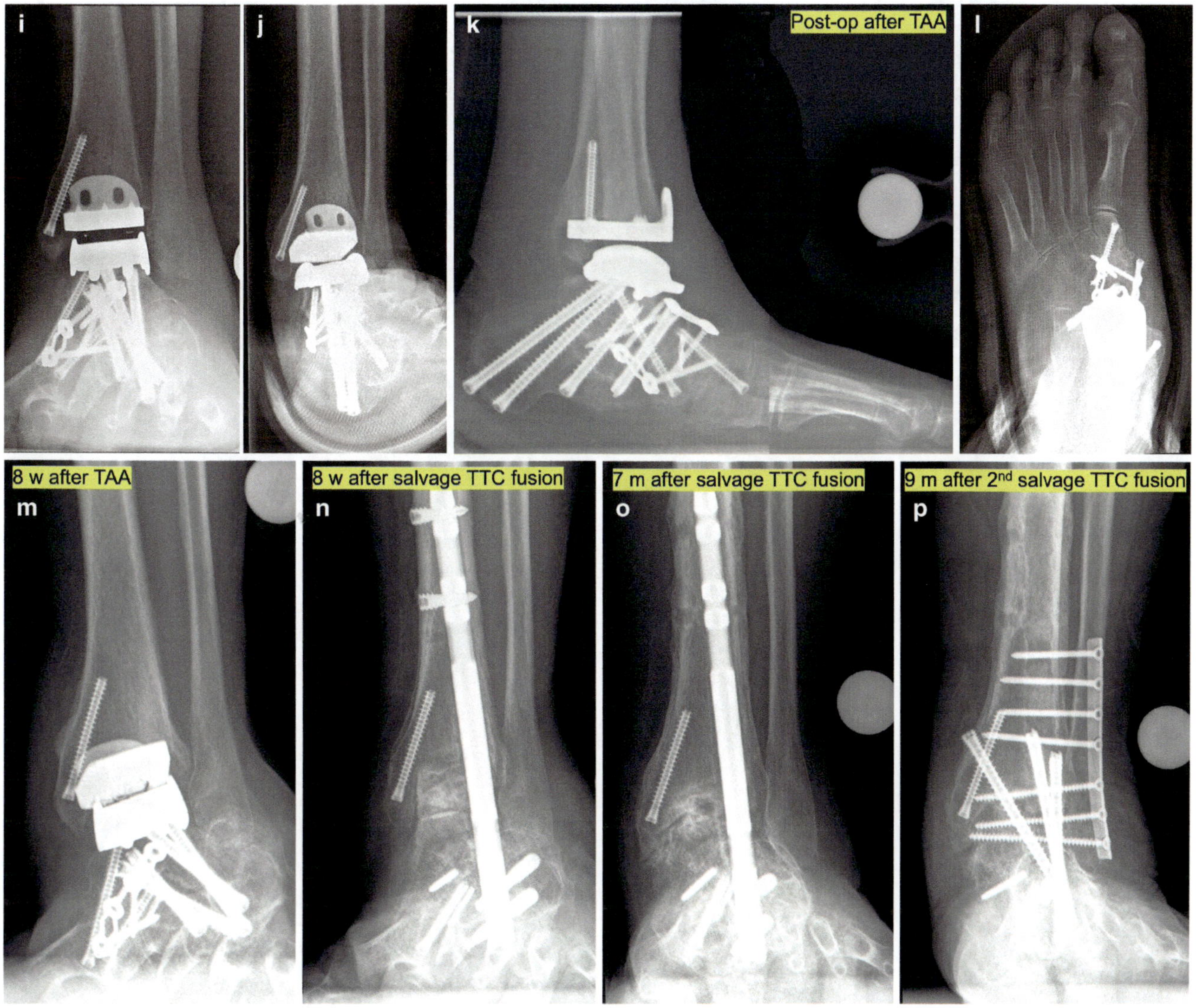

Fig. 11.5 (continued)

11.3 The Widened Ankle Mortise

A widened ankle mortise can be related to post-traumatic osteoarthritis (particularly after external rotation-abduction fractures of the ankle), and valgus and flatfoot deformities. Consequently, the talus will lose its stability in the coronal plane, which may result in tilting or translational movements (Figs. 11.6 and 11.7).

The Authors' Experience

A stable ankle mortise with appropriate closure of the medial and lateral gutters is paramount in obtaining a stable ankle, especially when using a mobile-bearing ankle that allows free translational movement along its second interface between the flat undersurface of the tibial component and the polyethylene insert. Though not proven, a syndesmotic fusion is the most efficient to achieve this goal. It also stabilizes the talus in the sagittal plane.

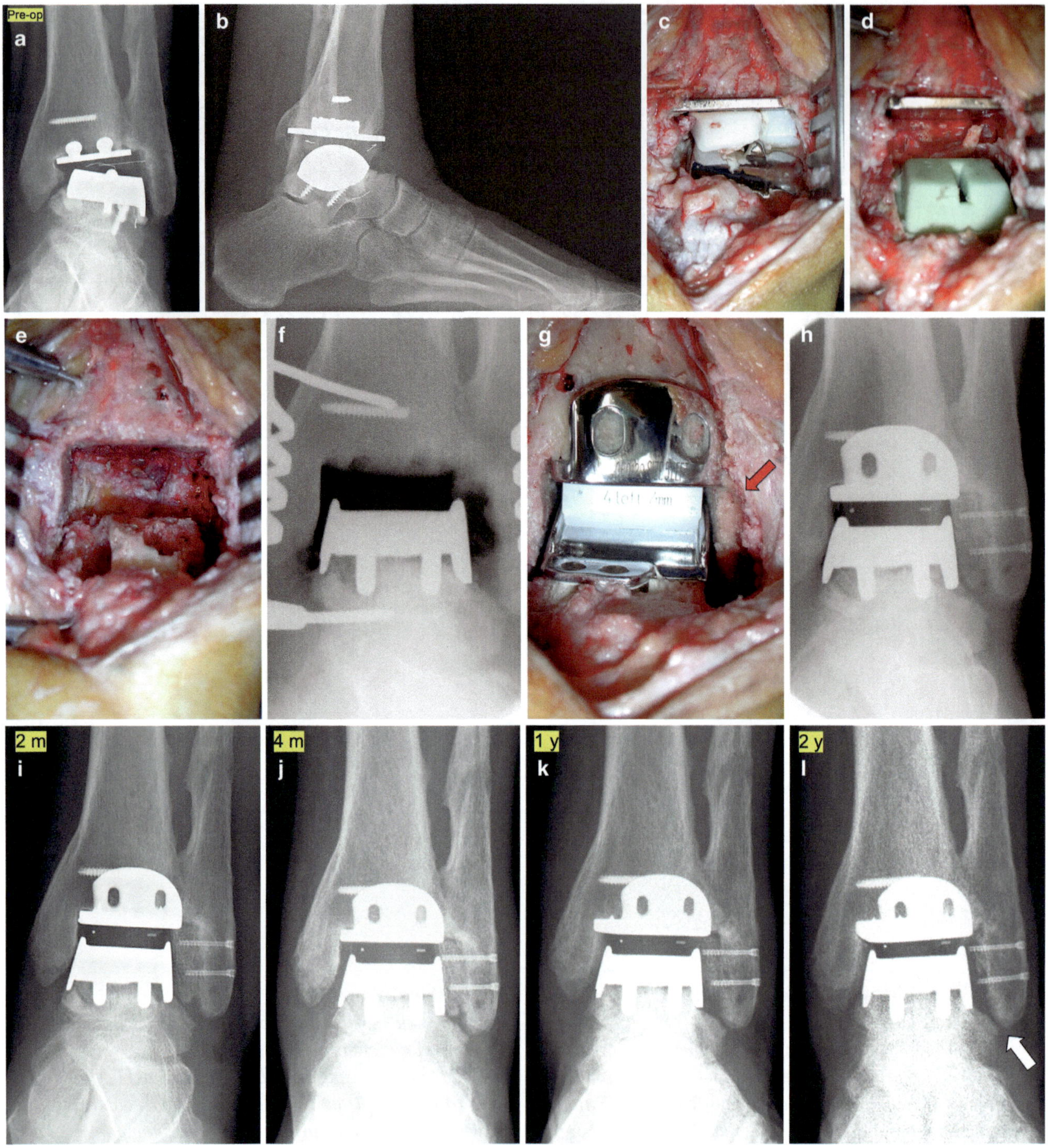

Fig. 11.6 Management of the widened ankle mortise with allograft. A 64-year-old gardener, 11.5 years after a total ankle replacement with a mobile ankle for post-traumatic osteoarthritis, complains of pain in his medial ankle. He felt a cracking some months ago and has observed a tilt of the heel into the varus. (**a**) AP view showing a varus tilt of the talus within the widened ankle mortise associated with synostosis of the distal tibiofibular joint and a dislocation of the polyethylene insert. (**b**) The tilt of the talus can also be seen in the lateral view. (**c**) After exposure of the ankle, a fracture of the polyethylene insert is found. (**d**) The talar component was fixed by bone cement. (**e**) Significant bone defects on the talus are seen after the bone cement removal. (**f**) After a revision talar implant is inserted, a significant bone defect on the inner side of the fibula is seen. (**g**) The defect is filled by an allograft (arrow) and fixed by screws inserted percutaneously, as shown under fluoroscopy (**h**). (**i–l**) Series of AP views showing the evolution of the graft incorporation. Though some progressive resorption is seen after 1 year, the talus was kept in place, indicating that the graft could keep the talus in place during the postoperative scarring process and bone formation in the distal tibiofibular joint (arrow)

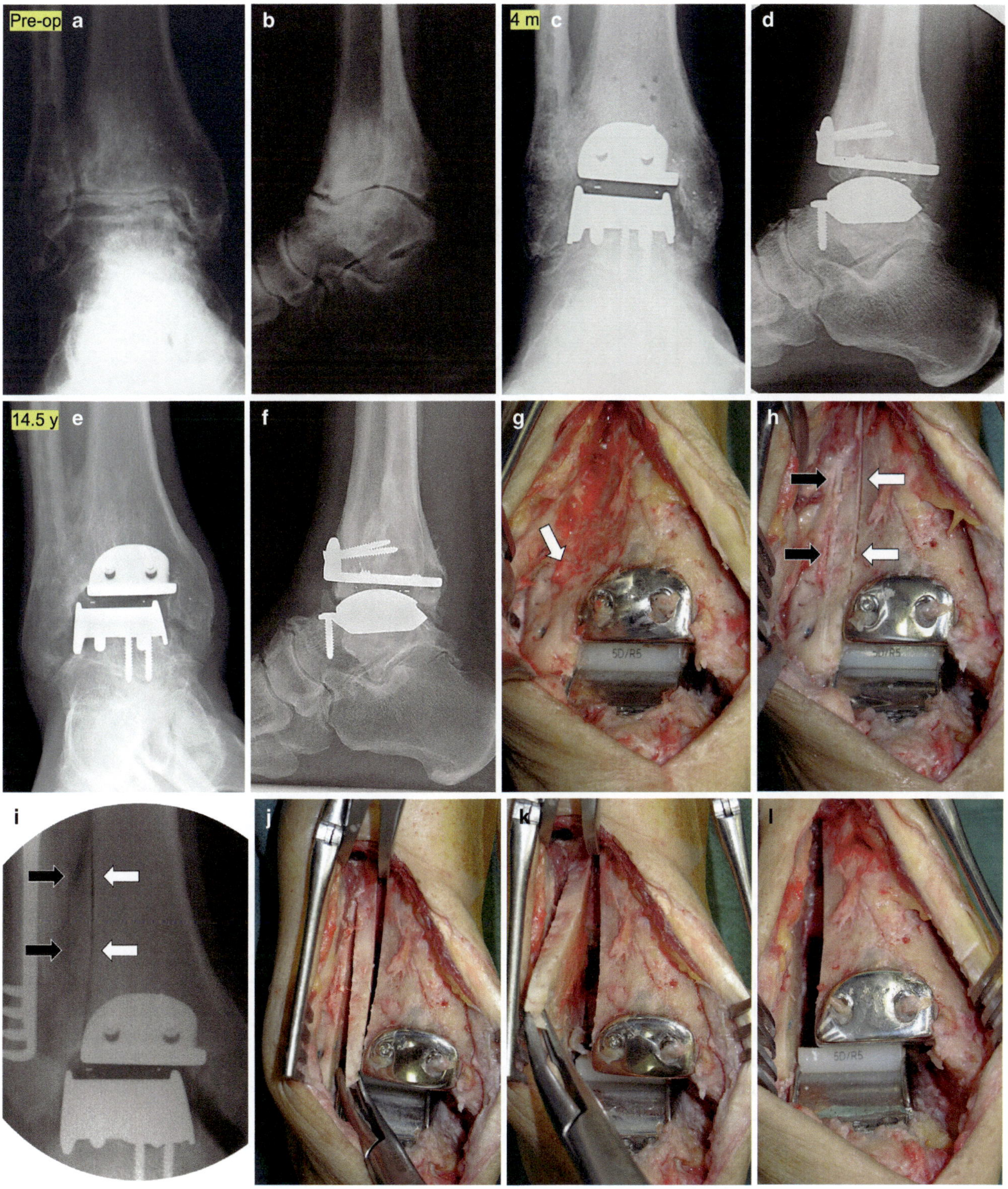

Fig. 11.7 Management of the widened ankle mortise (synostosis) with resection osteotomy. A 59-year-old lawyer underwent 14.5 y ago total ankle arthroplasty for post-traumatic osteoarthritis. (**a**, **b**) Preoperative situation before the total ankle arthroplasty. (**c**, **d**) The ankle looks well-aligned 4 months after the surgery, with a slightly widened medial gutter. (**e**) The patient presents shortly before his 15-year control because he noticed a strange rub in his ankle. The AP view shows a lateral displacement of the talus within the widened mortise as fixed by synostosis. (**f**) The lateral view shows stable implants but some ossifications. (**g**) After ankle exposure, synostosis can be seen (arrow). (**h**) An osteotomy is made along the original tibia border (white arrows) and the border of the original fibula (black arrows). (**i**) The osteotomies are shown under fluoroscopy (arrows). (**j**, **k**) The created gap is opened with a lamina spreader, allowing the removal of the bone slice. (**l**) The situation after the bone removal. (**m**) The fibula is pressed with a clamp against the tibia, closing the gap. (**n**) To avoid a crash of the fibula during this maneuver, the clamp is positioned in the screw of a short third-fibular plate. (**o**) After the insertion of four screws to achieve high compression at the osteotomy site, the clamp and the distal screws are removed, and the construct is seen to be stable, as shown also under fluoroscopy (**p**). AP views show a stable construct with the talus well centralized within the mortise after 4 months (**q**) and 2 years, respectively (**r**)

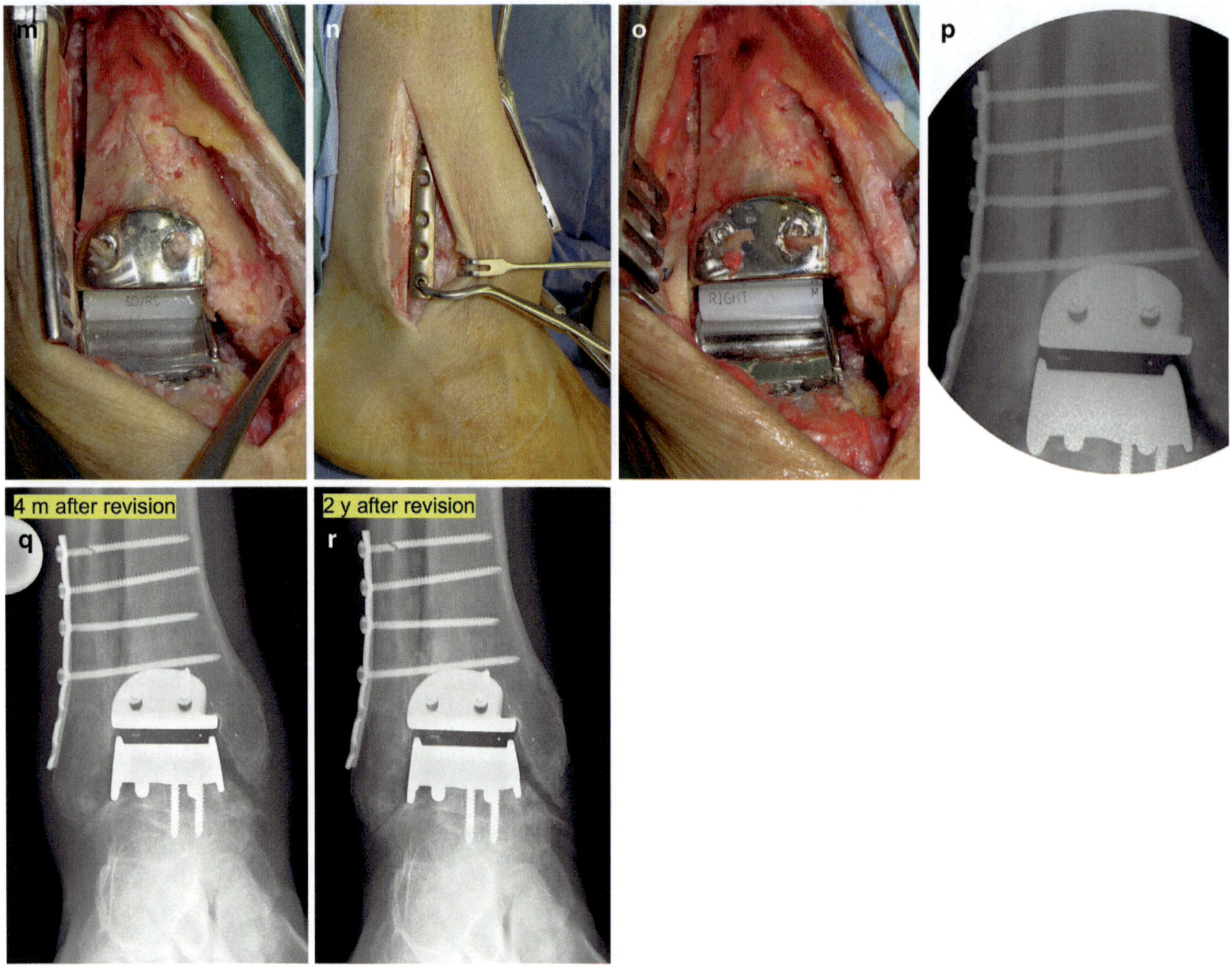

Fig. 11.7 (continued)

11.4 The Ankle After Septic Arthritis

Septic arthritis of the ankle typically affects the subtalar and, in some instances, the talonavicular joints, resulting in a stiff hindfoot. Therefore, a total ankle replacement is superior to a tibiotalar fusion as the patient gains motion. Complete healing of the infection is mandatory, however. Another challenging problem may be the condition of the soft tissues, which are often scarred and weak (Fig. 11.8).

The Authors' Experience

The risk of recurrent infection after total ankle arthroplasty has not increased after septic arthritis in the past. Special attention must be paid to the soft tissues. If critical, a flap should be considered to cover critical scarred areas. Analogously, bone defects should be filled with vascularized bone grafts.

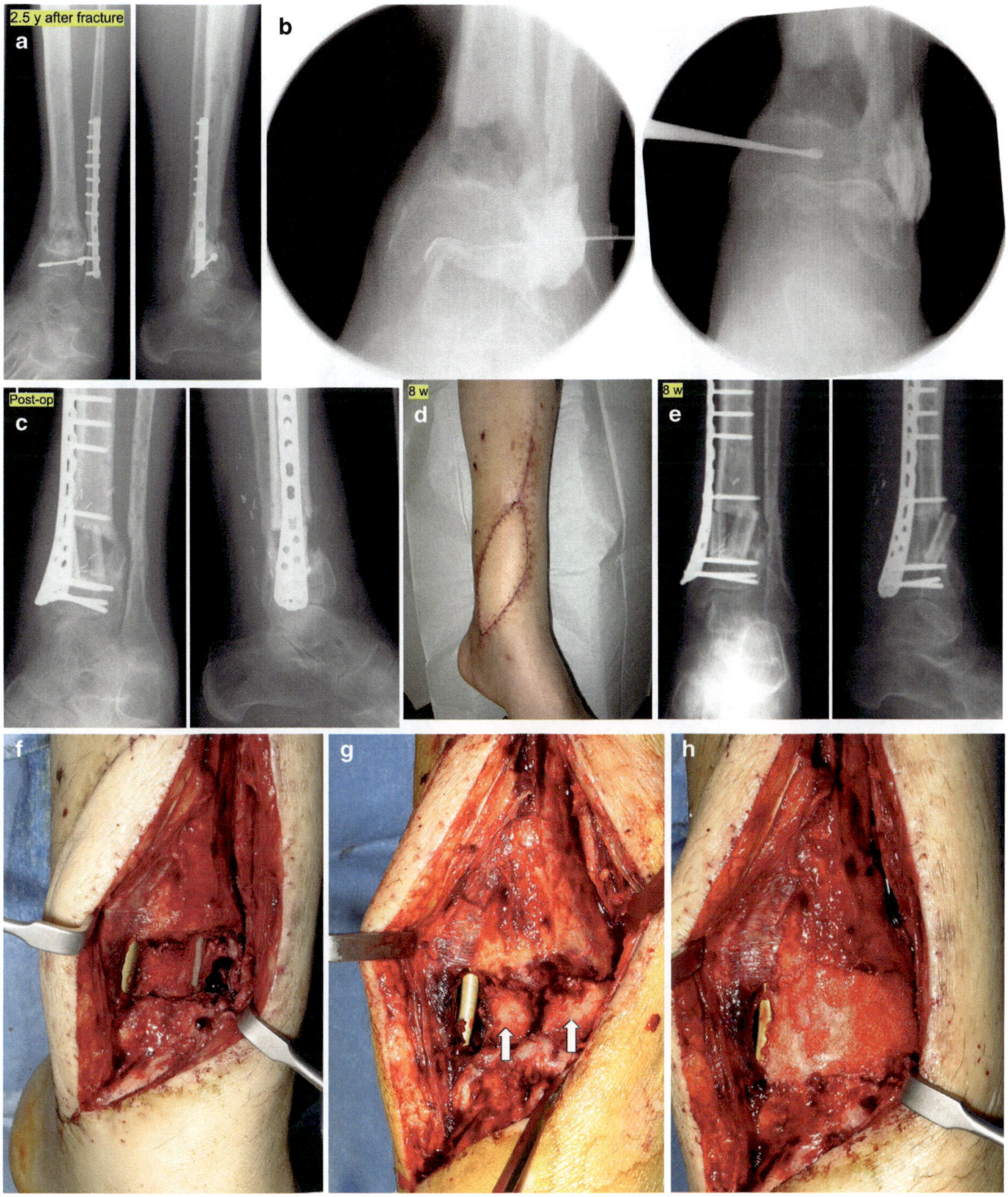

Fig. 11.8 Infected pseudarthrosis of distal tibia treated with vascularized bone graft and total ankle arthroplasty. A 42-year-old constructor manager, after an open distal tibia fracture for 2.5 years treated by internal fixation complains of a painful and stiff ankle 2.5 years after an open distal tibia fracture. (**a**) The standard radiographs show a non-union of the distal tibia. (**b**) First, the implants are removed, and probes are taken at the pseudarthrosis site. Intraarticular injection of contrast medium shows communication with the pseudarthrosis area. Staphylococcus aureus is identified in the probes; thus, specific antibiotic therapy is done. Surgical reconstruction included segmental resection of the pseudarthrosis area by two bone cuts and stabilization of the tibia with a plate. The intermediate part of the contralateral fibula is harvested as a free vascularized bone graft with a soft tissue flap and used as an interposition graft for the bone and a cutaneous flap to accomplish the soft tissue defect (not shown). (**c**) Postoperative radiographs showing the fibular grafts well in place. (**d**) At 8 weeks of control, the flap is well integrated. (**e**) The radiographs show a dislocation of one bone graft. (**f**) Therefore, the fracture area is approached along the anterior border of the soft tissue graft. (**g**) The two bone grafts (arrows) are repositioned, and cancellous bone is also used to fill the defect (**h**). (**i**) Series of AP views showing the evolution. Notice the remodeling process of the fibular graft seen already at 4 months, though the revision 2 months before because of the graft dislocation. The implant is removed after 1 year. Total ankle arthroplasty was performed 20 months after the reconstruction. 16 months later, the ankle is revised due to stiffness, with the exchange of polyethylene insert and tibial screw removal. (**j**) At 15-year follow-up control, the patient is delighted with his ankle, allowing him to fully accomplish his construction manager work despite the limited range of motion for dorsi-/plantar flexion to 3°-0°-25°

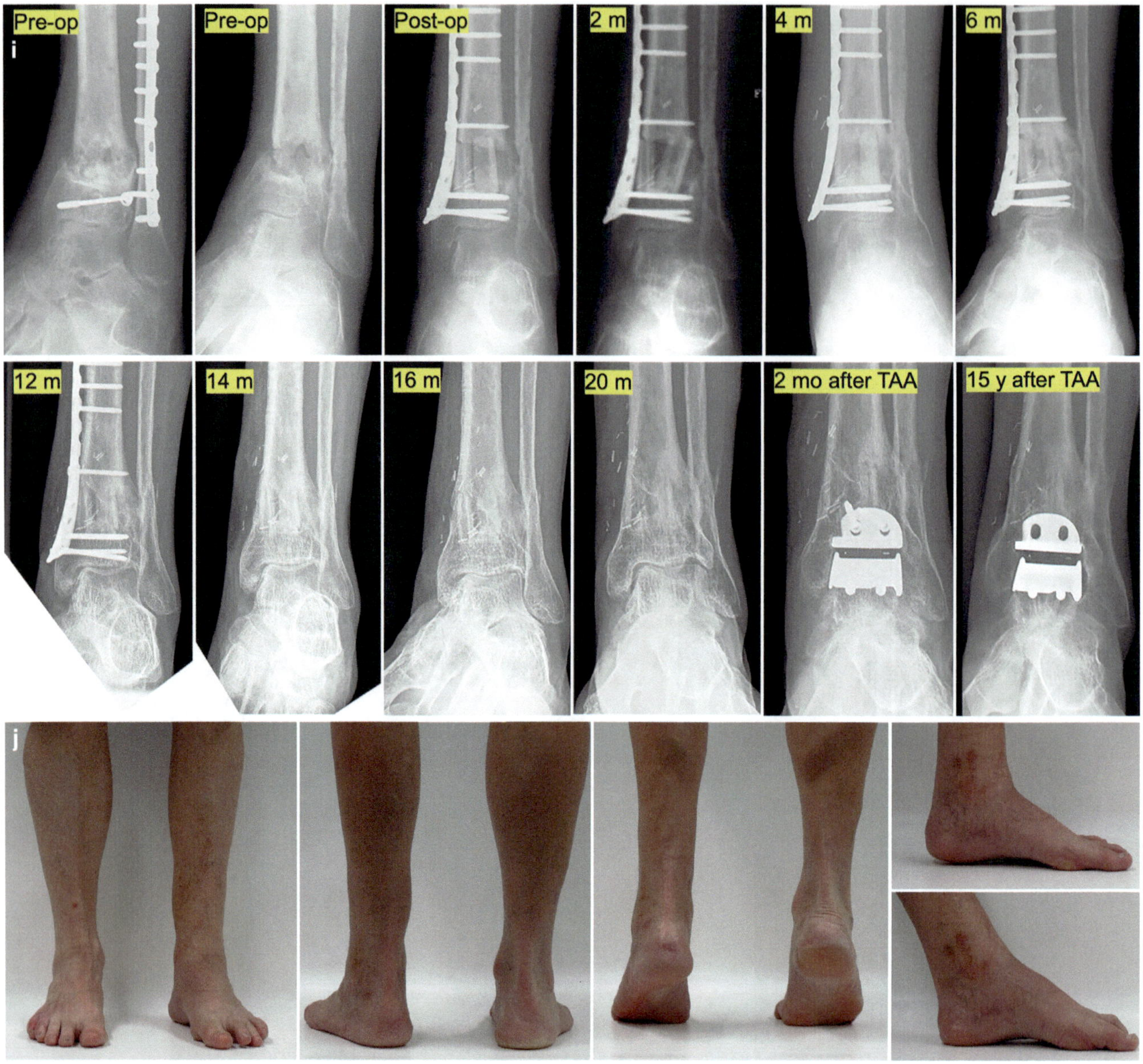

Fig. 11.8 (continued)

11.5 Neurologic Disorders

Neurologic disorders are generally considered contraindications for replacement surgeries of the osteoarthritic ankle. This is undoubtedly true for conditions associated with spasms and uncontrolled muscular contractures. Paralytic situations limited to the foot may be an exception. In most instances, fusions and osteotomies are necessary to obtain a plantigrade and stable foot position. Tendon transfers may improve foot function, especially a transfer of the posterior tibial tendon to the dorsal aspect of the foot or the peroneal tendons (Fig. 11.9).

The Authors' Experience

In selected cases, total ankle arthroplasty for treating end-stage osteoarthritis associated with neurologic disorders can be an excellent option for obtaining a plantigrade and stable foot. However, appropriate ligament balancing and addressing deforming forces are mandatory for success. In particular, the inversion force of the posterior tibial muscle must be removed when overpowering the dysfunctional peroneal and extensor muscles. Our experience is limited to using a mobile-bearing ankle in the long term.

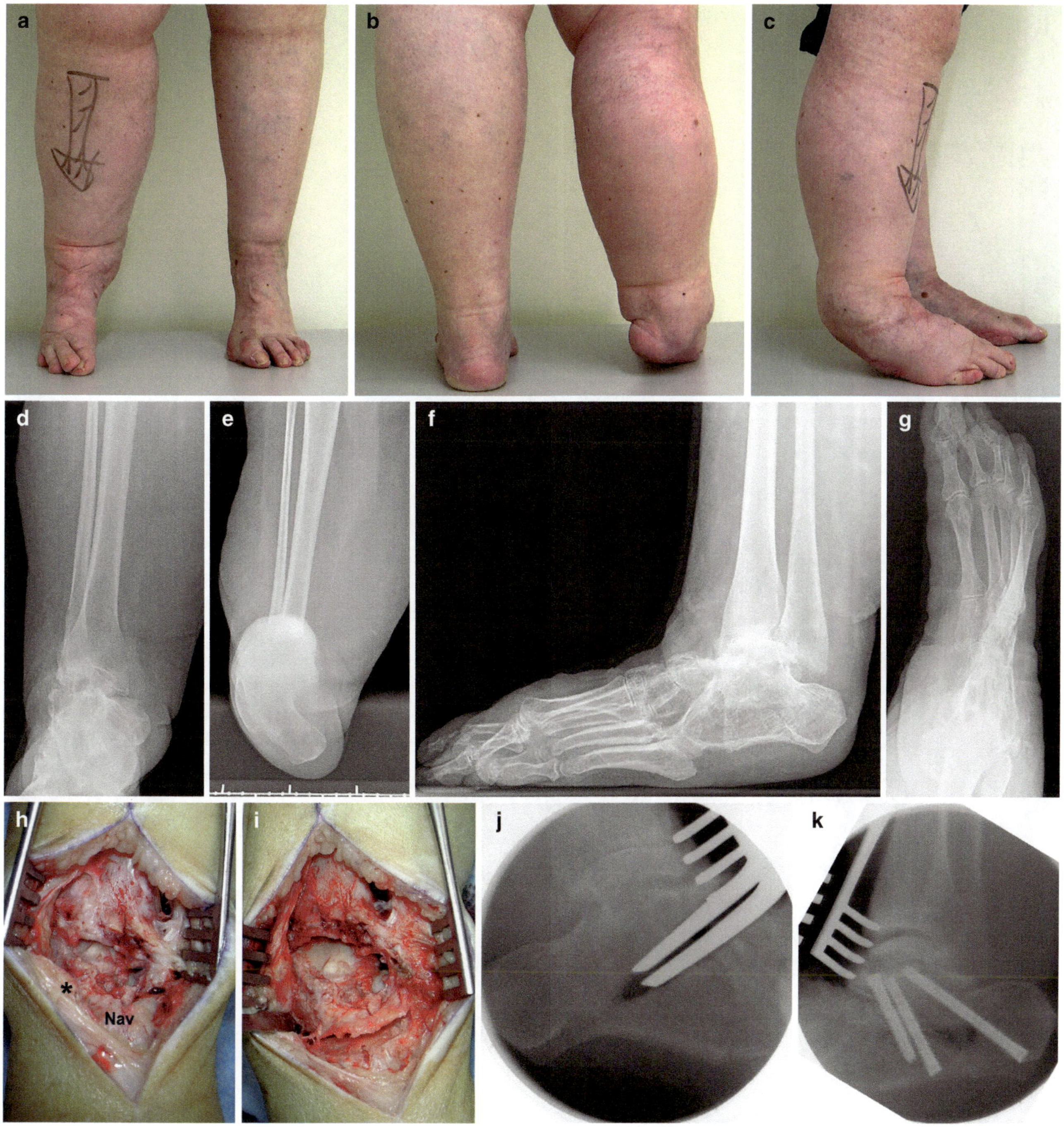

Fig. 11.9 Correcting osteotomy with total ankle arthroplasty in a polio foot. A 53-year-old female patient suffering from polio resulting in end-stage ankle osteoarthritis associated with a fixed varus-supinatus deformity and polio after a hindfoot fusion in adolescence. She complains of massive pain beneath her lateral foot with imminent ulceration. She wore special braces over the years, but the situation worsened, and she is looking for a solution. She was counseled to go for a tibiotalocalcaneal fusion in a slightly plantarflexed position, but she was not willing to follow this proposal for fear of continuation of the forefoot problems. (**a–c**) Clinical views showing the shortening of the affected leg, the fixed varus-supinatus deformity of the foot with critical soft tissues beneath her lateral midfoot. (**d–g**) Standard radiographs showing the complex three-dimensional deformity after a hindfoot fusion. (**h**) After exposure of the ankle joint, the talar head (star) is seen to be malunited to the navicular (Nav). (**i**) An open wedge osteotomy with the apex at dorsolateral aspect of the foot is performed, as seen in the fluoroscopy (**j**). (**k**) This allowed to evert and pronate the foot, combined with some abduction, and to fix it in the gained position. (**l**) The obtained alignment and plantigrade position of the foot can be seen in the AP view. (**m–o**) Fluoroscopies to show the result in all three planes after total ankle arthroplasty. 2.8 years after surgery, the patient sustained a tibial shaft fracture while falling on the stairs that was fixed with an intramedullary nail. (**p–s**) At 5-year control, the foot is well aligned, with a balanced ankle with stable implants. (**t–w**) No changes are seen 10 years later, at 15-year control. The patient is extremely pleased because she can still walk with adapted shoes but without a brace as before the surgery

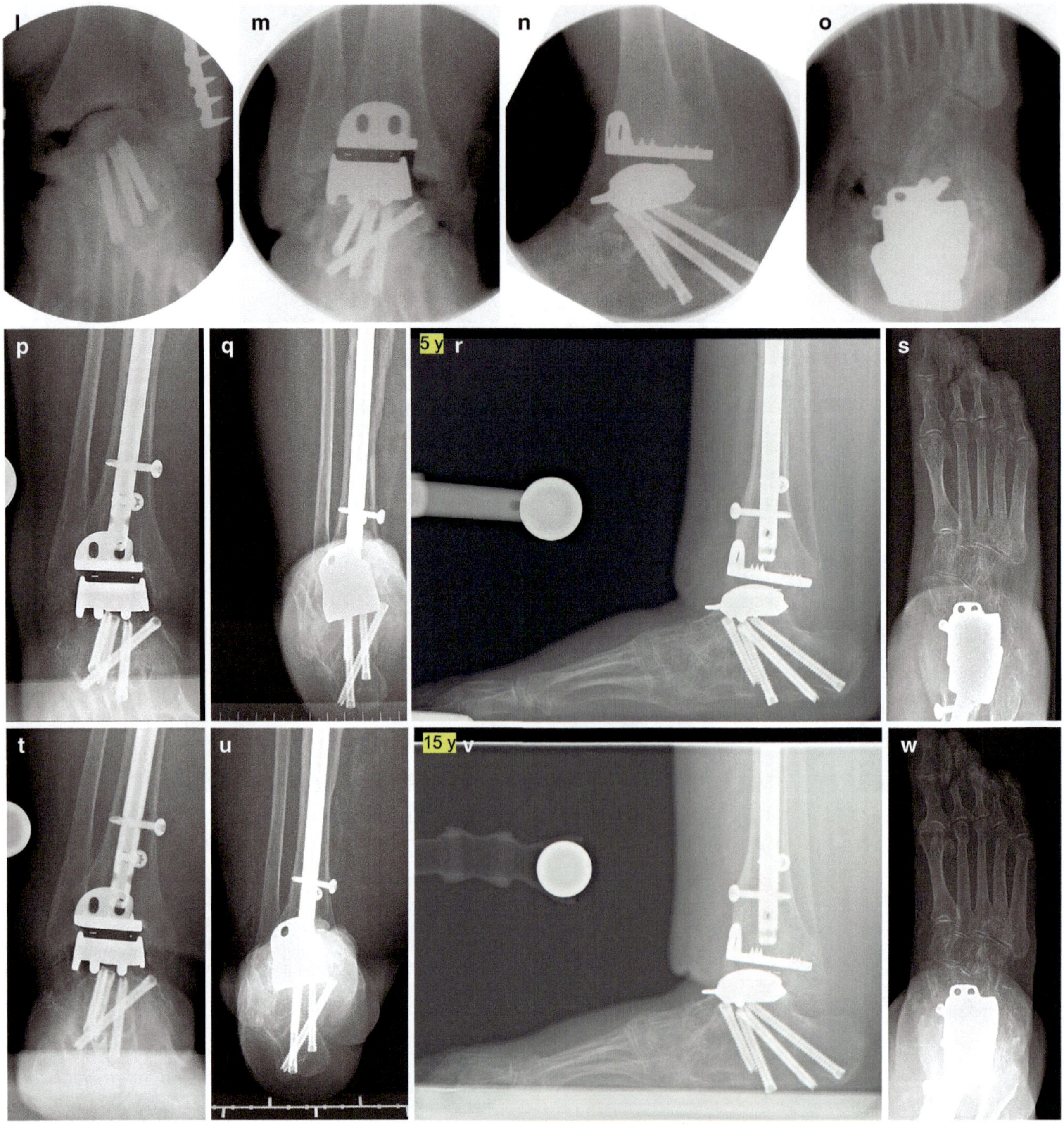

Fig. 11.9 (continued)

11.6 Addressing Implant Failures

Implants can fail because of osteolysis and subsequent subsidence. In some instances, surrounding bone is strong enough to resist subsidence, typically resulting in a cavity beneath the implant. This can be explained by the remodeling process of the bone in the fight against failing. Therefore, the remaining circumferential bone around the defect should be preserved and not weakened. Revision arthroplasty using a bulky implant that needs additional bone resection might thus be critical. Analogously, stem fixation of a new component might not be ideal as its stability would rely on the weak intramedullary bone instead of the peripheric solid bone (Fig. 11.10).

The Authors' Experience

The resurfacing concept also works for failed ankles with significant bone defects as long as the remaining circumferential bone is strong enough to support the implant. This is the case in most instances because of the remodeling process. However, caution must be paid to preserve the remaining bone, and an implant that uses the whole remaining bone as a support should be used. The platform must also be strong enough to withstand torsional forces.

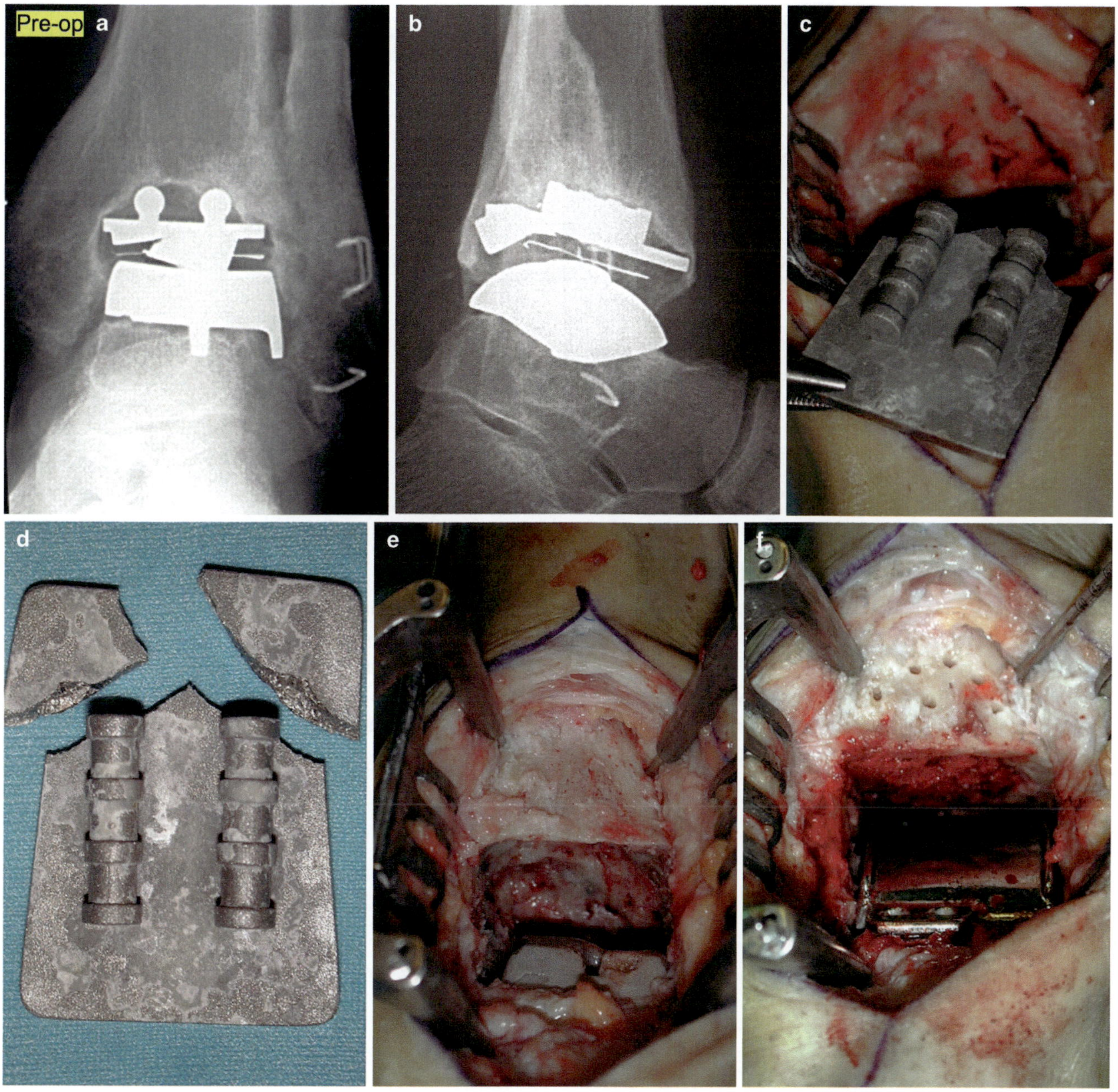

Fig. 11.10 Implant failure with central bone defect management with a flat resurfacing implant. A 54-year-old housekeeper suffering from post-traumatic osteoarthritis after an open ankle fracture treated 4.7 years before with total ankle arthroplasty using a STAR implant. During strenuous work, he felt a strange cracking in his replaced ankle, associated with pain. (**a**) The AP view shows a fracture of the tibial implant and a central defect in the tibial metaphysis. (**b**) The lateral view demonstrates the load transfer between the implant and the tibia limited to the circumferential cortex while the center of the tibia is empty due to osteolysis. (**c**) The broken implant is removed. (**d**) Its size is large, with a 2.2-mm-thick platform. (**e**) Visual inspection of the central defect while the circumferential cortex is well preserved. (**f**) The cortex is flattened with the saw with less than 1 mm bone resection, and the cavity is filled with autologous cancellous bone from the iliac crest. After that, a flat implant with a 4-mm-thick platform is inserted (not shown). (**g–j**) Ankle series showing the evolution from preoperatively to 22 years. The component remained stable without subsidence. At the latest follow-up, 22 years after the revision surgery, the still active patient was delighted with his ankle, allowing him an everyday life

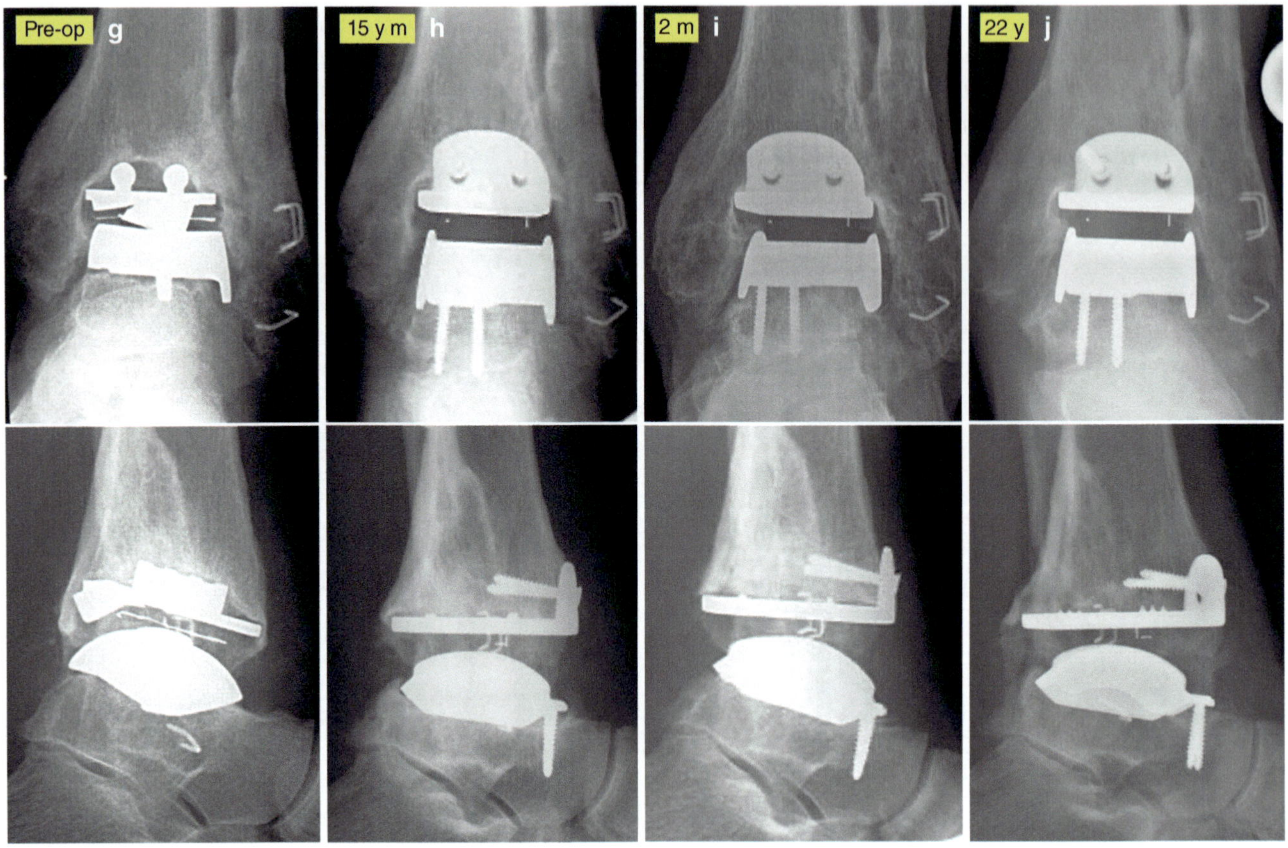

Fig. 11.10 (continued)

11.7 Conclusions

- Total ankle arthroplasty has become a viable alternative to ankle fusion in treating complex disorders and deformities of the foot and ankle.
- Requirements for its success include the achievement of a well-balanced and stable ankle and the removal of deforming forces.
- The limits still need to be defined.

12 Results and Efficacy of Total Ankle Arthroplasty

Ankle arthrodesis has, for many years, been the gold standard in the treatment of end-stage osteoarthritis. However, it is well documented that tibiotalar fusions lead to deficits in function and may cause or exacerbate adjacent joint arthritis, particularly in the subtalar joint [1–3]. Ankle arthroplasty preserves motion at the ankle joint while still achieving the primary goal of pain relief. However, the results from the first generations of total ankle replacement were disappointing because of poor clinical outcomes and high rates of aseptic loosening [4–7]. They discouraged many foot and ankle surgeons from performing arthroplasty surgery for many years. Perception has slowly changed with the reintroduction of modern, more anatomically designed, and better-engineered total ankle implants. Initially seen as a novel technique with potential benefits, there needed to be validated proof in the literature to support its use. Fortunately, improvements in prosthetic design and a better understanding of operative techniques have allayed most of these concerns, and the literature has produced promising early clinical results [8–16].

This section summarizes the most current literature on the outcomes of the currently used total ankle replacement prostheses.

12.1 International Registry Data

National joint registry data on total ankle replacements provide essential information and surveillance on the outcomes of total ankle arthroplasty. It must be recognized, however, that these data have limitations. There needs to be more clarity on how accurately the data reflect current practice, the need for patient-reported outcome measures PROMs, and the incomplete capture of the accurate picture, with somewhat hard endpoints. A report by Muir in 2017 [17] identified several issues with registry data for ankle replacements, including data confounders and data capture problems, especially with underreporting of revision procedures. Similarly, in a recent observational study including 17,648 patients after joint replacement surgery based on the Swedish orthopedic registry, missing patient-reported data was identified to be a problem for the registers, as only three of the five registers reached a 60% follow-up rate [18].

12.1.1 The Swedish Ankle Registry

This registry (available at www.swedankle.se) started in 1993. Of 1226 prostheses, 226 (22%) had been revised by December 31, 2016 [19]. Overall prosthetic survival rate at 5 years was 0.85 (95% CI 0.83–0.87), at 10 years 0.74 (CI 0.70–0.77), at 15 years 0.63 (CI 0.58–0.67), and at 20 years 0.58 (CI 0.52–0.65). For early prosthetic designs, the 5- and 10-year survival rates were 0.81 (CI 0.78–0.84) and 0.69 (CI 0.64–0.73), respectively, while the corresponding rates for current designs were 0.88 (CI 0.85–0.91) and 0.84 (CI 0.79–0.88). Current prosthetic designs had better survival (log-rank test $p < 0.001$).

12.1.2 The Norwegian Arthroplasty Register

This registry (available at http://nrlweb.ihelse.net/) started in 1994. The most common causes for revision of a primary prosthesis were a proximal (tibial) component (26%; 109/413), a loose distal (talar) component (20%; 83/413), malalignment (16%; 66/413), instability (9.7%; 40/413), and deep infection (8%; 33/413).

12.1.3 The New Zealand Joint Registry

This registry (available at https://nzoa.org.nz/nzoa-joint-registry) started in 2000. Data suggested a 5- and 10-year overall survivorship of 90.4% and 82.8%, respectively. The registry previously used a nonvalidated PROMS that was replaced by the Manchester- Oxford Foot Questionnaire toward the end of 2015. As such, there were no significant PROMS data available.

B. Hintermann, R. Ruiz, *Total Ankle Replacement*, https://doi.org/10.1007/978-3-031-56810-7_12

12.1.4 The Australian National Joint Replacement Registry

This registry (available at https://aoanjrr.sahmri.com/annual-reports) started in 2007. For osteoarthritis, the cumulative percent revision at five years was 10.4%, and for rheumatoid arthritis was 6.5%. Loosening was the most common cause for revision primary ankle replacements. This accounted for 27.7% of all revisions. Following this, lysis accounted for 10.5%, and instability accounted for 9.9% of revisions. Infection was the fourth most common cause of revision, occurring in 8.9%.

12.1.5 National Joint Registry for England, Wales, Northern Ireland, and the Isle of Man

This registry (available at www.njrcentre.org.uk) started in 2010 and constitutes the largest collection of primary ankle arthroplasty of all the registers. The overall estimate of cumulative percentage probability of the first revision was 6.93 (95% CI, 6.0–8.0) at five years, increasing to 8.70 (95% CI, 7.41–12.0) at seven years. The first revision was found to be more likely in individuals younger than age 65.

12.2 Single-Center Studies

Results from single-center specialized units are often better than those reported from national registries [20] but have yet to be reproduced in countries where national registry data are available. Several studies report 15-year survival rates between 0.64 and 0.76. This may be due to larger volumes of total ankle arthroplasties per surgeon and case mix, supporting the notion that ankle replacement surgery takes a long time to master [21, 22].

Prosthetic survival rates from national registries and high-volume units are summarized in Table 12.1.

Table 12.1 Prosthetic survival rates from national registries and high-volume units[a]

Study	Period of primary surgery	TAA (n)	Mean	Max	Revisions (n)	5-year	10-year	15-year	20-year	Prosthesis
Registry studies										
Fevang et al. (2007) [23]	1994–2005	257	3	12	27	0.89	0.76			
Henricson et al. (2007) [24]	1993–2005	531			101	0.78				
Henricson et al. (2011) [25]	1993–2010	780	6	10	168	0.81	0.69			
Unden et al. (2019) [19]	1993–2016	1′226	7	24	268	0.85	0.74	0.63	0.58	
Henricson et al. (2015) [26]	1993–1999	118			58	0.71	0.61			STAR single coat
	1999–2007	206			67	0.82	0.7			STAR double coat
Skytta et al. (2010) [27]	1997–2006	515	3	10	59	0.83				
Hosman et al. (2007) [28]	2000–2005	202	2	6	14	0.86				
www.nzoa.org.nz	2000–2017	728		11	50		0.83			
Dagneaux et al. (2022) [29]	2010–2019	4748	5	10	817	0.84	0.78			
Non-registry studies										
Kitaoka and Patzer (1996) [6]	1974–1988	204	9	17	57	0.79	0.65	0.61		Mayo
Buechel et al. (2004) [30]	1981–1988	40	12	20					0.74	BB flat sulcus
		75	5	12			0.92			BB deep sulcus
Kofoed (2004) [31]	1986–1989	33	9	15	9					STAR cemented
	1990–1995	25	9	12	1					STAR
Krishnapillai et al. (2019) [32]	1993–2010	101	17		31		0.86	0.74		BB
Clough et al. (2019) [33]	1993–2000	200	16	24	32	0.9	0.83	0.76		STAR

Table 12.1 (continued)

Study	Period of primary surgery	TAA (n)	Mean	Max	Revisions (n)	5-year	10-year	15-year	20-year	Prosthesis
Bedard et al. (2021) [34]	1993–2000	200	7	13	24	0.93	0.8			STAR
Frigg et al. (2017) [35]	1996–2006	50	15	16	12		0.78	0.7	0.55[b]	STAR
Brunner et al. (2013) [36]	1996–2000	72	11	15	35	0.93	0.64	0.46		STAR
Koivu et al. (2017) [37]	1997–2002	34	13	17	15	0.95	0.87	0.64		STAR
Bonnin et al. (2011) [38]	1997–2000	98	9	11	12		0.85			Salto
Mann et al. (2011) [15]	1997–2002	34		17	15	0.94	0.87	0.64		AES
Jastifer et al. (2015) [39]	1998–2003	41	10	13	7		0.95[a]			STAR
Palanca et al. (2018) [40]	1998–2000	84	9	11	9	0.96	0.9			STAR
Wood and Deakin (2003) [41]	1998–2000	84	16	18	15			0.73		STAR
Kerkhoff et al. (2016) [42]	1999–2008	134	9	15	20		0.78			STAR
Barg et al. (2013) [43]	2000–2010	722	6	10	61	0.94	0.84			Hintegra
Kvarda et al. (2022) [12]	2000–2010	638	13	20	126	0.93	0.86	0.82	0.74	Hintegra
Di Iorio et al. (2017) [44]	2003–2006	50	9	13	29		0.57			AES
Zafar et al. (2020) [45]	2004–2016	322			60	0.75	0.68			Hintegra
Van Es et al. (2022) [46]	2004–2012	254	8	14	94		0.71			CCI
Yoon et al. (2022) [47]	2006–2011	213	11	17	43		0.93[d]			Hintegra
Harston et al. (2017) [48]	2007–2011	149	6	10		0.91				Inbone I

a = 58% lost; *b* = at 19 y; *c* = minimal 20 y; *d* = at 11.3 y

12.3 Meta-Analyses and Systematic Reviews

In 2007, Haddad et al. [13] reported a systematic literature review, including 852 total ankle arthroplasties. The 5-year implant survival rate was 78% (95% confidence interval, 69.0–87.6%), and the 10-year survival rate was 77% (95% confidence interval, 63.3–90.8%). The revision rate following total ankle arthroplasty was 7% (95% confidence interval, 3.5–10.9%), with the primary reason for the revisions being loosening and/or subsidence (28%).

In 2013, Zaidi et al. [49] published the results of a meta-analysis including 58 studies, with 7942 total ankle arthroplasties. The mean age at operation was 60 years, ranging from 17 to 95 years. The overall 10-year survivorship was 89%, and the annual failure rate of 1.2% (95% CI, 0.7–1.6).

In 2018, Gross et al. [50], in a 27-year meta-analysis including 40 studies, with a total of 4835 total ankle arthroplasties, reported 5- and 10-year survival rates of 86% (P = 0.001) and 76% (P = 0.53), respectively. The revision rate was 9.6% (P = 0.10), more than a third of which was caused by component loosening. There were no differences in survival rates between second- and third-generation implants. However, the third-generation implants' functional scores, range of motion, and overall patient outcomes were significantly higher. To clarify, most second-generation implants were two-component, fixed-bearing systems with a polyethylene-bearing surface incorporated into the talar or tibial component, with a preference for press-fit designs. Third-generation prostheses were characterized by adding a third component, a polyethylene, mobile-bearing meniscus, with more significance placed on ligaments to retain stability.

In 2020, in a systematic review and meta-analysis, Onggo et al. [19] reported on 17 studies, with 1127 and 262 ankles in the 5- and 10-year minimum follow-up groups, respectively. At 5 years minimum follow-up, pooled proportion of prostheses revision for any reason other than polyethylene exchange was 0.122 (95% CI, 0.084–0.173), all-cause revision was 0.185 (95% CI, 0.131–0.256), unplanned reoperation was 0.288 (95% CI, 0.204–0.390), and all infection was 0.033 (95% CI, 0.021–0.051). At 10 years minimum follow-up, pooled proportion of prostheses revision for any reason other than polyethylene exchange was 0.202 (95% CI, 0.118–0.325), all-cause revision was 0.305 (95% CI, 0.191–0.448), unplanned reoperation was 0.422 (95% CI, 0.260–0.603), and all infection was 0.029 (95% CI, 0.013–0.066). The authors concluded that, despite good intermediate- and long-term functional outcome measures, total ankle arthroplasty has relatively higher revision surgery prevalence with longer follow-up periods.

12.4 Total Ankle Arthroplasty *Versus* Ankle Arthrodesis

There is only one large, nonindustry sponsored prospective mid- to long-term study of total ankle arthroplasty outcomes compared with ankle arthrodesis, the only current alternative to total ankle replacement [51]. These results, although not stratified, show that even second-generation total ankle replacement implants have outcomes at least as good as arthrodesis. Further data have been presented to suggest that with third-generation implants, patient-reported outcomes for total ankle replacement may be superior to arthrodesis, with both having similar mid-term revision rates.

In a prospective study, Goldberg et al. [33] reported on 281 patients randomly assigned to total ankle arthroplasty (fixed-bearing prosthesis) or ankle fusion. At one year, the mean MOXFQ-W/S scores improved for both groups. The adjusted difference in the change in MOXFQ-W/S scores from baseline was −5.6 (95% CI, −12.5 to 1.4), showing that total ankle arthroplasty improved more than ankle fusion. Still, the difference was not considered clinically or statistically significant. The number of adverse events was similar between the groups (109 vs. 104), but there were more wound healing issues in the total ankle arthroplasty group and more thromboembolic events and nonunion in the ankle fusion group. The symptomatic nonunion rate for ankle fusion was 7%. A post hoc analysis suggested the superiority of fixed-bearing total ankle arthroplasty over ankle fusion (−11.1 [CI, −19.3 to −2.9]).

Biomechanical and clinical studies have shown improved movement transfer in the ankle joint complex and better pain relief and postoperative function in a replaced ankle than in a fused ankle [52, 53]. Consequently, midtarsal joints are preserved from nonphysiological and subsequent degenerative changes, possibly affecting long-term clinical outcomes [54].

12.5 Conclusions

- End-stage ankle arthritis has a significant effect on function and quality of life.
- Total ankle arthroplasty continues to emerge as a safe and effective treatment for arthritis.
- With encouraging outcomes and improved implant longevity, there has been a significant improvement in the results of first-generation implants.
- Although a total ankle replacement involves a surgical procedure predisposed to complications, the results of the current literature suggest that total ankle has become a viable alternative to ankle arthrodesis.

References

1. Fuchs S, Sandmann C, Skwara A, Chylarecki C. Quality of life 20 years after arthrodesis of the ankle. A study of adjacent joints. J Bone Joint Surg Br. 2003;85(7):994–8.
2. Coester LM, Saltzman CL, Leupold J, Pontarelli W. Long-term results following ankle arthrodesis for post-traumatic arthritis. J Bone Joint Surg Am. 2001;83(2):219–28.
3. Hendrickx RP, Stufkens SA, de Bruijn EE, Sierevelt IN, van Dijk CN, Kerkhoffs GM. Medium- to long-term outcome of ankle arthrodesis. Foot Ankle Int. 2011;32(10):940–7.
4. Hintermann B. Total ankle arthroplasty—historical overview, current concepts and future perspectives. Wien-New York: Springer; 2004. 195 p
5. Helm R, Stevens J. Long-term results of total ankle replacement. J Arthroplast. 1986;1(4):271–7.
6. Kitaoka HB, Patzer GL. Clinical results of the Mayo total ankle arthroplasty. J Bone Joint Surg Am. 1996;78(11):1658–64.
7. Bolton-Maggs BG, Sudlow RA, Freeman MA. Total ankle arthroplasty. A long-term review of the London Hospital experience. J Bone Joint Surg Br. 1985;67(5):785–90.
8. Adams SB Jr, Demetracopoulos CA, Queen RM, Easley ME, DeOrio JK, Nunley JA. Early to mid-term results of fixed-bearing total ankle arthroplasty with a modular intramedullary tibial component. J Bone Joint Surg Am. 2014;96(23):1983–9.
9. Bonnin M, Judet T, Colombier JA, Buscayret F, Graveleau N, Piriou P. Midterm results of the Salto total ankle prosthesis. Clin Orthop Relat Res. 2004;424:6–18.
10. Hintermann B, Valderrabano V, Dereymaeker G, Dick W. The HINTEGRA ankle: rationale and short-term results of 122 consecutive ankles. Clin Orthop Relat Res. 2004;424:57–68.
11. Valderrabano V, Hintermann B, Dick W. Scandinavian total ankle replacement: a 3.7-year average followup of 65 patients. Clin Orthop Relat Res. 2004;424:47–56.
12. Kvarda P, Peterhans US, Susdorf R, Barg A, Ruiz R, Hintermann B. Long-term survival of HINTEGRA total ankle replacement in 683 patients: a concise 20-year follow-up of a previous report. J Bone Joint Surg Am. 2022;
13. Haddad SL, Coetzee JC, Estok R, Fahrbach K, Banel D, Nalysnyk L. Intermediate and long-term outcomes of total ankle arthroplasty and ankle arthrodesis. a systematic review of the literature. J Bone Joint Surg Am. 2007;89(9):1899–905.
14. Hofmann KJ, Shabin ZM, Ferkel E, Jockel J, Slovenkai MP. Salto Talaris Total ankle arthroplasty: clinical results at a mean of 5.2 years in 78 patients treated by a single surgeon. J Bone Joint Surg Am. 2016;98(24):2036–46.

15. Mann JA, Mann RA, Horton E. STAR ankle: long-term results. Foot Ankle Int. 2011;32(5):S473–84.
16. Wood PL, Prem H, Sutton C. Total ankle replacement: medium-term results in 200 Scandinavian total ankle replacements. J Bone Joint Surg Br. 2008;90(5):605–9.
17. Muir D. Is there anything to learn from a National Joint Registry? Foot Ankle Clin. 2017;22(2):465–75.
18. Coster MC, Bremander A, Nilsdotter A. Patient-reported outcome for 17,648 patients in 5 different Swedish orthopaedic quality registers before and 1 year after surgery: an observational study. Acta Orthop. 2023;94:1–7.
19. Unden A, Jehpsson L, Kamrad I, Carlsson A, Henricson A, Karlsson MK, et al. Better implant survival with modern ankle prosthetic designs: 1226 total ankle prostheses followed for up to 20 years in the Swedish Ankle Registry. Acta Orthop. 2020;91(2): 191–6.
20. Labek G, Janda W, Agreiter M, Schuh R, Bohler N. Organisation, data evaluation, interpretation and effect of arthroplasty register data on the outcome in terms of revision rate in total hip arthroplasty. Int Orthop. 2011;35(2):157–63.
21. Henricson A, Cöster M, Carlsson A. The Swedish national ankle registry. Fuus Sprunggelenk. 2014;12(2):65–9.
22. Barg A, Wimmer MD, Wiewiorski M, Wirtz DC, Pagenstert GI, Valderrabano V. Total ankle replacement. Dtsch Arztebl Int. 2015;112(11):177–84.
23. Fevang BT, Lie SA, Havelin LI, Brun JG, Skredderstuen A, Furnes O. 257 ankle arthroplasties performed in Norway between 1994 and 2005. Acta Orthop. 2007;78(5):575–83.
24. Henricson A, Skoog A, Carlsson A. The Swedish ankle arthroplasty register: an analysis of 531 arthroplasties between 1993 and 2005. Acta Orthop. 2007;78(5):569–74.
25. Henricson A, Nilsson JA, Carlsson A. 10-year survival of total ankle arthroplasties: a report on 780 cases from the Swedish Ankle Register. Acta Orthop. 2011;82(6):655–9.
26. Henricson A, Carlsson A. Survival analysis of the single- and double-coated STAR ankle up to 20 years: long-term follow-up of 324 cases from the Swedish Ankle Registry. Foot Ankle Int. 2015;36(10):1156–60.
27. Skytta ET, Koivu H, Eskelinen A, Ikavalko M, Paavolainen P, Remes V. Total ankle replacement: a population-based study of 515 cases from the Finnish Arthroplasty Register. Acta Orthop. 2010;81(1):114–8.
28. Hosman AH, Mason RB, Hobbs T, Rothwell AG. A New Zealand national joint registry review of 202 total ankle replacements followed for up to 6 years. Acta Orthop. 2007;78(5):584–91.
29. Dagneaux L, Nogue E, Mathieu J, Demoulin D, Canovas F, Molinari N. Survivorship of 4748 contemporary total ankle replacements from the French discharge records database. J Bone Joint Surg Am. 2022;104(8):684–92.
30. Buechel FF Sr, Buechel FF Jr, Pappas MJ. Twenty-year evaluation of cementless mobile-bearing total ankle replacements. Clin Orthop Relat Res. 2004;424:19–26.
31. Kofoed H. Scandinavian total ankle replacement (STAR). Clin Orthop Relat Res. 2004;424:73–9.
32. Krishnapillai S, Joling B, Sierevelt IN, Kerkhoffs G, Haverkamp D, Hoornenborg D. Long-term follow-up results of Buechel-Pappas ankle arthroplasty. Foot Ankle Int. 2019;40(5):553–61.
33. Goldberg AJ, Chowdhury K, Bordea E, Hauptmannova I, Blackstone J, Brooking D, et al. Total ankle replacement versus arthrodesis for end-stage ankle osteoarthritis: a randomized controlled trial. Ann Intern Med. 2022;175(12):1648–57.
34. Bedard N, Saltzman CL, Den Hartog T, Carlson S, Callaghan J, Alvine G, et al. The agility total ankle arthroplasty: a concise follow-up at a minimum of 20 years. Foot Ankle Int. 2021;42(10): 1241–4.
35. Frigg A, Germann U, Huber M, Horisberger M. Survival of the Scandinavian total ankle replacement (STAR): results of ten to nineteen years follow-up. Int Orthop. 2017;41(10):2075–82.
36. Brunner S, Barg A, Knupp M, Zwicky L, Kapron AL, Valderrabano V, et al. The Scandinavian total ankle replacement: long-term, eleven to fifteen-year, survivorship analysis of the prosthesis in seventy-two consecutive patients. J Bone Joint Surg Am. 2013;95(8):711–8.
37. Koivu H, Kohonen I, Mattila K, Loyttyniemi E, Tiusanen H. Long-term results of scandinavian total ankle replacement. Foot Ankle Int. 2017;38(7):723–31.
38. Bonnin M, Gaudot F, Laurent JR, Ellis S, Colombier JA, Judet T. The Salto total ankle arthroplasty: survivorship and analysis of failures at 7 to 11 years. Clin Orthop Relat Res. 2011;469(1):225–36.
39. Jastifer JR, Coughlin MJ. Long-term follow-up of mobile bearing total ankle arthroplasty in the United States. Foot Ankle Int. 2015;36(2):143–50.
40. Palanca A, Mann RA, Mann JA, Haskell A. Scandinavian total ankle replacement: 15-year follow-up. Foot Ankle Int. 2018;39(2):135–42.
41. Wood PL, Deakin S. Total ankle replacement. The results in 200 ankles. J Bone Joint Surg Br. 2003;85(3):334–41.
42. Kerkhoff YR, Kosse NM, Metsaars WP, Louwerens JW. Long-term functional and radiographic outcome of a mobile bearing ankle prosthesis. Foot Ankle Int. 2016;37(12):1292–302.
43. Barg A, Zwicky L, Knupp M, Henninger HB, Hintermann B. HINTEGRA total ankle replacement: survivorship analysis in 684 patients. J Bone Joint Surg Am. 2013;95(13):1175–83.
44. Di Iorio A, Viste A, Fessy MH, Besse JL. The AES total ankle arthroplasty analysis of failures and survivorship at ten years. Int Orthop. 2017;41(12):2525–33.
45. Zafar MJ, Kallemose T, Benyahia M, Ebskov LB, Penny JO. 12-year survival analysis of 322 Hintegra total ankle arthroplasties from an independent center. Acta Orthop. 2020;91(4):444–9.
46. van Es LJM, van der Plaat LW, Sierevelt IN, Hoornenborg D, Haverkamp D. Long-term Follow-up of 254 ceramic coated implant (CCI) evolution total ankle replacements. Foot Ankle Int. 2022;43(10):1285–94.
47. Yoon YK, Park KH, Park JH, Lee W, Han SH, Lee JW. Long-term clinical outcomes and implant survivorship of 151 total ankle arthroplasties using the HINTEGRA prosthesis: a minimum 10-year follow-up. J Bone Joint Surg Am. 2022;104(16):1483–91.
48. Harston A, Lazarides AL, Adams SB Jr, DeOrio JK, Easley ME, Nunley JA 2nd. Midterm outcomes of a fixed-bearing total ankle arthroplasty with deformity analysis. Foot Ankle Int. 2017;38(12):1295–300.
49. Zaidi R, Cro S, Gurusamy K, Siva N, Macgregor A, Henricson A, et al. The outcome of total ankle replacement: a systematic review and meta-analysis. Bone Joint J. 2013;95-B(11):1500–7.
50. Gross C, Haddad S, Morris J. A 27-year metaanalysis of ankle arthroplasty. Foot Ankle Orthop. 2018;3(3)
51. Pedersen E, Pinsker E, Younger AS, Penner MJ, Wing KJ, Dryden PJ, et al. Outcome of total ankle arthroplasty in patients with rheumatoid arthritis and noninflammatory arthritis. A multicenter cohort study comparing clinical outcome and safety. J Bone Joint Surg Am. 2014;96(21):1768–75.
52. Mousavian A, Baradaran A, Schon LC, Daniel J, Pedowitz D, Kachooei AR. Total ankle replacement outcome in patients with inflammatory versus noninflammatory arthritis: a systematic review and meta-analysis. Foot Ankle Spec. 2022:19386400221136591.
53. Valderrabano V, Hintermann B, Nigg BM, Stefanyshyn D, Stergiou P. Kinematic changes after fusion and total replacement of the ankle: Part 2: Movement transfer. Foot Ankle Int. 2003;24(12):888–96.
54. Sokolowski M, Krahenbuhl N, Wang C, Zwicky L, Schweizer C, Horn Lang T, et al. Secondary subtalar joint osteoarthritis following total ankle replacement. Foot Ankle Int. 2019;40(10):1122–8.

Complications in Total Ankle Arthroplasty

13

Despite improvements in implant design and techniques, total ankle arthroplasty is still plagued by numerous complications. Some complications are minor and easily treatable, while others significantly impact the patient and the longevity of the prosthesis. Patients with new-onset or persistent pain after total ankle arthroplasty should be approached systematically to identify the cause: infection, fracture, loosening/subsidence, cysts/osteolysis, impingement, and nerve injury [1]. The alignment of the foot and ankle must also be reassessed, as malalignment or adjacent joint pathology can contribute to pain and failure of the implant. Advanced imaging techniques, including single-photon emission computed tomography and metal-subtraction magnetic resonance imaging, are helpful and accurate in identifying pathology.

The overall postoperative complication rate for total ankle arthroplasty surgery varies widely from 13.5% to 54.5% in the literature [2–16]. This chapter aims to comprehensively review potential complications associated with total ankle arthroplasty, with a summation of the previously reported data.

13.1 Intraoperative Complications

13.1.1 Malpositioning/Technical Error

Any technical error may be related to surgical inexperience, the type of implant used, or the jigs used. Intraoperative fluoroscopy may help to reduce this rate by allowing accurate placement of the cutting blocks, but a proportion will be due to surgeon inexperience. This learning curve is known to be particularly steep for total ankle arthroplasty and can affect implantation quality (Fig. 13.1) [8, 17]. The longevity and function of total ankle arthroplasty depend primarily on achieving a well-fixed, aligned, and stable prosthesis (Fig. 13.2). Achieving this depends on implant and instrument design and the surgeon's ability to correct any preoperative deformity and achieve ligament balancing. The reported rate for malpositioning of implants varies from 5.2% to 6% [8, 9]. It was found to be the second most typical complication in the series by Gadd et al. [4].

13.1.2 Intraoperative Fractures

The type of implant used and the cutting jigs used may impact the rate of intraoperative fractures. They have been reported more frequently with the mobility system than with others [8]. There may also be an association with poor visualization of the surgical field, possibly obscured by the jig itself, and the inadvertent use of the saw blade. Another factor that may lead to intraoperative fracture is the oversizing of the prosthesis (Fig. 13.3). Press-fit implantation of the tibial component creates high compressive loads on the medial malleolus, and using an oversized tibial component increases the risk of intraoperative fracture. The surgeon must be cognizant of this complication and actively prevent it. Measures such as attention to saw blade excursion, careful preoperative templating, infrequent implant manipulations, and prophylactic pinning may significantly reduce the incidence of this potentially disastrous problem.

An avulsion fracture of the medial malleolus can also occur by enforced mobilizing the replaced ankle (Fig. 13.4).

Overall, the reported rate of intraoperative fractures of the medial malleolus varies between 3.1% and 9% [4–6], whereas it is lower for the lateral malleolus with a rate between 0.05% and 2.1% [6, 7]. There is a steep learning curve with total ankle arthroplasty; intraoperative fractures have been reported higher with surgeons' earlier procedures [17, 18].

B. Hintermann, R. Ruiz, *Total Ankle Replacement*, https://doi.org/10.1007/978-3-031-56810-7_13

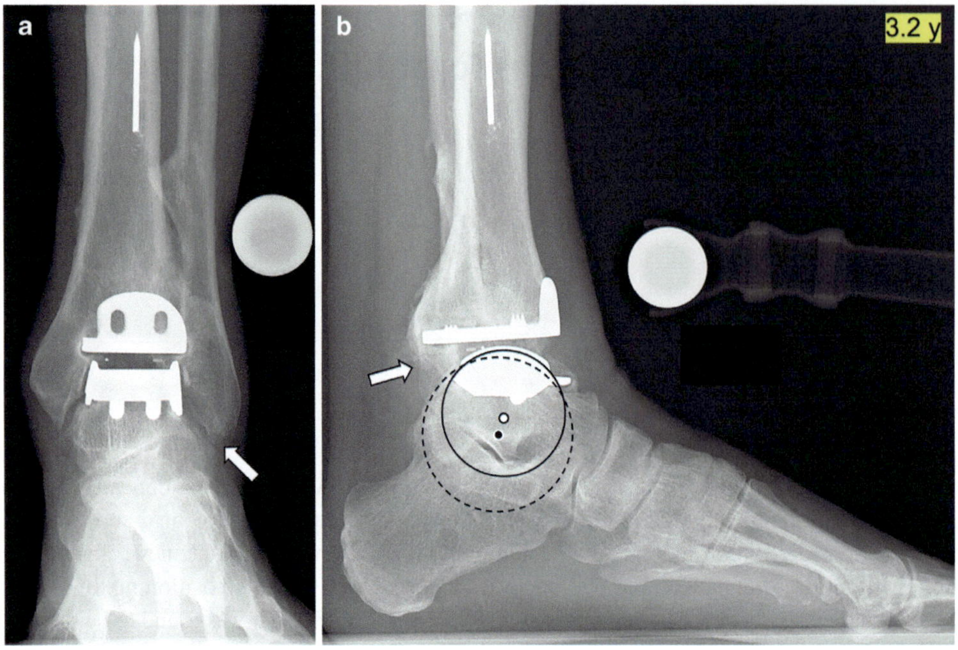

Fig. 13.1 Painful dysfunction after malpositioning of talar component. This 56-year-old teacher complains about pain and limited motion since total ankle arthroplasty 3.2 years ago. (**a**) The AP view shows an undersized talar component with bone formation in the medial and lateral gutters. The original talofibular space is increased as a sign of overstuffing the ankle (arrow). (**b**) The too-high positioning of the too-small talar component is seen on the lateral view. The dotted circle indicates the contours of the original talus. The periarticular ossifications, especially on the posterior aspect of the ankle (arrow), might result from overstuffing and the malpositioning of the too-small talar component

Intraoperative fractures are managed with surgical stabilization through the anterior approach used for total ankle arthroplasty, usually with screws. Lateral malleolar fractures, in contrast, are better fixed through a separate lateral incision with a plate and screw. This complication is entirely innocent when recognized intraoperatively and stabilized, with little untoward long-term sequelae [5].

13.1.3 Nerve Injuries

The anterior approach to the ankle places the superficial and deep peroneal nerves at risk, and being aware of the nerve's anatomy and path may help reduce the risk. Inadvertent or prolonged use of a retractor during surgery may cause neurapraxia. The posterior tibial nerve can be injured during the tibial resection, directly with the saw or indirectly by the heat produced during the cut.

Primadi et al. [19] reported a 6% incidence of the posterior tibial nerve, a 4% incidence of the deep peroneal nerve, a 4% incidence of the superficial nerve, a 0.7% incidence of the saphenous nerve, and a 0.7% incidence of sural nerve involvement with total ankle arthroplasty surgery. The nerve injury spontaneously recovered in 57% of cases, a partial recovery in 39% of cases, and no recovery in 4% of cases.

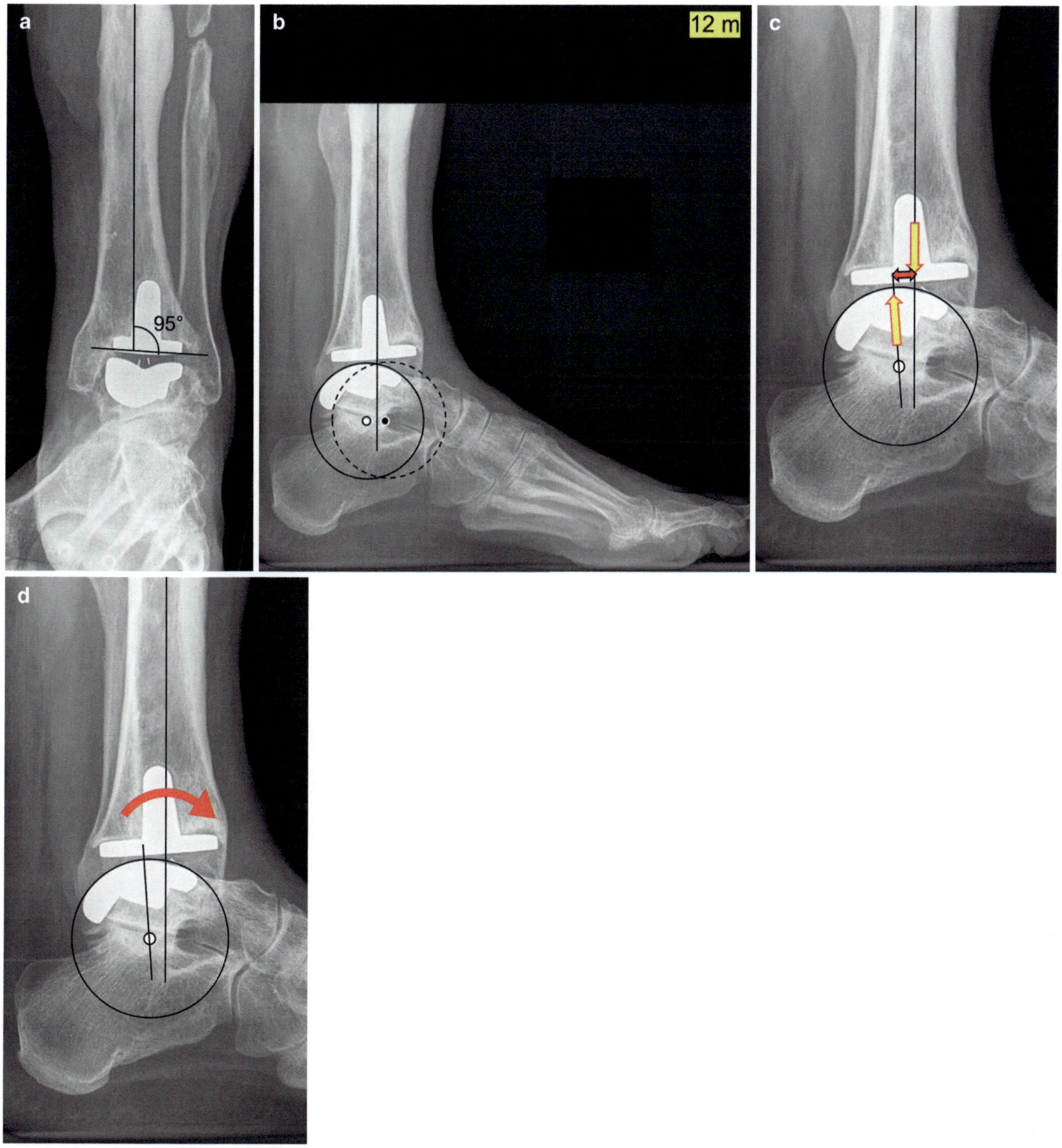

Fig. 13.2 Primary loosening of the tibial component due to malpositioning of talar component. This 40-year-old female patient, 12 months after total ankle arthroplasty for posttraumatic osteoarthritis, complains about pain when loading the ankle and limited plantarflexion. (**a**) AP view showing the tibial component in a 5°-varus position with a slightly too-medial positioning of the talar component. (**b**) Besides lucency lines along the tibial component, the lateral view shows a too-posterior positioning of the talar component; the axis of rotation of the created ankle is moved markedly posterior to the longitudinal axis of the tibia. (**c**) As a consequence, the load transfer from the talus to the tibia (yellow arrows) occurs significantly posteriorly to its center (red arrow). (**d**) The resulting tilting force to the tibial component might be the main cause of primary loosening

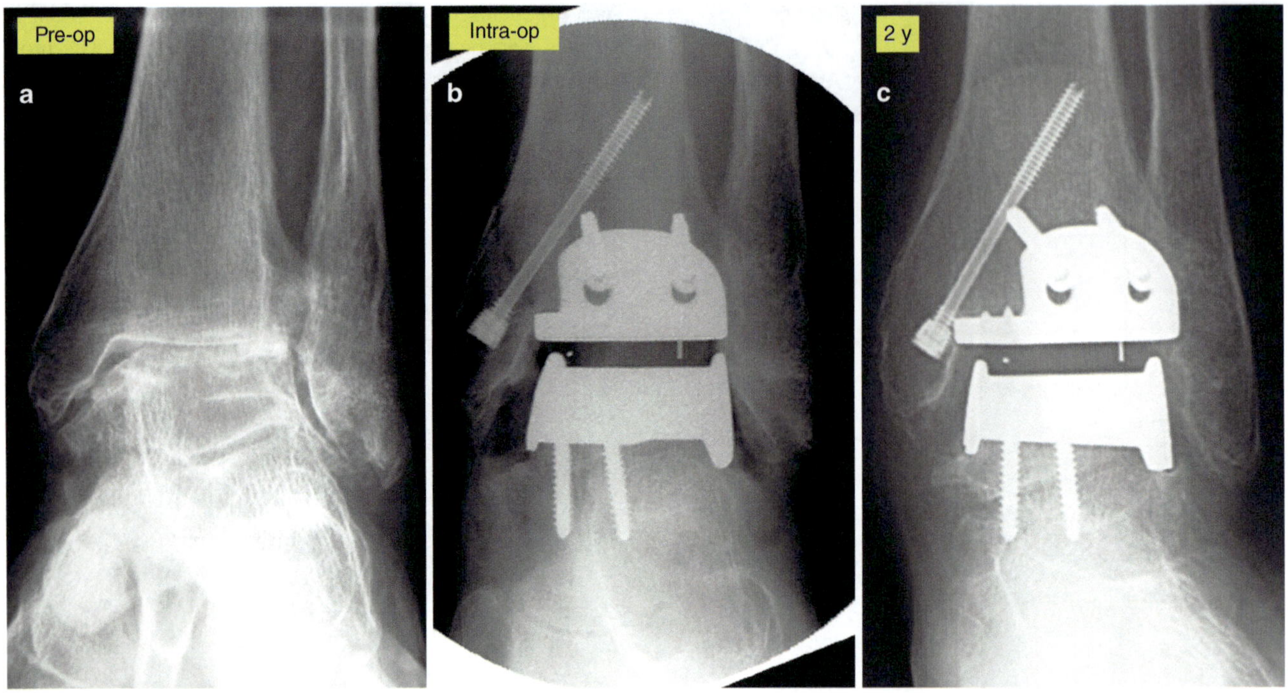

Fig. 13.3 Intraoperative fracture of medial malleolus due to oversized implant. (**a**) AP view preoperatively of this valgus osteoarthritic ankle. Notice the decreased bone density of the medial malleolus. (**b**) A vertical-type fracture of the medial malleolus is created while impacting an oversized tibial component. (**c**) The fracture healed uneventfully using the standard postoperative protocol after percutaneous fixation

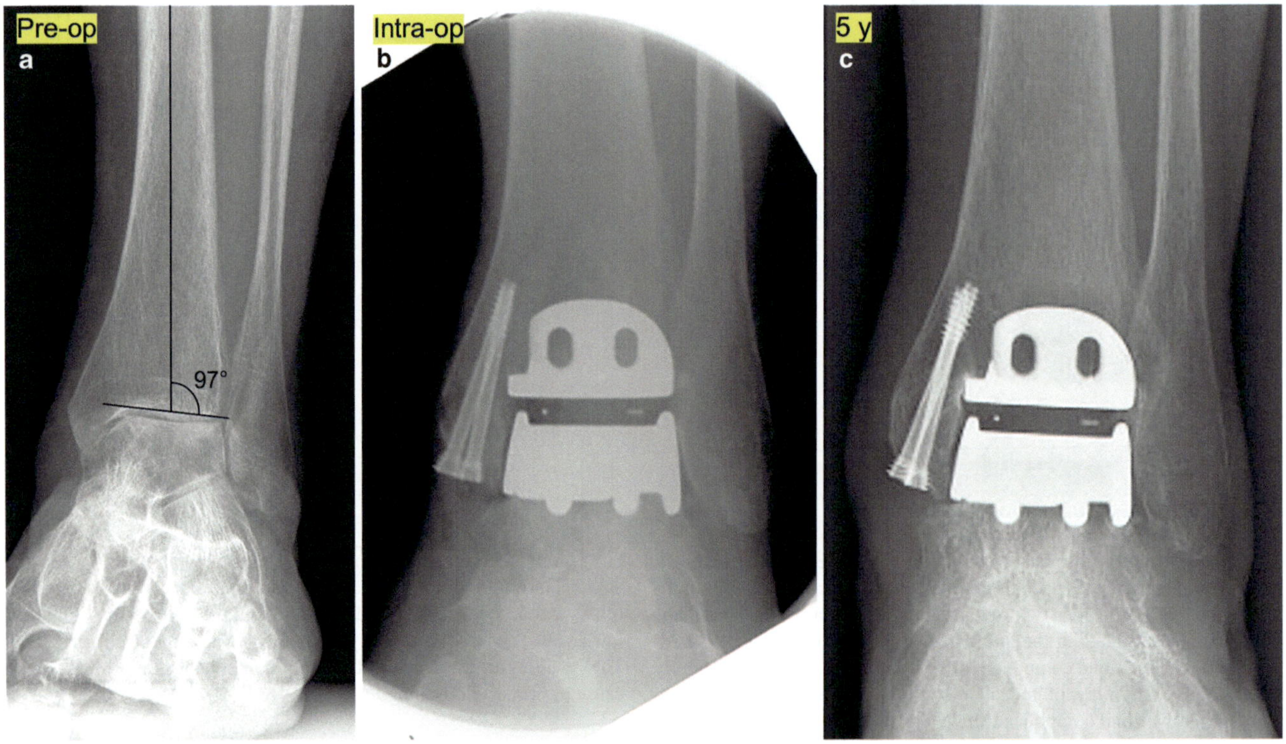

Fig. 13.4 Intraoperative avulsion of medial malleolus due to overstuffing. (**a**) AP view preoperatively of a varus osteoarthritic ankle (LDTA = 97°) with fixed equinus position at 3° in a 74-year-old female patient. (**b**) While, after the replacement, the ankle was manually mobilized into maximal dorsiflexion, an avulsion fracture of the medial malleolus occurred, resulting in a significantly increased dorsiflexion. Accepting the new position as the result of "balancing" the ankle, the fracture was fixed percutaneously with two screws in the displaced position. The fracture healed uneventfully using the standard postoperative protocol. (**c**) At 5-year follow-up control, the patient was pain-free with a preserved dorsiflexion of >10°. Notice the changed medial malleolus to the preoperative situation

13.2 Postoperative Complications

13.2.1 Wound Healing Problems

Wound healing problems are a significant complication of total ankle arthroplasty (Fig. 13.5) [20–23]. The soft tissue envelope surrounding the ankle joint is thin, and previous surgery in the area can cause scarring and increase the risk of delayed healing. Wound healing problems can occur due to patient factors and surgeon factors. Patient factors include inflammatory connective tissue disease, predominantly rheumatoid arthritis, that carries a 14-fold risk of requiring further surgery following a total ankle arthroplasty for wound problems [24], due to the condition's immunosuppressive effect and its medications. Patients on oral steroids, or those with diabetes, mainly if poorly controlled, also carry an increased risk [24]. Obesity (body mass index over 30 kg/m^2), on its own, is not a risk factor for wound healing problems [25]. Surgical risk factors include poor tissue handling and prolonged use of self-retainers in the wound. These factors mainly seem to relate to the level of surgeons' experience. Haskell et al. [13] reported more than a 50% reduction in wound problems, from 34% to 14%, after the surgeons' first five total ankle arthroplasties. Overall reported rates of wound healing problems vary from 0.9% to 14.7% [3–5, 17].

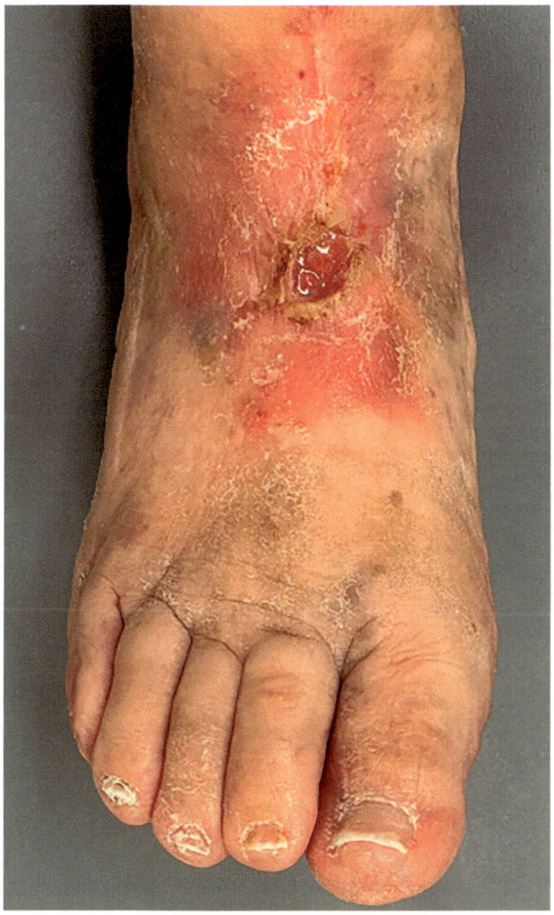

Fig. 13.5 Delayed wound healing. The wound shows a superficial defect 4 months after a revision arthroplasty through an anterior approach. Conservative treatment was continued as the tendon sheath of the anterior tibial tendon was not opened. It healed 3 months later uneventfully

13.2.2 Superficial Infection

Most superficial infections respond to appropriate oral antibiotic therapy. For rheumatoid arthritis, a prevalence of 6.5% has been reported [24]. In contrast, for diabetes, the risk of complications, including infection and the need for wound debridement, is double that of non-diabetics [26]. The major concern of superficial infection is progression to deep infection, potentially resulting in failure and revision surgery (Fig. 13.6). The incidence varies from 1.3% to 3.8% [6].

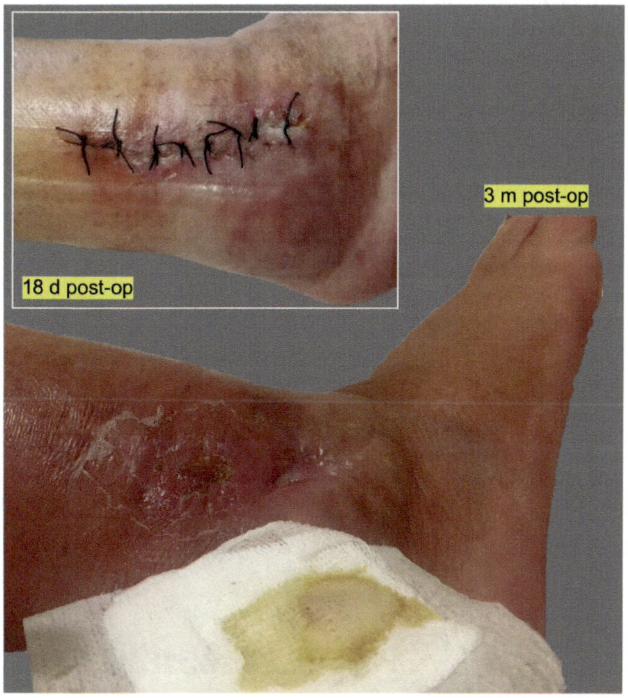

Fig. 13.6 Superficial infection progressing to deep infection. Wound healing problem after total ankle arthroplasty through a lateral approach. 18 days postoperatively, the wound was leaking. The stitches were removed 1 week later. Three months postoperatively, there was a fistula communicating with the joint

13.2.3 Periprosthetic (Deep) Infection

Periprosthetic (deep) joint infection can be a devastating and costly complication of arthroplasty (Fig. 13.7) [27, 28]. This complication carries a poor prognosis, as it generally requires significant revision surgery. Furthermore, it leads to prolonged recovery, impaired joint function, and lower quality of life [29]. Many of the deep infection risk factors identified in the literature are the same as for surgical site infection, such as male gender, abnormal body mass index (BMI), smoking, diabetes mellitus, steroid use, rheumatoid arthritis, immunosuppression, prolonged operative time, and previous joint surgery [30–33]. Despite technical advances, the deep joint infection rate following total ankle arthroplasty has persisted. In a systematic review of 6977 total ankle arthroplasties, deep joint infection rates ranged from 3.0% to 4.8% from 2005 to 2012 [34].

Hematogenous deep infection features a sudden onset of joint infection after the index arthroplasty is asymptomatic (Fig. 13.8). Still, the interval between arthroplasty and its diagnosis varies in clinical studies, from 30 days to 2 years [35]. In many studies, the interval was set for at least 3 months after arthroplasty [36, 37]. Hematogenous deep infection is associated with the frequency of bacteremia. No risk factors have been firmly established for hematogenous periprosthetic joint infection [36, 38, 39].

13.2.4 Thromboembolism

Multiple comorbidities were found to lead to a higher risk for pulmonary embolism. The use of thromboprophylaxis was found to be controversial, with patients developing pulmonary embolisms even when protected with both chemical and mechanical prophylaxis [40]. The incidence of venous thromboembolism (Fig. 13.9) after total ankle arthroplasty is reported to vary between 0% and 4.8%. In their systematic review, Feld [41] Zaidi et al. [6] reported a mean venous thromboembolism incidence of 0.3%. A recent study in the United Kingdom using NJR data reported a 0.51% incidence of pulmonary embolism within 90 days of surgery [40], although none were fatal.

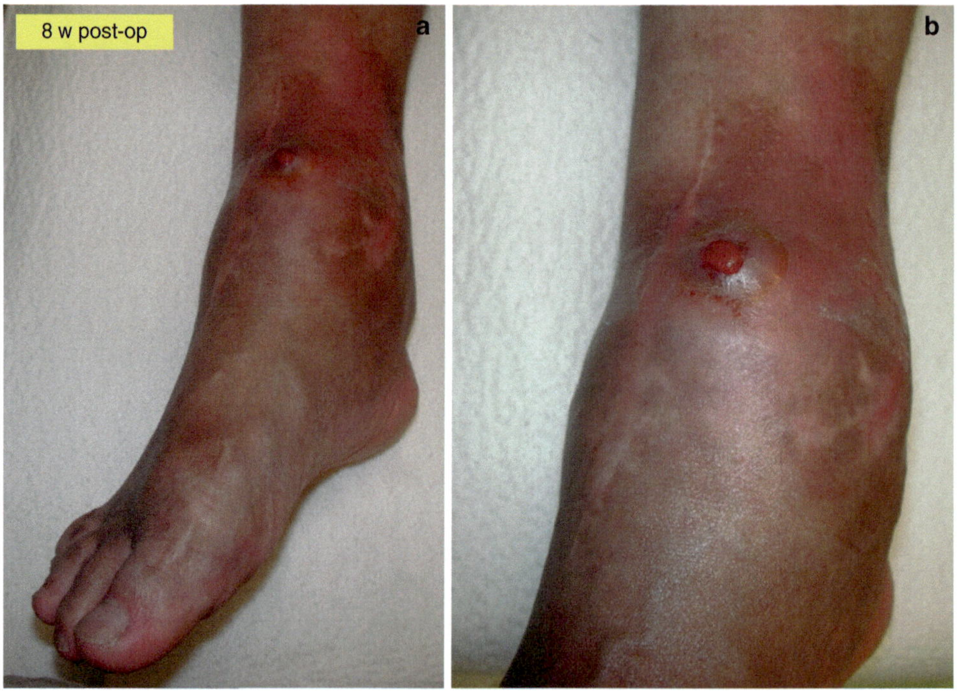

Fig. 13.7 Periprosthetic (deep) infection. 61-year-old male patient, smoker, post-traumatic osteoarthritis. Though the wound healed uneventfully after the replacement surgery, the ankle remained swollen and painful. Eight weeks postoperatively, the patient showed up after the wound started to leak. A deep infection was confirmed clinically and by probes

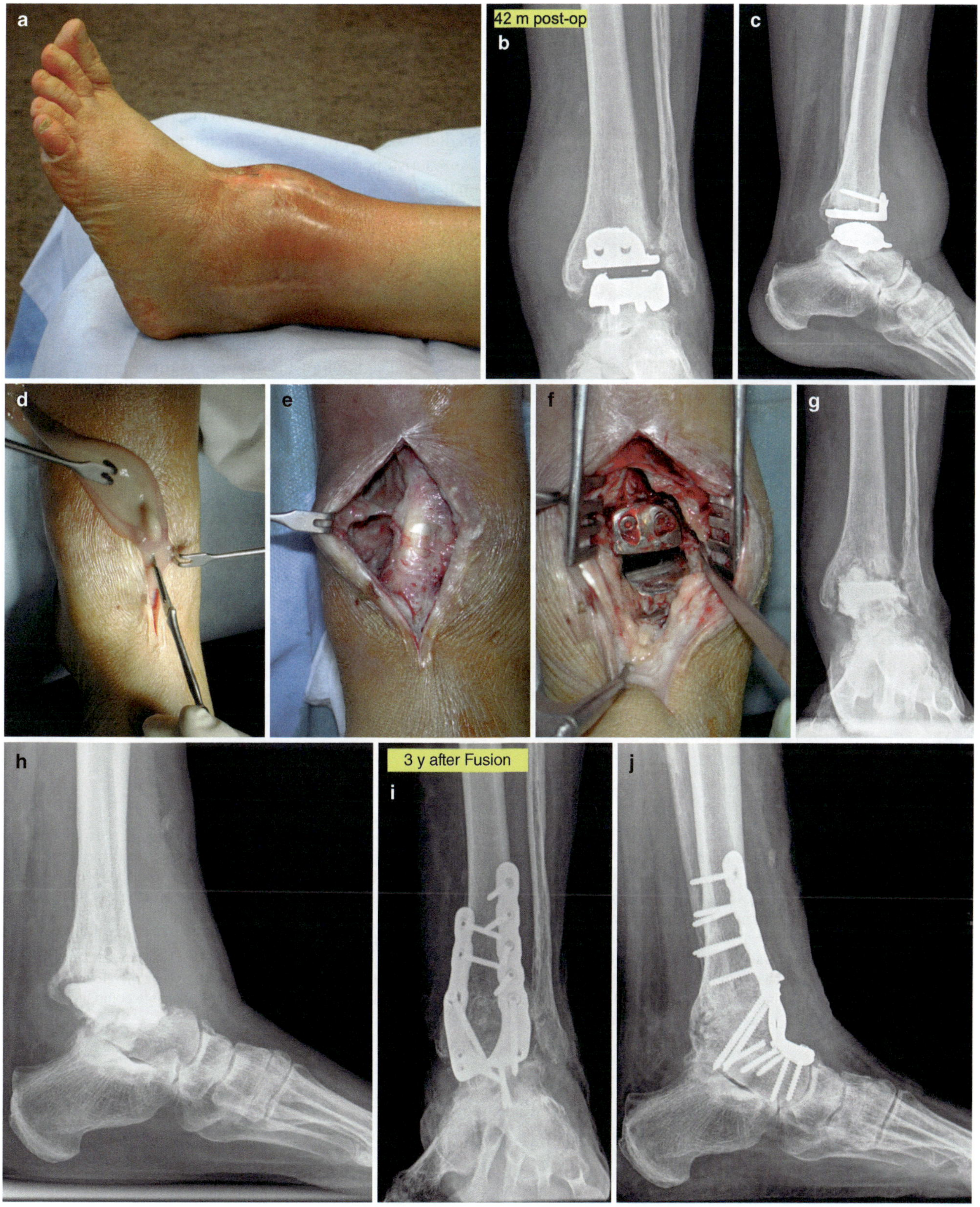

Fig. 13.8 Hematogenous deep infection. 46-year-old female teacher with no risk factors, 42 months after total ankle arthroplasty for post-traumatic osteoarthritis. The postoperative evolution was uneventful, and the patient was delighted with the result, permitting her unlimited activities in her daily life and profession. She was treated 3 weeks before for a urinal infection. (**a**) Clinical presentation of a painful, swollen, tendered ankle. Radiographs showing the immense periarticular swelling indicating fluid collection; (**b**) AP view; (**c**) lateral view. (**d**) Pus is evacuated after skin incision. (**e**) Periarticular cavity formation due to pus retention. (**f**) Exposure of the prosthesis showing the periprosthetic infection. (**g, h**) Radiographs showing the antibiotic cement spacer after explanation of the prosthesis. The ankle was fused 24 days later using a fresh-frozen femoral head allograft. (**i, j**) Radiographs 3 years later showing a solid tibiotalar fusion

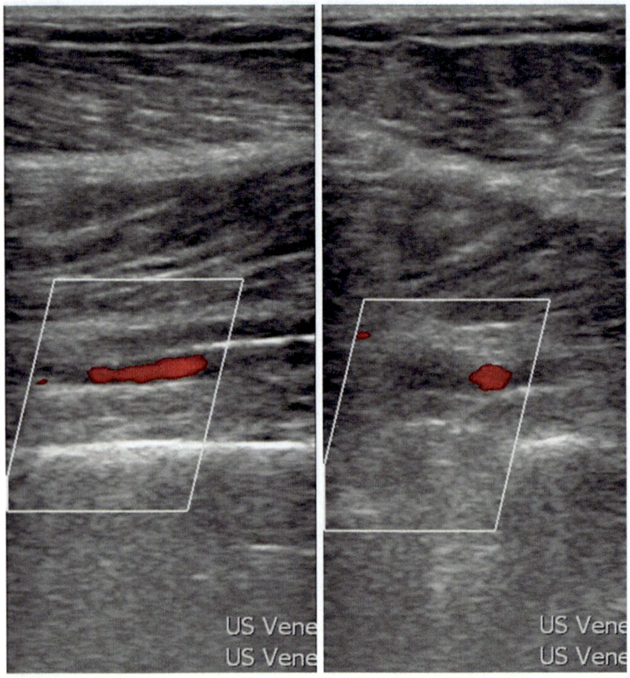

Fig. 13.9 Deep venous thrombosis. A deep venous thrombosis was confirmed by sonography 5 weeks after the surgery in this patient despite chemical prophylaxis

13.2.5 Postoperative Fractures

A postoperative fracture can occur after sufficient trauma (Fig. 13.10) or represent a stress fracture (Fig. 13.11) [41]. Stress fractures are typically located at the medial malleolus or further cranially at the medial shoulder of the distal tibial metaphysis. They can occur because of varus malpositioning during prosthesis implantation, which increases mechanical load. Signs indicative of increased mechanical loading on the medial malleolus due to a varus-implanted tibial component are reactive periosteal appositional bone growth and medial malleolar pain. However, valgus malpositioning during implantation can also result in medial malleolar stress fractures due to increased traction of the deltoid ligament complex on the medial malleolus [42]. Medial malleolar stress fractures can also result from talar medialization, either after fusion of the distal tibiofibular joint or secondary to using an oversized talar component with varus malpositioning [12].

Surgical fixation of the fracture is often required to prevent progressive hindfoot drift, together with consideration of further surgery to restore the mechanical axis. The incidence of late malleolar fractures due to stress has been reported to be between 2% and 5% [2, 7, 43].

13.2.6 Complex Regional Pain Syndrome (CRPS)

Complex Regional Pain Syndrome (CRPS) can occur postoperatively and is viewed as a complication of the surgery. Very little has been published on the incidence of CRPS following foot and ankle surgery, and nothing explicitly follows total ankle arthroplasty.

Fig. 13.10 Periprosthetic fracture after total ankle arthroplasty and supramalleolar osteotomy. A 47-year-old patient with rheumatoid arthritis sustained in the past a stress fracture of the tibia and fibula that resulted in a severe valgus deformity. (**a–c**) Preoperative radiographs showing the intraarticular valgus deformity in combination with a peritalar subluxation and severe valgus malalignment of the heel. (**d–f**) Weight-bearing CT scan showing the segmental destabilization into valgus with subsequent subfibular impingement (**g–I**). The intraoperative fluoroscans show a well-balanced replaced ankle after supramalleolar correcting osteotomy, subtalar fusion, and medial sliding osteotomy. (**j–l**) Radiographs taken 2.5 months postoperatively evidence a periprosthetic fracture of the distal tibia at the level of the previous osteotomy, with tilting into a varus malalignment. The implants look firmly osteointegrated. The patient did not complain of pain. The medial plate was removed and replaced by a longer one, correcting the malalignment. (**m–o**) The radiographs 1 year postoperatively show that the fracture healed in a correct position with stable components

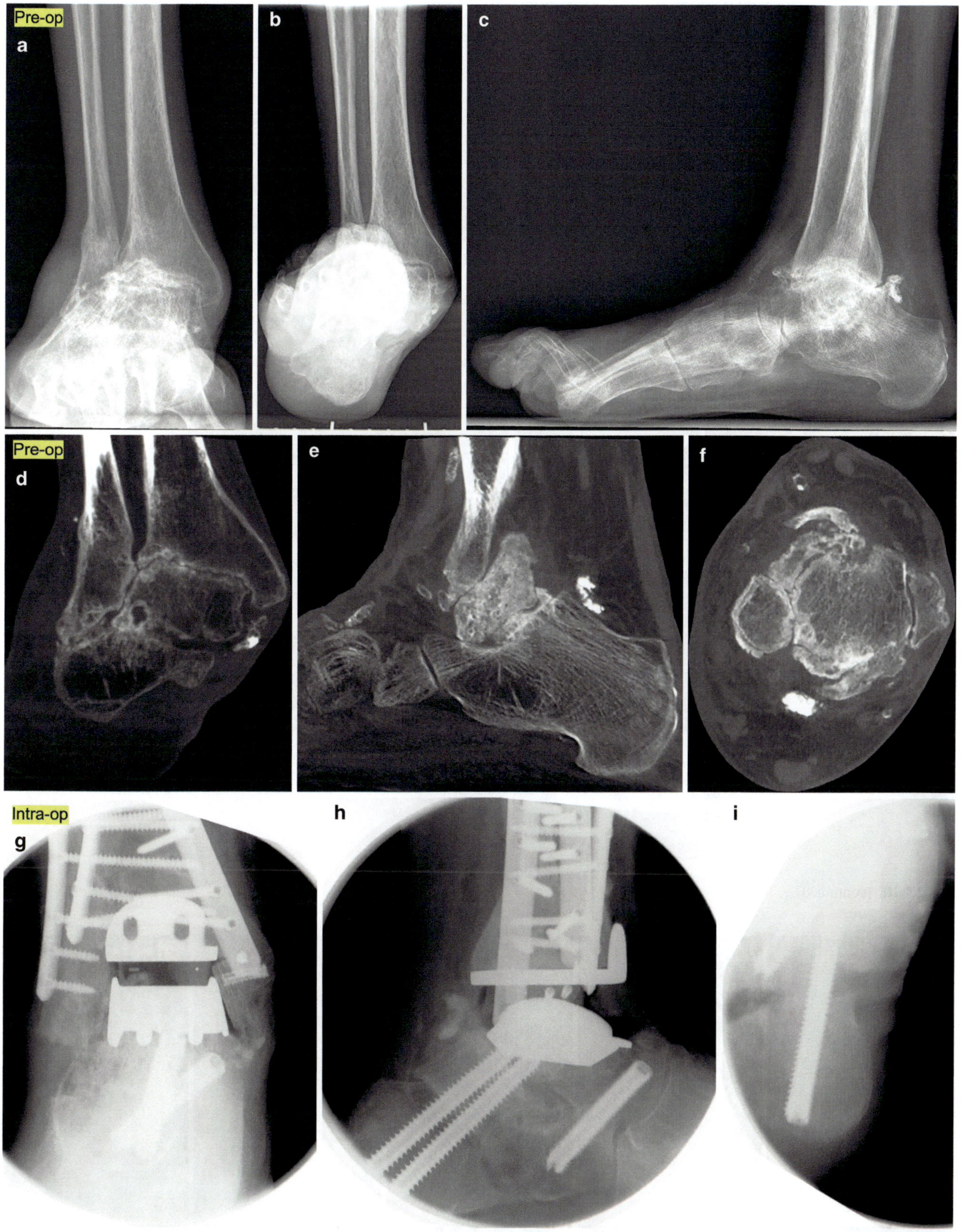
Pre-op
a
b
c
Pre-op
d
e
f
Intra-op
g
h
i

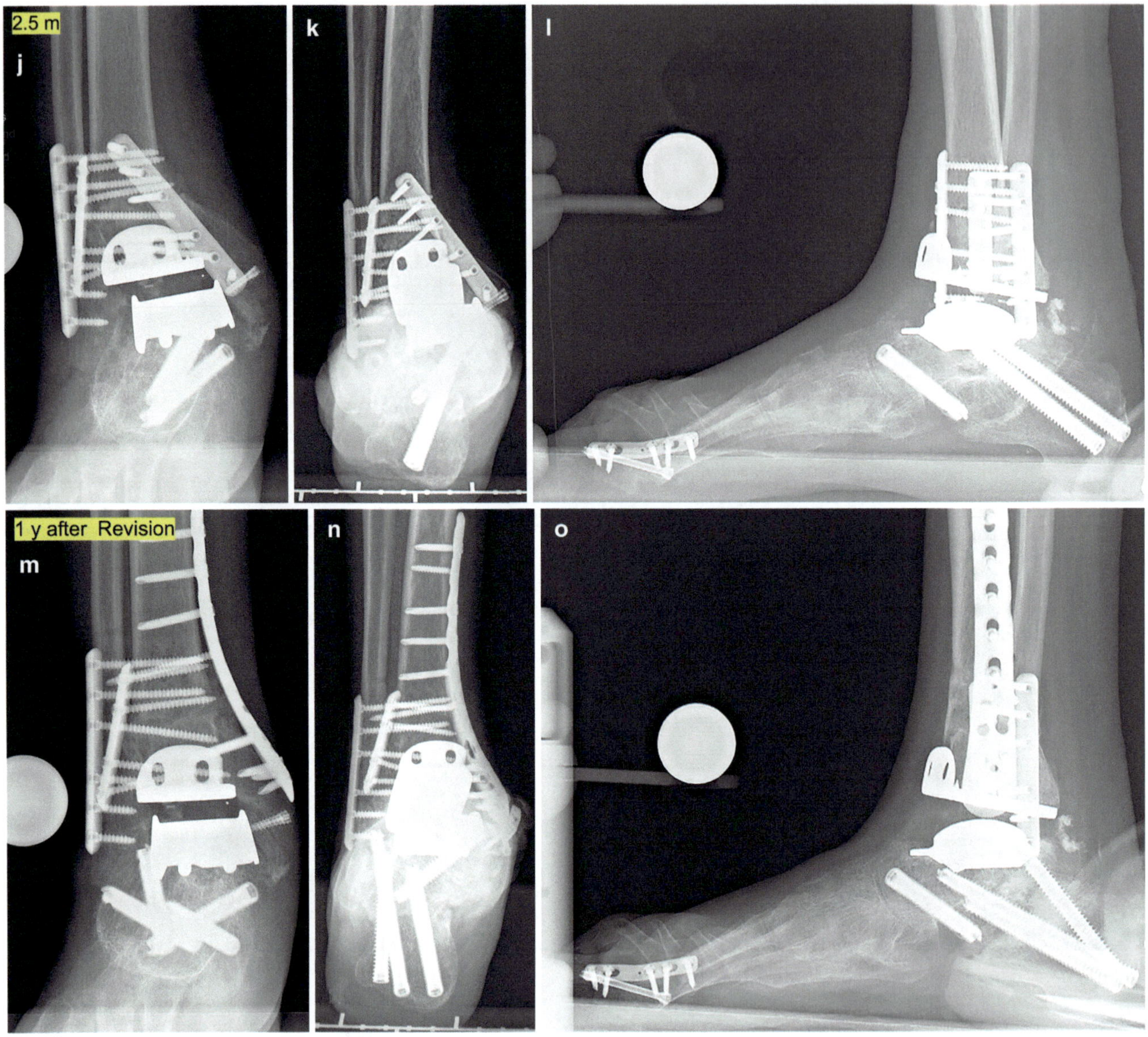

Fig. 13.10 (continued)

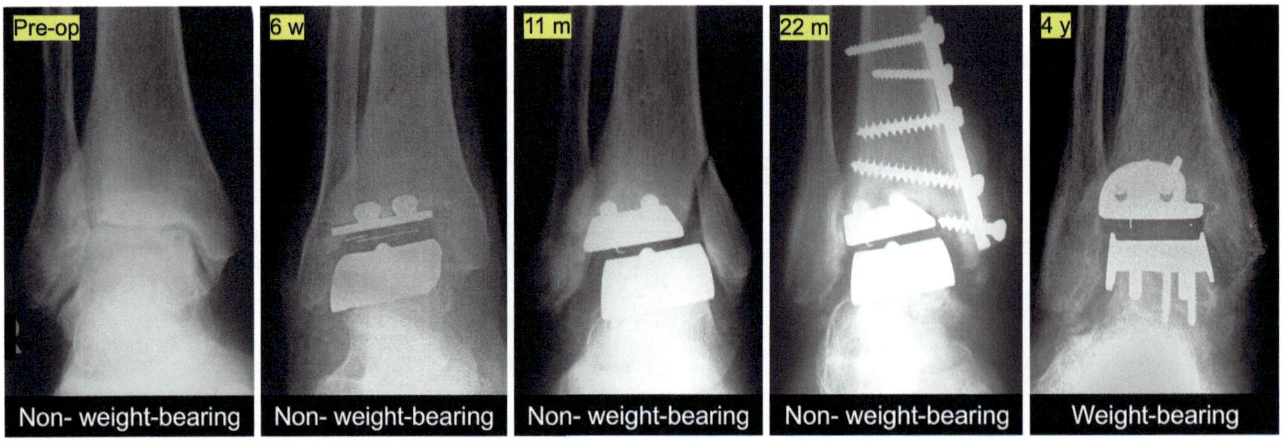

Fig. 13.11 Stress fracture after malpositioned implant. A 56-year-old patient presented with a medial malleolus stress fracture 11 months after total ankle arthroplasty with malpositioning of the tibial component in a varus position. The radiograph 11 months after internal fixation shows a persistent stress reaction explaining the pain. After revision arthroplasty, the ankle was balanced, and the stress reaction disappeared. Two years after that, meaning 4 years after index surgery, the patient was pain-free

13.3 Late Complications

13.3.1 Instability

In a varus ankle, inadequate soft tissue release about the ankle is usually associated with either instability or recurrence of deformity postoperatively. An overzealous release, in contrast, may produce instability on the contracted side of the joint or an increased joint space, which may lead to ankle instability of an implant or dislocation of the polyethylene due to exceeding the tibiotalar gap (Fig. 13.12).

In a valgus ankle, insufficient correction of malalignment or progressive destabilization of the medial hindfoot and arch may cause incompetence of the deltoid ligament due to the overload (Fig. 13.13).

13.3.2 Aseptic Loosening

Loosening and osteolysis of the tibial or talar component are responsible for most failures in total ankle arthroplasty [2–4].

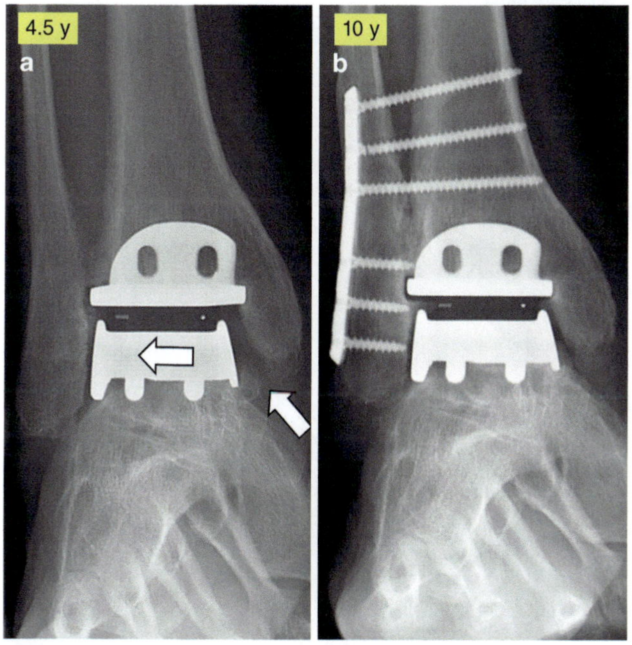

Fig. 13.12 Coronal plane instability after deltoid release. A 56-year-old female patient with progressive pain over the syndesmosis 4.5 years after total ankle arthroplasty. Her surgeon noted in the surgery protocol that he had problems with the medial soft tissue contracture in this moderate varus ankle, so he was forced to do an extended release of the deltoid ligament. (**a**) AP view showing the lateral translation of the talus with gapping of the medial gutter. (**b**) 5.5 years after syndesmotic fusion through a lateral approach, the ankle mortise was stable, and the patient was pain-free

Early loosening of the uncemented implant is mostly caused by excessive implant–bone micromotion (>50 ηm), which may hamper proper initial fixation between implant and bone (Fig. 13.14). Late loosening of the uncemented component is caused due to excessive bone density loss due to strain shielding and wear-induced osteolysis (Fig. 13.15) [44]. On one hand, the improper orientation of the implant may alter strain distribution in the bone, implant–bone micromotion, contact pressure at the bearing surface, and generation of wear. On the other hand, the proper combination of implant material (bearing material) also plays a crucial role in reducing strain shielding, contact pressure, and wear. Despite the recent trend for metal on UHMW polyethylene of total ankle arthroplasty, the long-term clinical effects of metal ion release and high polyethylene wear rate are still unclear and require an investigation for other low-wear bearing couples [45].

Osteolysis can be induced by the insertion of an implant into the bone [46]. This may result in localized, adjacent tissue necrosis caused by the approach, preparation of surfaces, and local effect of the implant on tissue. As a response, a natural envelope to enclose the implant is formatted by reparative granulomatous tissue. The thicker this reparative tissue coat is, the more likely bone formation around the implant may be suppressed, resulting in implant failure [47]. This is evident because this tissue envelope, also called pseudomembrane, includes large amounts of foreign body macrophage and giant-cell responses to wearing material with variable lymphocyte reactions [48]. In an inflammatory cascade, macrophages become activated, which activate osteoclasts and thus initiate bone resorption [49]. Polyethylene particles become phagocytosed by macrophages. As a result, cytokines are released, which modulate osteoblast and osteoclast activity, stimulating further osteolysis [48].

Component positioning may also impact component loosening (Fig. 13.5). Espinosa et al. [50] found that predicted average contact stresses reached the yield stress of polyethylene when the implant was oriented version misalignments more than 5°. Mondal and Gosh [51], also based on 3D-finite element models, reported that optimally positioned implants could reduce strain shielding effect in the tibia bone, implant–bone micromotion, contact pressure, and wear depth. Previously, it has been indicated that ligaments and muscle forces influence load transfer across the ankle joint [51–53].

Besides poor component alignment and an incongruent polyethylene articulation, often due to recurrent hindfoot or ankle malalignment, the designs of total ankle arthroplasty may play a role (Fig. 13.16) [54]. Currier et al. [55], analyzing 70 retrieved components, reported that loosening could be more of a problem in fixed-bearing devices than mobile-bearing devices. Bony ingrowth did not occur substantially,

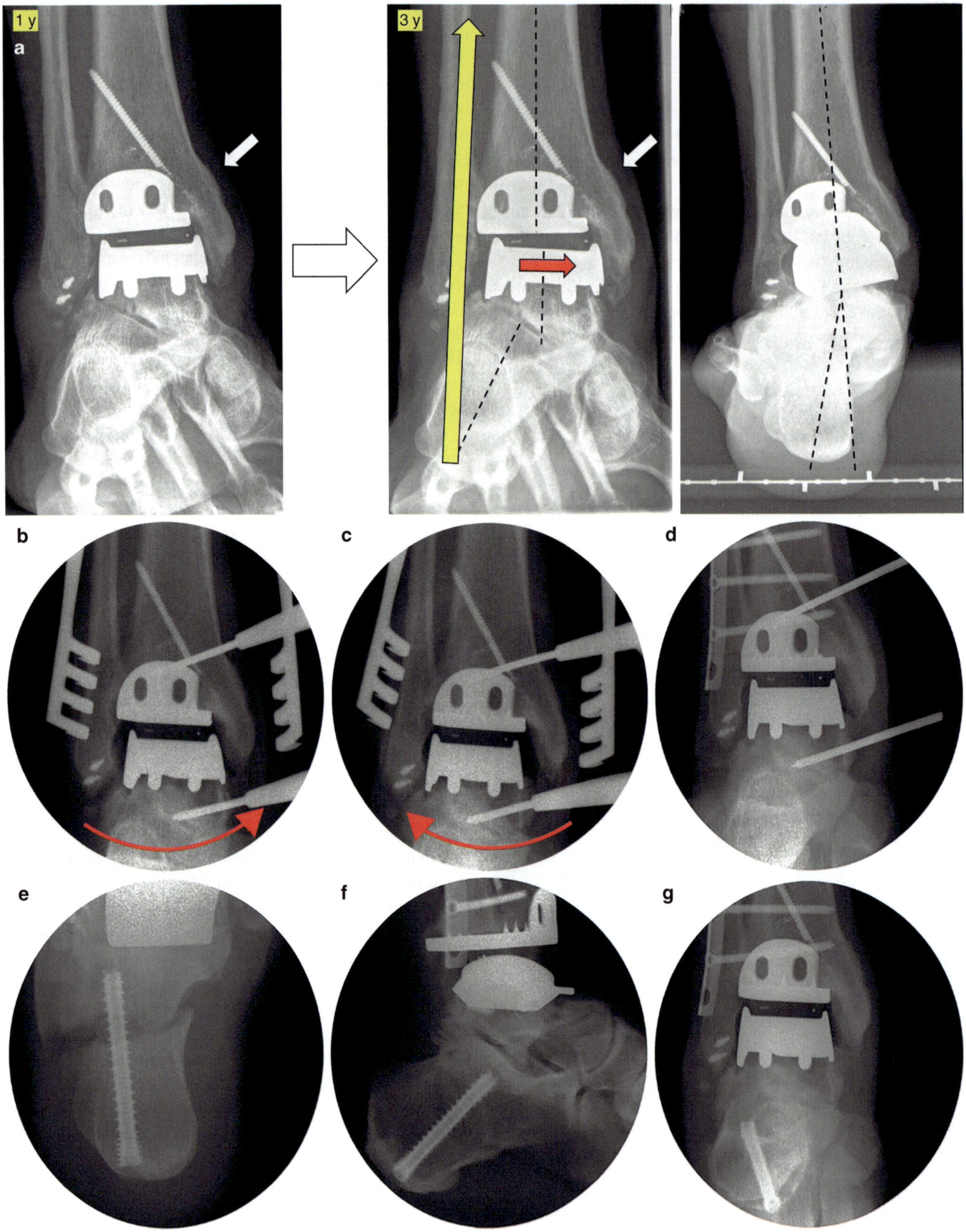
1 y
a
3 y
b
c
d
e
f
g

Fig. 13.13 Progressive deltoid incompetence in a valgus ankle. (**a**) One year after total ankle arthroplasty, this 62-year-old former soccer player complained of medial pain. A stress reaction can be seen at the shoulder of the medial malleolus (arrow). The patient refused the proposed medial sliding osteotomy. Two years later, he presents with increasing pain involving the lateral side. The X-rays evidence an increase in valgus destabilization with some joint gapping. Notice the increased bone density of the medial malleolus due to the stress concentration. The alignment view shows the significant valgus malalignment of the heel. Fluoroscans showing the coronal plane play of the talus while applying medial (**b**) and lateral (**c**) stress. Notice the parallelism of the component, indicating that the polyethylene insert was intact (**d**). Therefore, a periarticular correction without revision of the prosthesis was decided with a fusion of the distal tibiofibular joint to narrow the ankle mortise and a medial sliding osteotomy to realign the hindfoot (**e**, **f**). (**g**) Final situation showing a balanced and aligned ankle. (**h**–**j**) Seven years later, the patient was pain-free at the 10-year follow-up control, and the ankle was still well-balanced and stable. As the stress disappeared, the bone density of the medial malleolus normalized

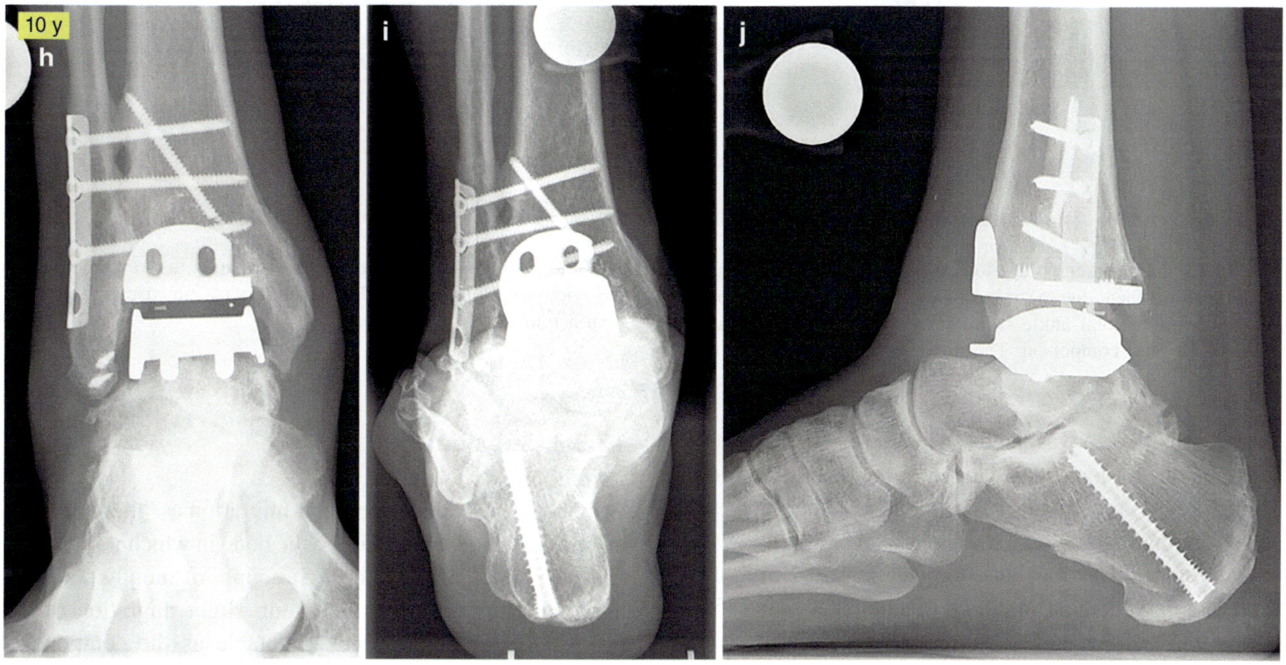

Fig. 13.13 (continued)

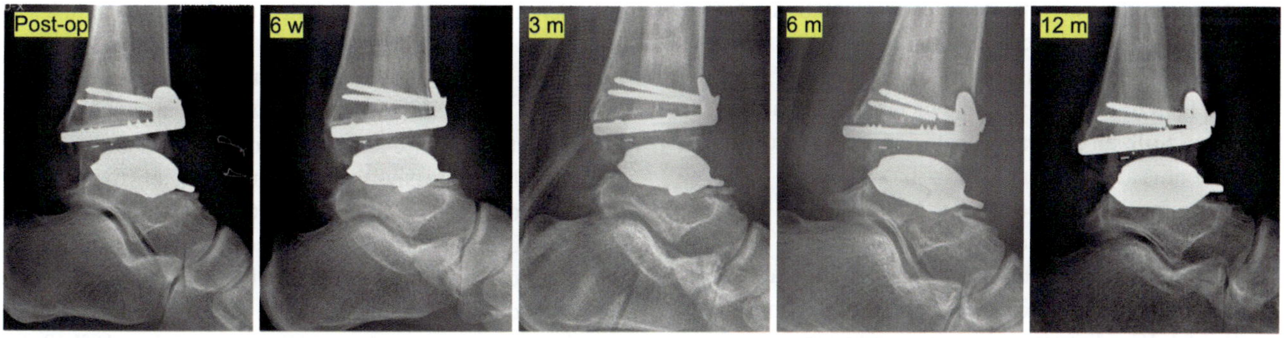

Fig. 13.14 Early loosening due to micromotion. Primary loosening of the tibial component in a 54-year-old female patient. The implant of this generation (second generation of the Hintegra ankle) used a porous coat by CoCr and flat pyramidal peaks; thus, screw fixation was used to enhance the primary stability

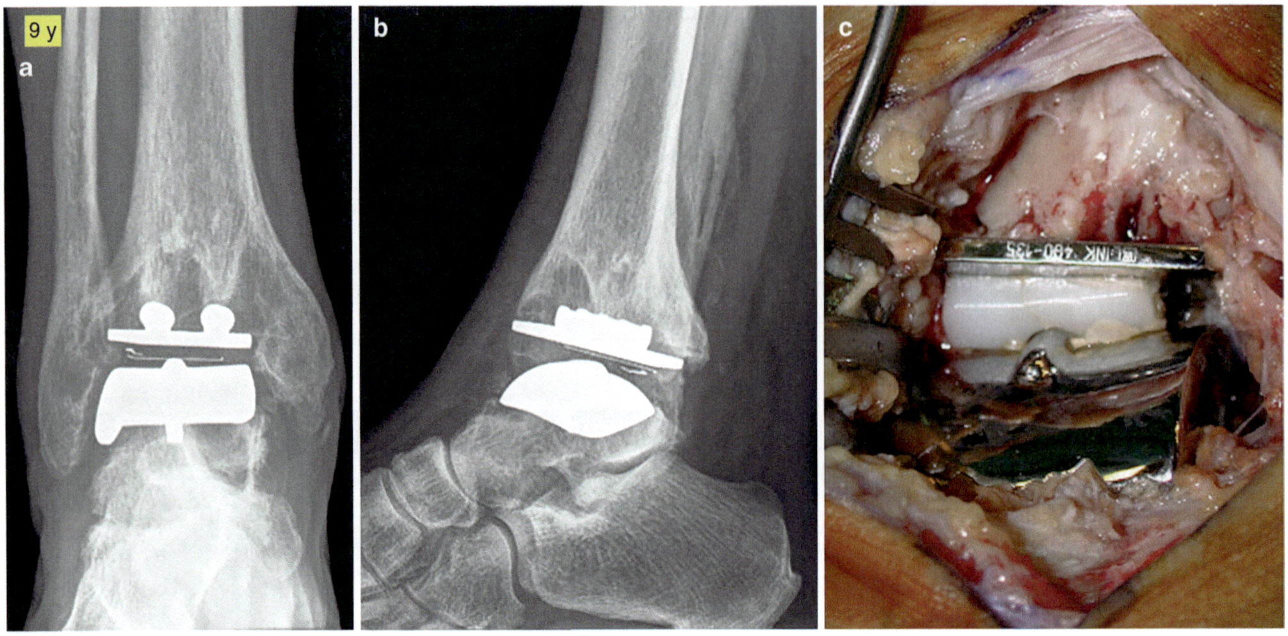

Fig. 13.15 Late loosening due to strain shielding. Late loosening of the tibial component due to strain-shielding and wear-induced osteolysis 9 years after total ankle arthroplasty. Notice the osteolysis also beneath the talar component. The implant of this generation (STAR ankle) used only a single coat of hydroxyapatite. (**a**) AP view; (**b**) lateral view. (**c**) Intraoperatively, significant asymmetric polyethylene wear is found

whether the device was fixed- or mobile-bearing, in most of the revisions for loosening. However, the time to revision for loosening was much longer for mobile-bearing devices than fixed-bearing ones.

Micromotion at the bone-implant interface might promote the development of periprosthetic osteolysis [56, 57]. The initial stability and alignment achieved during surgery are vital to reduce micromotion and avoid premature loosening (Fig. 13.17) [46, 58]. The process is analogous to fracture healing: Stability ensures proper fracture healing and mechanical strength. However, assessing micromotion at the interfaces in the early phase after implantation of a total ankle arthroplasty is challenging. Nowadays, computed tomography (CT) or single-photon emission CT (SPECT)–CT can help to evaluate possible metabolic alterations at the interface. Still, an accurate conclusion could be drawn only 6–12 months after surgery [59].

Loosening will be seen as a periprosthetic lucency or demarcation on radiographs (Figs. 13.16 and 13.17) [60]. Zaidi et al. [6] in their meta-analysis, reported a 21% incidence of radiographic lucencies adjacent to the tibial component and 1.4% adjacent to the talar component at a mean of 4.4 years, further reporting that 9.4% of these required revisions. Gadd et al. [4] and Glazebrook et al. [5], in contrast, found this complication to have a much poorer long-term prognosis, with an 85% and 70.3% risk of requiring revision surgery, respectively.

13.3.3 Subsidence

Fong et al. [43] defined implant migration as "the longitudinal movement of an implant to the bone in which it is embedded over time." During the first couple of months after the total ankle arthroplasty placement, slight migration of the components is regular and acceptable as the components reach their final positions and achieve a solid combination with the bone; this movement is slight and can be considered physiologic prosthetic component migration (Fig. 13.18) [43, 61]. In contrast, subsequent continuous migration is considered to be pathologic, with much larger magnitudes of migration.

Several factors may contribute to subsidence, including poor bone ingrowth (Fig. 13.19), insufficient bone support (osteoporotic bone), cyst formation beneath the prosthesis (Fig. 13.20), progressive avascular necrosis, and overstuffing or overloading the joint [4, 5, 17, 62, 63]. Stress shielding may also lead to bone resorption and component subsidence [64]. This can be related to the quality of the bone or technical errors during implantation. The reported rate of subsidence in the literature varies widely from 0.9% to 46% [3–5]. This complication carries a poor long-term prognosis for the prosthesis, with estimates of revision rates from 32% to 100% [4, 5].

Management of talar component subsidence is challenging because there is always bone loss and sometimes massive loss, which can be caused by direct mechanical erosion, peri-

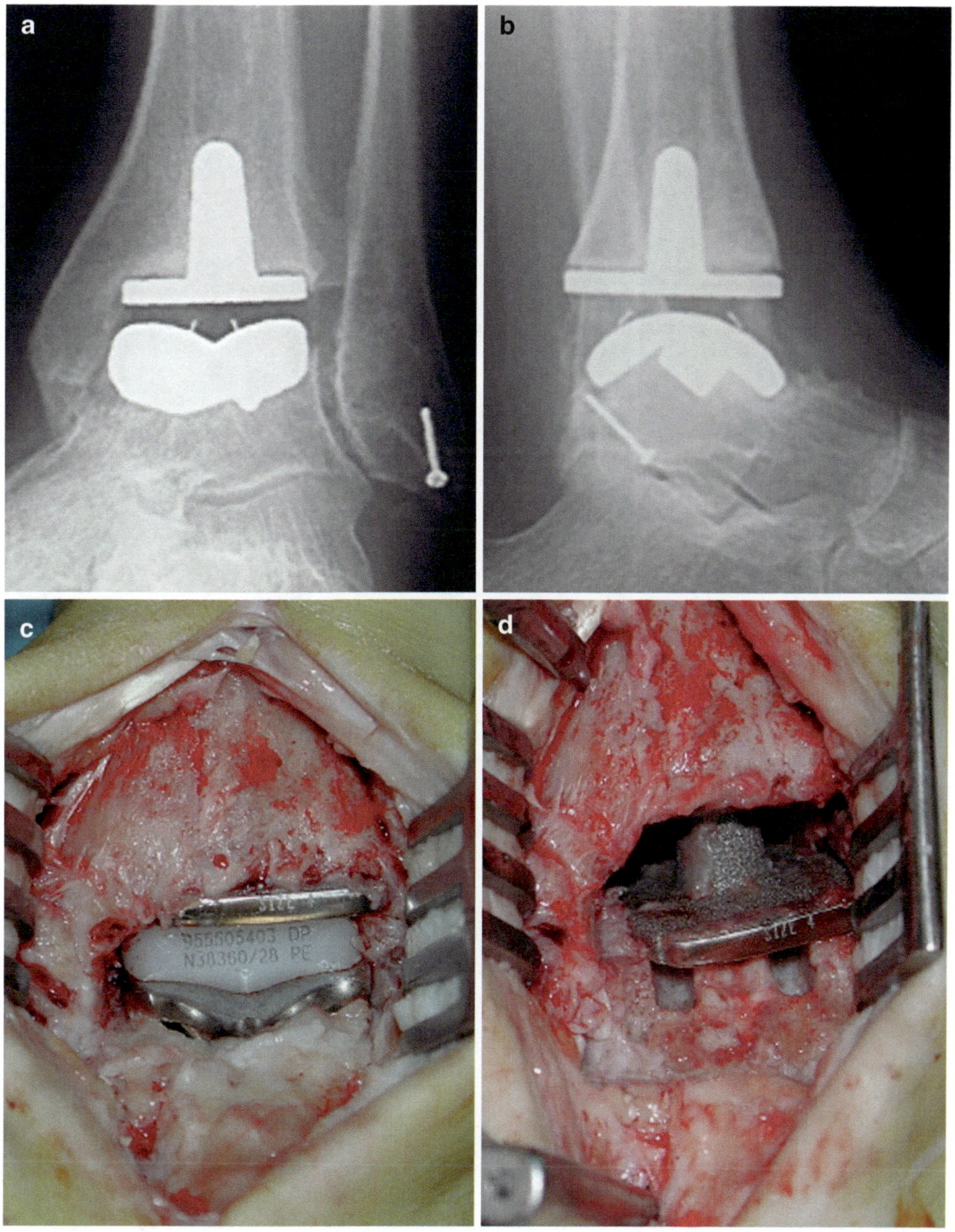

Fig. 13.16 Design-related micromotion resulting in loosening. Single central stem fixation is critical in providing primary stability against rotational forces. (**a**, **b**) Despite adequate positioning with regular transmission forces in this 62-year-old female patient, the tibial component, as the lucency lines along the plateau, was unstable. (**c**) Surgical exploration confirmed the instability. (**d**) The implant was covered by connective tissue without a sign of osteointegration

prosthetic osteolysis, or necrotic changes of the underlying trabecular bone. The subsidence can be severe, with complete erosion of the talar body and migration of the talar component into the subtalar joint, which may be difficult, if not impossible, to correct [65].

13.3.4 Cyst Formation

Periprosthetic bone cysts are common following total ankle arthroplasty. Cysts can range from small asymptomatic to large cysts, so-called "ballooning osteolysis," causing total ankle arthroplasty catastrophic failure. Along with implant loosening and subsidence, periprosthetic bone cysts can result in persistent pain and periprosthetic fracture (Fig. 13.20).

The cause of periprosthetic bone cysts after total ankle arthroplasty is not entirely understood. The most described process of periprosthetic bone cyst formation is osteolysis secondary to polyethylene wear (Fig. 13.15), as seen with total hip and knee arthroplasties [60, 66]. Phagocytosis of debris from polyethylene wear by macrophages can stimulate cytokine release, activating osteoclasts and causing bone resorption and cyst formation [46, 67]. The polyethylene wear rate can be affected by the type of polyethylene implanted. Conventional polyethylene may produce increased wear particles when compared with highly cross-linked polyethylene [68, 69]. In addition, implant design

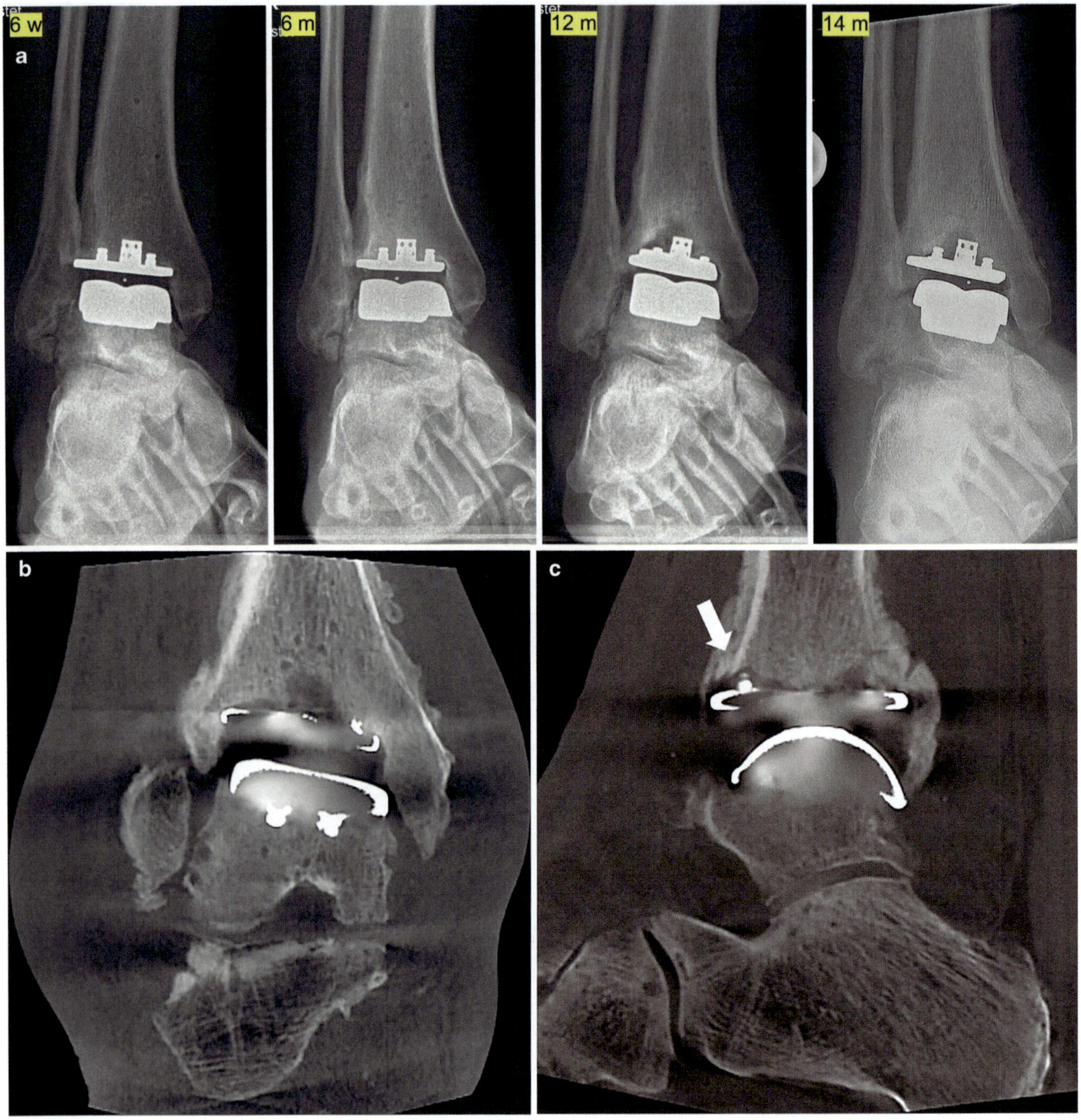

Fig. 13.17 Micromotion promoting periprosthetic osteolysis. The tibial implant of this ankle uses a central crone and three peripheric pegs for fixation. (**a**) Given that the primary stability was not provided in the ankle of this 75-year-old patient, the development of periprosthetic osteolysis was promoted, resulting in asymmetric subsidence of the component with progressive tilting into valgus. (**b**, **c**) A CT scan confirmed the osteolytic process around the central crone. The anteromedial peg was seen in conflict with the cortex (arrow), which may have counteracted the symmetric initial subsidence of the component

may contribute to polyethylene wear. Adding a second interface in a mobile-bearing prosthesis could increase polyethylene wear, given the admitted translational and rotational movement that may result in edge loading (Fig. 13.21). Increased periprosthetic bone cysts with mobile-bearing implants were reported [70–73].

In a cohort of 31 patients with a syndesmotic overload in a three-component total ankle arthroplasty, Ruiz et al. [74] found polyethylene wear in 10 ankles (32%). It always occurred on the tibial-polyethylene interface. Cyst formation prevalence was not associated with polyethylene wear. However, while extending this study with the inclusion of 46

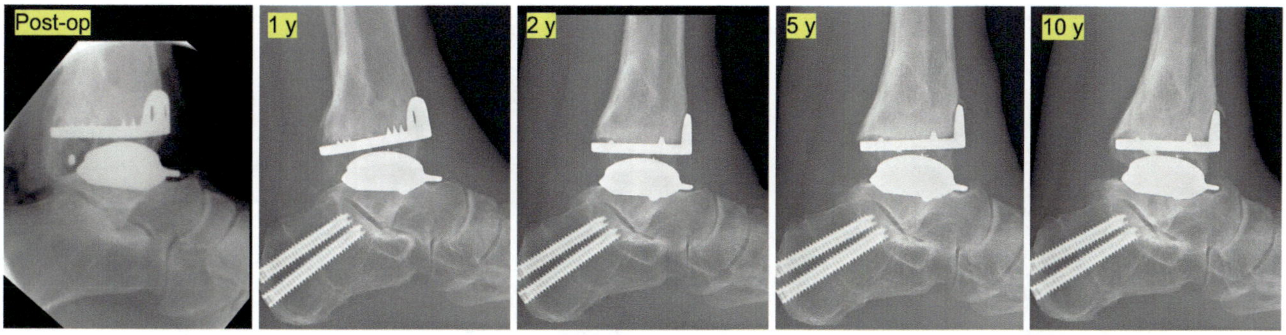

Fig. 13.18 Physiological primary migration with delayed osteointegration. The osteointegration process of the tibial component took exceptionally long in the ankle of this 69-year-old postman. As he didn't experience pain at no stage after the total ankle arthroplasty, no revision was considered. The patient was delighted with the result at the 10-year follow-up control

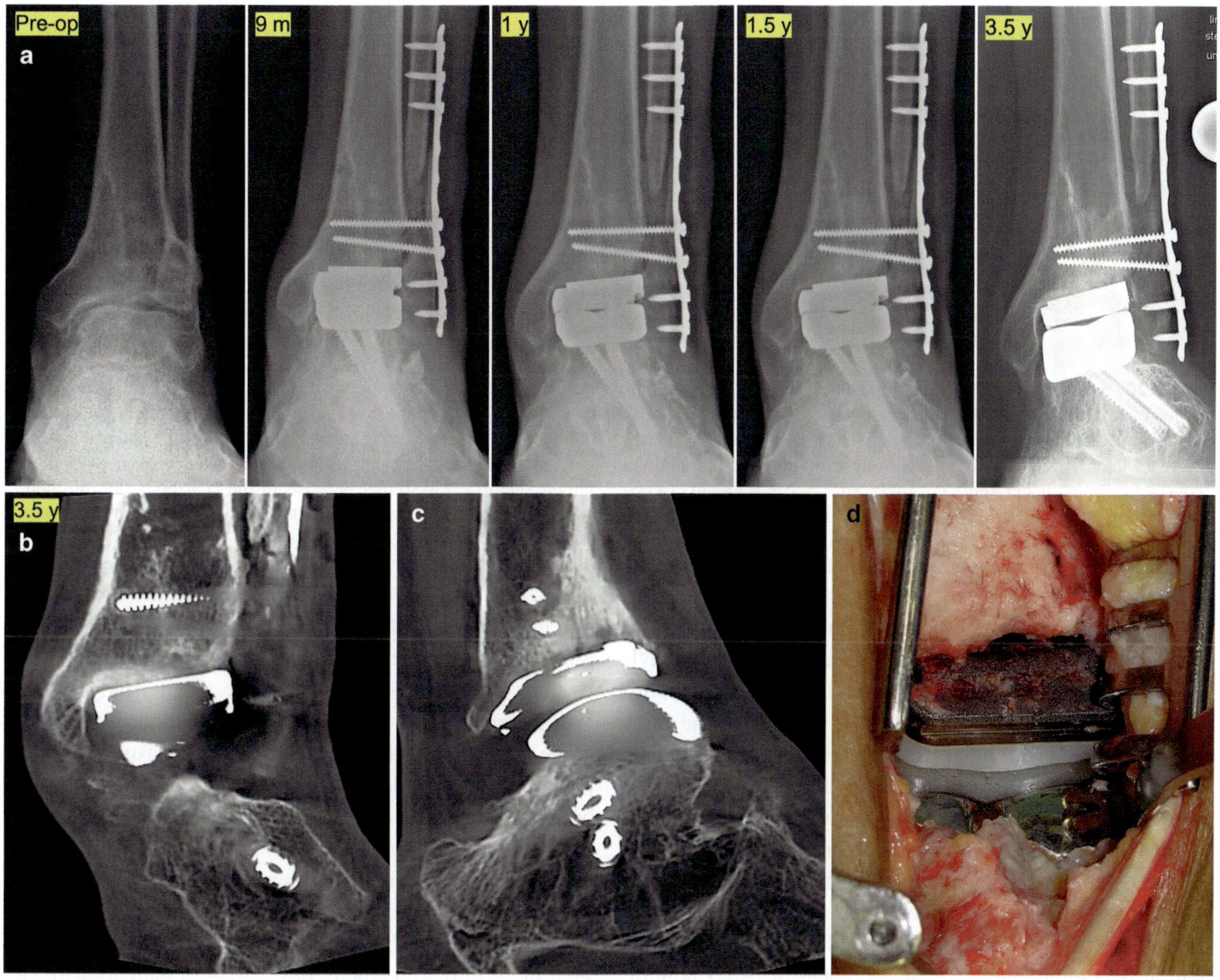

Fig. 13.19 Subsidence associated with poor bone ingrowth and malalignment. The ankle series of a 47-year-old very active merchant showed initial posttraumatic osteoarthritis with malunited lateral tibial pilon. (**a**) The ankle was inserted through a lateral approach. The fibula was fixed with a solid plate but didn't heal. Despite the trabecular metal coat, osteointegration didn't occur, resulting in asymmetric subsidence of the tibial component, as provoked by the valgus malalignment and the weak bone of lateral tibial pilon. (**b–c**) The missing osteointegration of the tibial component was confirmed by CT scan and (**d**) intraoperatively. Notice the connective tissue covering the implant

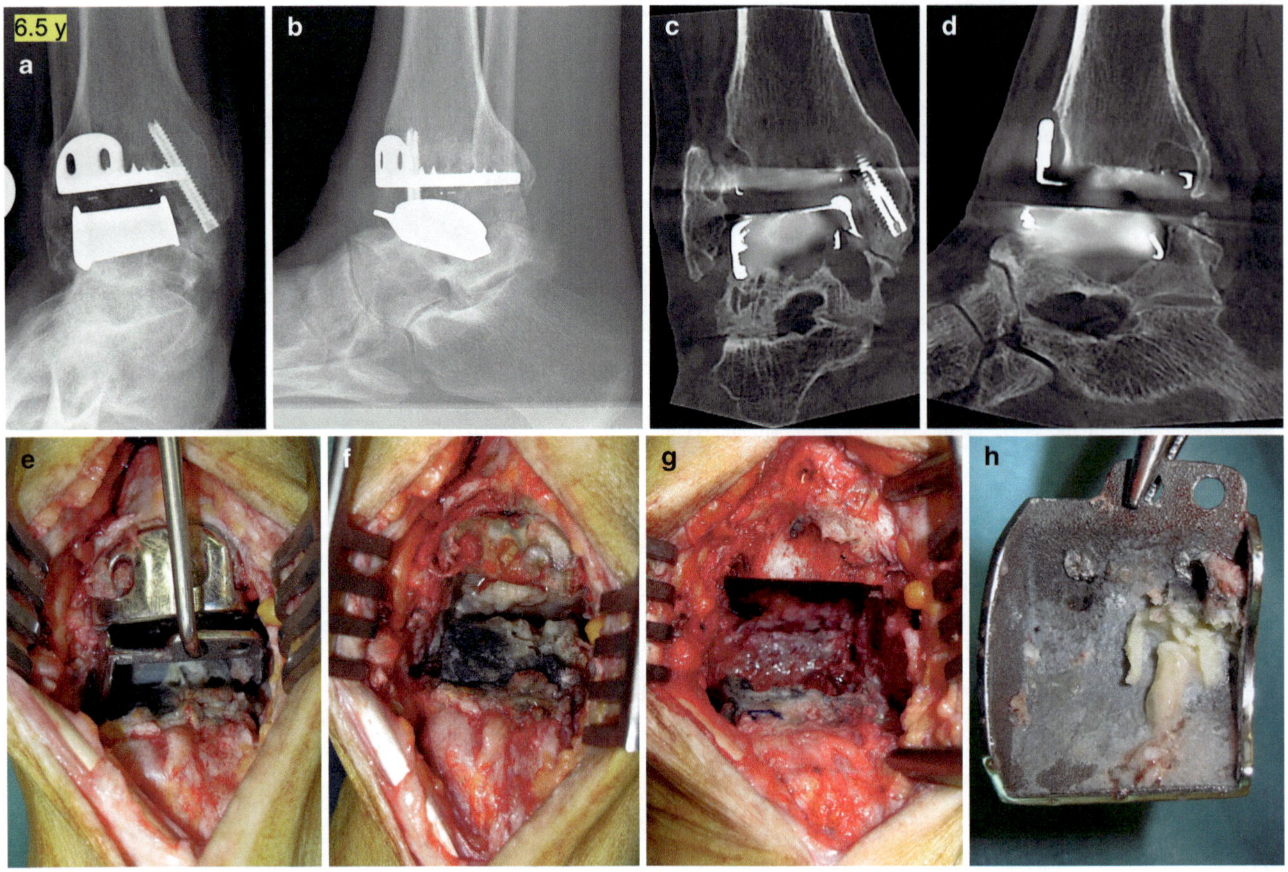

Fig. 13.20 Subsidence of the talar component associated with avascular necrosis. This 55-year-old female secretary, who sustained a talar dislocation fracture 11 years ago, underwent total ankle arthroplasty 4.5 years later. After initially uneventfully evolving, she complained about acute pain in her replaced ankle after a car accident. (**a**, **b**) Standard radiographs showed the subsidence of the talar component. (**c**, **d**) CT scans evidenced gross cyst formation, especially beneath the talar component. (**e**) Intraoperatively, the tibial component was found stable, but not the talar component, which could easily be lifted. (**f**) The extent of cyst formation can be seen after component removal and cyst debridement (**g**). Notice the sclerotic bone left at the anterior aspect of the cyst. (**h**) The retrieved component showed broken pegs due to fatigue due to the avascular necrosis of the talar body that resulted in excessive bending forces to the pegs firmly anchored in the sclerotic bone at the anterior aspect of the talus

other patients with syndesmotic incompetence, we found a correlation between coronal plane instability and polyethylene wear and cyst formation, respectively (Ruiz et al., unpublished data). Increased coronal plane shifting of the talus within the ankle mortise is detrimental to the polyethylene with subsequent wear and cyst formation (Fig. 13.22). We thus advocate considering a syndesmotic fusion when revising a total ankle arthroplasty because of cyst formation.

The results of several studies have indicated that factors other than polyethylene may contribute to periprosthetic cyst formation. Rodriguez et al. [75] hypothesized that cyst formation is comparable to the development of osteochondral lesions, possibly based on a sort of synovial inclusion (Fig. 13.23). In contrast, Bonnin et al. [76] suggested some cysts might have evolved from pre-existing arthritic cysts (Fig. 13.24). Jacobs et al. [77] hypothesized that cyst formation might be related to overwhelming a local afferent transport mechanism with wear particles, accumulating wear particles in periprosthetic tissue. A recent study by von Wijngaarden et al. [78] indicated polyethylene does not cause osteolysis in failed total ankle arthroplasty. Dalat et al. [79] proposed that delamination of the coating and foreign-body reaction to wearing particles may result from insufficient primary fixation. In a study using histomorphometric, immunohistochemical, and elemental analysis of tissues, Sing et al. [80] found the odds of having ballooning osteolysis were 300 times higher in patients with calcium content >0.5 mg/g in periprosthetic tissue than in patients with calcium content ≤0.5 mg/g ($p < 0.001$). This data suggests that the hydroxyapatite coating of the implant may be a contributory factor in ballooning osteolysis seen in failed total ankle arthroplasty.

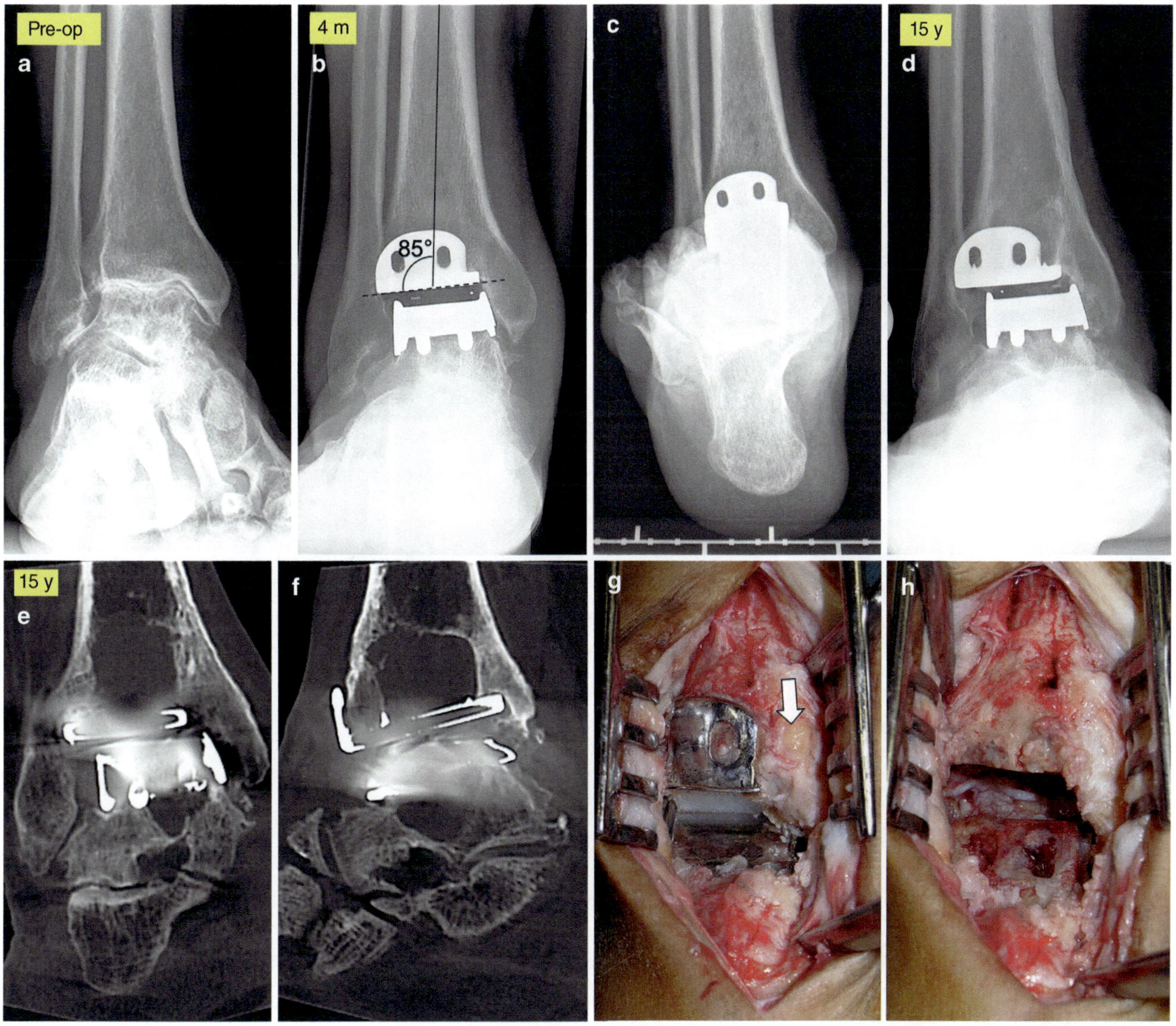

Fig. 13.21 Progressive cyst formation in a globally unstable ankle. This 49-year-old hunter sustained a polytrauma in a crash in the mountains. Six years later, he presented with end-stage osteoarthritis in a globally unstable ankle. (**a**) Preoperatively, the syndesmosis was widened, and the heel was in distinct valgus. (**b**) The AP view 4 months after the replacement surgery shows the tibial component in 5° of varus, but the ankle looked somehow balanced with an overall neutral alignment (**c**). (**d**) At 15-year follow-up control, the patient reported increasing instability and pain in the medial gutter of his ankle. The radiograph shows a widening of the ankle mortise with significant medialization of the talus and a narrowing of the joint space due to polyethylene wear. (**e**, **f**) CT scans show massive cyst formation at the tibial and talar sides, the implants being stable. (**g**) The surgical exploration confirmed the polyethylene wear and the edge loading, and it also shows the significant bone formation at the medial malleolus due to chronic overload (arrow). (**h**) After implant removal, the cystic changes in the center of the talus can be seen, while the circumferential bone contours are preserved

The Authors' Experience

- *Periprosthetic bone cysts are common after total ankle arthroplasty and can often be asymptomatic.*
- *The exact cause of bone cyst formation is likely multifactorial, with contributing factors including polyethylene wear, implant micromotion, and implant design (including coating).*
- *After the replacement surgery, the ankle should never be left with coronal plane instability and valgus malalignment, as they are detrimental to polyethylene wear and subsequent cyst formation.*
- *Synovial fluid penetration into the bone should be avoided by completely covering the resection surfaces with the implants and preserving the cortex.*

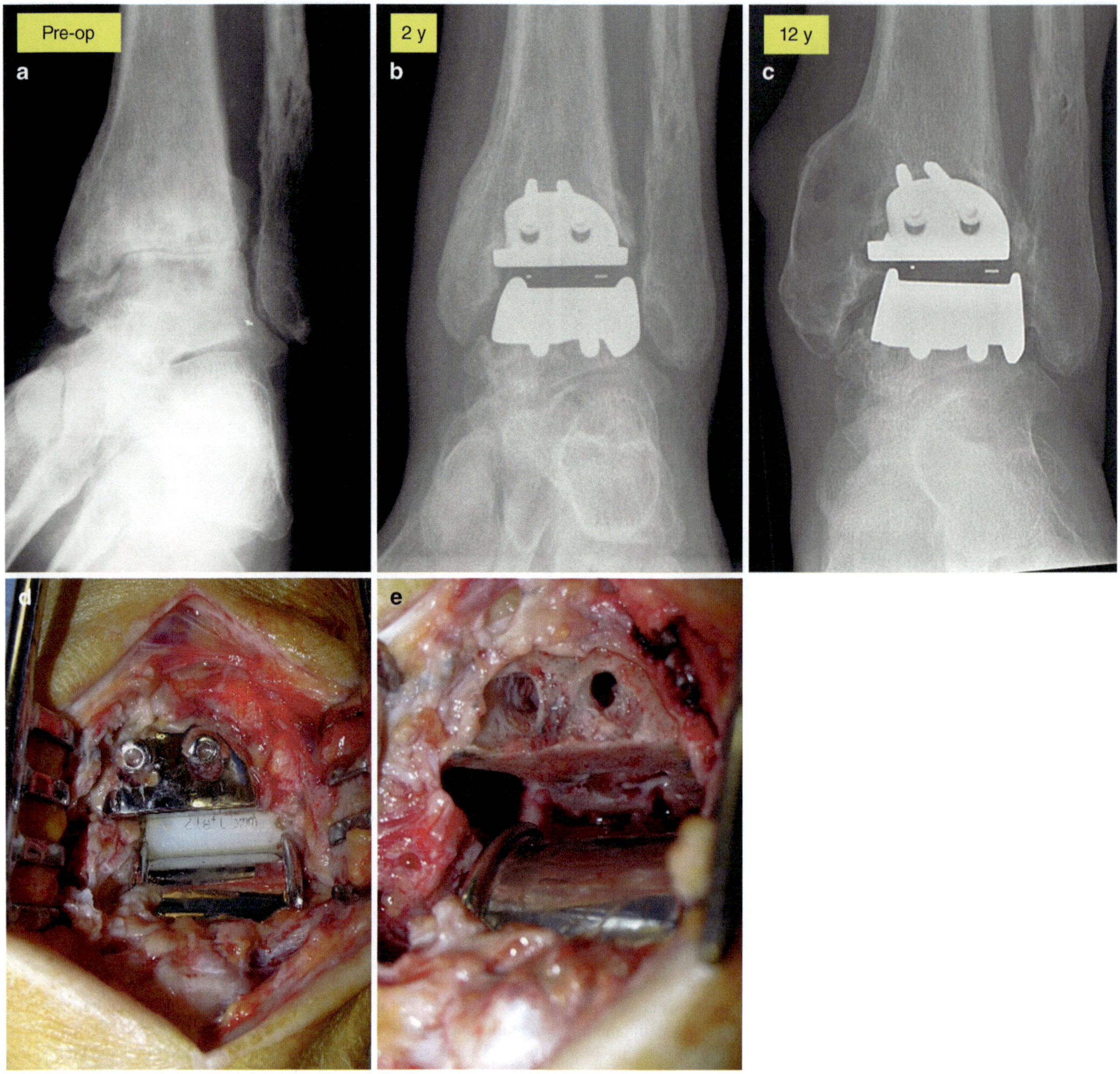

Fig. 13.22 Cyst formation due to coronal plane instability. A 56-year-old carpenter, 9 years after a tibial pilon fracture, underwent three surgeries after initial internal fixation due to an infection. (**a**) Preoperative AP view showing a diastasis of the fibula and the tibia. As the scarred syndesmosis was found somehow stable during the replacement surgery, no measures were taken for stabilization. (**b**) The patient was pain-free 2 years postoperatively, and the AP view shows a well-aligned and balanced ankle. (**c**) The patient showed up 12 years after the total ankle arthroplasty because he noticed a swelling on his medial ankle. The AP view evidenced ballooning cyst formation with lateralization of the talus in the widened ankle mortise and asymmetric wear of the polyethylene insert. (**d**) The surgical exploration confirmed the polyethylene wear and the edge loading while the talus moved laterally. (**e**) The vast cyst in the medial malleolus can be seen after removing the tibial component

13.3.5 Implant Failures

Fracture or dislocation of the mobile-bearing polyethylene insert is rarely reported through case series, suggesting that it is a rare complication [2]. Indeed, it was not reported as a complication in two recent meta-analyses [5, 6]. In contrast, Brunner et al. [10] reported an incidence of 14% in their series of 72 patients with STAR implants and felt it was more likely if the preoperative coronal malalignment was greater than 5° (Fig. 13.25). Scott and Nunley [81] reported that thinner inserts were more likely to fracture and fail. Dislocation of the mobile-bearing implant has been reported to occur if ligament laxity of the ankle is not addressed at the time of surgery [63].

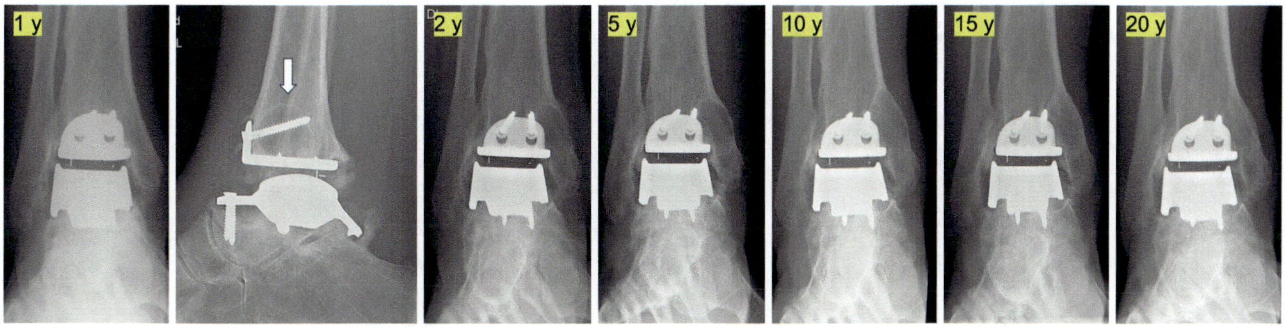

Fig. 13.23 Intermediate cyst formation due to synovial fluid. A 46-year-old female clerk was treated with a custom-made talar implant for avascular necrosis of the talus after a fracture. One year postoperatively, a cyst formation (arrow) can be detected at the tibial side caused by synovial fluid penetration along the screw. One year later, the cyst is seen to have progressed to the medial malleolus. After a further progression of 3 years, it is seen to become stable, disappearing step by step

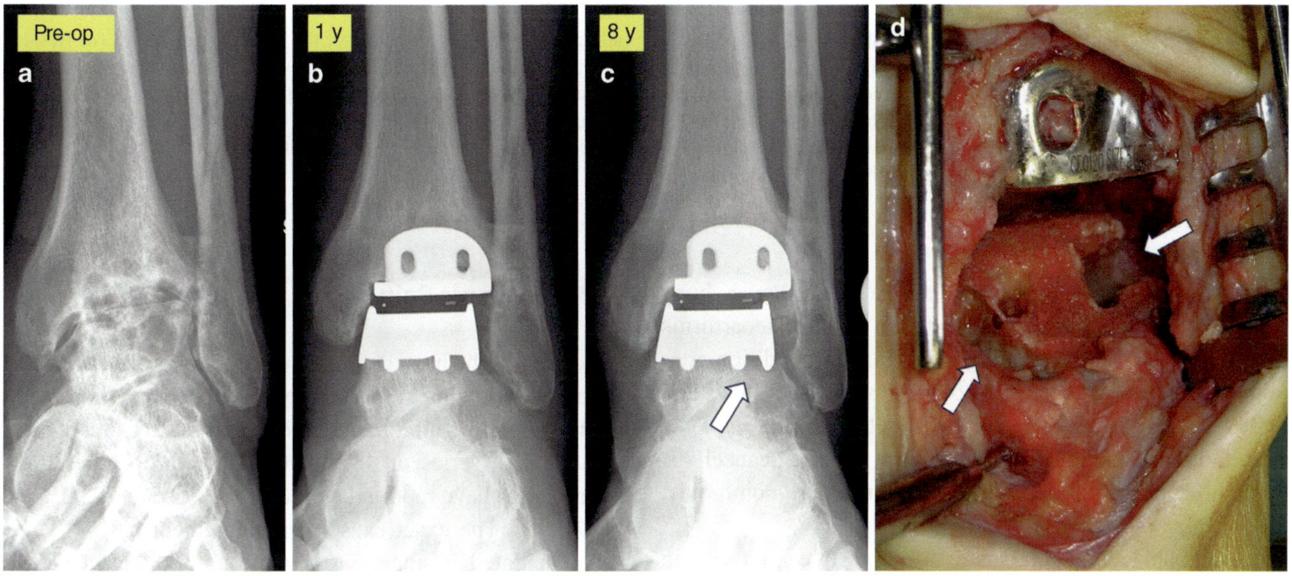

Fig. 13.24 Cyst evolvement from pre-existing arthritic cysts. (**a**) A 60-year-old patient with primary ankle osteoarthritis associated with multiple cyst formation. (**b**) One year postoperatively, the talus is slightly medially positioned in the ankle mortise. (**c**) While the medialization of the talus progressed, the re-appearance of the cysts in the talus can be seen (arrow). (**d**) The cysts are exposed after removing the talar component (arrows)

Another cause associated with polyethylene failure is edge-loading caused by remaining ligament imbalance or inappropriate placement of implants during surgery (Fig. 13.21 and 13.26). Preoperative coronal plane deformity of >10° has been associated with a tenfold risk of progressive edge loading of the polyethylene compared with congruent joints [17]. A systematic review on survival of the STAR prosthesis that included 16 studies (2088 patients) reported 18% failure due to implant malalignment and edge loading of polyethylene [82].

There are several reasons for the failure of the total ankle arthroplasty implant. These can be related to implant design, surgeon, and patient factors. Meta-analyses of several implants reported a 90% survival rate at 5 years, a survival rate between 73% and 89% at 10 years, a wide variability between different implants and centers, and an annual failure rate of around 1.5% [3]. The Hintegra prosthesis in 722 ankles (684 patients) has been reported to show 93%, 86%, and 82% implant survival at five, ten, and 15 years, respectively [83]. However, the incidence of polyethylene failure was not reported.

13.3.6 Stiffness

Postoperative formation of proliferative bone and heterotopic ossifications is more likely in patients with posttraumatic ankle osteoarthritis and may occur posteriorly [84, 85]

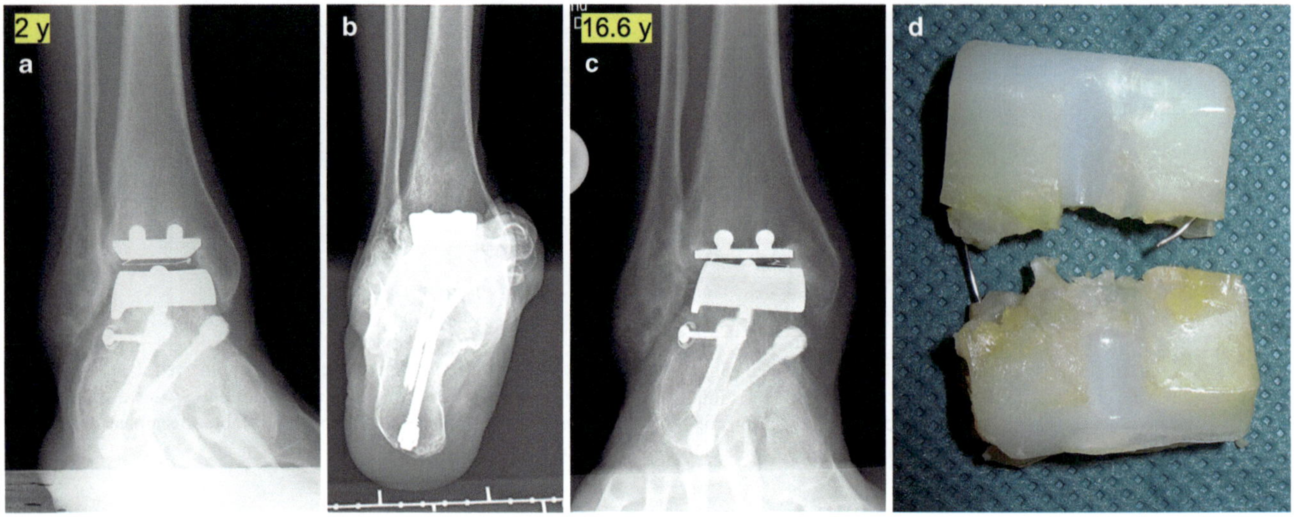

Fig. 13.25 Polyethylene fracture in a malaligned STAR ankle. A 54-year-old ranger with valgus osteoarthritis of the ankle and subtalar joint after a non-anatomic lateral ligament reconstruction underwent simultaneous total ankle arthroplasty and subtalar fusion. (**a**, **b**) As shown in the 2-year follow-up, the valgus was not sufficiently addressed. (**c**) 16.6 years after the surgery, he felt a popping in his ankle. The AP radiograph evidences a fracture of the polyethylene insert. (**d**) Besides the fracture, the polyethylene liner shows significant wear damage. The patient underwent an exchange of the polyethylene insert and a medial sliding osteotomy of the calcaneus (not shown), and he passed his 25-year follow-up recently, still delighted with his ankle

and anteriorly [86]. The proliferative periarticular bony growth in patients with posttraumatic ankle osteoarthritis may also represent an ongoing inflammatory condition after total ankle arthroplasty predisposing this group to gutter disease (Fig. 13.27) [87–90]. Most currently available implants result in some residual exposure of raw, bleeding cancellous bone after implantation on the tibial and, more commonly, on the talar side (Fig. 13.28) [63].

A stiff ankle after total ankle arthroplasty can be seen in the early stage of recovery [91], but also a progressive process several years after total ankle arthroplasty [10, 11]. It may be associated with significant pain and restrictions in daily activities; however, most surprisingly, stiffness could be well tolerated by many patients, mainly if they had limited motion before the total ankle arthroplasty. Generally, surgical treatment should only be recommended in patients with substantial pain and functional impairment.

Although not proven, based on our experience, the better a total ankle arthroplasty is balanced, the less likely scar and heterotopic bone formation will occur postoperatively [63, 92]. In patients with a stiff and painful ankle replacement, a detailed preoperative diagnostic workup is mandatory to fully understand the underlying pathologic process and plan the best appropriate treatment. As a principle, all underlying causes should be addressed appropriately, including malpositioning and oversized implants, loosening of implants, cyst formation, hindfoot malalignment, soft tissue contractures, and hypertrophic bone formation.

13.3.7 Chronic Pain

Gutter pain is the most common, usually noticeable from 3 to 6 months following surgery. The incidence of symptomatic medial or lateral gutter pain requiring surgical reintervention was 7% in a series of 489 total ankle arthroplasties [90], other studies have reported an incidence of 2% to 23.5% [7, 89, 92–95]. The exact cause of impingement has yet to be fully elucidated but appears to be multifactorial [95]. Possible inciting factors include prosthesis design [7, 96], oversized tibial and talar components [7, 63, 97, 98], undersized talar component [99, 100], uncontrolled varus or valgus thrust [1, 92, 101, 102], component loosening [14, 98], residual gutter debris after total ankle replacement [7, 102–105], undersized polyethylene thickness, and talar subsidence [5, 99]. It has been speculated that implants, where the talar component has metallic medial or lateral surfaces may be prone to causing symptoms, as the component can encroach on either malleolus [102]. Other causes for gutter pain include a progression of the natural arthritic change in the medial gutter of the ankle and localized bone cyst formation. This latter complication is classically caused by polyethylene wear. However, other factors include joint fluid penetrating bone, pre-existing enlarging subchondral cysts, and disease-specific cysts (rheumatoid arthritis or hemochromatosis) [89, 95].

Our experience with the primary use of mobile-bearing ankles is that most gutter impingement is caused by insufficient ankle balancing due to malalignment left or secondary

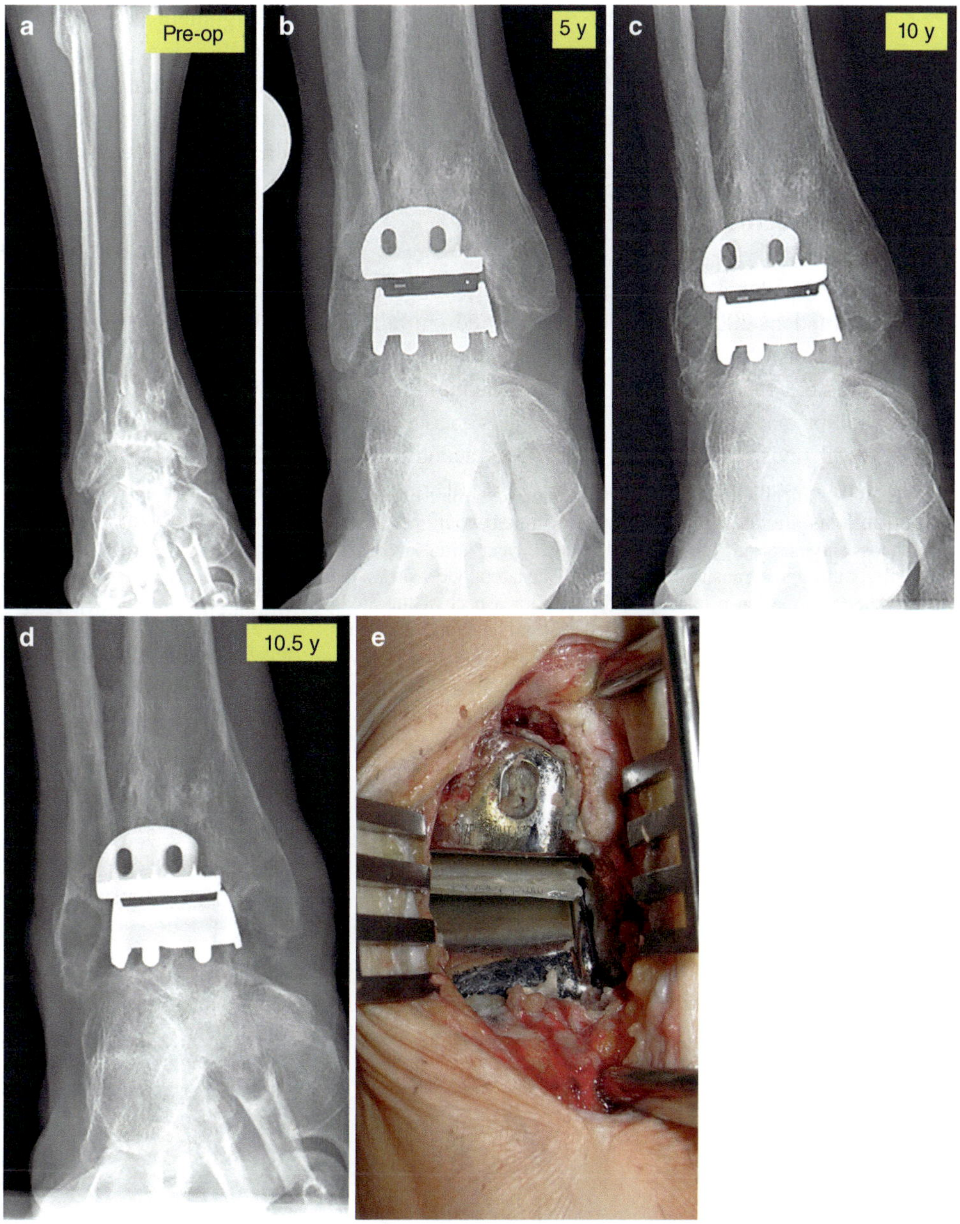

Fig. 13.26 Polyethylene fracture due to remaining ligament imbalance. A 61-year-old policeman with post-traumatic osteoarthritis after a Weber Type C fracture in the past. (**a**) The preoperative AP view shows the valgus and lateralized position of the talus in the widened ankle mortise. The syndesmosis was stable after the replacement surgery; thus, no additional measures were taken. (**b**) The ankle was well-aligned 5 years after the surgery, with adequately positioned components. (**c**) At 10-year control, the polyethylene insert was narrowed, and the fibula had a cyst. As the patient had imminent holiday plans and no pain, he refused the proposed revision. (**d**) Six months later, the insert was broken, as seen on X-ray, with cyst formation also on the medial malleolus. (**e**) Intraoperative exploration showing the failed polyethylene insert

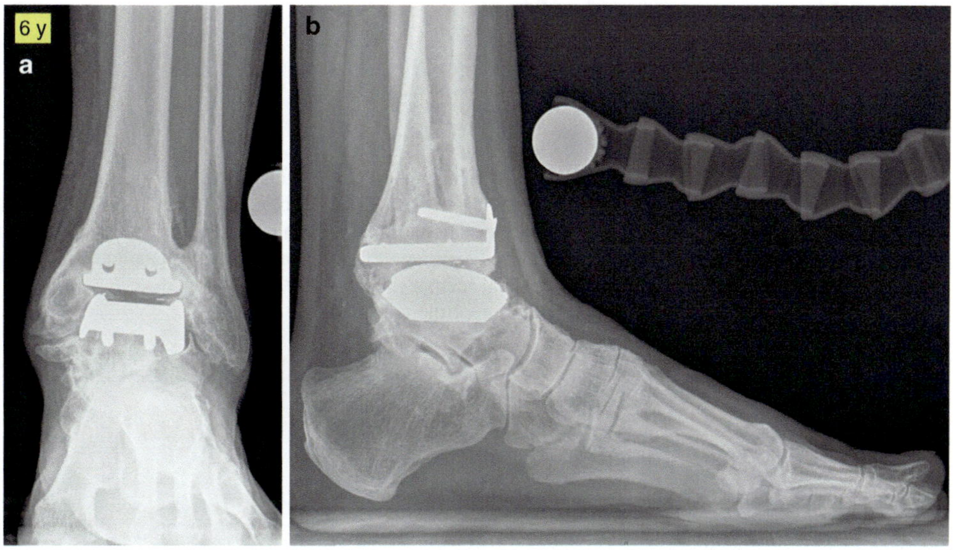

Fig. 13.27 Proliferative periarticular bony growth in post-traumatic osteoarthritis. A 57-year-old roofer 6 years after total ankle arthroplasty for post-traumatic osteoarthritis. (**a**) The AP view shows massive ossifications, including the gutters and the syndesmosis. (**b**) In the lateral view, the involvement of the posterior ankle can be seen

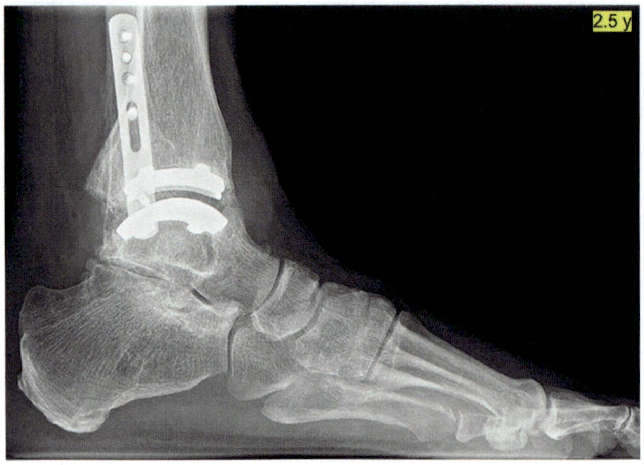

Fig. 13.28 Ossification associated with residual exposure of cancellous bone. A 56-year-old female patient complained about progressive motion loss and increasing anterior ankle pain 2.5 years after total ankle arthroplasty through a transfibular approach. The lateral view shows the massive bone formation primarily at the anterior aspect of the ankle caused by undersized implants, having left raw and bleeding cancellous bone uncovered after the replacement surgery

malalignment due to the progression of the deformity, as typically seen in a flatfoot configuration (Fig. 13.29). Similarly, a malpositioning of the tibial component in the coronal plane provokes a medial or lateral shift of the talus when loading the ankle.

13.3.8 Adjacent Joint Disease

Pain after total ankle arthroplasty may also be caused by adjacent joint disease. Although total ankle arthroplasty protects adjacent joints from aberrant motion and arthritic changes more than an ankle fusion, adjacent joint pathology can still occur [106]. In a series of more than 900 TAR patients, 4% underwent secondary subtalar fusion due to osteoarthritis (Fig. 13.30), instability, talar osteonecrosis, or cystic change [107]. In a 15-year follow-up of 84 STAR total ankle arthroplasties, one patient (1.2%) required subsequent subtalar fusion [108]. In a series of more than 1000 TARs, nearly 3% of patients returned to the operating room for a subtalar, talonavicular, double, or triple arthrodesis [109].

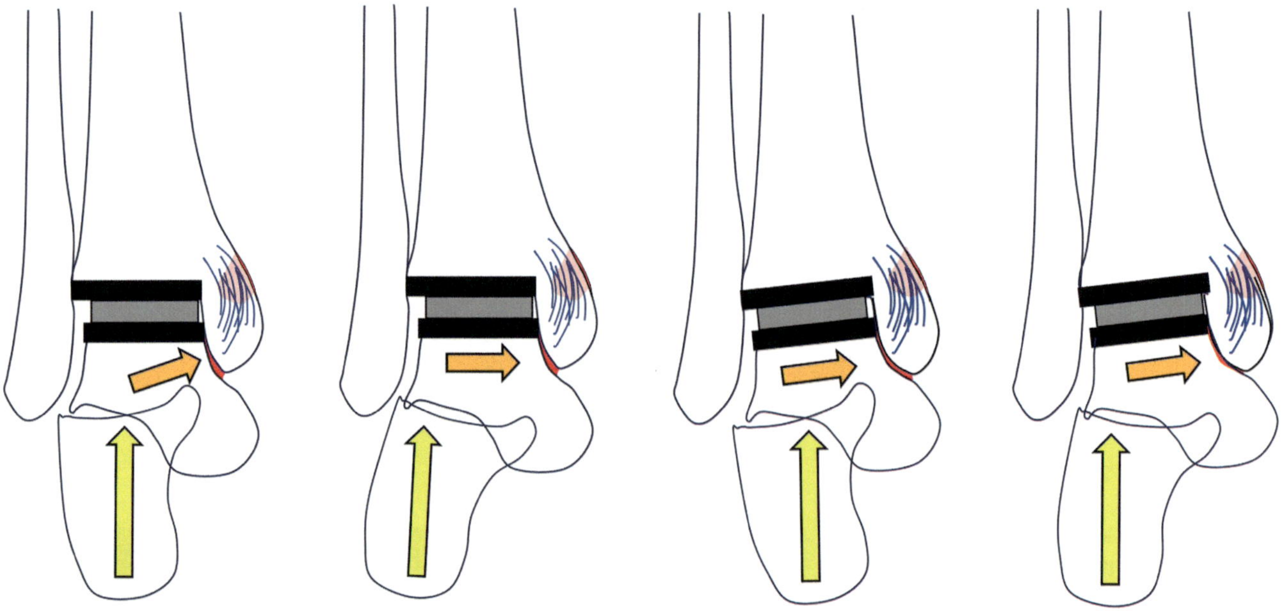

Fig. 13.29 Classification of medial gutter pain ("medial pain syndrome"). The underlying cause is a peritalar instability with a medial talus slide on the calcaneus, resulting in a medial translational force to the talus during push-off. It is increased with increasing valgus malalignment of the heel. A varus malpositioned tibial component additionally increases the effect on the medial translation of the talus and subsequent stress reaction at the medial malleolus. Type I, neutral heel alignment; Type II, valgus malalignment; Type III, neutral heel alignment and varus malpositioning of the tibial component; and Type IV, valgus heel malalignment and varus malpositioning of the tibial component

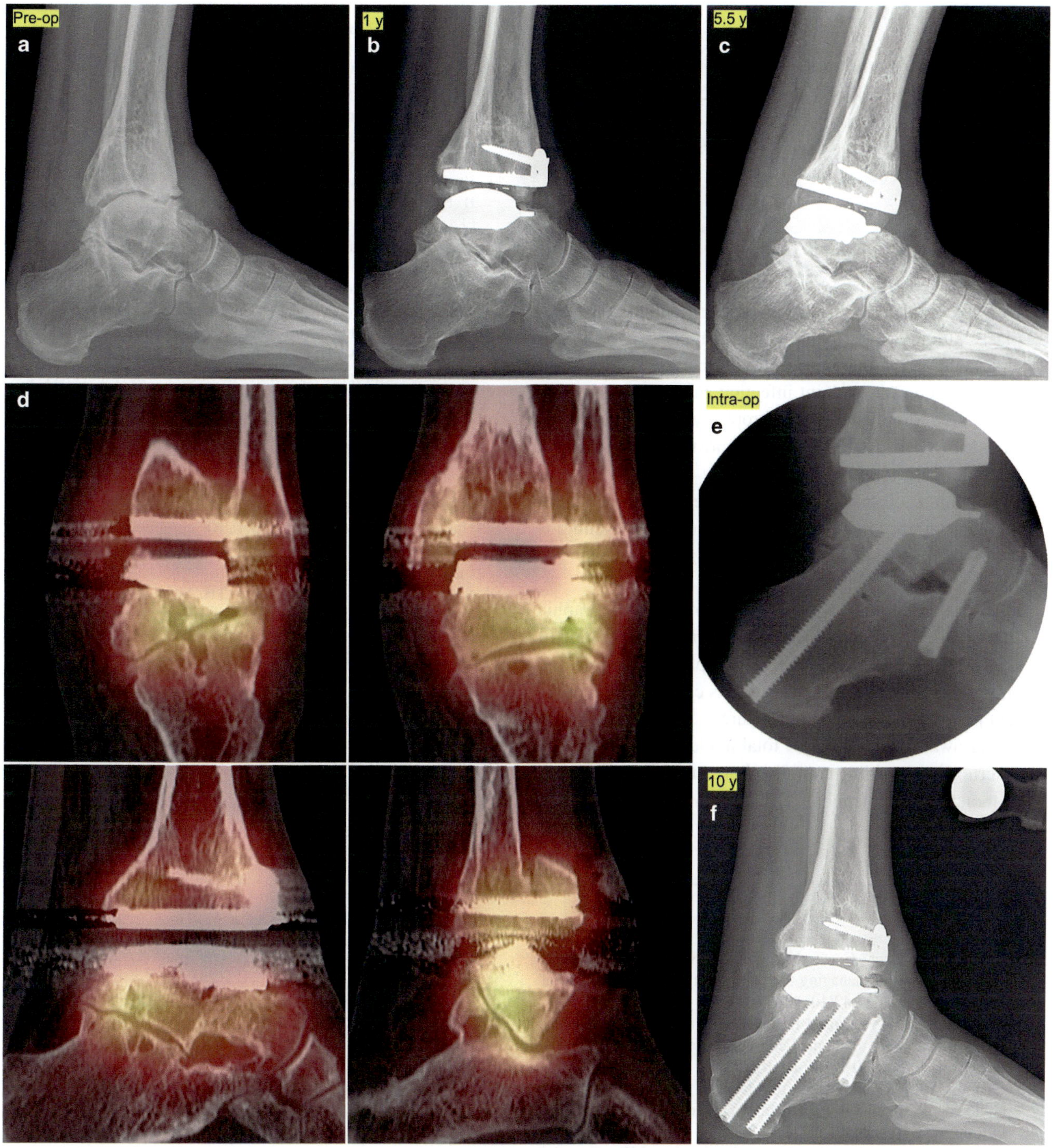

Fig. 13.30 Subtalar osteoarthritis after total ankle replacement requiring a fusion. A 55-year-old patient was treated 11 years ago with a supramalleolar osteotomy for a varus osteoarthritis. (**a**) The preoperative lateral view evidences some morphologic changes and degenerative disease of the subtalar joint. A fusion of this joint during the total ankle replacement surgery was not considered because there was no pain. (**b**) One year after the surgery, the patient was pain-free. Radiographically, the subtalar joint looks improved, and its position changed from a pronated position to a more neutral one, as seen by the opening of the sinus tarsi. (**c**) However, 5.5. y after the replacement surgery, the patient complains about significant pain in the subtalar joint. Radiographically, the degenerative disease of the subtalar joint has increased, and in the Spect CT, cyst formation with focal activity is seen (**d**). The range of motion for dorsi–/plantarflexion is as high as 15°-0°-30°; thus compensatory overstress of the joint cannot be the underlying cause. (**e**) Therefore, a subtalar fusion in a neutral position is performed. (**f**) Ten years later, the patient is still pain-free, and he is delighted with the result, though the range of motion has decreased. This case raises the question of whether secondary osteoarthritis after a total ankle arthroplasty is effectively a complication, as it is evident that the same progression might have occurred without the replacement surgery or after a fusion instead

13.3.9 Amputation

As with any lower-limb surgery of this magnitude and complexity, there is a risk of catastrophic complications, ultimately requiring below-knee amputation. However, this should be explained to the patient preoperatively; fortunately, the reported incidence is <1% [3, 4].

13.4 Conclusions

- Despite a higher complication rate for total ankle arthroplasty surgery, most complications appear to be minor and do not affect the final clinical outcome.
- Periprosthetic (deep) joint infection can be a devastating and costly complication of arthroplasty.
- Loosening and osteolysis are the most common reasons for failures in total ankle arthroplasty. However, the reasons behind loosening still need to be fully understood; there is evidence that the time to revision for loosening is significantly longer for mobile-bearing devices than for fixed-bearing devices.
- Periprosthetic bone cysts are a common radiographic finding after total ankle arthroplasty with a wide range of clinical consequences; along with implant loosening and subsidence, periprosthetic bone cysts can result in persistent pain and periprosthetic fracture.
- Being aware of the risks of total ankle arthroplasty may be crucial in avoiding complications, and, if encountered, to treat them adequately.

References

1. Henry JK, Rider C, Cody E, Ellis SJ, Demetracopoulos C. Evaluating and managing the painful total ankle replacement. Foot Ankle Int. 2021;42(10):1347–61.
2. Clough TM, Alvi F, Majeed H. Total ankle arthroplasty: what are the risks?: a guide to surgical consent and a review of the literature. Bone Joint J. 2018;100-B(10):1352–8.
3. Gougoulias N, Khanna A, Maffulli N. How successful are current ankle replacements? A systematic review of the literature. Clin Orthop Relat Res. 2010;468(1):199–208.
4. Gadd RJ, Barwick TW, Paling E, Davies MB, Blundell CM. Assessment of a three-grade classification of complications in total ankle replacement. Foot Ankle Int. 2014;35(5):434–7.
5. Glazebrook MA, Arsenault K, Dunbar M. Evidence-based classification of complications in total ankle arthroplasty. Foot Ankle Int. 2009;30(10):945–9.
6. Zaidi R, Cro S, Gurusamy K, Siva N, Macgregor A, Henricson A, et al. The outcome of total ankle replacement: a systematic review and meta-analysis. Bone Joint J. 2013;95-B(11):1500–7.
7. Rippstein PF, Huber M, Naal FD. Management of specific complications related to total ankle arthroplasty. Foot Ankle Clin. 2012;17(4):707–17.
8. Lee KT, Lee YK, Young KW, Kim JB, Seo YS. Perioperative complications and learning curve of the mobility total ankle system. Foot Ankle Int. 2013;34(2):210–4.
9. Myerson MS, Shariff R, Zonno AJ. The management of infection following total ankle replacement: demographics and treatment. Foot Ankle Int. 2014;35(9):855–62.
10. Brunner S, Barg A, Knupp M, Zwicky L, Kapron AL, Valderrabano V, et al. The Scandinavian total ankle replacement: long-term, eleven to fifteen-year, survivorship analysis of the prosthesis in seventy-two consecutive patients. J Bone Joint Surg Am. 2013;95(8):711–8.
11. Barg A, Zwicky L, Knupp M, Henninger HB, Hintermann B. HINTEGRA total ankle replacement: survivorship analysis in 684 patients. J Bone Joint Surg Am. 2013;95(13):1175–83.
12. Wood PL, Deakin S. Total ankle replacement. The results in 200 ankles. J Bone Joint Surg Br. 2003;85(3):334–41.
13. Simonson DC, Roukis TS. Incidence of complications during the surgeon learning curve period for primary total ankle replacement: a systematic review. Clin Podiatr Med Surg. 2015;32(4):473–82.
14. Spirt AA, Assal M, Hansen ST Jr. Complications and failure after total ankle arthroplasty. J Bone Joint Surg Am. 2004;86(6):1172–8.
15. Mercer J, Penner M, Wing K, Younger AS. Inconsistency in the reporting of adverse events in total ankle arthroplasty: a systematic review of the literature. Foot Ankle Int. 2016;37(2):127–36.
16. Endstrasser F, Lindtner RA, Landegger A, Wagner M, Eichinger M, Schonthaler H, et al. Midterm results of AAA ankle arthroplasty. Foot Ankle Int. 2023;10711007231186375
17. Haskell A, Mann RA. Perioperative complication rate of total ankle replacement is reduced by surgeon experience. Foot Ankle Int. 2004;25(5):283–9.
18. Sung KS, Ahn J, Lee KH, Chun TH. Short-term results of total ankle arthroplasty for end-stage ankle arthritis with severe varus deformity. Foot Ankle Int. 2014;35(3):225–31.
19. Primadi A, Xu HX, Yoon TR, Ryu JH, Lee KB. Neurologic injuries after primary total ankle arthroplasty: prevalence and effect on outcomes. J Foot Ankle Res. 2015;8:55.
20. Conti SF, Wong YS. Complications of total ankle replacement. Clin Orthop Relat Res. 2001;391:105–14.
21. Hintermann B, Valderrabano V. Total ankle replacement. Foot Ankle Clin. 2003;8(2):375–405.
22. Borenstein TR, Anand K, Li Q, Charlton TP, Thordarson DB. A review of perioperative complications of outpatient total ankle arthroplasty. Foot Ankle Int. 2018;39(2):143–8.
23. Saito GH, Sanders AE, de Cesar NC, O'Malley MJ, Ellis SJ, Demetracopoulos CA. Short-term complications, reoperations, and radiographic outcomes of a new fixed-bearing total ankle arthroplasty. Foot Ankle Int. 2018;39(7):787–94.
24. Raikin SM, Kane J, Ciminiello ME. Risk factors for incision-healing complications following total ankle arthroplasty. J Bone Joint Surg Am. 2010;92(12):2150–5.
25. Gross CE, Lampley A, Green CL, DeOrio JK, Easley M, Adams S, et al. The effect of obesity on functional outcomes and complications in total ankle arthroplasty. Foot Ankle Int. 2016;37(2):137–41.
26. Schipper ON, Jiang JJ, Chen L, Koh J, Toolan BC. Effect of diabetes mellitus on perioperative complications and hospital outcomes after ankle arthrodesis and total ankle arthroplasty. Foot Ankle Int. 2015;36(3):258–67.
27. Tubb CC, Polkowksi GG, Krause B. Diagnosis and prevention of periprosthetic joint infections. J Am Acad Orthop Surg. 2020;28(8):e340–e8.
28. Zhang Z, Chien BY, Noori N, Day J, Robertson C, Schon L. Application of the Mayo periprosthetic joint infection risk score for total ankle arthroplasty. Foot Ankle Int. 2023;44(5):451–8.
29. Hintermann B, Zwicky L, Knupp M, Henninger HB, Barg A. HINTEGRA revision arthroplasty for failed total ankle prostheses. J Bone Joint Surg Am. 2013;95(13):1166–74.
30. Kunutsor SK, Whitehouse MR, Blom AW, Beswick AD, Team I. Patient-related risk factors for periprosthetic joint infection after total joint arthroplasty: a systematic review and meta-analysis. PLoS One. 2016;11(3):e0150866.

31. Ong KL, Kurtz SM, Lau E, Bozic KJ, Berry DJ, Parvizi J. Prosthetic joint infection risk after total hip arthroplasty in the medicare population. J Arthroplast. 2009;24(6 Suppl):105–9.
32. Zhu Y, Zhang F, Chen W, Liu S, Zhang Q, Zhang Y. Risk factors for periprosthetic joint infection after total joint arthroplasty: a systematic review and meta-analysis. J Hosp Infect. 2015;89(2):82–9.
33. Kessler B, Sendi P, Graber P, Knupp M, Zwicky L, Hintermann B, et al. Risk factors for periprosthetic ankle joint infection: a case-control study. J Bone Joint Surg Am. 2012;94(20):1871–6.
34. Althoff A, Cancienne JM, Cooper MT, Werner BC. Patient-related risk factors for periprosthetic ankle joint infection: an analysis of 6977 total ankle arthroplasties. J Foot Ankle Surg. 2018;57(2):269–72.
35. Balato G, Ascione T, de Matteo V, Lenzi M, Amato M, de Giovanni R, et al. Debridement and implant retention in acute hematogenous periprosthetic joint infection after knee arthroplasty: a systematic review. Orthop Rev (Pavia). 2022;14(2):33670.
36. Shohat N, Goswami K, Tan TL, Fillingham Y, Parvizi J. Increased failure after irrigation and debridement for acute hematogenous periprosthetic joint infection. J Bone Joint Surg Am. 2019;101(8):696–703.
37. Wouthuyzen-Bakker M, Sebillotte M, Arvieux C, Fernandez-Sampedro M, Senneville E, Barbero JM, et al. How to handle concomitant asymptomatic prosthetic joints during an episode of hematogenous periprosthetic joint infection, a multicenter analysis. Clin Infect Dis. 2021;73(11):e3820–e4.
38. Honkanen M, Jamsen E, Karppelin M, Huttunen R, Eskelinen A, Syrjanen J. Periprosthetic joint infections as a consequence of bacteremia. Open Forum Infect Dis. 2019;6(6):ofz218.
39. Kessler B, Knupp M, Graber P, Zwicky L, Hintermann B, Zimmerli W, et al. The treatment and outcome of peri-prosthetic infection of the ankle: a single cohort-centre experience of 34 cases. Bone Joint J. 2014;96-B(6):772–7.
40. Zaidi R, MacGregor A, Cro S, Goldberg A. Pulmonary embolism and mortality following total ankle replacement: a data linkage study using the NJR data set. BMJ Open. 2016;6(6):e011947.
41. Manegold S, Haas NP, Tsitsilonis S, Springer A, Mardian S, Schaser KD. Periprosthetic fractures in total ankle replacement: classification system and treatment algorithm. J Bone Joint Surg Am. 2013;95(9):815–20. S1–3
42. Steck JK, Anderson JB. Total ankle arthroplasty: indications and avoiding complications. Clin Podiatr Med Surg. 2009;26(2):303–24.
43. Fong JW, Veljkovic A, Dunbar MJ, Wilson DA, Hennigar AW, Glazebrook MA. Validation and precision of model-based radiostereometric analysis (MBRSA) for total ankle arthroplasty. Foot Ankle Int. 2011;32(12):1155–63.
44. Engh CA, O'Connor D, Jasty M, McGovern TF, Bobyn JD, Harris WH. Quantification of implant micromotion, strain shielding, and bone resorption with porous-coated anatomic medullary locking femoral prostheses. Clin Orthop Relat Res. 1992;285:13–29.
45. Mondal S, Ghosh R. Effects of implant orientation and implant material on tibia bone strain, implant-bone micromotion, contact pressure, and wear depth due to total ankle replacement. Proc Inst Mech Eng H. 2019;233(3):318–31.
46. Espinosa N, Klammer G, Wirth SH. Osteolysis in total ankle replacement: how does it work? Foot Ankle Clin. 2017;22(2):267–75.
47. Jonitz-Heincke A, Lochner K, Schulze C, Pohle D, Pustlauk W, Hansmann D, et al. Contribution of human osteoblasts and macrophages to bone matrix degradation and proinflammatory cytokine release after exposure to abrasive endoprosthetic wear particles. Mol Med Rep. 2016;14(2):1491–500.
48. Athanasou NA. The pathobiology and pathology of aseptic implant failure. Bone Joint Res. 2016;5(5):162–8.
49. Archibeck MJ, Jacobs JJ, Roebuck KA, Glant TT. The basic science of periprosthetic osteolysis. Instr Course Lect. 2001;50:185–95.
50. Espinosa N, Walti M, Favre P, Snedeker JG. Misalignment of total ankle components can induce high joint contact pressures. J Bone Joint Surg Am. 2010;92(5):1179–87.
51. Mondal S, Ghosh R. A numerical study on stress distribution across the ankle joint: effects of material distribution of bone, muscle force and ligaments. J Orthop. 2017;14(3):329–35.
52. Reggiani B, Leardini A, Corazza F, Taylor M. Finite element analysis of a total ankle replacement during the stance phase of gait. J Biomech. 2006;39(8):1435–43.
53. Ozen M, Sayman O, Havitcioglu H. Modeling and stress analyses of a normal foot-ankle and a prosthetic foot-ankle complex. Acta Bioeng Biomech. 2013;15(3):19–27.
54. Yoon HS, Lee J, Choi WJ, Lee JW. Periprosthetic osteolysis after total ankle arthroplasty. Foot Ankle Int. 2014;35(1):14–21.
55. Currier BH, Hecht PJ, Nunley JA 2nd, Mayor MB, Currier JH, Van Citters DW. Analysis of failed ankle arthroplasty components. Foot Ankle Int. 2019;40(2):131–8.
56. Goodman SB, Huie P, Song Y, Lee K, Doshi A, Rushdieh B, et al. Loosening and osteolysis of cemented joint arthroplasties. A biologic spectrum. Clin Orthop Relat Res. 1997;337:149–63.
57. Lee GW, Seo HY, Jung DM, Lee KB. Comparison of preoperative bone density in patients with and without periprosthetic osteolysis following total ankle arthroplasty. Foot Ankle Int. 2021;42(5):575–81.
58. Collier JP, Mayor MB, Chae JC, Surprenant VA, Surprenant HP, Dauphinais LA. Macroscopic and microscopic evidence of prosthetic fixation with porous-coated materials. Clin Orthop Relat Res. 1988;235:173–80.
59. Kohonen I, Koivu H, Pudas T, Tiusanen H, Vahlberg T, Mattila K. Does computed tomography add information on radiographic analysis in detecting periprosthetic osteolysis after total ankle arthroplasty? Foot Ankle Int. 2013;34(2):180–8.
60. Mehta N, Serino J, Hur ES, Smith S, Hamid KS, Lee S, et al. Pathogenesis, evaluation, and management of osteolysis following total ankle arthroplasty. Foot Ankle Int. 2021;42(2):230–42.
61. Carlsson A, Markusson P, Sundberg M. Radiostereometric analysis of the double-coated STAR total ankle prosthesis: a 3-5 year follow-up of 5 cases with rheumatoid arthritis and 5 cases with osteoarthrosis. Acta Orthop. 2005;76(4):573–9.
62. Morgan SS, Brooke B, Harris NJ. Total ankle replacement by the ankle evolution system: medium-term outcome. J Bone Joint Surg Br. 2010;92(1):61–5.
63. Hintermann B. Total ankle arthroplasty—historical overview, current concepts and future perspectives. Wien-New York: Springer; 2004. 195 p
64. Mulcahy H, Chew FS. Current concepts in total ankle replacement for radiologists: complications. AJR Am J Roentgenol. 2015;205(6):1244–50.
65. Li SY, Myerson MS. Management of talar component subsidence. Foot Ankle Clin. 2017;22(2):361–89.
66. Hur ES, Mehta N, Lee S, Bohl DD. Management of periprosthetic bone cysts after total ankle arthroplasty. Orthop Clin North Am. 2023;54(1):109–19.
67. Besse JL. Osteolytic cysts with total ankle replacement: frequency and causes? Foot Ankle Surg. 2015;21(2):75–6.
68. Schipper ON, Haddad SL, Fullam S, Pourzal R, Wimmer MA. Wear characteristics of conventional ultrahigh-molecular-weight polyethylene versus highly cross-linked polyethylene in total ankle arthroplasty. Foot Ankle Int. 2018;39(11):1335–44.
69. Bischoff JE, Fryman JC, Parcell J, Orozco Villasenor DA. Influence of crosslinking on the wear performance of polyethylene within total ankle arthroplasty. Foot Ankle Int. 2015;36(4):369–76.
70. Assal M, Kutaish H, Acker A, Hattendorf J, Lubbeke A, Crevoisier X. Three-year rates of reoperation and revision following mobile versus fixed-bearing total ankle arthroplasty: a cohort of 302 patients with 2 implants of similar design. J Bone Joint Surg Am. 2021;103(22):2080–8.

71. Gaudot F, Colombier JA, Bonnin M, Judet T. A controlled, comparative study of a fixed-bearing versus mobile-bearing ankle arthroplasty. Foot Ankle Int. 2014;35(2):131–40.
72. Nunley JA, Adams SB, Easley ME, DeOrio JK. Prospective randomized trial comparing mobile-bearing and fixed-bearing total ankle replacement. Foot Ankle Int. 2019;40(11):1239–48.
73. Arcangelo J, Guerra-Pinto F, Pinto A, Grenho A, Navarro A, Martin OX. Peri-prosthetic bone cysts after total ankle replacement. A systematic review and meta-analysis. Foot Ankle Surg. 2019;25(2):96–105.
74. Ruiz R, Susdorf R, Krahenbuhl N, Barg A, Hintermann B. Syndesmotic overload in 3-component total ankle replacement. Foot Ankle Int. 2020;41(3):275–85.
75. Rodriguez D, Bevernage BD, Maldague P, Deleu PA, Tribak K, Leemrijse T. Medium term follow-up of the AES ankle prosthesis: High rate of asymptomatic osteolysis. Foot Ankle Surg. 2010;16(2):54–60.
76. Bonnin M, Gaudot F, Laurent JR, Ellis S, Colombier JA, Judet T. The Salto total ankle arthroplasty: survivorship and analysis of failures at 7 to 11 years. Clin Orthop Relat Res. 2011;469(1):225–36.
77. Jacobs JJ, Hallab NJ, Urban RM, Wimmer MA. Wear particles. J Bone Joint Surg Am. 2006;88(Suppl. 2):99–102.
78. van Wijngaarden R, van der Plaat L, Nieuwe Weme RA, Doets HC, Westerga J, Haverkamp D. Etiopathogenesis of osteolytic cysts associated with total ankle arthroplasty, a histological study. Foot Ankle Surg. 2015;21(2):132–6.
79. Dalat F, Barnoud R, Fessy MH, Besse JL, French Association of Foot Surgery A. Histologic study of periprosthetic osteolytic lesions after AES total ankle replacement. A 22 case series. Orthop Traumatol Surg Res. 2013;99(Suppl. 6):S285–95.
80. Singh G, Reichard T, Hameister R, Awiszus F, Schenk K, Feuerstein B, et al. Ballooning osteolysis in 71 failed total ankle arthroplasties. Acta Orthop. 2016;87(4):401–5.
81. Scott AT, Nunley JA. Polyethylene fracture following STAR ankle arthroplasty: a report of three cases. Foot Ankle Int. 2009;30(4):375–9.
82. Zhao DH, Huang DC, Zhang GH, Fan YP, Yu J, Wang SB, et al. Talar dome investigation and talocrural joint axis analysis based on three-dimensional (3D) models: implications for prosthetic design. Biomed Res Int. 2019;2019:8634159.
83. Kvarda P, Peterhans US, Susdorf R, Barg A, Ruiz R, Hintermann B. Long-term survival of HINTEGRA total ankle replacement in 683 patients: a concise 20-year follow-up of a previous report. J Bone Joint Surg Am. 2022;
84. Choi WJ, Lee JW. Heterotopic ossification after total ankle arthroplasty. J Bone Joint Surg Br. 2011;93(11):1508–12.
85. Lee KB, Cho YJ, Park JK, Song EK, Yoon TR, Seon JK. Heterotopic ossification after primary total ankle arthroplasty. J Bone Joint Surg Am. 2011;93(8):751–8.
86. Jung HG, Lee SH, Shin MH, Lee DO, Eom JS, Lee JS. Anterior heterotopic ossification at the talar neck after total ankle arthroplasty. Foot Ankle Int. 2016;37(7):703–8.
87. Hintermann B, Ruiz R, Barg A. Dealing with the stiff ankle: preoperative and late occurrence. Foot Ankle Clin. 2017;22(2):425–53.
88. Devos Bevernage B, Deleu PA, Birch I, Gombault V, Maldague P, Leemrijse T. Arthroscopic debridement after total ankle arthroplasty. Foot Ankle Int. 2016;37(2):142–9.
89. Kim BS, Choi WJ, Kim J, Lee JW. Residual pain due to soft-tissue impingement after uncomplicated total ankle replacement. Bone Joint J. 2013;95-B(3):378–83.
90. Schuberth JM, Babu NS, Richey JM, Christensen JC. Gutter impingement after total ankle arthroplasty. Foot Ankle Int. 2013;34(3):329–37.
91. Hintermann B, Valderrabano V, Knupp M, Horisberger M. The HINTEGRA ankle: short- and mid-term results. Orthopade. 2006;35(5):533–45.
92. Barg A, Suter T, Zwicky L, Knupp M, Hintermann B. Medial pain syndrome in patients with total ankle replacement. Orthopade. 2011;40(11):991–2. 4–9
93. Zhao HM, Yang YF, Yu GR. Complications in total ankle arthroplasty: a meta analysis. Zhonghua Wai Ke Za Zhi. 2011;49(8):737–40.
94. Valderrabano V, Hintermann B, Dick W. Scandinavian total ankle replacement: a 3.7-year average followup of 65 patients. Clin Orthop Relat Res. 2004;424:47–56.
95. Kurup HV, Taylor GR. Medial impingement after ankle replacement. Int Orthop. 2008;32(2):243–6.
96. Hintermann B, Valderrabano V, Dereymaeker G, Dick W. The HINTEGRA ankle: rationale and short-term results of 122 consecutive ankles. Clin Orthop Relat Res. 2004;424:57–68.
97. Saltzman CL, Mann RA, Ahrens JE, Amendola A, Anderson RB, Berlet GC, et al. Prospective controlled trial of STAR total ankle replacement versus ankle fusion: initial results. Foot Ankle Int. 2009;30(7):579–96.
98. Younger A, Penner M, Wing K. Mobile-bearing total ankle arthroplasty. Foot Ankle Clin. 2008;13(3):495–508. ix–x
99. Cerrato R, Myerson MS. Total ankle replacement: the agility LP prosthesis. Foot Ankle Clin. 2008;13(3):485–94. ix
100. Knecht SI, Estin M, Callaghan JJ, Zimmerman MB, Alliman KJ, Alvine FG, et al. The agility total ankle arthroplasty. Seven to sixteen-year follow-up. J Bone Joint Surg Am. 2004;86(6):1161–71.
101. Hintermann B, Barg A, Knupp M, Valderrabano V. Conversion of painful ankle arthrodesis to total ankle arthroplasty. Surgical technique. J Bone Joint Surg Am. 2010;92(Suppl. 1 Pt. 1):55–66.
102. Hsu AR, Haddad SL, Myerson MS. Evaluation and management of the painful total ankle arthroplasty. J Am Acad Orthop Surg. 2015;23(5):272–82.
103. Raikin SM, Myerson MS. Avoiding and managing complications of the agility total ankle replacement system. Orthopedics. 2006;29(10):930–8.
104. Ryssman D, Myerson MS. Surgical strategies: the management of varus ankle deformity with joint replacement. Foot Ankle Int. 2011;32(2):217–24.
105. Wood PL, Prem H, Sutton C. Total ankle replacement: medium-term results in 200 Scandinavian total ankle replacements. J Bone Joint Surg Br. 2008;90(5):605–9.
106. SooHoo NF, Zingmond DS, Ko CY. Comparison of reoperation rates following ankle arthrodesis and total ankle arthroplasty. J Bone Joint Surg Am. 2007;89(10):2143–9.
107. Sokolowski M, Krahenbuhl N, Wang C, Zwicky L, Schweizer C, Horn Lang T, et al. Secondary subtalar joint osteoarthritis following total ankle replacement. Foot Ankle Int. 2019;40(10):1122–8.
108. Palanca A, Mann RA, Mann JA, Haskell A. Scandinavian total ankle replacement: 15-year follow-up. Foot Ankle Int. 2018;39(2):135–42.
109. Gross CE, Lewis JS, Adams SB, Easley M, DeOrio JK, Nunley JA 2nd. Secondary arthrodesis after total ankle arthroplasty. Foot Ankle Int. 2016;37(7):709–14.

14 Addressing Complications After Total Ankle Arthroplasty

Total ankle arthroplasty has a wide range of complications. Some complications are minor and unrelated to the implants, thus mainly treatable without revising the components. The treatment of patients with a painful total ankle arthroplasty is complex and requires careful consideration of symptom history, workup, and nonsurgical and surgical treatment options. Workup for periprosthetic infection should be performed before that of other chronic pathologies. Ankle stiffness and limited range of motion are common complaints after total ankle arthroplasty. They may be influenced by preoperative motion, component sizing and positioning, soft tissue and/or bony impingement, and arthrofibrosis. Ankle stiffness may exacerbate pain in the subtalar joint, and this contribution must be discerned from other etiologies of total ankle arthroplasty failure. Progressive instability, as commonly seen after not fully addressed valgus and flatfoot configurations, may put the replaced ankle at risk too. Acute trauma may result in periprosthetic fractures.

14.1 Basic Considerations

Secondary surgery not concerning the prosthetic components was designated with different terms by different authors: further surgery [1, 2], subsequent surgery [3, 4], corrective surgery [5], additional procedures [6, 7], reoperations [6, 8], minor secondary operations [9], or revision [10].

Glazebrook et al. [11] found nine main complications in the literature: intraoperative fracture, postoperative fracture, wound healing problems, deep infection, aseptic loosening, nonunion, implant failure, subsidence, and technical error. They proposed a classification system based on the failure rate for a given complication. Intraoperative bone fracture and wound healing problems are considered low-grade and unlikely to cause failure. Technical error, subsidence, and postoperative bone fracture are classified as medium-grade and lead to failure less than 50% of the time. Deep infection, aseptic loosening, and implant failure are considered high-grade and lead to failure of total ankle arthroplasty more than 50% of the time.

With total ankle arthroplasty, documented complications can be categorized chronologically into intraoperative, postoperative, and late. Factors such as patient selection, surgeon experience, implant features, and prosthetic device selection can influence functional outcomes as well as the incidence of complications. Even with impeccable surgical technique and optimal patient selection, complications that require revision may still arise.

This section discusses the most common complications caused by factors other than the components, for which, in most instances, solutions without manipulating the metallic implants will be possible. The authors believe this is essential in the surgeon's process of analyzing the case and seeking the best solution.

14.2 Workup and Indications

Pain is the primary symptom that indicates early total ankle arthroplasty failure [8, 12]. Pain location, quality, and onset can provide useful information to clarify the underlying etiology and mechanism. Lack of any symptom relief after surgery may be indicative of an indolent deep infection, whereas progressive worsening of pain over time may point toward implant loosening and subsidence. Discomfort is often described as start-up or mechanical pain associated with increased physical activity. Intermittent periods of pain and swelling are more common in patients with limited preoperative range of motion who are gaining mobility after surgery. However, this pain is not typically located in the ankle joint but in periarticular structures that experience increased tension as motion improves.

The clinical examination should include an evaluation of the surgical incision, tibiotalar and subtalar range of

B. Hintermann, R. Ruiz, *Total Ankle Replacement*, https://doi.org/10.1007/978-3-031-56810-7_14

motion, ligamentous stability, alignment, gait, and tenderness to palpation about the ankle gutters. Gutter discomfort is typically seen in cases of chronic pain after total ankle arthroplasty, but it can also appear early in the postoperative period with inadequate gutter debridement, which leads to impingement. Static and dynamic assessments of varus and valgus malalignment should be performed, observing the patient from the front and back and during gait. Vascular examination should focus on signs of venostasis or vasculopathy because poor blood flow may indicate poor wound healing potential if a revision becomes necessary.

The most common early complications are ligament imbalance, component malpositioning, and impingement. These situations may necessitate revision surgery to reduce the risk of premature total ankle arthroplasty failure.

14.3 Solutions for Addressing Complications After Total Ankle Arthroplasty

14.3.1 Wound Healing Complications

To prevent wound healing problems, dissection without delamination of layers, maintaining tibialis anterior in its sheath, careful handling of soft tissue, and layered wound closure are recommended. If present, wound healing issues are typically managed with parenteral antibiotics, local wound care, or negative-pressure wound therapy (Fig. 14.1). Wound necrosis that has failed to heal with daily care or negative pressure wound therapy and with the exposed tendon (anterior tibial tendon or extensor hallucis longus tendon) requires rotational or free vascularized flap coverage [13–16]. Treating wounds aggressively and promptly is paramount to prevent a bacterial breach of the joint capsule that would lead to periprosthetic infection and the need for major revision.

14.3.2 Deep Periprosthetic Infection

Deep periprosthetic infection after total ankle arthroplasty is a serious complication, often requiring revision surgery, including revision arthroplasty, conversion to ankle arthrodesis, or even amputation.

14.3.2.1 Antimicrobial Therapy

Retention of prosthesis components and antimicrobial therapy can be considered in cases with the following findings [17]:

(1) Early postoperative infection with symptom duration of fewer than 4 weeks
(2) Absence of sinus tract communicating to any of prosthesis components
(3) Pathogens susceptible to antibiotic therapy identified before treatment
(4) Presence of adequate periarticular soft tissue envelope

Further indications for this treatment option are high perioperative risk due to significant comorbidities, low virulence

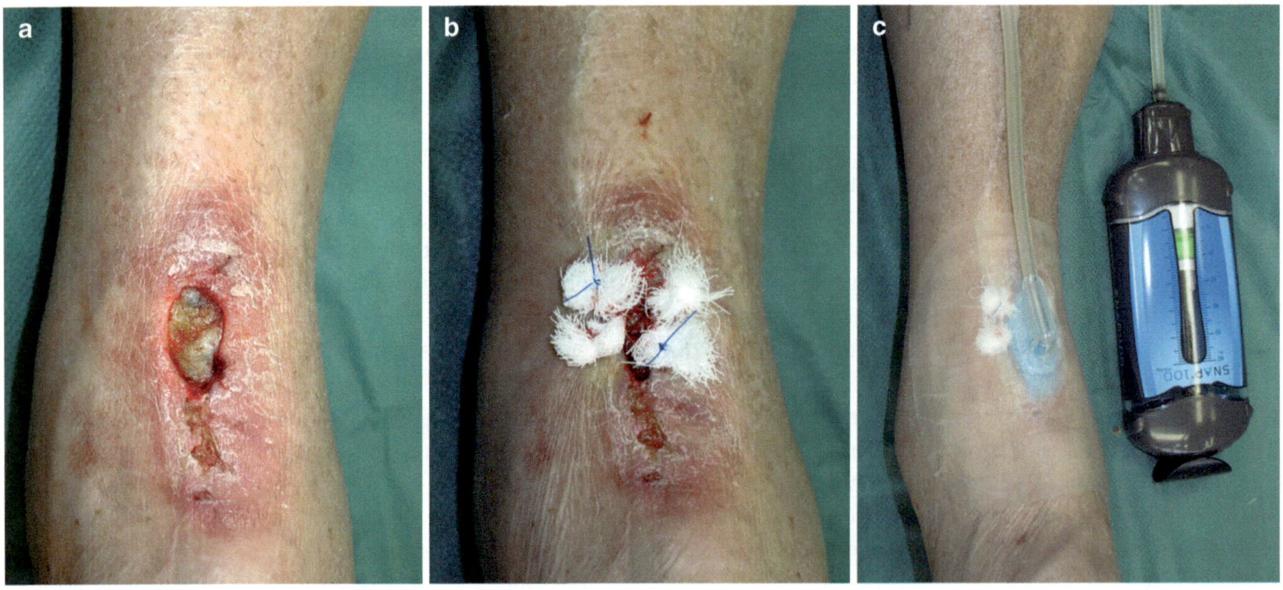

Fig. 14.1 Local wound care and negative-pressure wound therapy. A 69-year-old female patient, 9 weeks after revision arthroplasty for progressive cyst formation. (**a**) The wound is presenting with a defect after removal of the scab. As the extensor tendon sheath was not opened, conservative treatment was administered. (**b**) The wound was stabilized with some sutures and protected with a negative-pressure dressing (**c**)

organisms susceptible to well-tolerated antibiotic therapy, and mechanically stable components without lucencies at the prosthesis-bone interface.

14.3.2.2 Irrigation and Debridement With or Without Polyethylene Exchange

Irrigation and debridement with component retention remain controversial as a treatment option in patients with periprosthetic ankle infections [18]. In patients with infected hip arthroplasties, irrigation and debridement only resulted in a 20% success rate which increased to 70% when combined with jet lavage and change of all modular components of the hip prosthesis [17, 19]. In patients with infected knee arthroplasties, the therapy success rate was 45% and 55.1% in patients with irrigation and debridement without and with polyethylene exchange, respectively [20]. These results suggested that if irrigation and debridement should be the treatment option for a deep ankle infection, the polyethylene should also be exchanged [21].

14.3.2.3 Revision Ankle Arthroplasty

In patients with deep chronic infections, the formation of bacterial biofilms on prosthesis components may result in resistance to both host defense and antibiotic therapy. Therefore, a two-stage revision surgery, including removing all components, is the most successful surgical treatment in patients with periprosthetic ankle infections [22]. The most important critical points of treatment are the correct identification of the pathogenic organism, the appropriate planning of possibly multiple debridements, and the specific antimicrobial therapy. Revision ankle arthroplasty is a challenging surgical procedure [12, 23–25].

Surgical steps include removing all prosthesis components (polyethylene, tibial, and talar) and temporarily inserting an antibiotic-loaded polymethylmethacrylate cement spacer (Fig. 14.2). After all prosthesis components are removed, the underlying bone, including the previous bone-prosthesis interface, should be carefully debrided. Radical debridement is the key to reducing the intraarticular bacterial

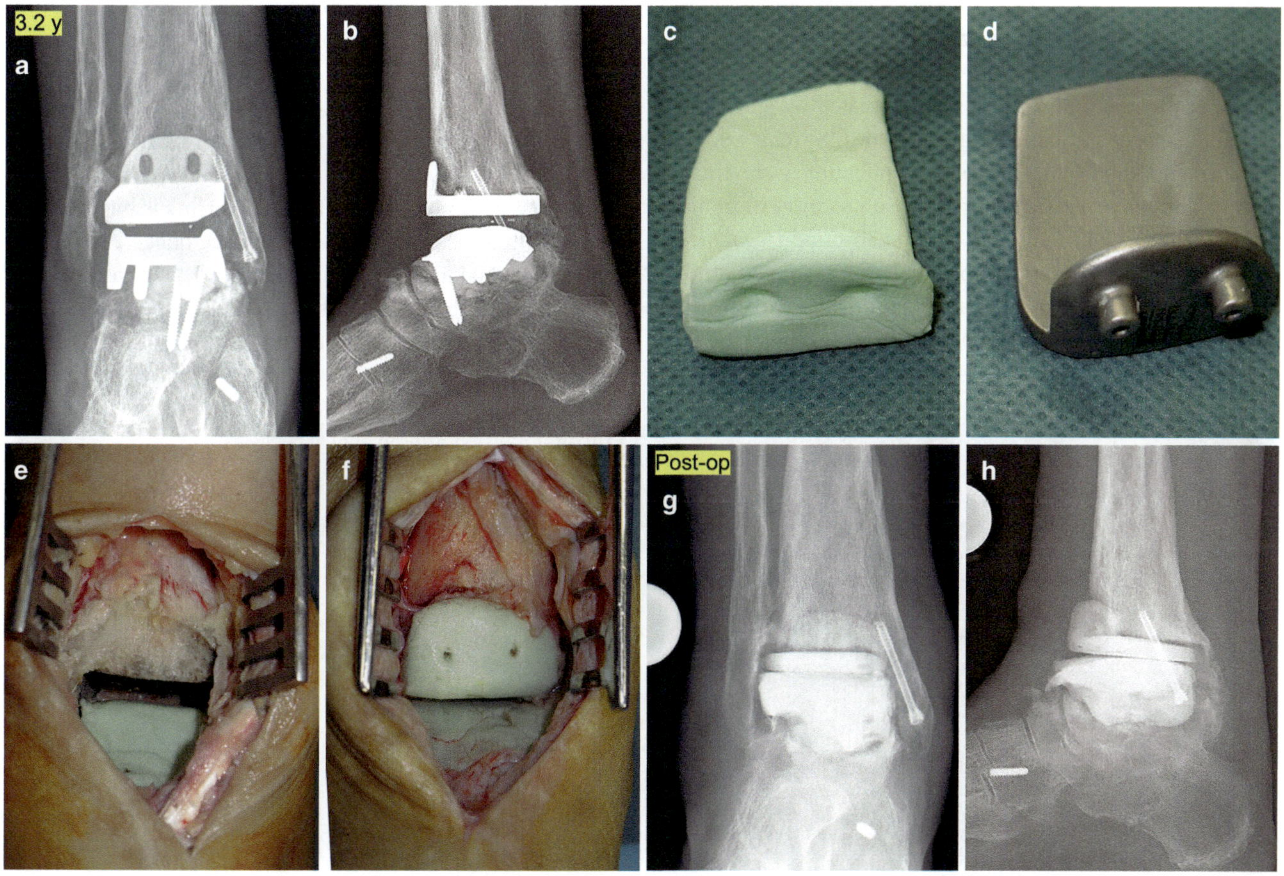

Fig. 14.2 Implant removal and insertion of an antibiotic-loaded cement spacer. A 64-year-old female patient, 3.2 years after taking down a painful arthrodesis and conversion in total ankle arthroplasty, presents with a periprosthetic infection. 14 months ago, a colon carcinoma was detected and treated with surgical resection and chemotherapy. After the last surgical intervention 9 weeks ago, she developed an infection. (**a**, **b**) Radiographs taken in the emergency department showing septic loosening of the tibial implant. (**c**) After removal of the implants and surgical debridement, a tibial component is formed with antibiotic-loaded cement, based on the form of a trial component (**d**). (**e**) At the same time, another piece of bone cement is inserted in the defect on the talar side, preparing a rounded surface on the top. (**f**) Once the cement is hardened, the created tibial component is also inserted, and the wound is closed. (**g**) Postoperative radiographs showing the spacers in place, (**g**) AP view, (**h**) lateral view

load. The removed implants should be sent for sonication analysis [26]. Antibiotics used in the polymethylmethacrylate cement spacer must be heat stable, available in lyophilized form, and effective against the microorganisms as identified by preoperative microbiologic testing. Intravenous antibiotic therapy guided by microbiologic cultures is recommended for 4–6 weeks after spacer implantation [27]. The cement spacer has two different functions:

(1) Prevention of soft tissue contracture by maintaining the ankle joint space
(2) Delivery of antibiotics locally to the bone and surrounding soft tissues by elution

The second stage, revision arthroplasty, should only be performed if the eradication of the infection is supported by clinical history and examination, serologic investigation, and synovial fluid aspiration (Fig. 14.3). If the soft tissues are critical, a flap procedure should be considered to ensure proper wound healing (Fig. 14.4).

14.3.2.4 Cement Spacer as a Definitive Treatment

Deep periprosthetic infections can be treated by leaving the antibiotic spacer in place. Myerson et al. [28] reviewed 613 replacements, and 7 of 19 cases of infection were treated with a permanent antibiotic spacer. Subluxation of cement was the only issue noted and is typically due to incorrect insertion. Their treatment protocol consists of maximum distraction during insertion with a lamina spreader and ensuring the cement fills all voids. Lee et al. [29] investigated the outcomes of cement arthroplasty as a primary salvage procedure in 16 patients: 9 had deep ankle infections, including three patients with previous total ankle arthroplasty. The cement spacers were retained without breakage for a mean of 39 months ranging from 14 to 100 months. One patient had osteolysis around the spacer. Another patient was diagnosed with subluxation. At the final follow-up, 9 of 16 patients did not require walking aids, 10 used no pain medication, and nine could walk continuously for more than an hour.

14.3.2.5 Conversion to Ankle Arthrodesis

Conversion to ankle arthrodesis can also salvage the failed total ankle arthroplasty (Figs. 16.1, 16.3, 16.4, and 16.6). However, this is a challenging surgery [30–32]. Furthermore, salvage ankle arthrodesis after failed total ankle arthroplasty resulted in impaired life quality, reduced function, and significantly higher pain than primary ankle arthrodesis [33].

14.3.2.6 Below-the-Knee Amputation

Below-the-knee amputation should be considered an ultimate solution after other limb salvage procedures have failed [28, 34, 35].

14.3.3 Malalignment/Malposition of the Tibia

The most common cause of alignment errors is misinterpreting the tibial axis during the replacement surgery [5]. Component malalignment can also result from asymmetric physiological subsidence in the first months postoperatively. Implant orientation affects strain distributions in the tibia,

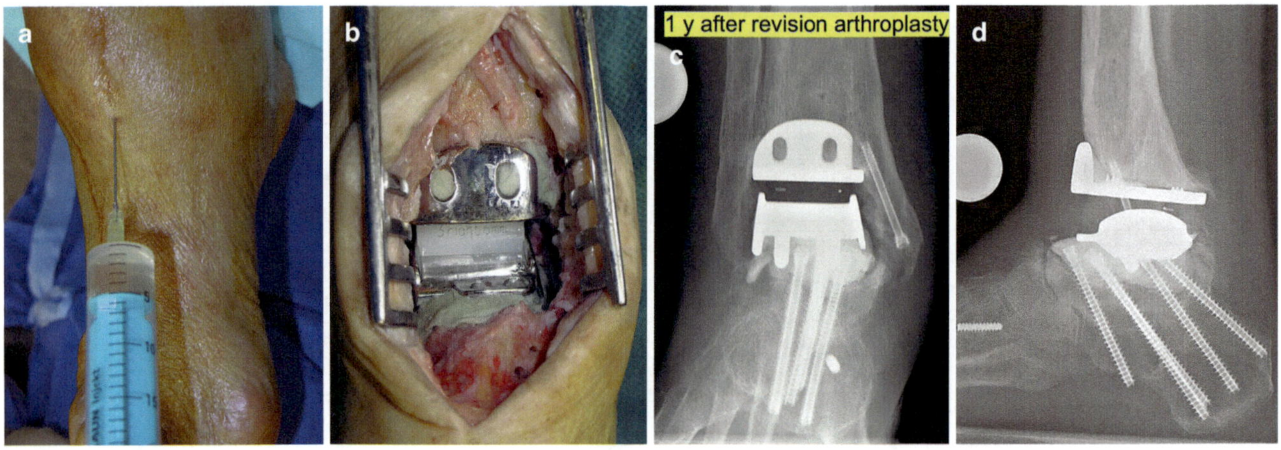

Fig. 14.3 Revision arthroplasty after septic arthritis and spacer treatment. (**a**) To complete testing whether the eradication of the infection was successful, a synovial fluid analysis is done before considering revision arthroplasty. (**b**) The cement spacers are removed, and revision arthroplasty is performed, using, in this case, bone cement for implant fixation because of the poor bone quality. (**c**, **d**) Radiographs 1 year after the revision surgery showing stable implants. No recurrent infection was observed, and antibiotic therapy was stopped 6 months after the surgery

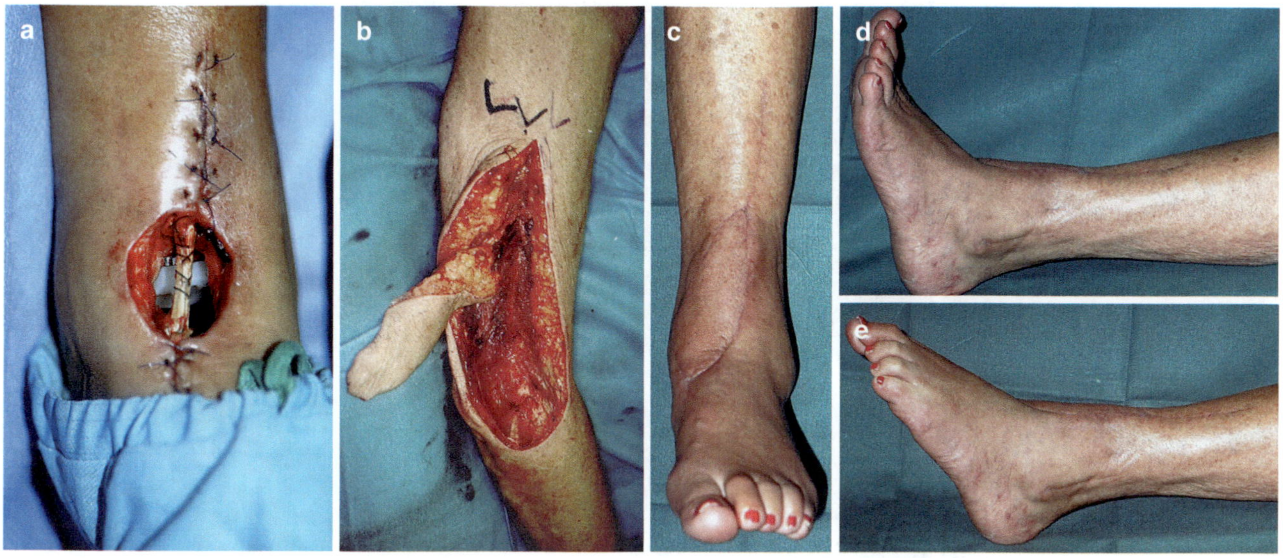

Fig. 14.4 Flap procedure for soft tissue defect. (**a**) Soft tissue defect six days after revision total ankle arthroplasty. The wound was excised, and the anterior tibial tendon was reconstructed using a free plantaris tendon graft. (**b**) A free flap was harvested from the lateral upper arm. (**c**–**e**) Six months after the surgery, the flap is well integrated but slightly swollen. The extensor function is also found to work well

especially in the region away from the implant vicinity [36]. Furthermore, implant-bone micromotion increased in valgus and varus orientations [36, 37]. To which extent the load transfer from the component to the bone may be reduced with a mobile-bearing ankle has yet to be elucidated in detail. However, recent research indicated that talar translation in the coronal plane might lead to medial or lateral impingement over time [38–41].

If malalignment is found, it usually requires revision, as the imbalance is progressive and will lead to failure. A malpositioned tibial component can be revised by exchanging the component in association with a corrective resection cut to the distal tibia [42]. However, removing a well-anchored, stable component may damage the bone stock, making reinserting a component difficult or impossible. Furthermore, an additional corrective resection cut of the distal tibia would result in additional bone loss. Osteointegration of the new implant into potentially damaged bone stock may be compromised. In addition, such revision arthroplasty may damage the soft tissue and result in reactive scarring with loss of function. An alternative to the exchange of the tibial component is a corrective osteotomy of the distal tibia above the stable implant [43]. This strictly extraarticular procedure would preserve the integrity of the replaced joint.

14.3.3.1 Medial Gutter Pain

Medial gutter impingement can be caused by insufficient ankle balancing due to malalignment left (Fig. 13.29). Similarly, a varus malpositioning of the tibial component provokes a shift of the talus toward the medial when loading the ankle, particularly when associated with the heel left in the valgus [44]. The malalignment of the tibial component can be addressed with a supramalleolar osteotomy (Fig. 14.5) [43, 45] or an exchange with repositioning of the tibial component (Fig. 14.6) [23]. In the latter case, a shortening osteotomy of the fibula might be necessary for proper balancing of the ankle, however. The inframalleolar malalignment can be addressed with a calcaneal osteotomy [44, 46]. Such correction should always be done before considering a surgical gutter debridement [47–51]. Medial gutter pain can also result from a varus deformity above the ankle requiring a high tibial osteotomy for correction (Fig. 14.7).

14.3.3.2 Lateral Gutter Pain

Lateral gutter impingement can be caused by insufficient ankle balancing due to malalignment left or secondary malalignment due to the progression of the deformity, as typically seen in a flatfoot configuration. Similarly, a valgus malpositioning of the tibial component provokes a shift of the talus toward the lateral when loading the ankle [43, 44]. The subsequent overload of the syndesmotic ligaments may result in pain and progressive incompetence. While the malalignment of the tibial component can be addressed with a supramalleolar osteotomy [43, 45] or an exchange with repositioning of the tibial component [23], the inframalleolar malalignment can be addressed with a calcaneal osteotomy or subtalar fusion [44, 46]. Also, a distal tibiofibular fusion should be considered for managing symptomatic syndesmotic incompetence (Fig. 9.46) [52].

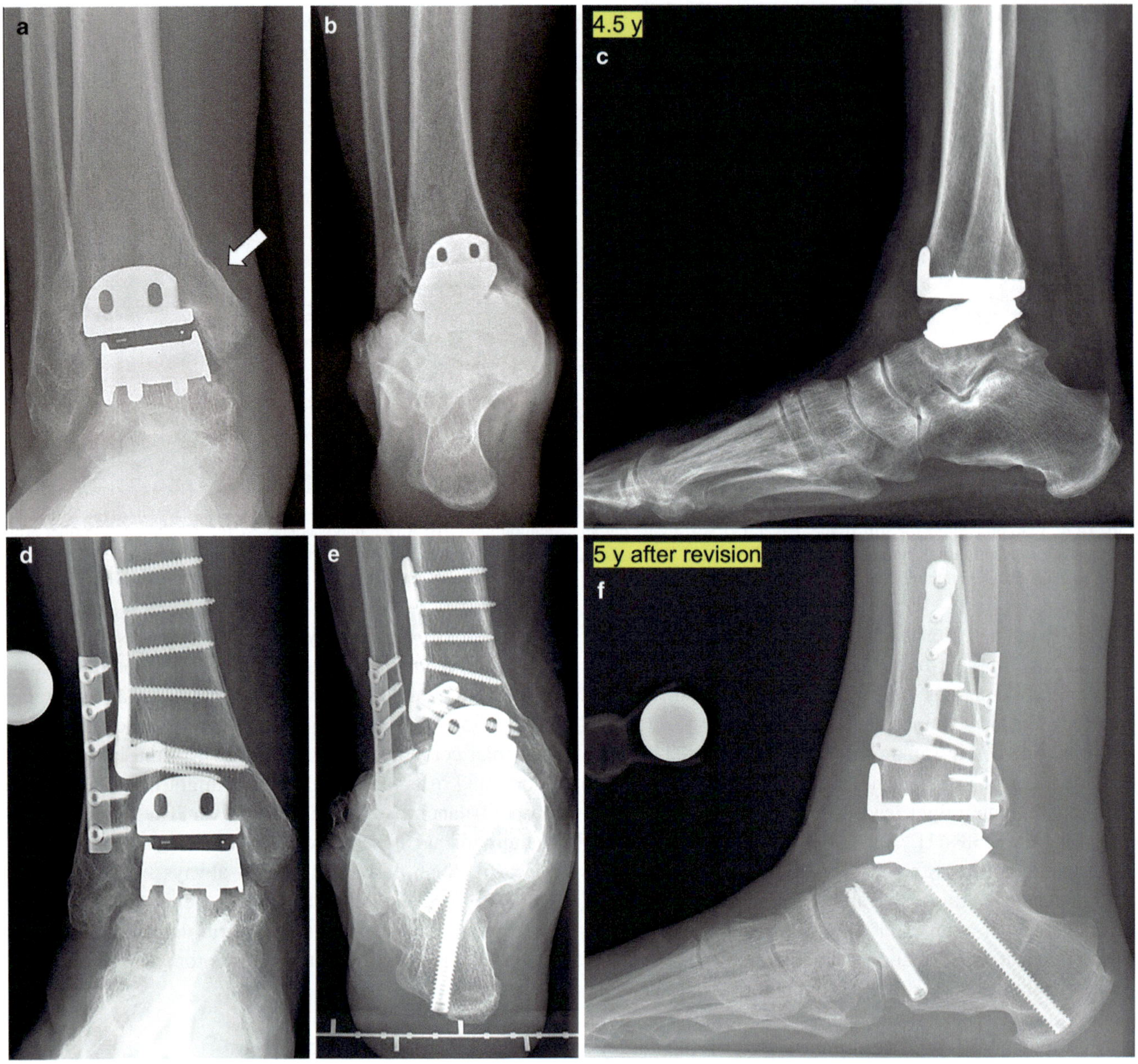

Fig. 14.5 Medial pain syndrome in a varus mispositioned ankle (addressed with supramalleolar osteotomy). A 54-year-old female patient, 4.5 years after total ankle arthroplasty, complained of tremendous pain over the medial malleolus. (**a**) The AP view evidences an 8°-varus malpositioning of the tibial component and a stress reaction over the medial malleolus (arrow). (**b**) The hindfoot alignment view shows a neutral heel alignment due to compensatory pronation at the subtalar joint, as seen in the lateral view by the closure of sinus tarsi (**c**). The patient was pain-free 5 years after supramalleolar lateral closing wedge osteotomy, subtalar fusion, and medial sliding osteotomy. The radiographs show a well-balanced ankle, and the stress reaction on the medial malleolus has disappeared. (**d**) AP view; (**e**) hindfoot alignment view, and (**f**) lateral view

14.3.4 Malalignment/Malposition of the Talus

The talar component can be malpositioned on the body, or the whole talus can be translated anteriorly, posteriorly, or rotated externally or internally. Every condition affects the relationship of each component. Patients may subsequently present with pain in the ankle or loss of range of motion. A lateral radiograph will typically reveal the deformity. In a more complex deformity, primarily to assess a rotational malposition of the talus, a weight-bearing CT scan will help assess the deformity [53, 54].

14.3.4.1 Anterior Malposition of Talar Component

If an anterior approach is used and the ankle is stiff, the error may be to place the talar component too anterior (Fig. 4.19). Equally, if the posterior talus needs to be better visualized with the correct gap between the tibia and talus, the talar

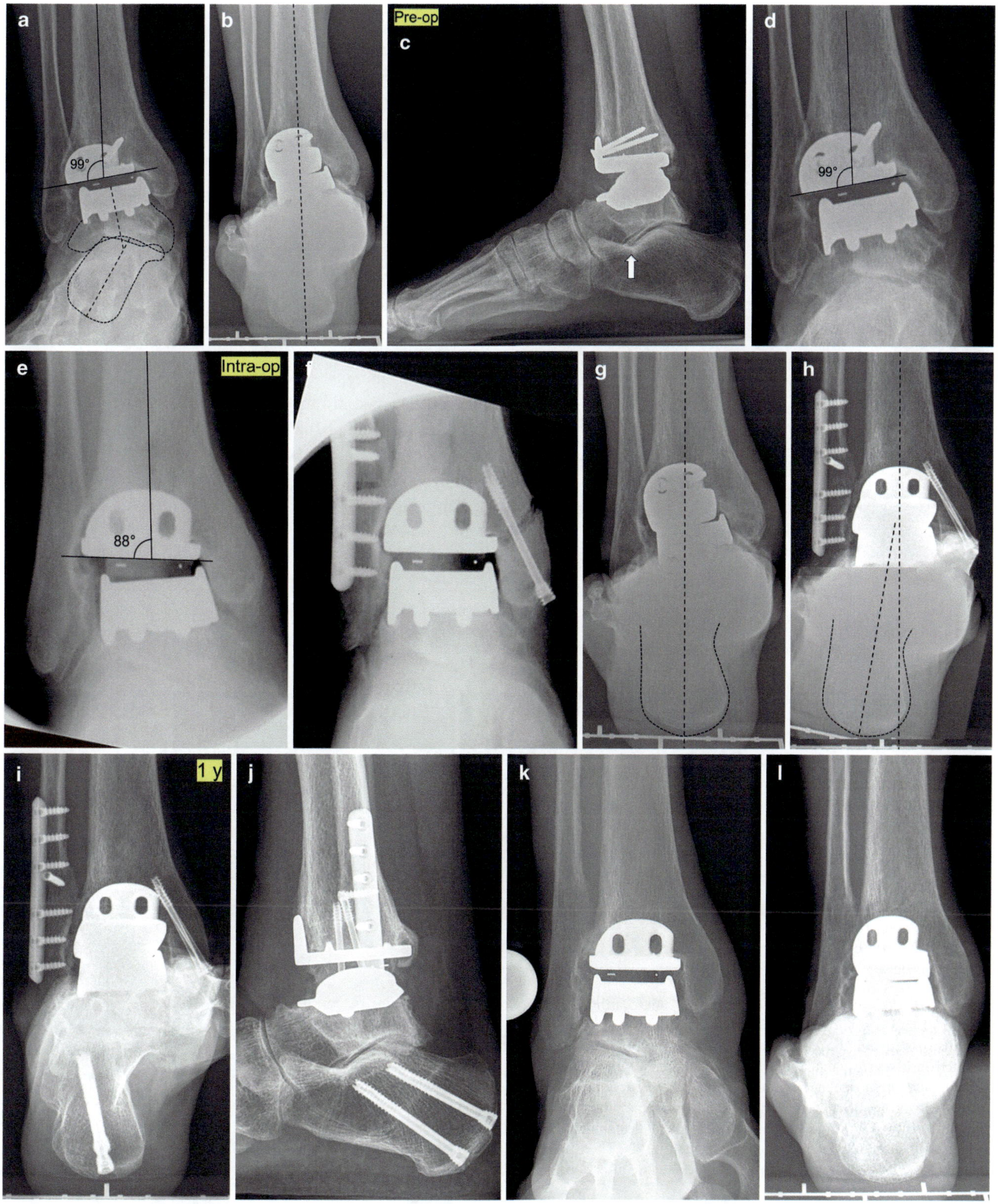

Fig. 14.6 Medial pain syndrome in a varus mispositioned ankle (addressed with revision arthroplasty). A 52-year-old female physiotherapist, 3.5 years after total ankle arthroplasty, complained of continuous medial ankle pain after four revision surgeries (medial gutter debridement) and lateral ankle pain. (**a**)The AP view evidences a 9°-varus malpositioning of the tibial component associated with compensatory pronation at the subtalar joint, which results in a neutral heel alignment (**b**). (**c**) The lateral view shows the pronation position of the subtalar joint with subsequent sinus tarsi impingement (arrow). (**e**) As the patient was scared about the proposed supramalleolar correction, a revision of the tibial component was done, in combination with a shortening osteotomy of the fibula and a flip osteotomy of the medial malleolus to balance the ankle (**f**). Compared with the preoperative neutral alignment of the heel (**g**), these measures created a valgus malalignment (**h**). Therefore, a medial sliding osteotomy was performed to realign the heel, as shown in the hindfoot alignment (**i**) and lateral views (**j**). (**k–m**) Radiograph series at the 15-year follow-up control, showing a well-balanced ankle. The patient was delighted with the result, with no limitations in her daily life and sports activities. The clinical inspection shows an appropriate ankle alignment (**n–p**) with satisfactory motion (**q–s**)

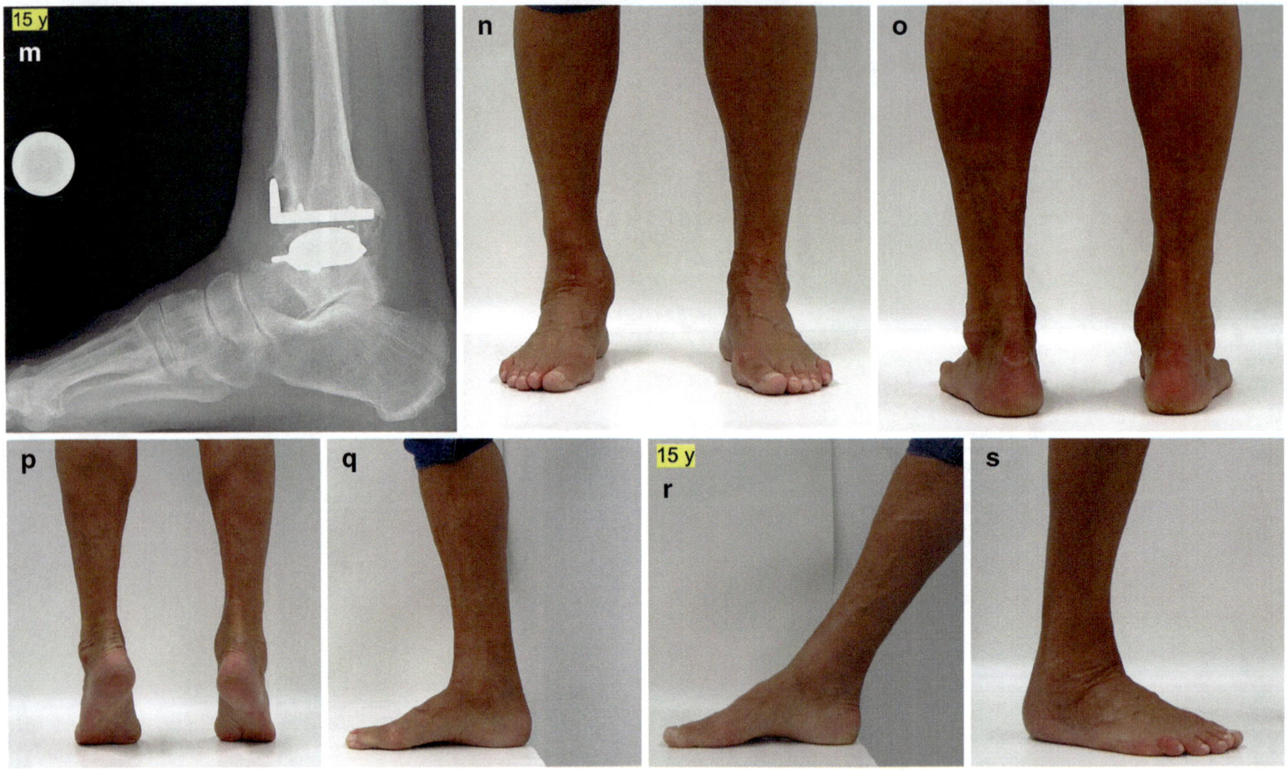

Fig. 14.6 (continued)

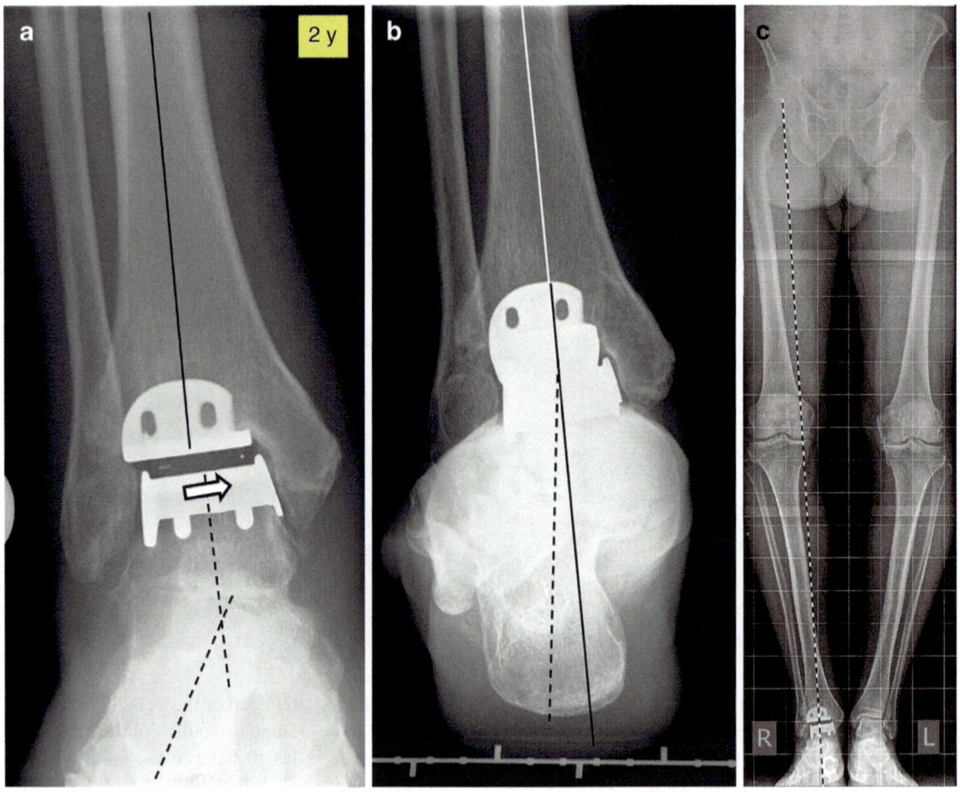

Fig. 14.7 Medial pain syndrome caused by a deformity above the ankle needing a leg correction. A 54-year-old bank clerk complains of medial ankle pain 2 years after the total ankle arthroplasty. (**a**) The implants and the ankle look well aligned in the AP view, with a slightly compensatory valgus (pronation) at the subtalar joint (**b**). (**c**) The underlying cause of the translation force of the talus toward medially causing the painful medial gutter pain is a varus deformity above the ankle. The medial ankle pain disappeared after a high tibial correcting osteotomy (not shown)

guide may be placed too anteriorly. A laterally placed ankle may be less prone to anterior translation of the talar component. A too-anterior placed talar component requires an exchange (Fig. 14.8). A flat revision component will facilitate this procedure. In an overstuffed ankle, the tibial component must be exchanged as well.

14.3.4.2 Anterior Translation of the Talus

In a mobile-bearing ankle, the tibial component's anterior slope (extension) can result in an anterior glide of the talar component [55]. An anterior tibial osteotomy or a tibial component revision can correct the deformity by combining a posteriorly directed ankle joint force and a translation of the foot on the tibia (Fig. 14.8).

A tight posterior capsule or tight posterior structures can result in an equinus deformity with the anterior translation of the talus on the tibia (Fig. 9.54). This tightness may exist after trauma, causing fibrosis of the posterior structures that may not have been sufficiently addressed at the index arthroplasty or after too-long immobilization. A posterior release will be required to correct the deformity (Fig. 9.51).

A similar appearance can exist with an overstuffed ankle, resulting in loss of dorsiflexion range and anterior translation of the talar component to the tibial axis. An exchange of the polyethylene liner for a smaller one or additional bone resection may be required to relax the capsular-ligamentous structures.

After a long-standing instability with anterolateral extrusion of the talus out of the mortise, the talar position may not be correctable because of secondary osteophyte formation. If this deformity is not corrected at the time of index arthroplasty, then the ankle joint will remain deformed. Resection of osteophytes and extended soft tissue reconstruction will be required to stabilize and balance the ankle joint, including lateral ligament reconstruction and peroneus longus to brevis tendon transfer. Often a medial soft tissue is also required.

14.3.4.3 Posterior Malposition of Talar Component

A posterior malpositioning of the talar component during index arthroplasty is very rare and may result in substantial dysfunction of the replaced ankle (Fig. 13.2). In particular, plantarflexion might be limited.

14.3.4.4 Medio-Lateral Malposition of Talar Component

Talar components that cover only the tibiotalar surface but not the medial and lateral talus are prone to be placed too medially or laterally, particularly if the surgeon needs to expose the medial gutter before placing the talar resection block (Figs. 4.20 and 4.21). In the case of pain and dysfunction, an exchange of the talar component will be required to normalize the load transfer and joint function.

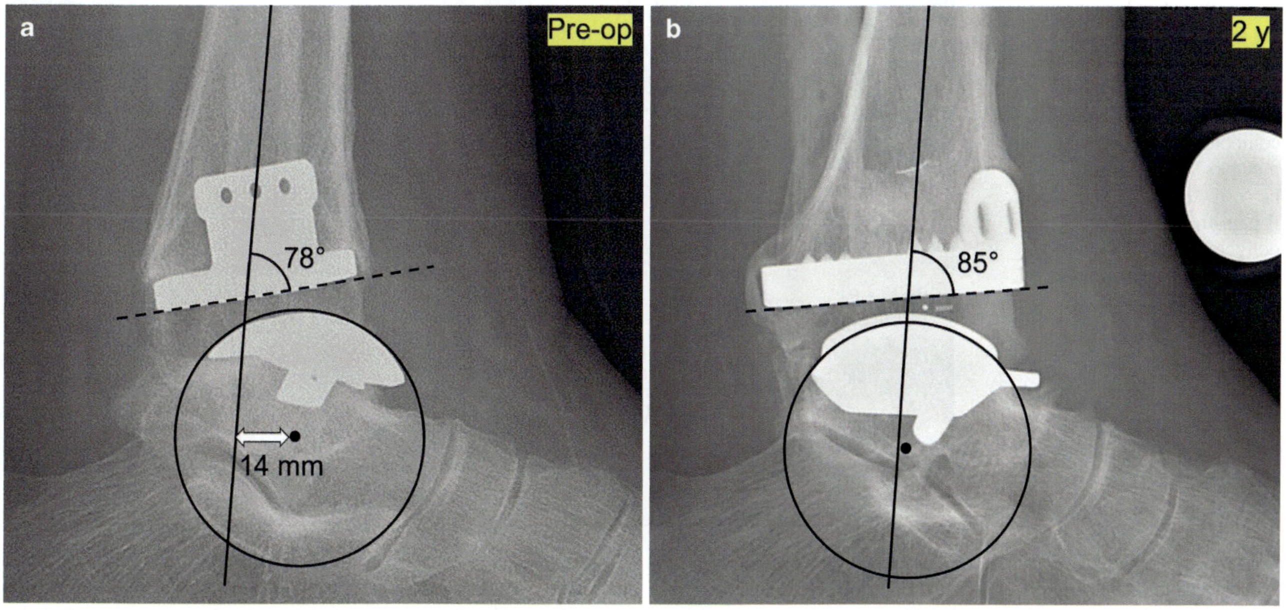

Fig. 14.8 Pain due to a too-anterior position of talar component. A 61-year-old female patient complains of painful dysfunction and stiffness 20 months after the total ankle arthroplasty. Pain mainly occurs when loading the foot. The motion is limited to dorsi-/plantarflexion of 0°-0°-25°. (**a**) The lateral view shows a too-anteriorly positioned talar component. In addition, it reveals a too-high slant of the tibial component. With loading the foot, the posterior tilt of 12° might create a translational force to the talus anteriorly, further displacing the center of rotation anteriorly and thus causing painful dysfunction with limited dorsiflexion. Therefore, the tibial component was also exchanged. (**b**) Two years after revision arthroplasty, the ankle is well balanced. The pain completely disappeared, and the range for dorsi-/plantarflexion increased to 8°-0°-30°

14.3.4.5 Rotational Malposition of Talar Component

Little is known about the impact of rotational malposition of the talar component on ankle function. It is suggested that an internally malpositioned component has a higher impact on a valgus ankle than a varus ankle. In contrast, an externally malpositioned component affects a varus ankle. A rotational malpositioned talar component may have a higher impact on a fixed-bearing ankle than a mobile-bearing ankle (Fig. 14.9). However, specific studies are needed to bring more insight into this problem.

14.3.5 The Unstable Ankle

The longevity and function of total ankle arthroplasty depend primarily on achieving a well-fixed, aligned, and stable prosthesis. Achieving this depends on implant and instrument design and the surgeon's ability to correct any preoperative deformity and achieve ligament balancing. The soft tissues remain overused if a globally unstable ankle is not sufficiently addressed at index arthroplasty. This is especially true for mobile-bearing ankles. Subsequent translational and rotational movements at the liner-tibial component interface will increase polyethylene wear. In the worst scenario, dislocation may occur.

14.3.5.1 The Varus Ankle

Complications in varus ankles mainly occur when the deforming forces are not sufficiently addressed at index arthroplasty or when the lateral ankle ligaments fail due to chronic overload (Fig. 14.10). Therefore, additional measures for lateral ligament reconstruction are necessary to successfully revise the total ankle arthroplasty, such as tendon transfer and fusions [56].

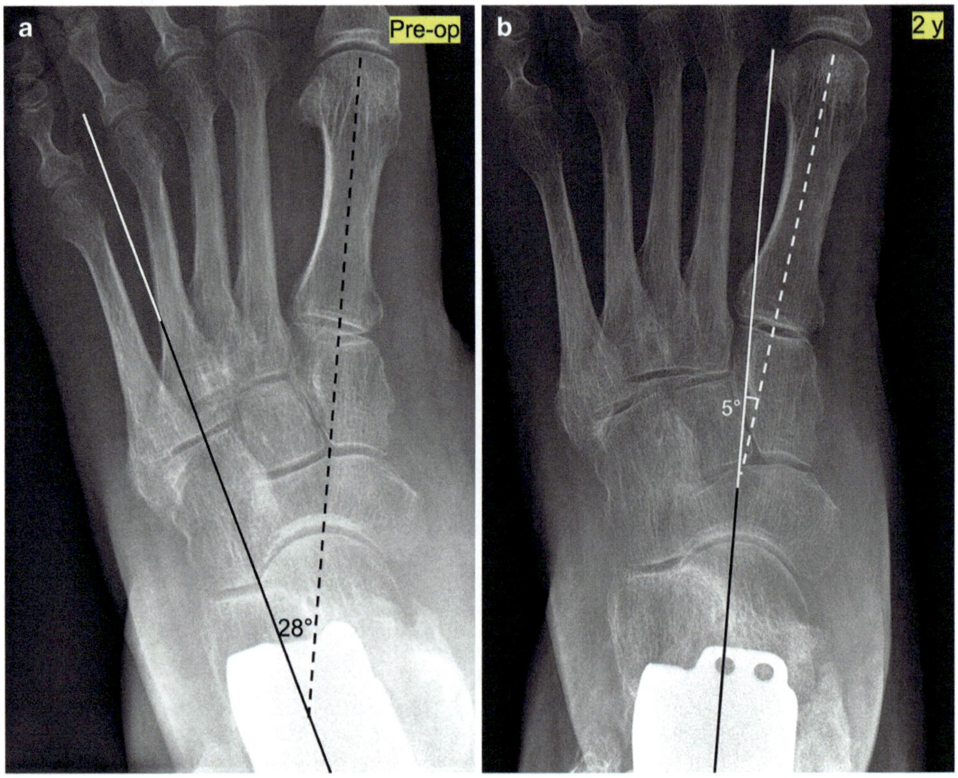

Fig. 14.9 Externally malrotated talar component. A 66-year-old retired businessman complains of painful dysfunction and pain 32 months after the total ankle arthroplasty. He describes the discomfort as an overload of the lateral foot, especially when walking downhill. (**a**) DP view showing the externally rotated position of the talar component, and a talo-first metatarsal angle of 28° is measured. (**b**) Two years after the revision of the components, the talo-first metatarsal angle is found to be corrected to 5°. The patient is pain-free, and he is delighted as the discomfort feeling has disappeared

Fig. 14.10 Polyethylene dislocation due to recurrent varus instability. A 58-year-old female sports teacher suffering from varus osteoarthritis of her right ankle. (**a**) The preoperative AP view shows a varus deformity with incongruency, overlength fibula, and short dysplastic medial malleolus. (**b**) Total ankle arthroplasty was performed without addressing the medial contracture and the overlength fibula. At 6 weeks of control, the polyethylene is dislocated. (**c**) Clinical views showing the varus deformity of the ankle. The revision surgery included an exchange of the polyethylene insert, a flip osteotomy of the medial malleolus, lateral ligament reconstruction, and a peroneus longus to brevis tendon transfer. (**d**) 12 months after that, the ankle was stable but with a continuous tendency to recurrent varus deformity, as seen with asymmetric wear of the polyethylene insert. (**e**) The persistent varus deformity can also be seen clinically. (**f**) Radiographs of the contralateral ankle also show an ongoing varus osteoarthritis, mainly of the medial compartment, as typically seen in high intrinsic varus forces, which may explain the failure of the primary replacement surgery of the right ankle. Complementary measures, as taken in the revision surgery, could have avoided this complication

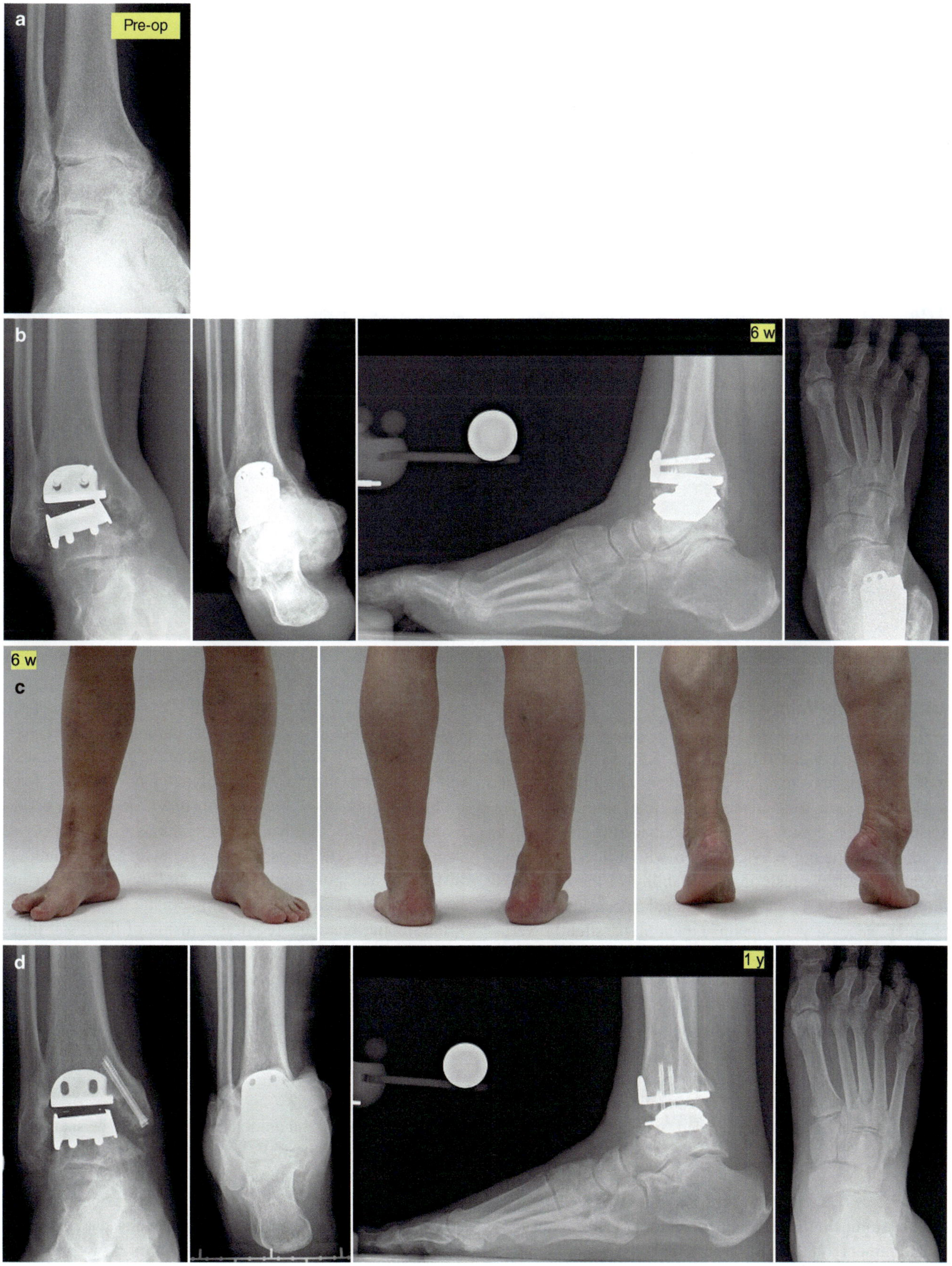
a
Pre-op
b
6 w
6 w
c
d
1 y

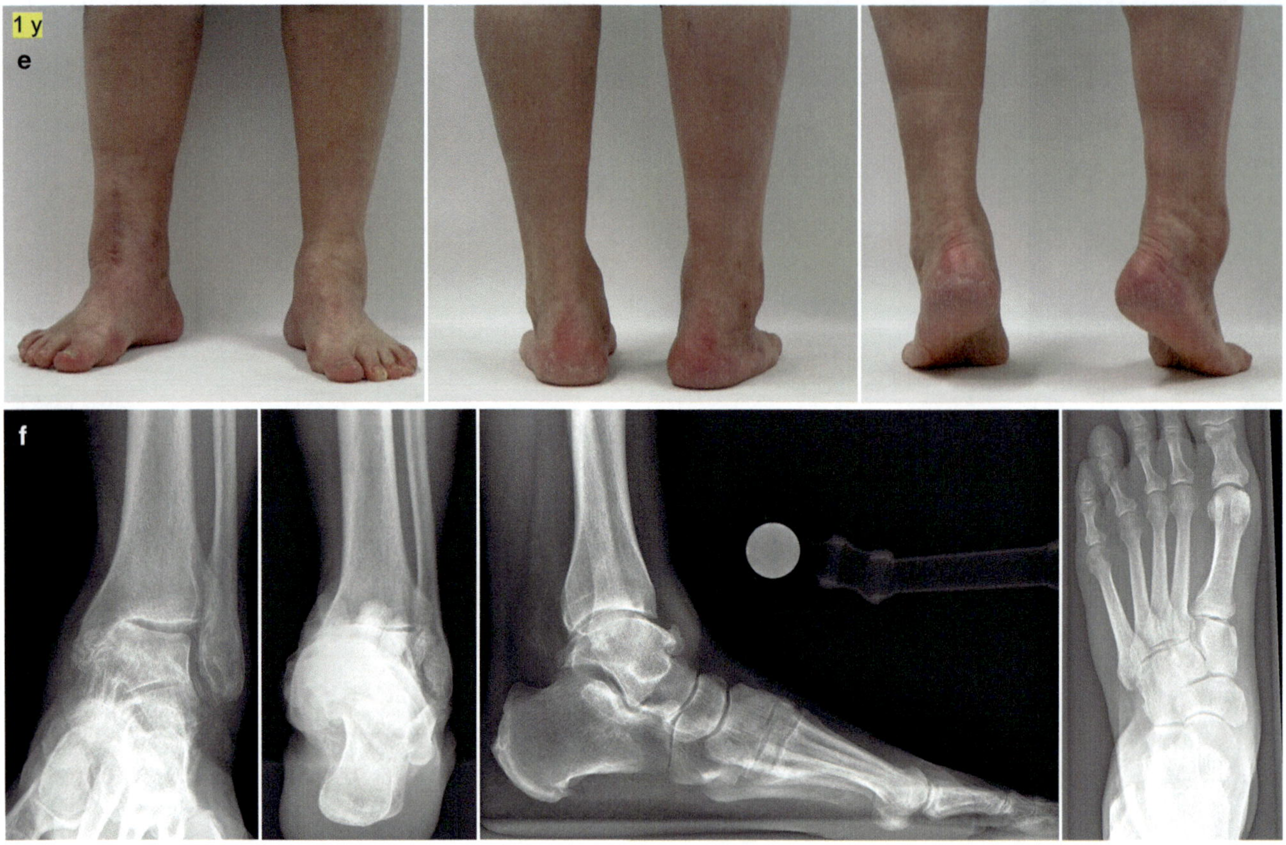

Fig. 14.10 (continued)

14.3.5.2 The Valgus Ankle

The conflicting problem in treating valgus osteoarthritic ankles is that associated incompetence of the medial arch at index arthroplasty may progress even when the foot and ankle were seen well aligned after tightening the deltoid-spring ligament complex [57]. In subtle medial instability, an exchange of the polyethylene insert with a thicker one may be appropriate for restoring the stability of the total ankle arthroplasty (Fig. 14.11). An additional calcaneal osteotomy is often necessary to obtain a neutral or slightly varus-positioned heel. In greater instability with a medial gapping of the ankle of >5mm, a deltoid ligament reconstruction might also be required to distract the ankle with a thicker polyethylene insert. In any case, the medial arch needs to be stabilized with plantar flexing osteotomy or fusions (Fig. 14.12). As the concomitant peritalar instability might be the origin of the progressive destabilizing process, a subtalar joint fusion is recommended, especially in a medial gapping of >10mm.

14.3.5.3 The Incompetent Syndesmosis

Recent studies indicated that soft tissue overload caused by malalignment of the prosthesis components could induce pain [43, 58, 59]. This is especially true when associated with syndesmotic instability present before index total ankle arthroplasty [52]. Additional motion at the interface between the tibial component and the polyethylene insert, as for a mobile-bearing ankle, may also increase the load on periarticular ligaments, thus leading to ligamentous incompetence over time [41, 60]. An association of increased translational instability and polyethylene wear and cyst formation has been suggested (Fig. 14.13). Symptomatic instability of the syndesmotic ligaments requires a fusion of the distal tibiofibular joint (Figs. 9.43 and 14.14). To the authors' experience, simple stabilizing with position screws or tightrope does not sufficiently address the instability.

14.3.6 Stiffness

A stiff ankle after total ankle arthroplasty can be seen in the early stage of recovery [61], but also as a progressive process several years after the replacement surgery [62]. It may be associated with significant pain and restrictions in daily activities; however, most surprisingly, many patients could tolerate stiffness, especially if they had limited motion before

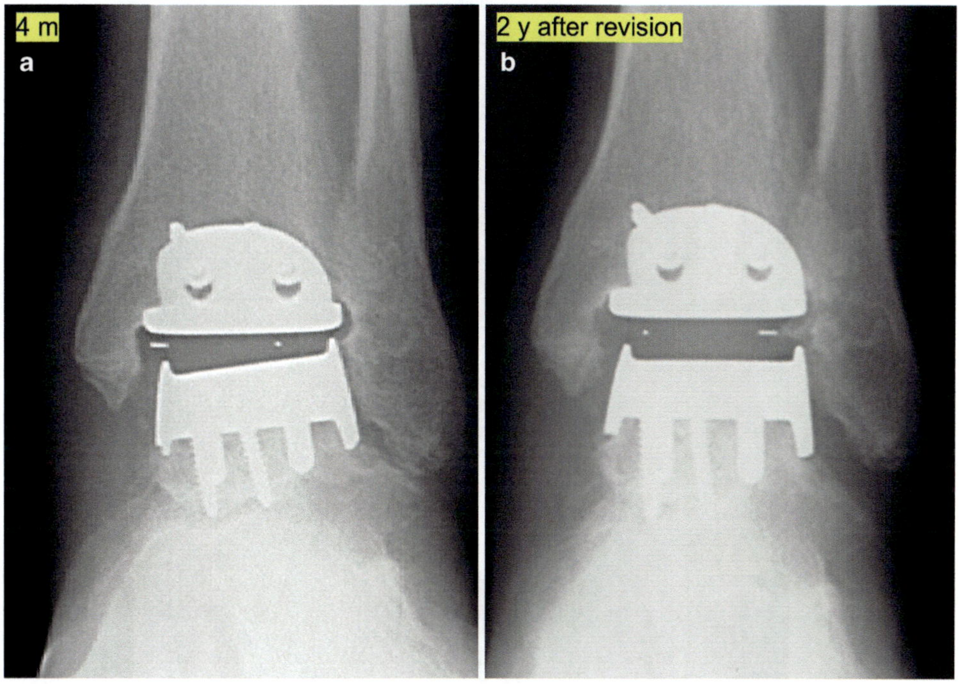

Fig. 14.11 Polyethylene dislocation of a valgus ankle addressed with thicker insert. A 62-year-old teacher underwent total ankle arthroplasty with a mobile-bearing prosthesis for valgus osteoarthritis. (**a**) At a 4-month follow-up, he was delighted with the result and was unaware of any adverse event. However, in the AP view, a gapping of the medial ankle was detected, with a dislocation of the polyethylene insert. (**b**) The ankle was stable and well-balanced 2 years after exchanging the polyethylene insert with a 2-mm-thicker one

the total ankle arthroplasty. Generally, surgical treatment should only be recommended in patients with substantial pain and functional impairment.

Joint stiffness after total ankle arthroplasty is often multifactorial. Prior trauma and previous surgery can cause the thin, soft tissue envelope to become scarred and stiff [6, 46, 63]. Prolonged immobilization, ineffective rehabilitation, poor soft tissue envelope, overstuffing the joint, inadequate soft tissue release, heterotopic bone growth, multiple operations, and previous infection can decrease range of motion [5, 23, 64]. Intraoperatively, surgeon experience determines the optimal thickness of the implant components to maximize the range of motion without sacrificing stability.

14.3.6.1 Diagnosis

In addition to standard radiographs, functional weight-bearing lateral radiographs can be performed in maximal dorsiflexion and plantar flexion. Alternatively, the true ankle motion in the sagittal plane can be assessed using fluoroscopy. A CT scan can help accurately assess the amount of extra bone formation. The degree of radiographic evidence of bony hypertrophy does not necessarily correlate with symptoms and/or physical examination findings. Single-photon emission computed tomography (SPECT CT) may help to identify areas of impingement in those patients with equivocal radiographic studies.

Accurately identifying the structures causing ankle pain and stiffness may be challenging owing to the proximity of the extrinsic tendons of the foot and ankle. Many patients had limited ankle range of motion before replacement surgery, and the resultant motion and excursion can cause pain in these dormant tendons. The most affected tendons are the posterior tibial and flexor hallucis longus tendons.

14.3.6.2 Treatment

A purely isolated anterior stiffness of the replaced ankle is rare and often presents with an incompetent heel cord. The clinical assessment typically reveals some degree of dorsiflexion but only minimal plantar flexion. Therefore, after debridement of the anterior ankle, including the medial and lateral gutter, the improvement in ankle range of motion should be assessed carefully. If there is no significant improvement in either dorsiflexion or plantar flexion, as a next step, the polyethylene insert should be removed, and the posterior ankle structures should be debrided (Fig. 14.15).

If clinical assessment demonstrates a hard stop against dorsiflexion, significant scarring and ossification of the posterior capsule should be expected. In this case, a posterior approach is considered for extended open debridement (Fig. 14.16). After complete posterior debridement, the ankle is mobilized manually into maximal dorsiflexion and plantar flexion. After that, if the achieved dorsiflexion is not satisfactory, an additional release of the heel cord should be considered (Fig. 14.17). However, concomitant triceps surae lengthening in total ankle arthroplasty may reduce the positive work at the ankle joint; thus, it should be done with cau-

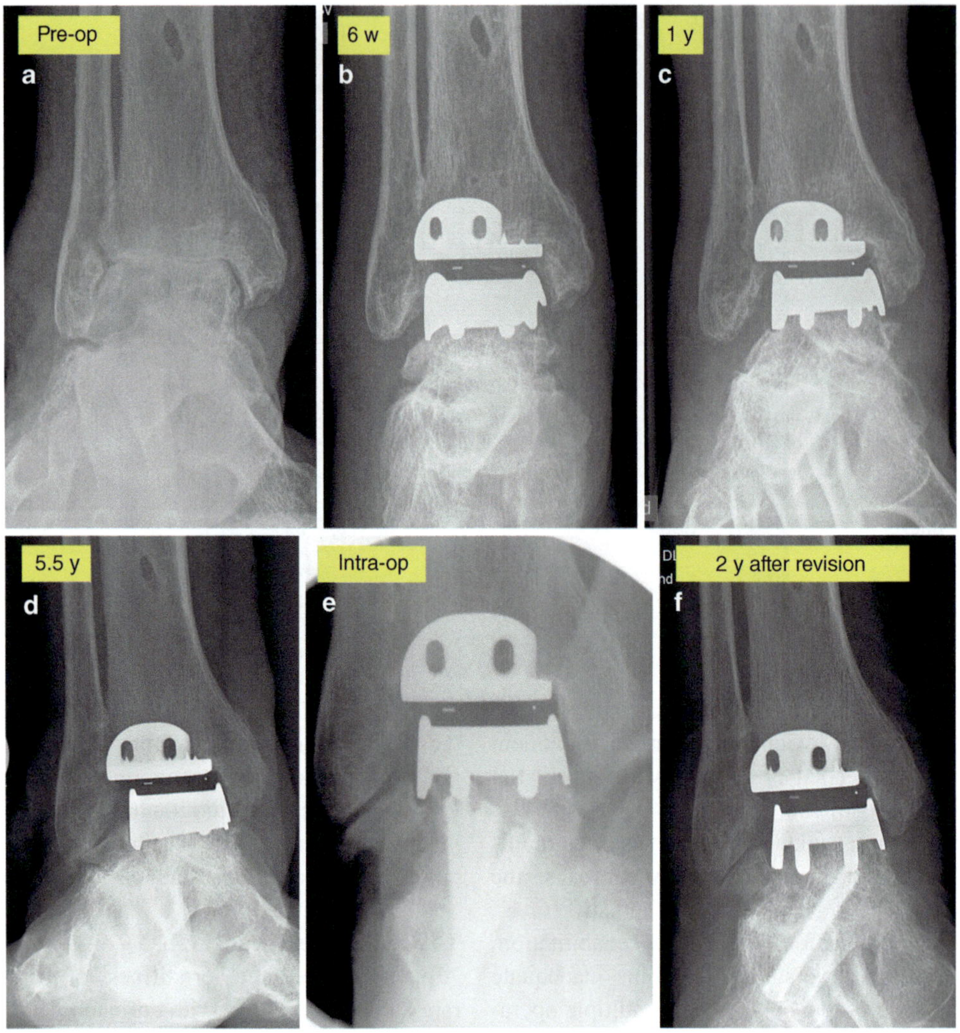

Fig. 14.12 Peritalar instability in a valgus ankle addressed with subtalar fusion. A 67-year-old patient with valgus osteoarthritis. (**a**) Preoperative AP-view showing valgus osteoarthritis of the ankle associated with some valgus at the subtalar joint ("valgus-valgus"-deformity. (**b**) Six weeks after total ankle arthroplasty, the ankle joint complex is seen well-aligned due to tensioning of the ligaments. (**c**) However, after 1 year, a recurrent valgus position of the calcaneus can be seen, associated with a medial translation of the talus, causing some medial gutter pain. (**d**) As the peritalar instability and medial gutter pain increased, a revision was considered after 5.5 years. (**e**) Intraoperative fluoroscopy after subtalar fusion and exchange of the polyethylene liner for a thicker one showing the ankle joint complex aligned. (**f**) Obviously, the screw fixation was not strong enough to resist the deforming forces, with some recurrent valgus deformity occurring until the subtalar fusion finally healed. At the 2-year control, the patient was pain free. He died 1.5 years later due to unrelated causes to the ankle

tion [65]. To prevent postoperative loss of dorsiflexion due to recurrent scarring, we consider the patient at risk of an external fixator for 4–6 weeks (Fig. 14.18).

A thinner polyethylene liner can increase dorsiflexion by removing osteophytes and Achilles tendon lengthening or gastrocnemius recession. When the talar component is too anterior malpositioned, an implant revision is mandatory to achieve an appropriate postoperative outcome.

14.3.7 Periprosthetic Fractures

Periprosthetic fractures following total ankle replacements are uncommon. A postoperative fracture should be categorized as having occurred after a trauma or representing a stress fracture [66–68]. The possibility of implant loosening should always be considered with these fractures.

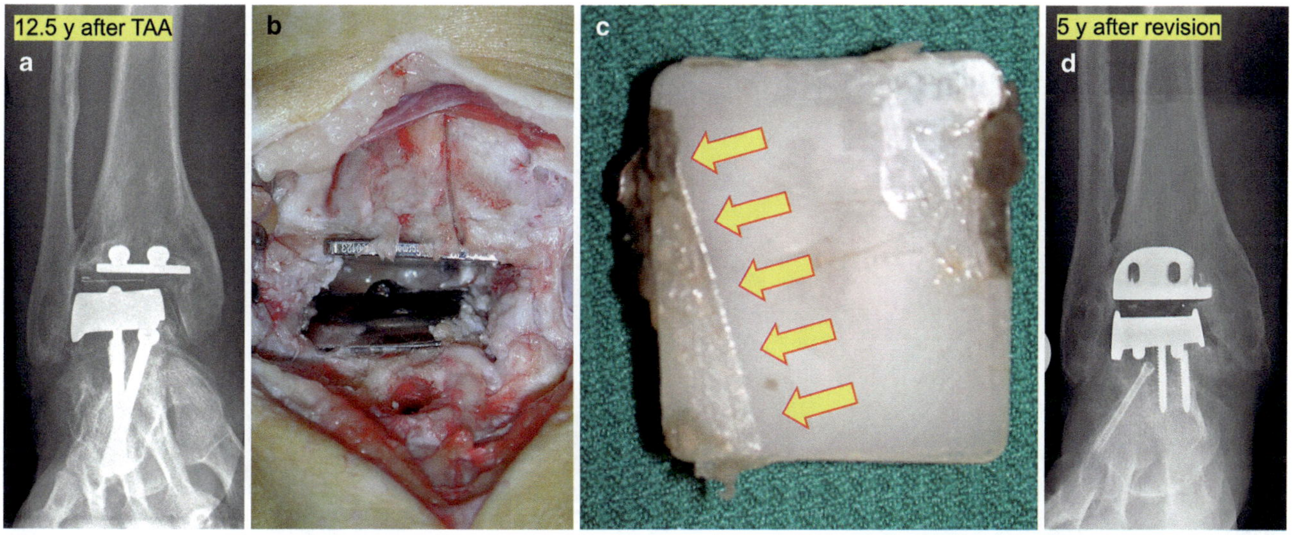

Fig. 14.13 Syndesmotic incompetence with widening of the ankle mortise and subsequent edge load. A 71-year-old former soccer player was treated for post-traumatic osteoarthritis associated with peritalar instability with total ankle arthroplasty and subtalar fusion. The patient complains of lateral ankle pain 12.5 years after total ankle arthroplasty. (**a**) AP view showing a widening of the ankle mortise with lateral translation and varus tilt of the talus due to asymmetric polyethylene wear. Notice the lateral position of the talar component, which may have further increased the edge load of the polyethylene insert. (**b**) Surgical exposure showing the talus's lateral translation and the joint space's asymmetric narrowing. (**c**) Retrieved polyethylene insert showing the wear due to the edge load (arrows). (**d**) The syndesmosis was found stable after the revision of the prosthesis; thus, no stabilization was necessary. At a 5-year follow-up, the ankle was found to be stable, with a well-aligned ankle

14.3.7.1 Trauma-Induced Fractures

Periprosthetic fractures after trauma are typically located at the distal tibia. Based on limited data, stemmed-type prostheses are more prone to sustain a periprosthetic fracture [69, 70]. The fractures should be treated with plate fixation as long as the component is not loose (Fig. 14.19). Periprosthetic fractures associated with component loosening require component revision (Fig. 14.20). In the worst scenario, a fusion may be considered (Fig. 14.21).

14.3.7.2 Stress Fractures

Periprosthetic stress fractures are typically located in the medial malleolus, with a vertical fracture line (Fig. 13.11) [71]. One cause may be a varus malpositioning of the tibial component, causing an increased mechanical load of the medial malleolus. Indicative signs are periosteal appositional bone growth and medial malleolar pain. In contrast, a valgus malpositioning of the component may result in increased traction of the deltoid ligament on the medial malleolus [3]. Theoretically, a medial malleolar stress fracture can also result from an oversized talar component, particularly associated with a varus malpositioning of the tibial component [50].

Identifying the underlying cause is essential for successfully treating periprosthetic stress fractures. Supra- and inframalleolar osteotomies may be considered to eliminate the stress. Vertical medial malleolus fractures should be treated using a compression plate, though they are not dislocated. The authors disagree with others [71] who advocated conservative treatment as the primary measure.

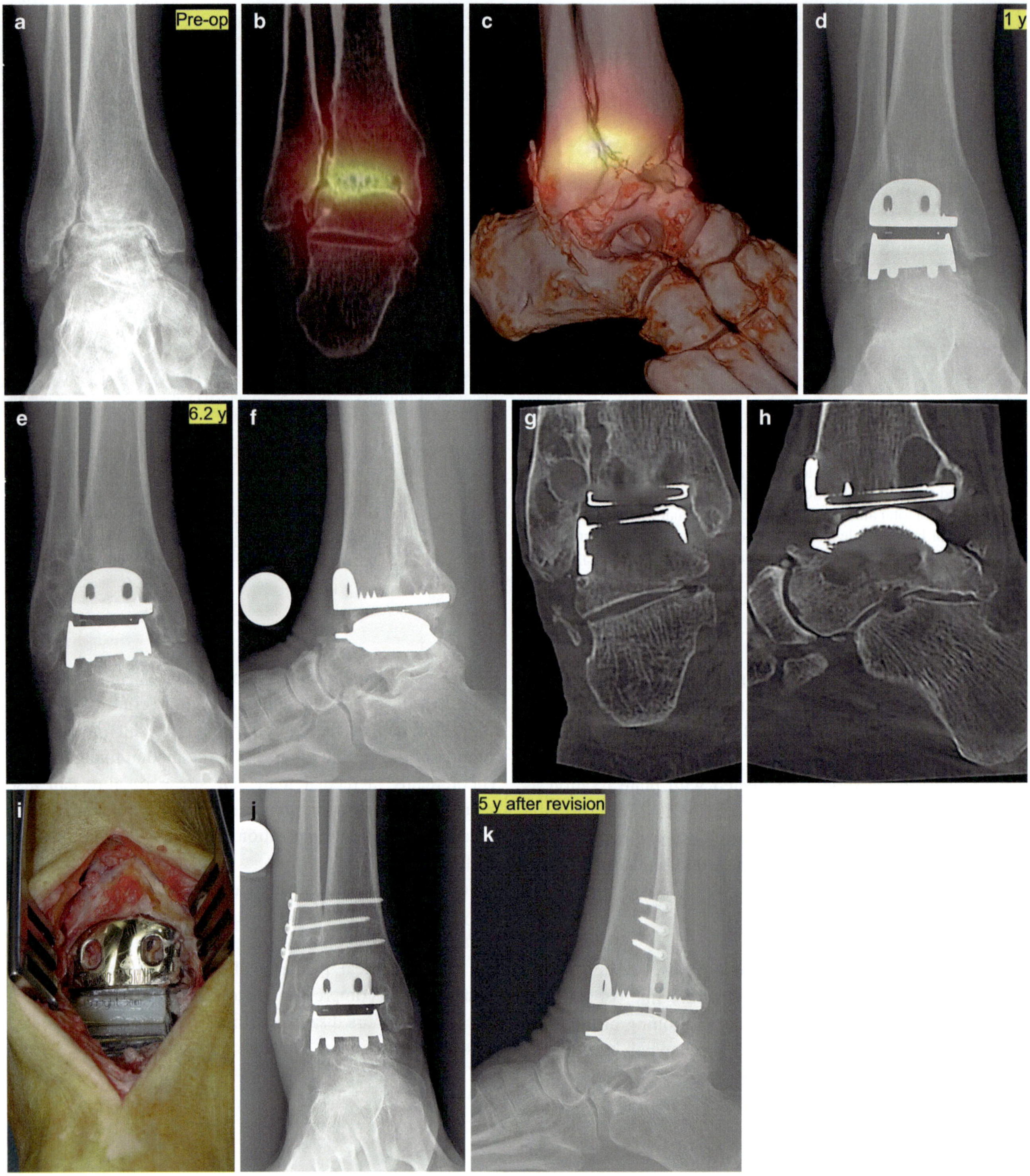

Fig. 14.14 Syndesmotic incompetence requiring a fusion. A 62-year-old manager suffered from posttraumatic osteoarthritis after an ankle fracture over 35 years ago. (**a**) AP view showing bipolar cystic lesions of the tibiotalar joint. (**b**) The spect CT confirms the activity process in this area and the syndesmotic area (**c**). (**d**) One year after the replacement surgery, the AP view shows the ankle well balanced. (**e**, **f**) After 6.2 years, an AP view taken because of sudden pain reveals multiple cyst formations, mainly in the syndesmotic area in the tibia and fibula, as well as lateralization of the talus and some asymmetric wear of the polyethylene insert on the medial side. (**g**, **h**) Weight-bearing CT scans show the extent of the cysts affecting the talar body. (**i**) The surgical exploration shows the polyethylene insert's wear and the talus's lateralization. (**j**, **k**) Five years after the implant exchange, the cysts' revision, and syndesmotic fusion, the ankle is well-aligned with firmly osteointegrated components and no signs of recurrent cyst formation

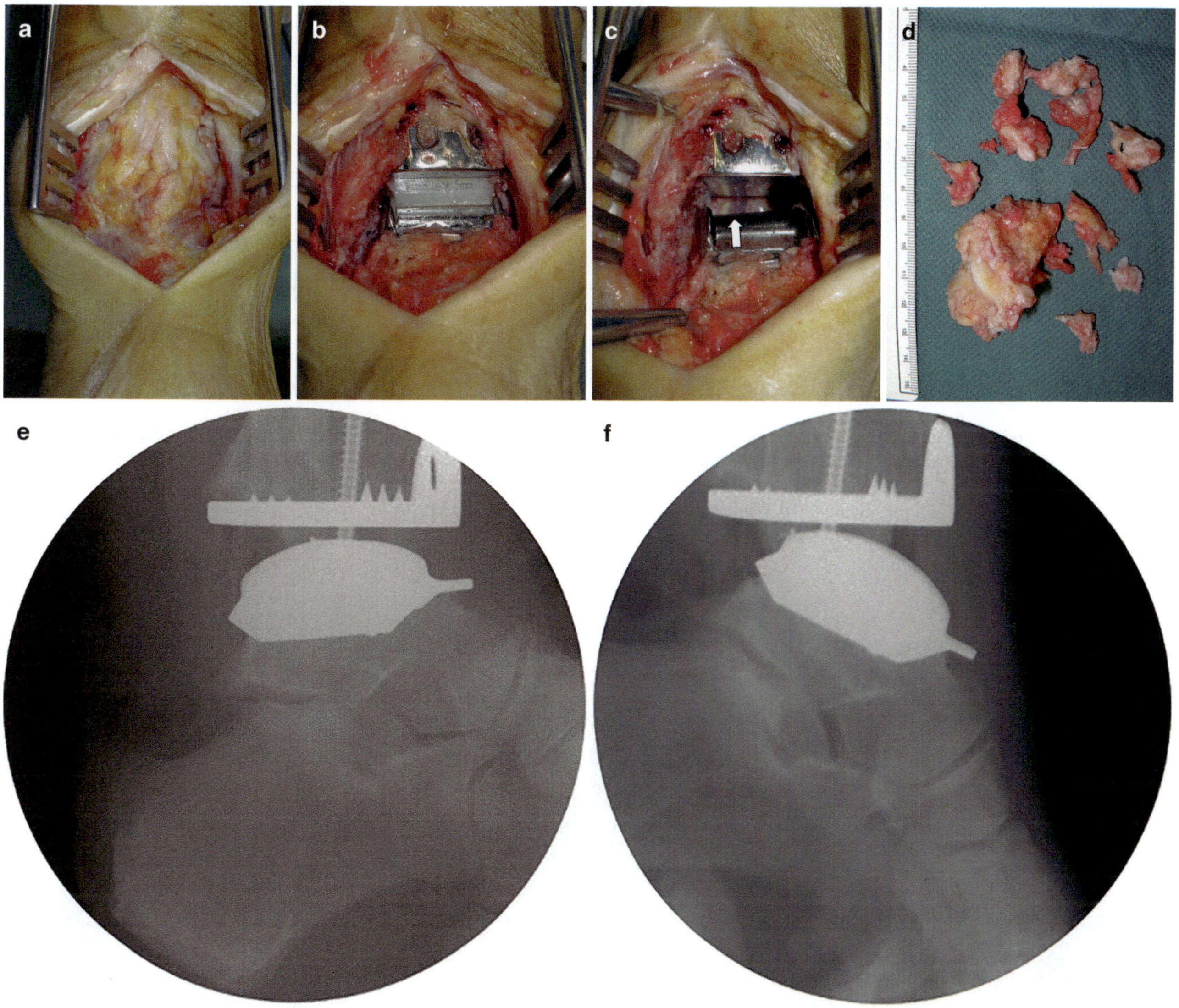

Fig. 14.15 Release of the anterior and posterior capsule through an anterior approach in a mobile-bearing ankle. (**a**) The anterior scarred capsule is exposed through the former anterior approach of index surgery. (**b**) After resection of the anterior scarred capsular structure and ossifications, the medial and lateral gutters are debrided. (**c**) While the ankle is distracted over two K-wires, the polyethylene insert is extracted, which allows access to the posterior capsular and ossification. After careful resection of the posterior scars and ossifications, the flexor hallucis tendon with its muscle can be seen (arrow). (**d**) The resected material includes scarred capsular structures and ossifications. After inserting a new polyethylene insert, the ankle is manually mobilized in maximal dorsiflexion. Gained motion at the ankle joint is checked by fluoroscopy. (**e**) Dorsiflexion; and (**f**) plantarflexion

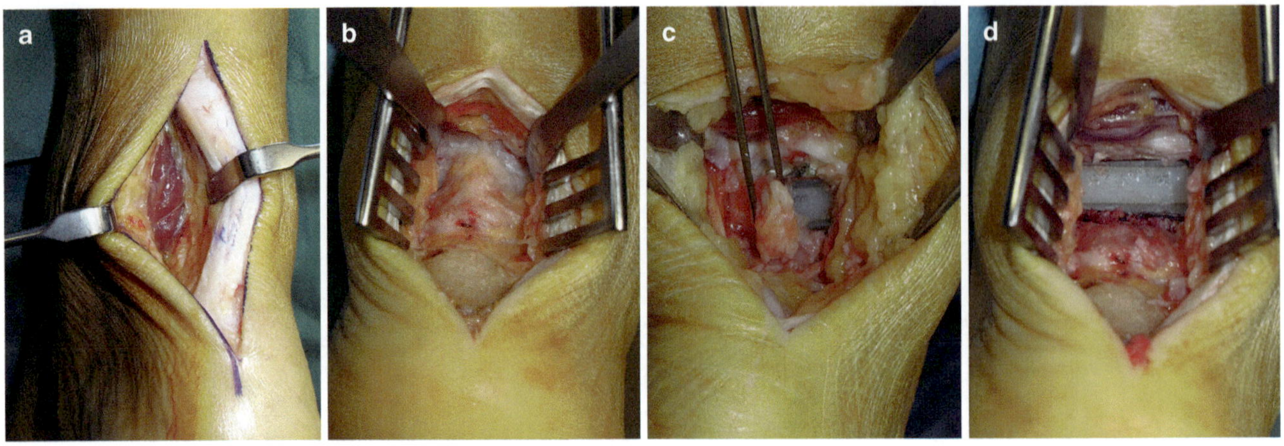

Fig. 14.16 Open release through a posterior approach. (**a**) After a longitudinal incision along the Achilles tendon, the flexor hallucis longus muscle is exposed. This can be done medially, laterally, or through a longitudinal splitting of the Achilles tendon. (**b**) While the flexor hallucis longus muscle is kept medially, the posterior capsule of the ankle is exposed. (**c**) It is step-by-step resected. (**d**) Final situation after complete debridement of posterior scars and ossifications

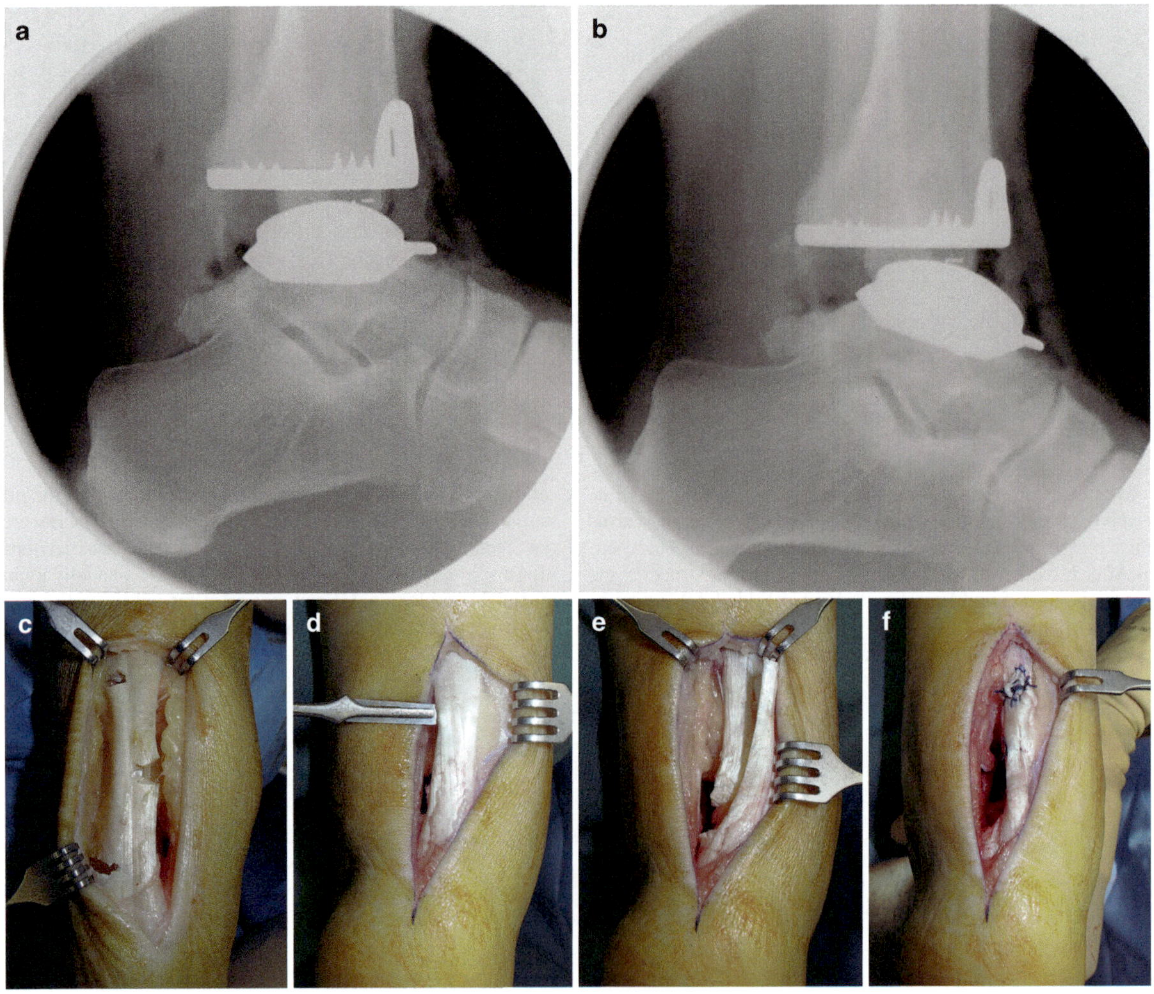

Fig. 14.17 Open release of the Achilles tendon. (**a**) If, after the release of the posterior capsule (Fig. 13.29), dorsiflexion is not, but the plantarflexion is satisfactory (**b**), a lengthening procedure of the Achilles tendon is considered. (**c**) The hemi-triple section technique is used for minor lengthening (<5 mm). (**d**) If a lengthening of >5 mm is needed, the tendon is split by approximately 5 cm in the coronal plane, and the anterior part is dissected at the distal end and the posterior one at the proximal end. (**e**) While dorsiflexion is applied to the foot, the two bundles are seen to glide along each other. (**f**) They are fixed in the wanted position by side-to-side sutures

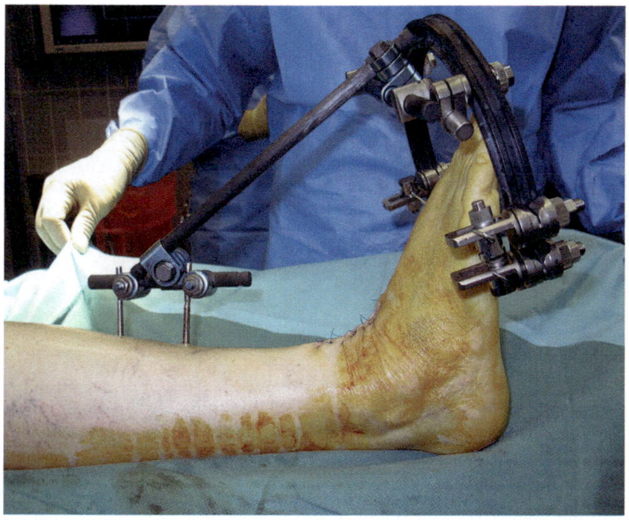

Fig. 14.18 Prevention of recurrent loss of dorsiflexion by an external fixator. An external fixator is used to keep the foot in slight dorsiflexion, thus preventing a loss of the gained dorsiflexion by scarring

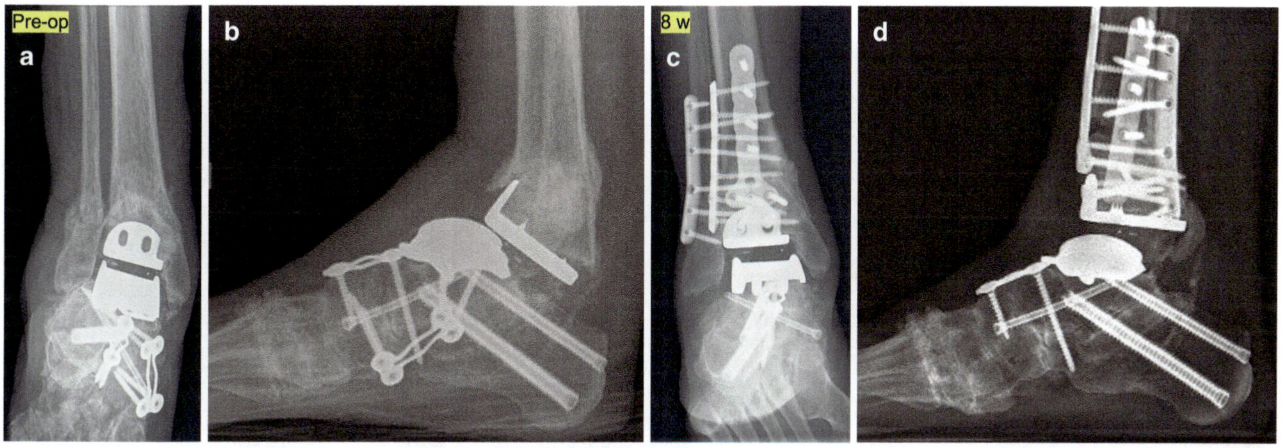

Fig. 14.19 Periprosthetic fracture after trauma without component loosening. This 63-year-old female patient, suffering from rheumatoid arthritis, sustained a periprosthetic right ankle fracture 9.2 years after replacement surgery. Initially unaware of the injury, she walked on her injured foot. (**a**) More than 1 month after the injury, she presented with a foot that deviated into valgus. (**b**) The lateral view shows the extraarticular fracture with impaction of the anterior tibia and an angulation of 40°. The tibia and fibula were mobilized at the fracture site and fixed by plates and screws. (**c**, **d**) After 8 weeks, the fracture is healed with correct ankle alignment

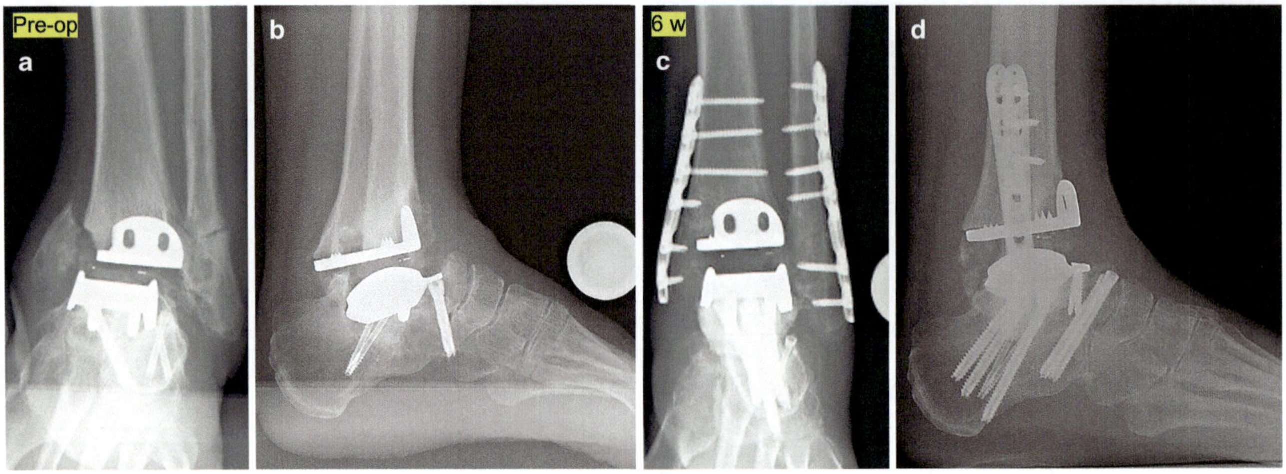

Fig. 14.20 Periprosthetic fracture after trauma with component loosening. This 56-year-old female patient sustained a periprosthetic fracture in a car accident 16.5 years after total ankle arthroplasty and subtalar fusion for post-traumatic osteoarthritis (Talus fracture Hawkins Type 3 at 21 years). (**a**) The AP view shows a bimalleolar fracture with disruption of the tibial component and impaction of the talar component into the talus. (**b**) The amount of subsidence of the talar component is seen in the lateral view. (**c**) Six weeks after internal fixation of the malleoli and exchange of the tibial component, the ankle is well-aligned in the coronal plane. (**d**) The lateral view shows the reconstruction of the talus with bone cement and screw fixation

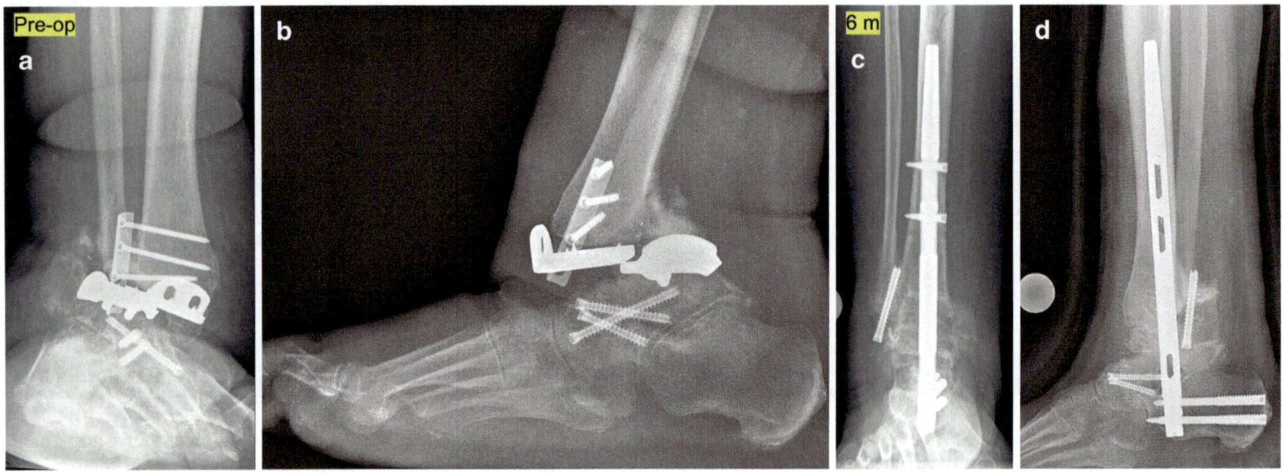

Fig. 14.21 Periprosthetic fracture after trauma revised with fusion. This 74-year-old obese female patient sustained a complex trauma at night while walking to the toilette 14 weeks after total ankle arthroplasty. (**a**, **b**) The AP view shows a tibial component disruption with a significant posterior distal tibia bone defect and a bimalleolar fracture with the translation of the talus in the posterolateral direction. (**c**, **d**) Six months after tibiotalar-calcaneal fusion with an intramedullary nail and fresh-frozen femoral head allograft, the ankle and the hindfoot are well-aligned and stable, permitting the patient to free walking. The further evolution was uneventful

14.4 Conclusions

- Careful clinical and radiographic assessment is mandatory for successful revision.
- Most critical are revision arthroplasties after periprosthetic infections.
- Complications can often be successfully treated without revision of the metallic components.
- Despite a slightly higher risk of failure and reoperation than primary replacement surgery, revision of primary total ankle arthroplasty can be an effective procedure with improved functional outcomes.

References

1. Knecht SI, Estin M, Callaghan JJ, Zimmerman MB, Alliman KJ, Alvine FG, et al. The agility total ankle arthroplasty. Seven to sixteen-year follow-up. J Bone Joint Surg Am. 2004;86(6):1161–71.
2. Whalen JL, Spelsberg SC, Murray P. Wound breakdown after total ankle arthroplasty. Foot Ankle Int. 2010;31(4):301–5.
3. Steck JK, Anderson JB. Total ankle arthroplasty: indications and avoiding complications. Clin Podiatr Med Surg. 2009;26(2):303–24.
4. Farber DC, Deorio JK. Oxygen tensiometry as a predictor of wound healing in total ankle arthroplasty. Acta Orthop Traumatol Turc. 2009;43(5):381–5.
5. Schuberth JM, Steck JK, Christensen JC. Ankle replacement arthroplasty. In: Southerland JTB, Boberg JS, Downey MS, editors. Mcglarmy's comprehensive textbook of foot and ankle surgery. 4th ed. Philadelphia: Wolters/Kluwer//Lippincott Williams & Wilkins Health; 2012. p. 717–56.
6. Conti SF, Wong YS. Complications of total ankle replacement. Foot Ankle Clin. 2002;7(4):791–807. vii
7. Raikin SM, Kane J, Ciminiello ME. Risk factors for incision-healing complications following total ankle arthroplasty. J Bone Joint Surg Am. 2010;92(12):2150–5.
8. Meeker J, Wegner N, Francisco R. Revision techniques in total ankle arthroplasty utilizing a stemmed tibial arthroplasty system. Tech Foot Ankle Surg. 2013;12(2):99–108.
9. Choi WJ, Lee JS, Lee M, Park JH, Lee JW. The impact of diabetes on the short- to mid-term outcome of total ankle replacement. Bone Joint J. 2014;96-B(12):1674–80.
10. Steck JK, Schuberth JM, Christensen JC, Luu CA. Revision total ankle arthroplasty. Clin Podiatr Med Surg. 2017;34(4):541–64.
11. Glazebrook MA, Arsenault K, Dunbar M. Evidence-based classification of complications in total ankle arthroplasty. Foot Ankle Int. 2009;30(10):945–9.
12. Hintermann B, Zwicky L, Knupp M, Henninger HB, Barg A. HINTEGRA revision arthroplasty for failed total ankle prostheses: surgical technique. JBJS Essent Surg Tech. 2014;3(2):e12.
13. Hallock GG. The role of free flaps for salvage of the exposed total ankle arthroplasty. Microsurgery. 2017;37(1):34–7.
14. Gross CE, Garcia R, Adams SB, DeOrio JK, Easley ME, Nunley JA 2nd. Soft tissue reconstruction after total ankle arthroplasty. Foot Ankle Int. 2016;37(5):522–7.
15. Fukui A, Tanaka Y, Inada Y, Samato N, Ito K, Oshima M, et al. Turndown retinacular flap for closure of skin fistula after total ankle replacement. Foot Ankle Int. 2008;29(6):624–6.
16. Yamamoto T, Saito T, Ishiura R, Iida T. Quadruple-component superficial circumflex iliac artery perforator (SCIP) flap: a chimeric SCIP flap for complex ankle reconstruction of an exposed artificial joint after total ankle arthroplasty. J Plast Reconstr Aesthet Surg. 2016;69(9):1260–5.
17. Trebse R, Pisot V, Trampuz A. Treatment of infected retained implants. J Bone Joint Surg Br. 2005;87(2):249–56.
18. D'Errico M, Morelli I, Castellini G, Gianola S, Logoluso N, Romanò D, Scarponi S, Pellegrini A. Is debridement really the best we can do for periprosthetic joint infections following total ankle replacements? A systematic review andinfections following total ankle replacements? A systematic review and meta-analysis. Foot Ankle Surg. 2022;28:697–708.
19. Triantafyllopoulos GK, Poultsides LA, Sakellariou VI, Zhang W, Sculco PK, Ma Y, et al. Irrigation and debridement for periprosthetic infections of the hip and factors determining outcome. Int Orthop. 2015;39(6):1203–9.
20. Triantafyllopoulos GK, Poultsides LA, Zhang W, Sculco PK, Ma Y, Sculco TP. Periprosthetic knee infections treated with irrigation and debridement: outcomes and preoperative predictive factors. J Arthroplasty. 2015;30(4):649–57.
21. Alrashidi Y, Galhoum AE, Wiewiorski M, Herrera-Perez M, Hsu RY, Barg A, et al. How to diagnose and treat infection in total ankle arthroplasty. Foot Ankle Clin. 2017;22(2):405–23.
22. Kessler B, Knupp M, Graber P, Zwicky L, Hintermann B, Zimmerli W, et al. The treatment and outcome of peri-prosthetic infection of the ankle: a single cohort-centre experience of 34 cases. Bone Joint J. 2014;96-B(6):772–7.
23. Hintermann B, Zwicky L, Knupp M, Henninger HB, Barg A. HINTEGRA revision arthroplasty for failed total ankle prostheses. J Bone Joint Surg Am. 2013;95(13):1166–74.
24. Horisberger M, Henninger HB, Valderrabano V, Barg A. Bone augmentation for revision total ankle arthroplasty with large bone defects. Acta Orthop. 2015;86(4):412–4.
25. Conti MS, Irwin TA, Ford SE, Jones CP, Anderson RB, Davis WH. Complications, reoperations, and patient-reported outcomes following a 2-stage revision total ankle arthroplasty for chronic periprosthetic joint infections. Foot Ankle Int. 2022;43(12):1614–21.
26. Trampuz A, Piper KE, Jacobson MJ, Hanssen AD, Unni KK, Osmon DR, et al. Sonication of removed hip and knee prostheses for diagnosis of infection. N Engl J Med. 2007;357(7):654–63.
27. Joseph TN, Chen AL, Di Cesare PE. Use of antibiotic-impregnated cement in total joint arthroplasty. J Am Acad Orthop Surg. 2003;11(1):38–47.
28. Myerson MS, Shariff R, Zonno AJ. The management of infection following total ankle replacement: demographics and treatment. Foot Ankle Int. 2014;35(9):855–62.
29. Lee HS, Ahn JY, Lee JS, Lee JY, Jeong JJ, Choi YR. Cement arthroplasty for ankle joint destruction. J Bone Joint Surg Am. 2014;96(17):1468–75.
30. Gross C, Erickson BJ, Adams SB, Parekh SG. Ankle arthrodesis after failed total ankle replacement: a systematic review of the literature. Foot Ankle Spec. 2015;8(2):143–51.
31. Espinosa N, Wirth SH. Revision of the aseptic and septic total ankle replacement. Clin Podiatr Med Surg. 2013;30(2):171–85.
32. Doets HC, Zurcher AW. Salvage arthrodesis for failed total ankle arthroplasty. Acta Orthop. 2010;81(1):142–7.
33. Rahm S, Klammer G, Benninger E, Gerber F, Farshad M, Espinosa N. Inferior results of salvage arthrodesis after failed ankle replacement compared to primary arthrodesis. Foot Ankle Int. 2015;36(4):349–59.
34. Patton D, Kiewiet N, Brage M. Infected total ankle arthroplasty: risk factors and treatment options. Foot Ankle Int. 2015;36(6):626–34.
35. Kamrad I, Henricson A, Magnusson H, Carlsson A, Rosengren BE. Outcome after salvage arthrodesis for failed total ankle replacement. Foot Ankle Int. 2016;37(3):255–61.
36. Mondal S, Ghosh R. Effects of implant orientation and implant material on tibia bone strain, implant-bone micromotion, contact pressure, and wear depth due to total ankle replacement. Proc Inst Mech Eng H. 2019;233(3):318–31.
37. Sopher RS, Amis AA, Calder JD, Jeffers JRT. Total ankle replacement design and positioning affect implant-bone micromotion and bone strains. Med Eng Phys. 2017;42:80–90.
38. Conti SF, Wong YS. Complications of total ankle replacement. Clin Orthop Relat Res. 2001;391:105–14.
39. Gaudot F, Colombier JA, Bonnin M, Judet T. A controlled, comparative study of a fixed-bearing versus mobile-bearing ankle arthroplasty. Foot Ankle Int. 2014;35(2):131–40.
40. Kurup HV, Taylor GR. Medial impingement after ankle replacement. Int Orthop. 2008;32(2):243–6.
41. Yi Y, Cho JH, Kim JB, Kim JY, Park SY, Lee WC. Change in talar translation in the coronal plane after mobile-bearing total ankle replacement and its association with lower-limb and hindfoot alignment. J Bone Joint Surg Am. 2017;99(4):e13.
42. Hintermann B, Barg A, Knupp M. Revision arthroplasty of the ankle joint. Orthopade. 2011;40(11):1000–7.

43. Deforth M, Krahenbuhl N, Zwicky L, Knupp M, Hintermann B. Supramalleolar osteotomy for tibial component malposition in total ankle replacement. Foot Ankle Int. 2017;38(9):952–6.
44. Barg A, Suter T, Zwicky L, Knupp M, Hintermann B. Medial pain syndrome in patients with total ankle replacement. Orthopade. 2011;40(11):991–2. 4–9
45. Franz AC, Krahenbuhl N, Ruiz R, Susdorf R, Horn-Lang T, Barg A, et al. Hindfoot balancing in total ankle replacement: the role of supramalleolar osteotomies. Int Orthop. 2020;44(9):1859–67.
46. Hintermann B. Total ankle arthroplasty—historical overview, current concepts and future perspectives. Wien-New York: Springer; 2004. 195 p
47. Haskell A, Mann RA. Perioperative complication rate of total ankle replacement is reduced by surgeon experience. Foot Ankle Int. 2004;25(5):283–9.
48. Schuberth JM, Babu NS, Richey JM, Christensen JC. Gutter impingement after total ankle arthroplasty. Foot Ankle Int. 2013;34(3):329–37.
49. Wood PL, Karski MT, Watmough P. Total ankle replacement: the results of 100 mobility total ankle replacements. J Bone Joint Surg Br. 2010;92(7):958–62.
50. Wood PL, Deakin S. Total ankle replacement. The results in 200 ankles. J Bone Joint Surg Br. 2003;85(3):334–41.
51. Simonson DC, Roukis TS. Incidence of complications during the surgeon learning curve period for primary total ankle replacement: a systematic review. Clin Podiatr Med Surg. 2015;32(4):473–82.
52. Ruiz R, Susdorf R, Krahenbuhl N, Barg A, Hintermann B. Syndesmotic overload in 3-component total ankle replacement. Foot Ankle Int. 2020;41(3):275–85.
53. Kim JB, Yi Y, Kim JY, Cho JH, Kwon MS, Choi SH, et al. Weightbearing computed tomography findings in varus ankle osteoarthritis: abnormal internal rotation of the talus in the axial plane. Skeletal Radiol. 2017;46(8):1071–80.
54. Kim JB, Park CH, Ahn JY, Kim J, Lee WC. Characteristics of medial gutter arthritis on weightbearing CT and plain radiograph. Skeletal Radiol. 2021;50(8):1575–83.
55. Veljkovic A, Norton A, Salat P, Abbas KZ, Saltzman C, Femino JE, et al. Sagittal distal tibial articular angle and the relationship to talar subluxation in total ankle arthroplasty. Foot Ankle Int. 2016;37(9):929–37.
56. Hintermann B, Ruiz R. Total replacement of varus ankle: three-component prosthesis design. Foot Ankle Clin. 2019;24(2):305–24.
57. Brunner SK, Knupp M, Hintermann B. Total ankle replacement for the valgus unstable osteoarthritic ankle. Foot Ankle Tech. 2010;9:174–9.
58. Hintermann B, Valderrabano V, Dereymaeker G, Dick W. The HINTEGRA ankle: rationale and short-term results of 122 consecutive ankles. Clin Orthop Relat Res. 2004;424:57–68.
59. Younger A, Veljkovic A. Current update in total ankle arthroplasty: salvage of the failed total ankle arthroplasty with anterior translation of the talus. Foot Ankle Clin. 2017;22(2):301–9.
60. Lewis G. Biomechanics of and research challenges in uncemented total ankle replacement. Clin Orthop Relat Res. 2004;424:89–97.
61. Hintermann B, Ruiz R, Barg A. Dealing with the stiff ankle: preoperative and late occurrence. Foot Ankle Clin. 2017;22(2):425–53.
62. Brunner S, Barg A, Knupp M, Zwicky L, Kapron AL, Valderrabano V, et al. The Scandinavian total ankle replacement: long-term, eleven to fifteen-year, survivorship analysis of the prosthesis in seventy-two consecutive patients. J Bone Joint Surg Am. 2013;95(8):711–8.
63. Johnson LG, Anastasio AT, Fletcher AN, Hendren S, Adams SB. Outcomes following total talus replacement: a systematic review. Foot Ankle Surg. 2022;28(8):1194–201.
64. Jonck JH, Myerson MS. Revision total ankle replacement. Foot Ankle Clin. 2012;17(4):687–706.
65. Deleu PA, Naaim A, Cheze L, Dumas R, Devos Bevernage B, Birch I, et al. Concomitant triceps surae lengthening in total ankle arthroplasty affects the mechanical work at the ankle joint. Foot Ankle Int. 2023;44(8):754–62.
66. Lundeen GA, Dunaway LJ. Etiology and treatment of delayed-onset medial malleolar pain following total ankle arthroplasty. Foot Ankle Int. 2016;37(8):822–8.
67. Zaidi R, Cro S, Gurusamy K, Siva N, Macgregor A, Henricson A, et al. The outcome of total ankle replacement: a systematic review and meta-analysis. Bone Joint J. 2013;95-B(11):1500–7.
68. Cody EA, Lachman JR, Gausden EB, Nunley JA 2nd, Easley ME. Lower bone density on preoperative computed tomography predicts periprosthetic fracture risk in total ankle arthroplasty. Foot Ankle Int. 2019;40(1):1–8.
69. Yang JH, Kim HJ, Yoon JR, Yoon YC. Minimally invasive plate osteosynthesis (MIPO) for periprosthetic fracture after total ankle arthroplasty: a case report. Foot Ankle Int. 2011;32(2):200–4.
70. Haendlmayer KT, Fazly FM, Harris NJ. Periprosthetic fracture after total ankle replacement: surgical technique. Foot Ankle Int. 2009;30(12):1233–4.
71. Manegold S, Haas NP, Tsitsilonis S, Springer A, Mardian S, Schaser KD. Periprosthetic fractures in total ankle replacement: classification system and treatment algorithm. J Bone Joint Surg Am. 2013;95(9):815–20. S1–3

Revision Arthroplasty for Failed Ankles

15

Over the past two decades, total ankle arthroplasty has become a viable and effective alternative to ankle fusion to treat end-stage osteoarthritis [1–9]. Biomechanical and clinical studies have shown improved movement transfer in the ankle joint complex and better pain relief and postoperative function in a replaced ankle than in a fused ankle [10, 11]. Consequently, midtarsal joints are preserved from non-physiologic load and subsequent degenerative changes, possibly affecting long-term clinical outcomes [12]. New implant designs and improvements in surgical techniques have widened the indication for total ankle arthroplasty to younger patients with more pronounced deformities, but overall implant survival after total ankle arthroplasty remains lower than after total hip arthroplasty and total knee arthroplasty [13–17]. As the number of ankle arthroplasties increases, so will the total number of patients requiring further surgery for failure.

15.1 Basic Considerations

The complexity of the procedure depends on the prosthetic design, instrumentation, indication, and the surgeon's experience and constitutes a great challenge for the foot and ankle surgeon. The long learning curve is well documented [18–20]. Deformity at or below the ankle joint or in combination can be challenging to handle and is one of the main reasons for failure [8, 21–25]. Altogether, the procedure of total ankle arthroplasty results in a substantial number of secondary procedures that may be named "revisions," "reoperations," or "additional procedures."

Anderson et al. [26] and Carlsson [19] used revision for any reason in their articles, but when scrutinizing their studies, it is evident that this concept includes the removal or exchange of one or more of the metallic components or exchange of the polyethylene meniscus in case of wear or fracture. Failed total ankle arthroplasty in the studies by Spirt et al. [27] and Hosman et al. [28] implies removing or replacing components, arthrodesis, or a below-knee amputation. It is generally accepted that revision constitutes manipulating one or two metal components [25, 29–33].

The most challenging issues in revision total ankle arthroplasty are achieving solid tibial and/or talar fixation on a residual bone stock without violating the subtalar joint, restoring ligamentous tensioning, and correcting hindfoot/forefoot alignment. The status of the soft-tissue envelope is a key aspect of revision surgery that directs the surgical approach to avoid potential wound complications. This section discusses the most common complications of failed total ankle arthroplasties with revision solutions constituting manipulation of metallic implants.

15.2 Indications

Factors that should be considered include the following: symptoms, pain, subsidence, alignment, bone stock, infection, and component integrity [34, 35]. The most common early complications are ligament imbalance or component: malpositioning, subsidence, and impingement. Typically, late complications are due to wear of the polyethylene liner, either from normal wear or malalignment, aseptic loosening and osteolysis, usually from polyethylene debris, or recurrent and or progressive frontal or sagittal plane deformity. Early recognition of these complications will lessen the complexity of the revision surgery necessary to yield a functional prosthesis.

15.3 Planning the Surgery

When faced with a failing or failed total ankle, the surgeon must decide between a complex revision arthroplasty, salvage procedures that include conversion to fusion, cement block interposition, and amputation [32, 36]. With significant bone loss, conversion to arthrodesis is difficult because

B. Hintermann, R. Ruiz, *Total Ankle Replacement*, https://doi.org/10.1007/978-3-031-56810-7_15

of the loss of structural bone support and the inability to place adequate fixation. This can be further complicated by nonunion and progressive arthritis of adjacent joints [21, 37–39]. If standard components are insufficient, a different prosthesis or larger components can be used with a bone graft [36, 37, 40]. Custom components can also be ordered to fit the anatomic constraints of revision better [41]. Recently, total talar replacement has also been proposed [42–44].

When the surgeon is considering revising a failed total ankle arthroplasty, a major challenge might be the loss of original references and bony contours, particularly in the presence of significant bone loss. Hodel et al. [45] used 3D triangular surface models of 96 paired lower legs that underwent a surface registration algorithm to superimpose the mirrored contralateral lower leg onto the original lower leg to approximate the original ankle joint line. The contralateral tibia and fibula reliably approximated the original ankle joint line. The contralateral distal fibular tip, anterior and posterior medial colliculi, anterior distal tibia angle (ADTA), and lateral distal tibia angle (LDTA) can be used reliably to plan revision total ankle arthroplasty with minor side-to-side differences reported.

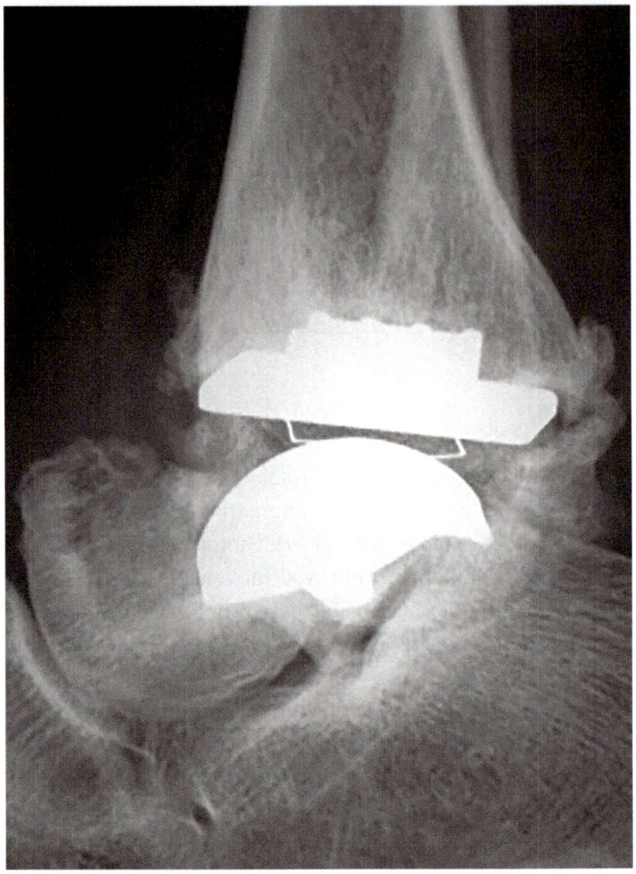

Fig. 15.1 Subsidence of talar component violating the subtalar joint. Lateral view of an ankle 12 years after total ankle arthroplasty with subsidence of talar component violating the subtalar joint

15.4 Solutions in Revision Arthroplasty

15.4.1 Subsidence

Subsidence is when a component migrates deeper into the osseous substrate [36, 39]. Minor subsidence is expected as a physiological process postoperatively and typically decreases at 3 months and stops at approximately 6 months. If component migration persists after 6 months, it usually indicates unstable bone-implant interfaces. On radiographs, component migration equal to or greater than 5 mm or 5° is considered unstable [46]. Talar component subsidence is more common than tibial component subsidence, probably due to decreased peripheral cortical coverage (Fig. 13.21). This can progress until the talar component violates the subtalar joint (Fig. 15.1). Tibial component subsidence is infrequent and will occur more posteriorly with osseous lipping surrounding the posterior edge of the implant (Fig. 15.2) [24]. This is particularly true with implants that do not cover the posterior cortex of the tibia.

Periprosthetic osteolysis can be asymptomatic but progressively increase in size and lead to component loosening, subsidence, and implant failure [47]. The cause of osteolysis can be mechanically related to stress shielding, biomechanically because of the wear particles of the prosthesis or biologically caused by remodeling. The design of total ankle arthroplasty is highly relevant to its biomechanical behavior and, therefore, influences overall results [48, 49]. Theoretically, any compromise of vascularity of the talus could lead to early component subsidence and malposition [50]. Another cause for subsidence is avascular necrosis of the talus. If a component is implanted on top of an avascular bone, it might fail because there will not be bone ingrowth into the prosthesis (Fig. 13.20). Therefore, inevitable loosening and subsidence will develop. Not sufficiently addressing malalignment and the component placement's malposition always leads to failure due to increased focal stress, edge loading, and subsidence risk [51].

15.4.1.1 Diagnosis

Revision surgery for subsidence must include a workup of why the subsidence occurred in the first place. The surgeon should be convinced that the underlying cause will be addressed before or during surgery.

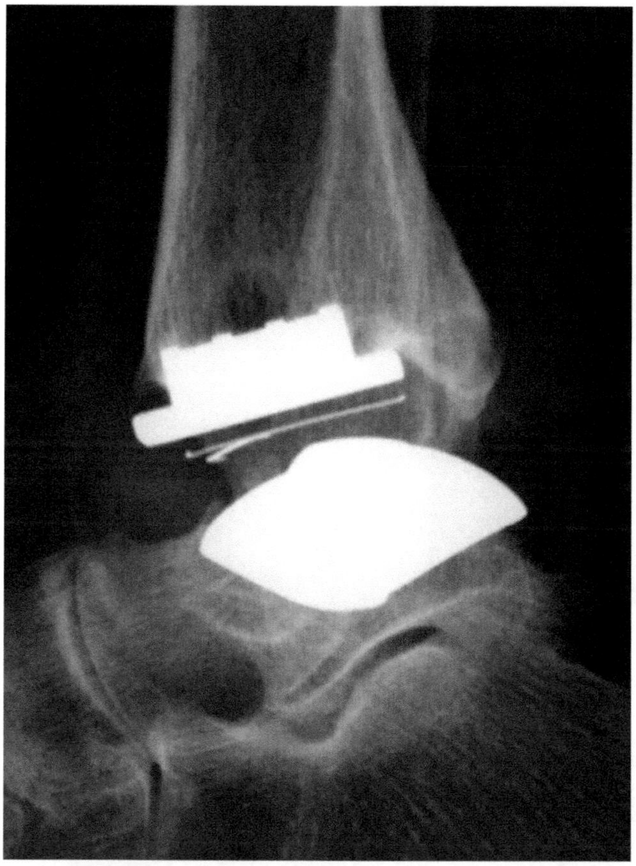

Fig. 15.2 Subsidence of tibial component. Lateral view of an ankle 8.5 years after total ankle arthroplasty with posterior subsidence of the tibial component. As it was undersized, there was not sufficient bone support on the posterior aspect

15.4.1.2 Treatment

Management of component subsidence is challenging because there is always bone loss and sometimes massive bone loss, which can be caused by direct mechanical erosion, periprosthetic osteolysis, or necrotic changes of the underlying trabecular bone [52]. With revision surgery, the joint line must be restored with a combination of bone graft (Fig. 15.3), cement (Fig. 15.4), and revision components that can replace the periarticular bone loss that is typically encountered. Limitations exist on revision components, and polyethylene thicknesses are also improved but limited. Therefore, the surgeon is usually left to devise a bone graft and cement plan to compensate for the bone loss caused by subsidence.

The Authors' Experience

As osteolysis and cyst formations are usually very slow processes, the simultaneous loss of bone support is compensated by remodeling the remaining bone, thereby ensuring the stability of the implant. When revising the ankle implants, it is thus of utmost importance to preserve the remodeled bone and use as much available genuine bone as possible to support the new implants. The defects must be carefully filled with auto- or allograft, and a bone matrix product may be used to seal the defects. Though not proven, there is evidence that penetration of synovial fluid can provoke recurrent cyst formation.

Alternatively, a custom-made talar component that compensates for bone loss and can preserve movement can be considered (Fig. 15.5) [41]. A total talar replacement was also recently proposed (Fig. 6.3) [43, 44, 53, 54].

The Authors' Experience

The meticulous reconstruction of the Chopart joint is paramount in treating a substantial loss of the talar body. Whenever possible, the talar head fragment should be preserved even when small and be used for getting a fusion to the calcaneus. This would also allow for a salvage tibiocalcaneal fusion without including the talonavicular joint, should the replacement surgery fail, a revision becomes necessary.

15.4.2 Polyethylene Wear and Aseptic Loosening

Aseptic loosening is one major cause of decreased longevity in total ankle arthroplasty. It can cause the implant to loosen prematurely [36, 55–57], with an incidence of 3.2–19% in the literature [58–61], which necessitates revision in 40–85% of cases [59, 60, 62, 63]. It is defined as noninfectious bone loss and is commonly used synonymously with osteolysis. Poor component alignment and an incongruent polyethylene articulation, often due to recurrent hindfoot or ankle malalignment, are thought to be the leading causes of osteolysis [64]. The rates of osteolysis can also vary significantly with different designs of total ankle arthroplasty. However, there can also be considerable variability in the progression rates of osteolysis, even in implants of the same design [64].

Multiple factors, including activity, quality, design of the insert, and placement, influence polyethylene wear rate [36]. In an analysis of 10 failed agility ankles, Vaupel et al. [65] noticed six wear patterns on polyethylene liners: burnishing, embedding, grooving/scratching, pitting, dishing, and abrasion. They called the area of the polyethylene liner with the most surface damage the "talar footprint," representing the area in which the talar component was primarily articulating. They also found titanium particles in the talar footprint of the retrieved liners demonstrating third body wear. Kobayashi et al. [66] analyzed polyethylene particles from synovial

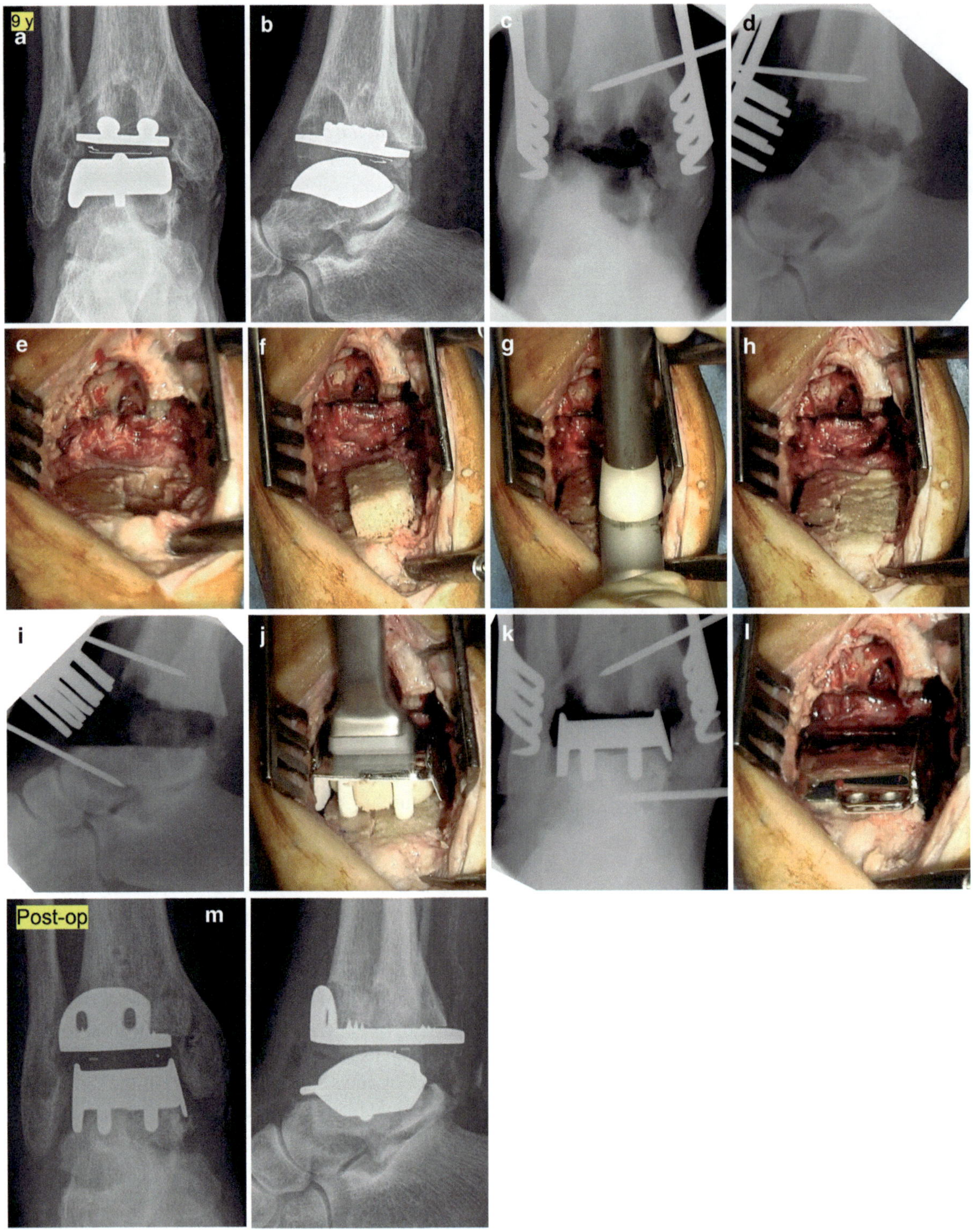

Fig. 15.3 Revision of subsided component with allograft augmentation. A 56-year-old heavy worker, 9 years after the total ankle arthroplasty, complained about some mild pain in his ankle. (**a**, **b**) The standard radiographs show significant osteolysis and cyst formation around both components and minor subsidence of the talar component. (**c**, **d**) The extent of bone loss becomes apparent after implant removal, reaching the talar head. (**e**) Remaining talar bone after flat resection and cyst debridement. Notice the preserved genuine bone that will be essential for supporting the implant. (**f**) An allograft bloc is shaped to be inserted into the defect. (**g**) Impaction of the allograft protected by a chisel. (**h**, **i**) Final situation after allograft impaction yield in a flat neo-surface. (**j**) The revision component with over some bone matrix is impacted and guided by the pegs. (**k**) The fluoroscopic control shows an appropriate press-fit contact of the implant to the bone. (**l**) Final position of the talar implant. The distal tibia is prepared using the same technique, and the implant is inserted using the same technique. (**m**–**q**) Ankle series showing the stable position of the talar implant and the osteointegration of the allograft over 5 years

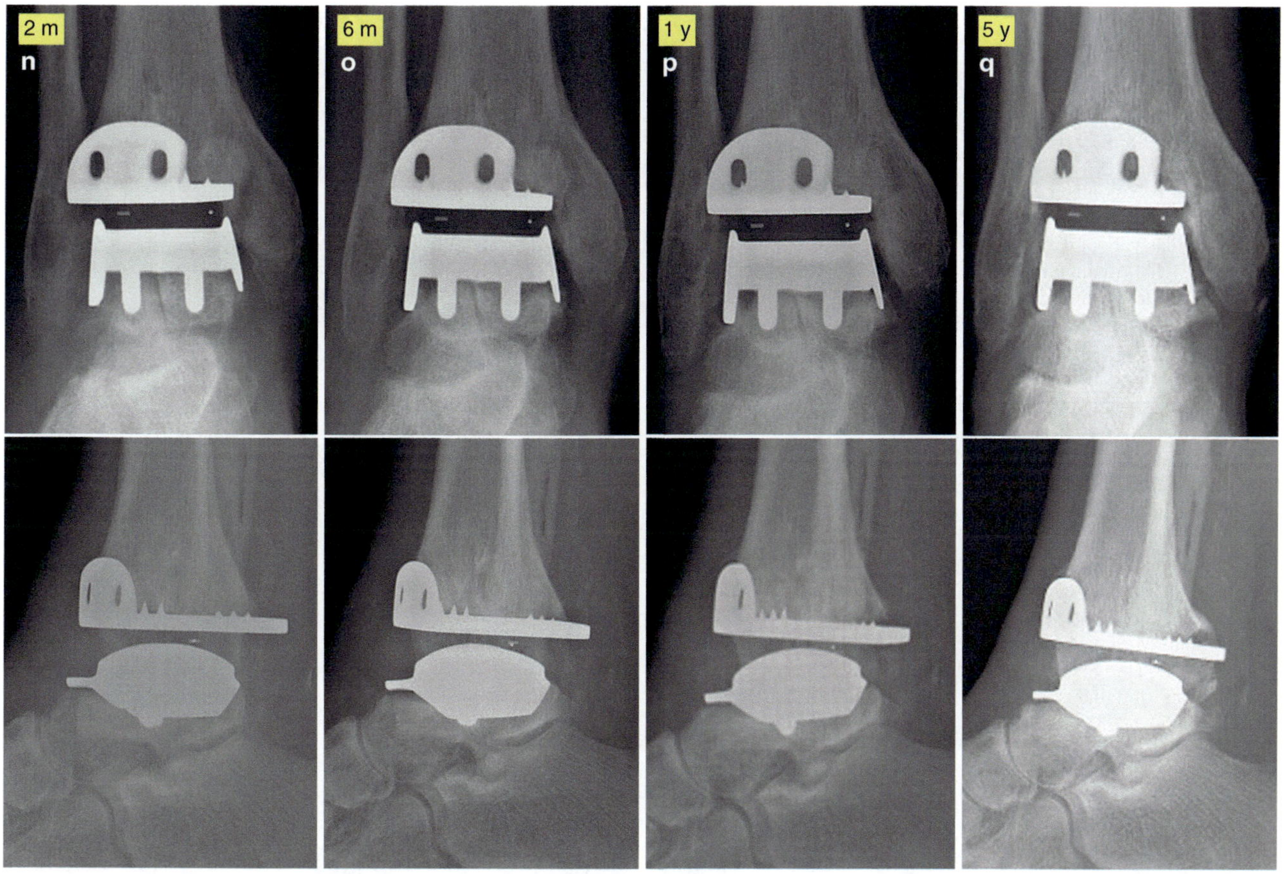

Fig. 15.3 (continued)

fluid from 15 patients with total ankle arthroplasties. They were comparable to 11 patients with posterior stabilized total knee arthroplasties at least 6 months postoperatively. Particulate polyethylene debris can incite a chronic inflammatory process that causes aseptic loosening.

Mobile bearings have been hypothesized to have better outcomes than fixed-bearing ankle designs because of their unconstrained biomechanical characteristics that better accommodate rotational forces in ankle articulation [4, 6, 22]. This was supported by the findings of a recent study of the MAUDE database, indicating that the mobile-bearing STAR ankle has a lower proportion of reported polyethylene wear than fixed-bearing total ankle arthroplasty but a higher reported proportion of polyethylene fractures and earlier revisions overall compared to fixed-bearing designs [67].

In 250 mobile-bearing Hintegra ankles, Lee et al. [68] found osteolysis in 79 ankles (31.6%) at a mean follow-up of 83.5 months (range, 36–182 months). Forty of these ankles were closely monitored without surgical treatment. Another 29 ankles underwent bone grafting, and exchange of the polyethylene inlay, and the remaining ten ankles underwent revision total ankle arthroplasty or arthrodesis. At the final follow-up, all clinical outcome variables were significantly lower in patients with osteolysis than those without ($p < 0.05$). The authors concluded that the prevention and appropriate treatment of osteolysis are crucial for the satisfactory long-term survival of total ankle arthroplasty.

15.4.2.1 Diagnosis

Diagnosis of aseptic loosening is predominantly made with plain radiographs and CT scans (Fig. 15.6). Most ankle arthroplasties will develop at least a focal region of osteolysis. Still, whether this leads to aseptic loosening must be evaluated, and we recommend follow-up annually for surveillance radiographs. The treatment goals are to restore bone stock, achieve stability, and correct any cause of poly wear, if possible.

15.4.2.2 Treatment

Asymptomatic aseptic loosening, diagnosed by a lucency line along the implant without progression, cortical erosion, and cyst formation, does not need treatment. This is typically

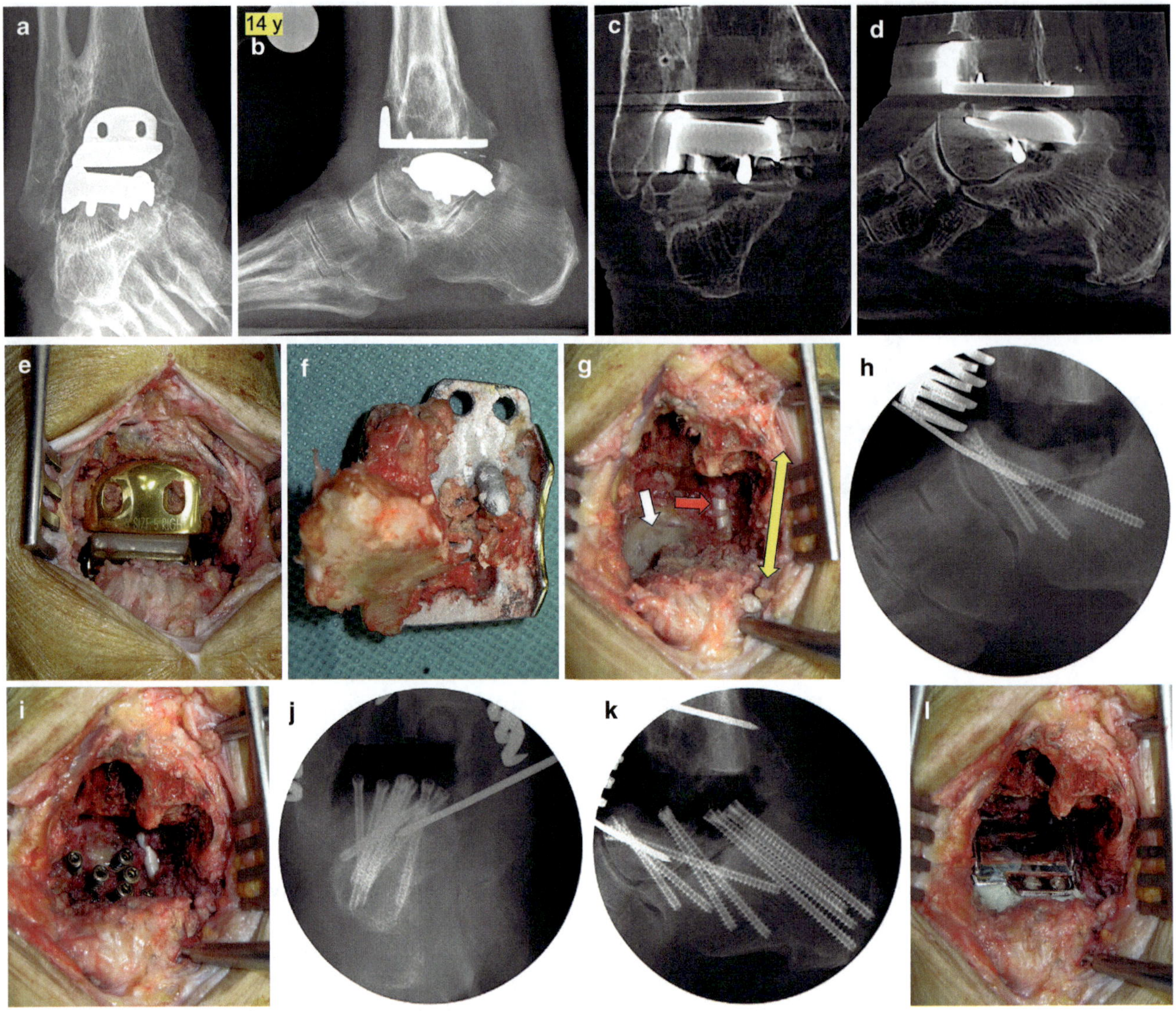

Fig. 15.4 Revision of subsided component with bone cement. A 77-year-old female patient, 14 years after total ankle arthroplasty, complained of pain in her ankle for 3 months. (**a**, **b**) Radiographs showing massive cyst formations and subsidence of the talar component with violation of the subtalar joint, shown in more detail in the CT scans (**c**, **d**). (**e**) The subsidence of the talar component is seen after ankle exposure. (**f**) A necrotic part of the talar body is extracted with the component. (**g**) Direct view of the calcaneus (white arrow) and the flexor hallucis longus tendon (red arrow). While a distraction is applied over two K-wires (yellow double arrow), the talar head is pushed against the navicular as much as needed to get the foot in a plantigrade position. (**h**) After preliminary fixation by K-wires, canulated screws are used to fix the talar head to the calcaneus. The fluoroscopy shows the correct position of the talar head and the adequate alignment of the Chopart joint. (**i**–**k**) While paying attention to keeping the space free for the pegs of the implant, six 5.0 mm screws are incompletely inserted into the calcaneus to serve as an anchorage for the bone cement. (**l**) The talar implant is then inserted using bone cement for fixation. (**m**–**n**) Fluoroscopies showing the final position of the talar implant over the bone cement-screw construct. (**o**) An allograft is used to fill the defects on the tibial side, providing stable support to the implant. (**p**–**r**) Fluoroscopies showing the final situation in three planes. (**s**, **t**) Radiographs 5 years after the arthroplasty revision show an unchanged and stable position of both implants. The patient is pain-free and pleased with her ankle

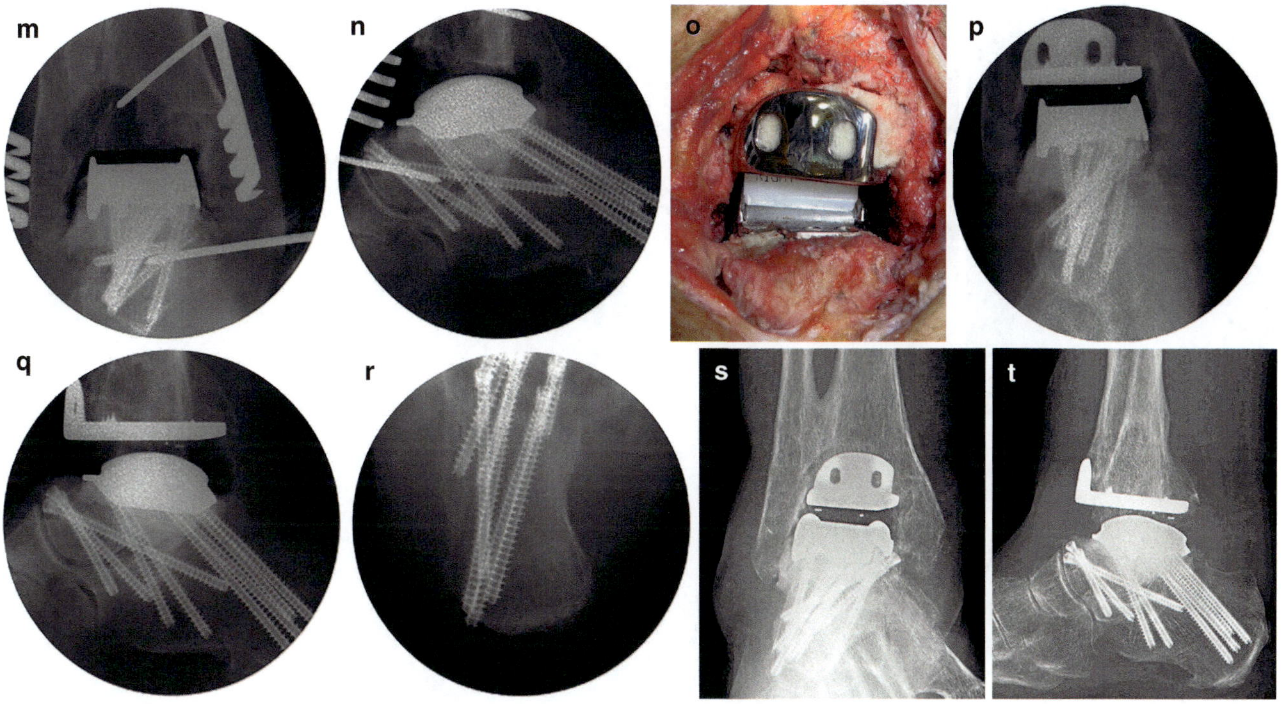

Fig. 15.4 (continued)

seen in implants with a single hydroxyapatite coating with the appearance of a cortical line along the lucency zone (Fig. 13.18). We call this phenomenon the "second line of defense." However, in the case of pain, progressive cyst formation, and subsidence of the component, revision of the component must be considered.

Often, in symptomatic aseptic loosening, the implant must be removed, and fresh cuts taken with bigger implants to fill up space from resected bone (Fig. 15.7). Cyst formation must be cleaned and filled with bone grafts (Fig. 15.8). Cement can be used for such defects but is much harder than bone and can stress shield; we prefer to use the impaction bone graft technique if possible.

15.4.3 Cyst Formation

Periprosthetic cysts have been correlated with total ankle arthroplasty failure when more than one-third of the bone-implant interface is compromised, or cortical lysis occurs, commonly reported with a mobile-bearing prosthesis, non-anatomic designs, hydroxyapatite coating, and malalignment [69–72]. Periprosthetic cysts are reported to occur in up to 95% of total ankle arthroplasty in the medium and long term, with an uncertain significance [1, 64, 73–84]. Kohonen et al. [77] reported that 34.6% of ankles had at least one periprosthetic cyst larger than 10 mm on radiographs at a mean follow-up of 43 months. They found that 68% of grafted cysts continued progressing despite bone grafting, which was disappointing. Of note is that 91% of patients had the AES implant, which was withdrawn from the market because of an excessively high rate of periprosthetic osteolysis. Their high rate of cyst progression may be directly related to the AES implant itself. In a CT-based analysis, Naude et al. [84] reported on the result of bone grafting of cysts greater than 15 mm in all planes (1.75 cm^3) that 89% (69–100%) incorporated. Others supported these results after cyst treatment with autograft; however, they didn't use CT scans to confirm integration and progression [1, 9, 64]. Lundeen et al. [85] reported on endoscopy-assisted curettage and bone grafting of periprosthetic cysts, which allows for better visualization and complete removal of cystic material, which could result in higher grafting fill and improved success of graft incorporation.

Another question to debate is which type of graft is preferable: autograft bone, allograft bone chips, calcium phosphate, or polymethylmethacrylate cement [70, 72, 86, 87]. These can be supplemented with mesenchymal stem cells, platelet-rich plasma, recombinant human bone morphogenic protein-2, and DBM [72, 86].

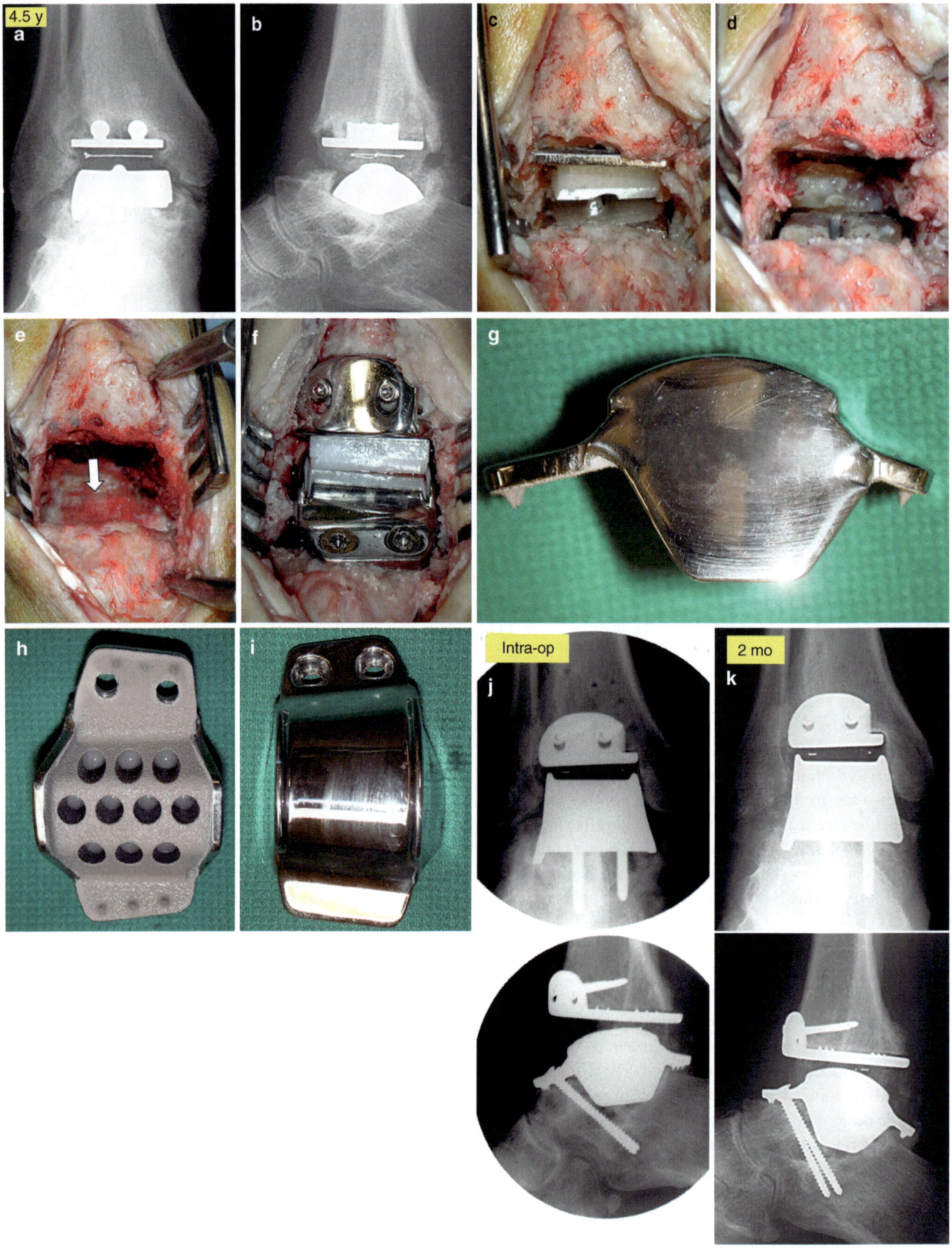
4.5 y
a
b
c
d
e
f
g
h
i
Intra-op
j
2 mo
k

Fig. 15.5 Revision of subsided component with custom-made implant. A 48-year-old farmer was treated for a talus Hawkins IV dislocation fracture with open reduction and primary subtalar fusion. 3.2 years later, he underwent total ankle arthroplasty for post-traumatic osteoarthritis. He complains of increasing pain 4.5 years after the replacement surgery, mainly beneath the malleoli. (**a**, **b**) Radiographs showing massive subsidence of the talar implant, which can also be seen after exposure of the ankle (**c**). (**d**) After removing the implants, the talar body is found necrotic. (**e**) The avascular necrosis extends to the calcaneus, as seen after the debridement (arrow). (**f**) Final result after the revision arthroplasty using a custom-made talar component as shown in figuress **g** to **i**. (**j**–**o**) The radiograph series shows the evolution over 21.5 years with stable implants and no significant polyethylene wear. The patient sustained a tibial shaft fracture 20.8 years after the replacement surgery, for which he was treated with an intramedullary nail fixation

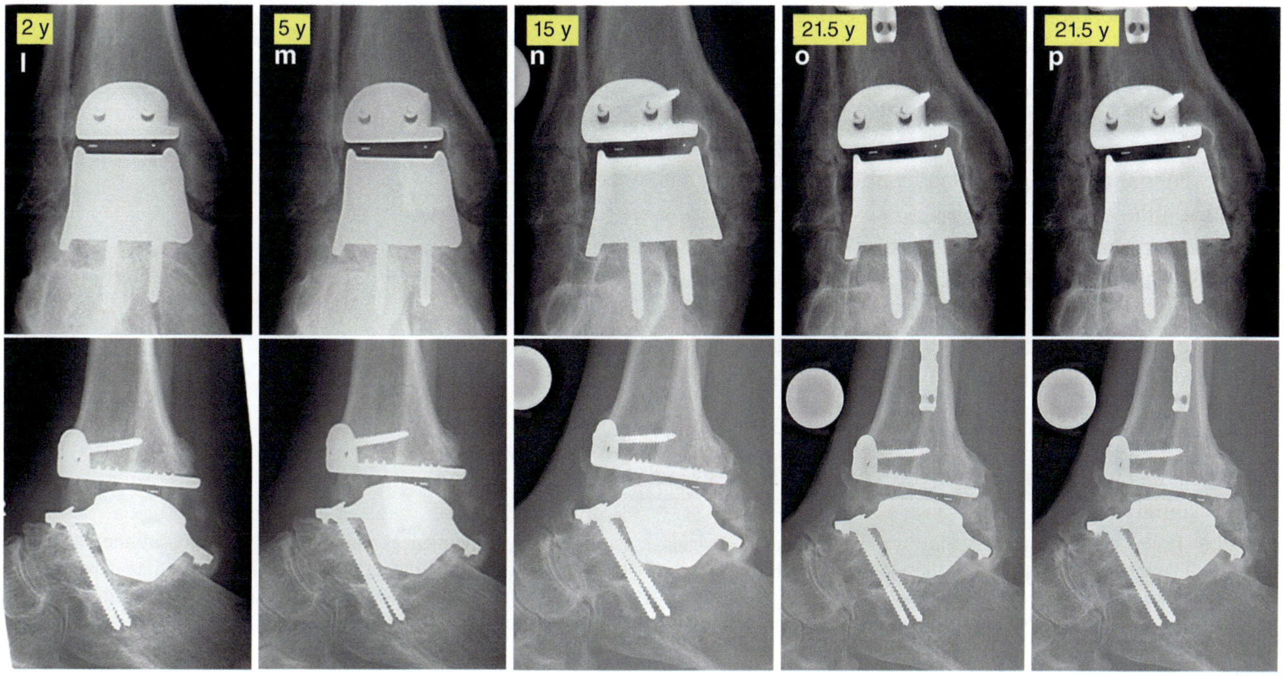

Fig. 15.5 (continued)

15.4.3.1 Diagnosis

Although periprosthetic cysts are most often diagnosed from plain radiographs (Fig. 15.9), CT scans are superior for early detection of—and more accurate in quantifying – ballooning osteolysis [75, 88, 89]. CT also allows more accurate preoperative planning before revision surgery, especially regarding residual bone stock (Fig. 15.10) [90].

15.4.3.2 Treatment

Nonoperative treatment is reserved for patients with small periprosthetic bone cysts without symptoms. These patients should be followed with clinical and radiographic observation and evaluated for symptoms such as startup pain development. The primary surgical treatment of isolated bone cysts without implant compromise is cyst debridement with grafting (Fig. 15.11) [91]. The goal of cyst debridement and grafting is the elimination of the cyst to relieve pain, provide implant stability, and prevent implant loosening or subsidence in the future. Also, accompanying polyethylene liner exchange has been recommended during cyst debridement and grafting, given concerns of polyethylene wear contributing to cyst formation [84].

Our treatment preference for the revision of symptomatic and progressive cysts is debridement associated with a component exchange (Figs. 15.12 and 15.13). Considering that bone remodeling has occurred around the cyst to resist the mechanical load of the component, our emphasis is to clean the cysts without damaging the remaining bone stock. Furthermore, we found the cysts consistently lined with a membrane. Stripping carefully down this membrane leaves the bone back with spots of bleeding, a sign of vitality. After that, we fill the cyst carefully with bone allograft and bone

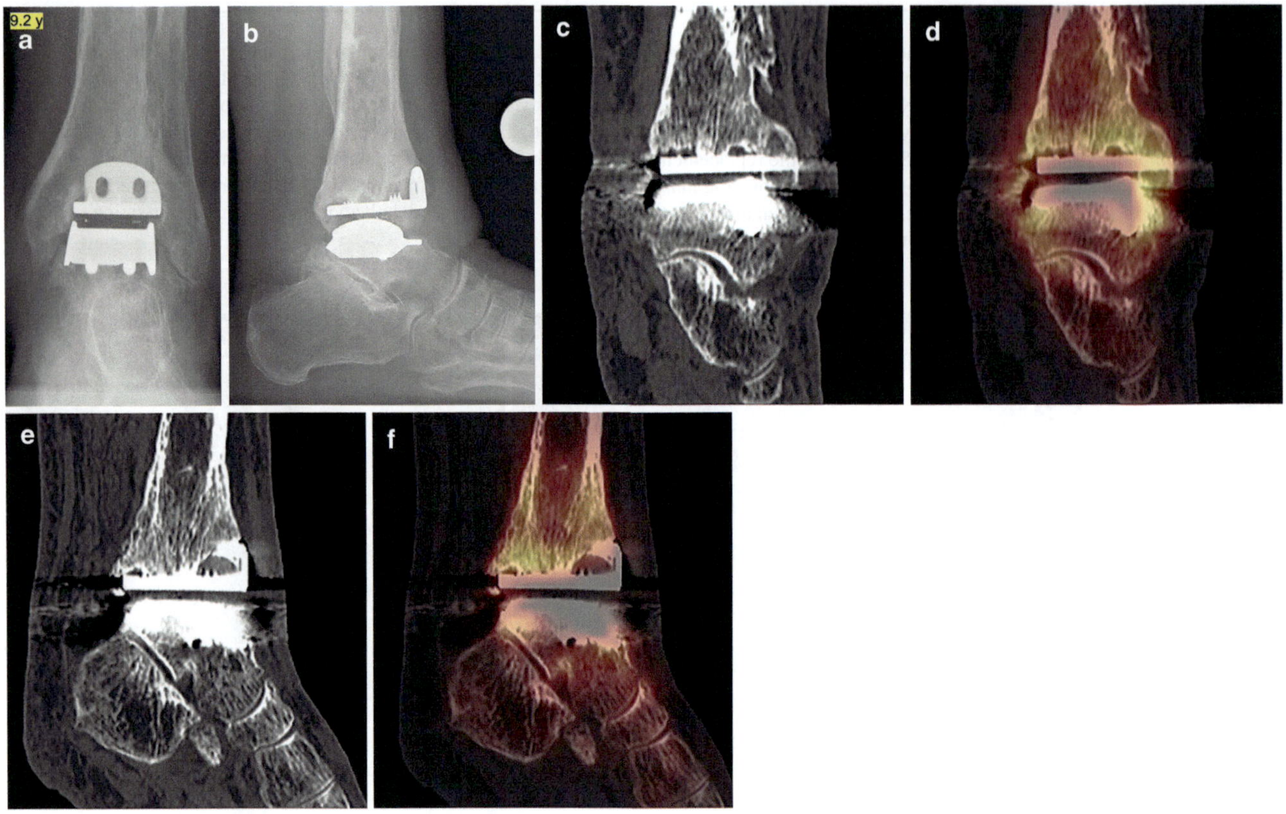

Fig. 15.6 Diagnosis of aseptic loosening by radiographs and CT scans. (**a**, **b**) Radiographs showing a lucency line along the tibial implant. The component has not moved yet because of small areas at the bone-implant interface left, with typical stress raisers. However, a destabilization of the component is imminent, as indicated by the pain when loading and unloading the ankle. (**c**–**f**) CT scans and associated Spect CT scans confirm the incomplete loosening of the implant with increased uptake in this area

matrix, paying attention to avoid damaging the genuine bone stock. Usually, the same type and size of the component can be used for the revision.

The Authors' Experience

- *Periprosthetic bone cysts are common after total ankle arthroplasty and can often be asymptomatic.*
- *The exact cause of bone cyst formation is likely multifactorial, with contributing factors including polyethylene wear, implant micromotion, and implant design; a significant role may play coronal plane instability of the talus due to incompetent syndesmotic and deltoid ligaments.*
- *Cysts do not always progress; therefore, they should be observed with annual clinical and radiographic follow-ups to assess cyst progression, implant stability, and patient symptoms.*
- *Operative treatment of isolated minor periprosthetic bone cysts without implant compromise may consist solely of cyst debridement and grafting. In contrast, treatments for potentially unstable implants in bone cysts should include revision of the implants or, if not possible, arthrodesis.*
- *There is no need for stemmed revision implants as long as standard implants can be firmly positioned on genuine bone.*
- *Bone incorporation occurs reliably on all three bones to substitute bone defects.*
- *If present, malalignment correction and stabilization procedures should be performed to get a well-balanced and stable ankle.*

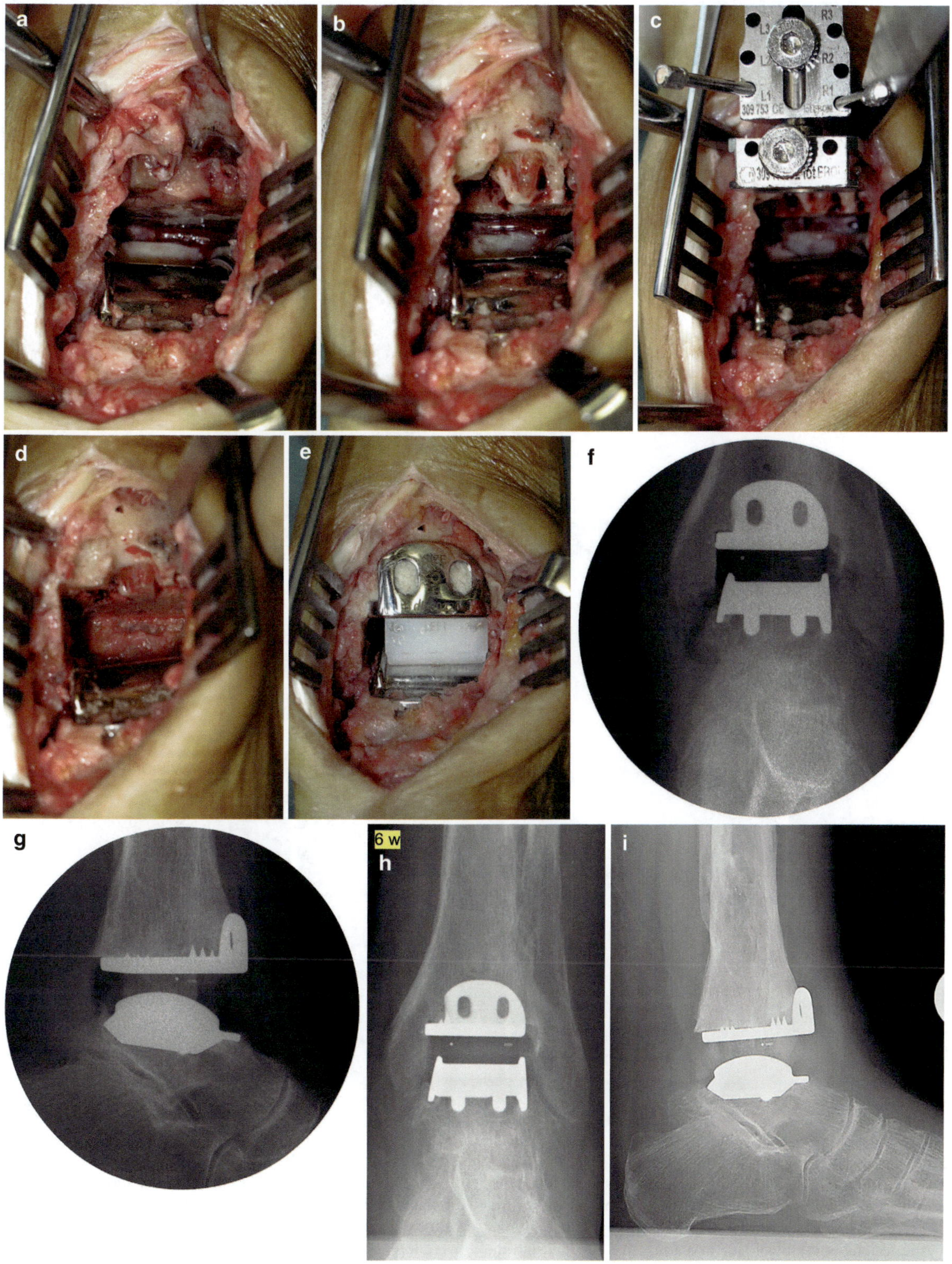

Fig. 15.7 Implant exchange with fresh bone cut for loosening. Same patient as Fig. 15.6. (**a**) After removing the tibial implant, the bone defects are seen filled with cystic material. (**b**) After meticulous cleaning, the remaining bone areas can be seen as solid pillars, typically sclerotic due to remodeling. (**c**) Minimal bone is aimed to preserve as much bone. (**d**) With the fresh cut, the created flat surface is prepared to receive the new implant, in most instances slightly bigger than the previous one, to achieve circumferential bone support. Bone grafts and bone matrix fill the remaining bone defects. (**e**) Final situation after insertion of the implants. Notice the bigger polyethylene insert and the bone matrix used for sealing the bone. (**f, g**) Intraoperative fluoroscans showing a perfect fit of components to the bone, confirmed by radiographs 6 weeks after the surgery (**h**, **i**)

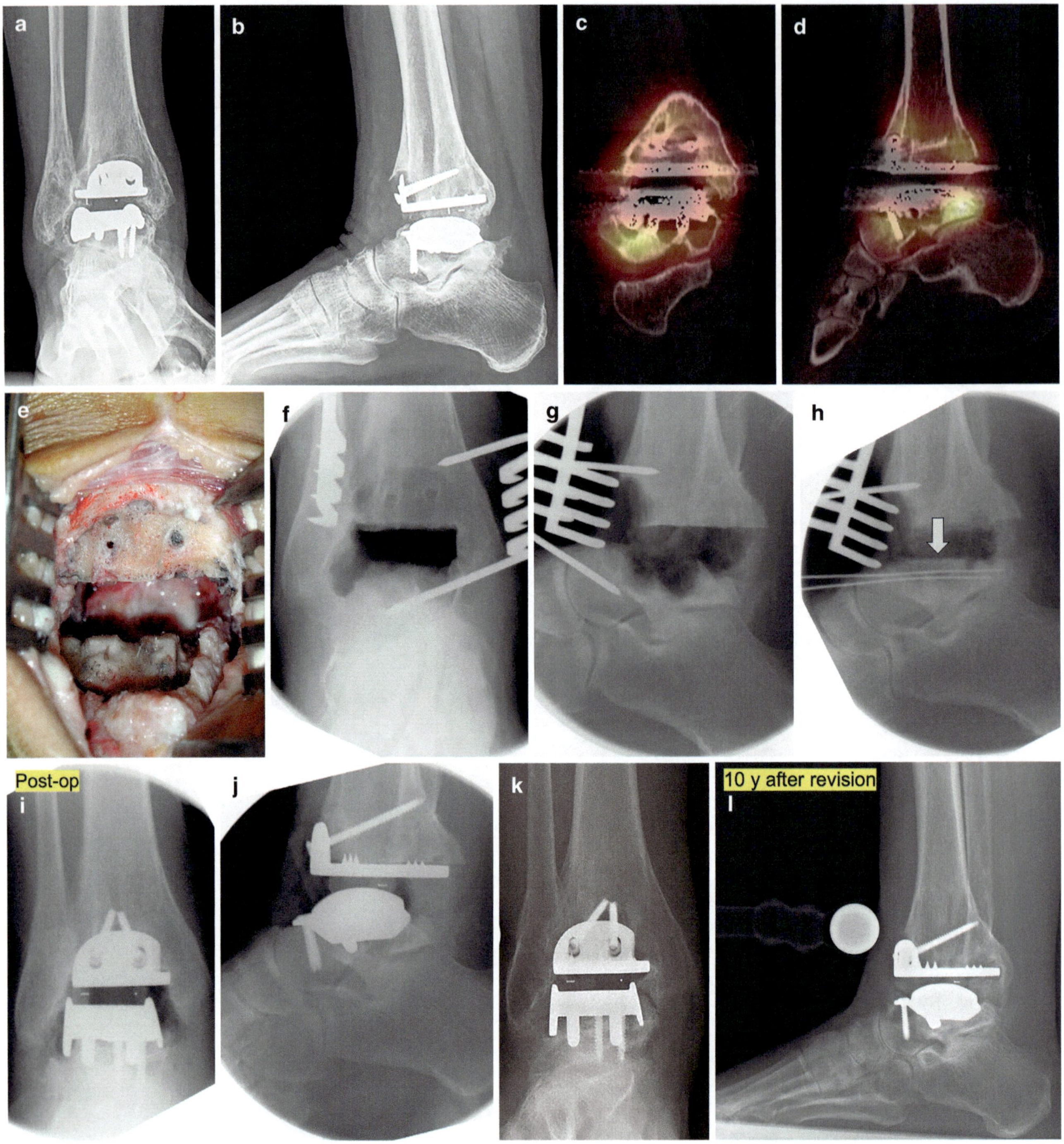

Fig. 15.8 Implant exchange with bone grafting for loosening. A 59-year-old female patient complains of acute pain onset and instability 7.5 years after a total ankle arthroplasty for post-traumatic osteoarthritis. (**a**) The AP view shows a wide ankle mortise. (**b**) The lateral view shows cystic lesions at the tibial side and a massive cyst beneath the talar implant, confirmed by the Spect CT (**c**, **d**). (**e**) Loosening of the talar component was confirmed intraoperatively, whereas the tibial component was stable. (**f**, **g**) Fluoroscans showing the extent of bone defect, most importantly, the posterior wall of the talus was preserved. This allowed us to fill the defect with an allograft preliminarily fixed by 2 K-wires (arrow) (**h**). (**i**, **j**) Final situation shows a regular fit of the implants to the bone; the wide medial gutter and the lateral translation of the talus due to incompetence of syndesmotic and deltoid ligaments were left non-addressed. (**k**, **l**) Recurrent cysts are seen at 10-year follow-up control, but the implants are stable and the patient pain-free. Therefore, an observing strategy was decided. This case shows the importance of restoring coronal plane stability during revision surgery

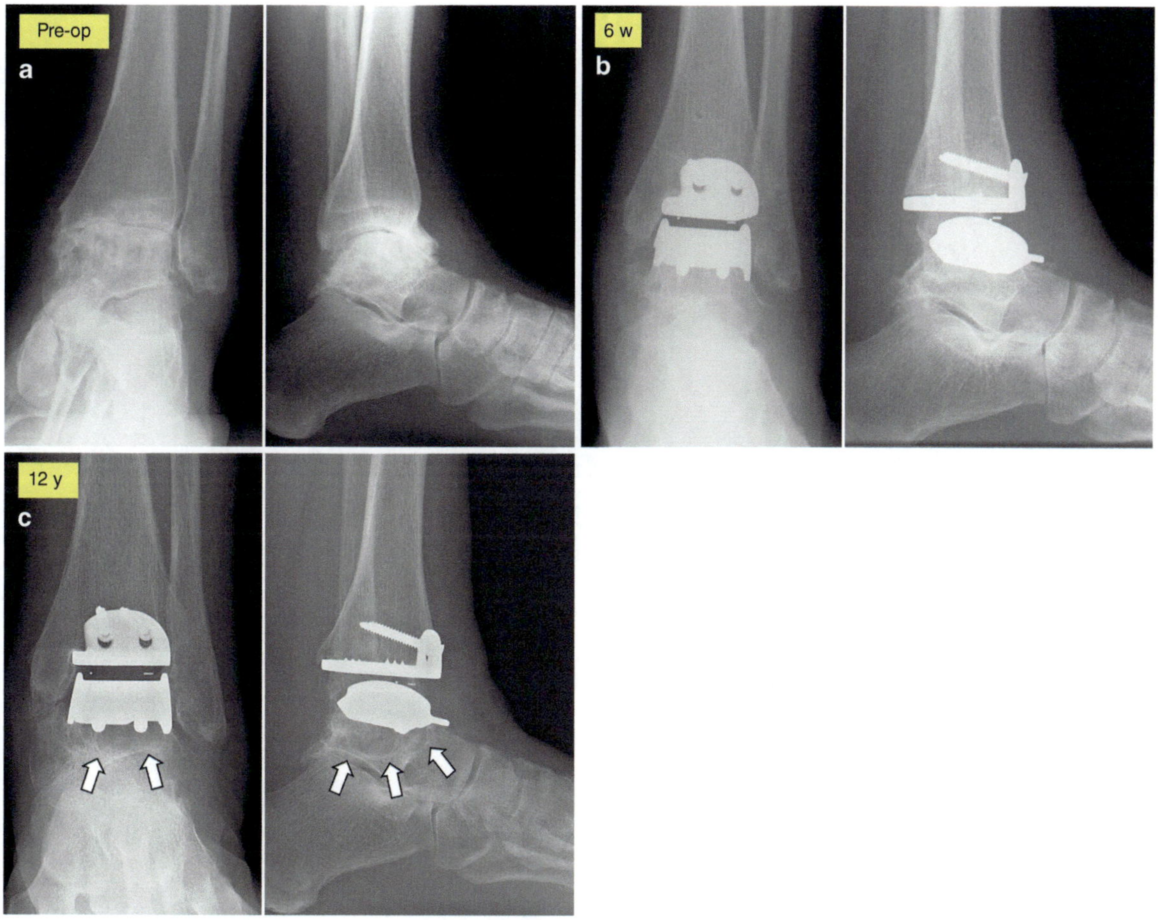

Fig. 15.9 Radiologic appearance of periprosthetic cysts. An osteoarthritic ankle of a 59-year-old female patient. (**a**) The preoperative radiographs show cystic lesions and sclerotic areas in the apex of the talar body. (**b**) During the total ankle arthroplasty, the cysts were debrided and filled with resected bone and bone matrix, and 6 weeks postoperatively, a regular fit of implants to the bone can be seen. (**c**) 12 years after the surgery, massive cyst formation can be seen beneath the talar implant, whereas the tibial bone does not show any cysts. The cysts are typically surrounded by a tinny cortical line (arrows). There are no signs of polyethylene wear

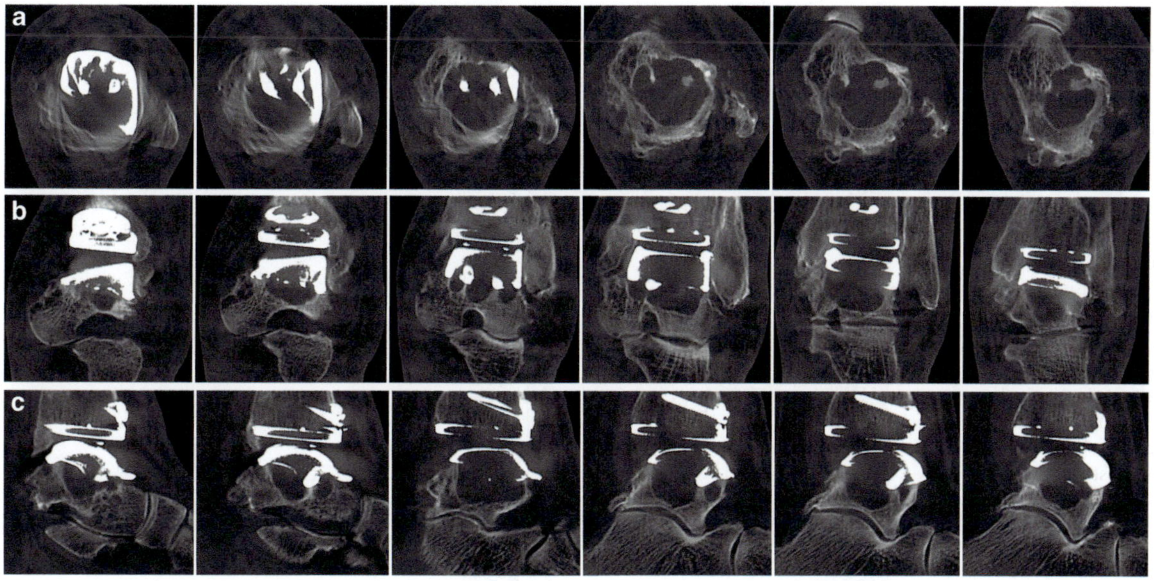

Fig. 15.10 CT scan for assessment of cyst formation. Same patient as Fig. 15.9. Weight-bearing scans showing the extent of the cysts beneath the talar implant. Notice the remodeling of the remaining bone with preserved bone circumferentially to the implant and the pegs as well. (**a**) Horizontal plane; (**b**) coronal plane; and (**c**) sagittal plane

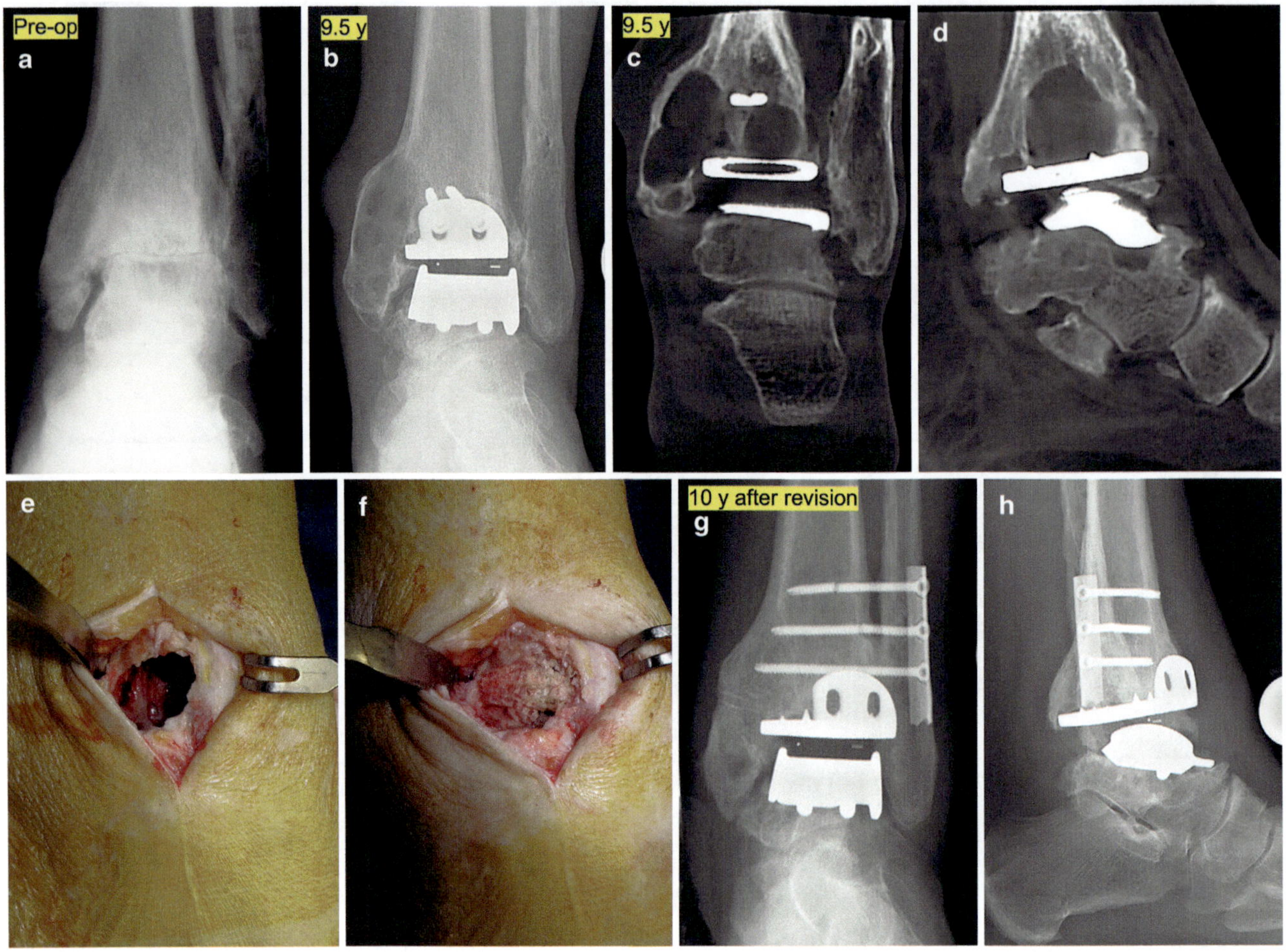

Fig. 15.11 Cyst debridement with grafting. A 59-year-old female patient with post-traumatic osteoarthritis 2.2 years after a bimalleolar fracture Weber Type C fixed by a plate (fibula) and screws (medial malleolus). Because of an infection, the implants were removed after 3 months. (**a**) Preoperative AP view showing a worn-out tibiotalar joint, slight shortening of the fibula, and some irregularity of the bone at the medial malleolus. (**b**) 9.5 years after the replacement surgery, she showed up because of a painful swelling over the medial malleolus. The AP view shows a bulky medial malleolus with massive cyst formation and a minor cyst in the center of the distal tibia; the component is stable, confirmed by the CT scans (**c**, **d**). (**e**) The cyst is approached through a short medial approach and cleaned. (**f**) After that, it is filled with allograft. In addition, the polyethylene insert is exchanged, and the distal tibiofibular joint is fused because of intraoperatively found instability (not shown). (**g**, **h**) Ten years after the revision surgery, the patient is pain-free and pleased with her ankle. The radiographs show stable implants, a solid tibiofibular fusion, and no recurrence of the cysts

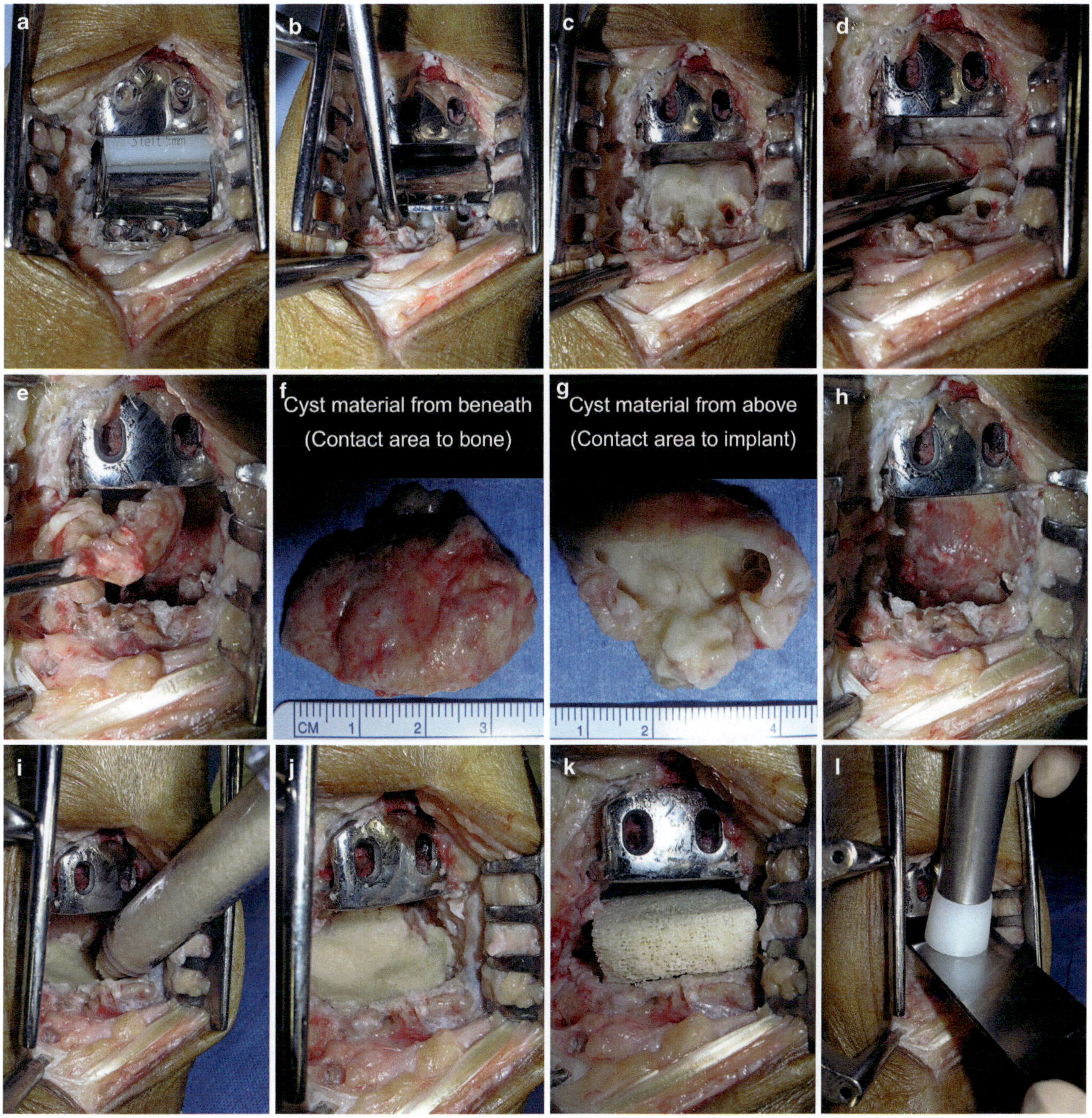

Fig. 15.12 Cyst debridement with grafting and talar implant exchange. Same patient as Figs. 15.9 and 15.10. (**a**) The polyethylene insert is confirmed to have no wear after the ankle exposure. (**b**) The screws on the tibial and the talar implant are carefully removed, followed by the removal of the talar component. (**c**) The huge cyst is exposed, extending all around to the border of the talus. (**d**) The cyst material is carefully removed in one piece. Typically, a solide membrane has formed along the bone (**e**, **f**), whereas the cyst tissue is open against the implant (**g**). (**h**) The bone is bleeding; thus, no further debridement is necessary. On the contrary, it would weaken the remaining bone that is very strong due to the previous remodeling process. (**i**, **j**) Bone matrix and cancellous bone fill the cavity on its bottom. (**k**) After that, an allograft is shaped and impacted by a flat chisel protection (**l**). (**m**) A lamina spreader with a big flat surface can also be used for impaction. (**n**) In this case, the allograft is left surpassing the surrounding genuine bone and shaped accordingly to the undersurface of a standard implant. If a revision implant with a flat undersurface is used, the allograft would be flattened to the surrounding genuine bone with an oscillating saw. (**o**) The holes of the pegs are made once the trial component is appropriately positioned, as verified visually and by fluoroscopy (not shown). (**p**) Bone matrix is mounted to the undersurface of the implant, and the implant is then inserted using the pegs as guidance (**q**). (**r**) The implant is impacted. Final situation before (**s**) and after (**t**) insertion of the polyethylene insert. The patient sustained a car accident 8.2 years after the revision surgery, the reason why she showed up for a check. The implants are found stable radiographically (**u**, **v**), and no recurrent cysts can be detected by the weight-bearing CT scans (**w**). However, the ankle mortise is found to be widened with subsequent lateralization of the talus and surpassing the polyethylene to the tibial implant, causing edge load. A distal tibiofibular (syndesmotic) fusion was proposed to the patient, but she, being 79 years old, preferred to wait and observe the evolution

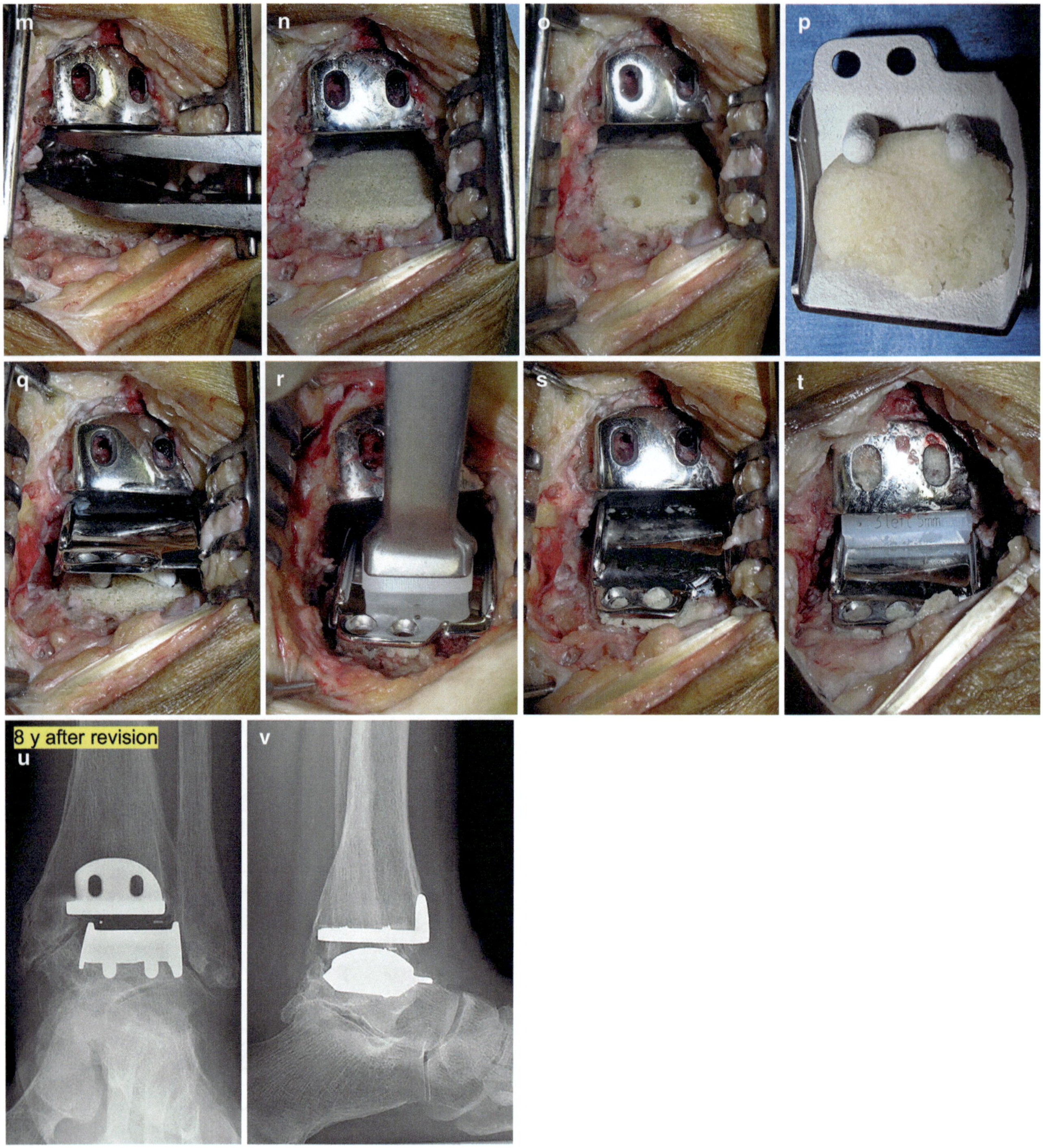

Fig. 15.12 (continued)

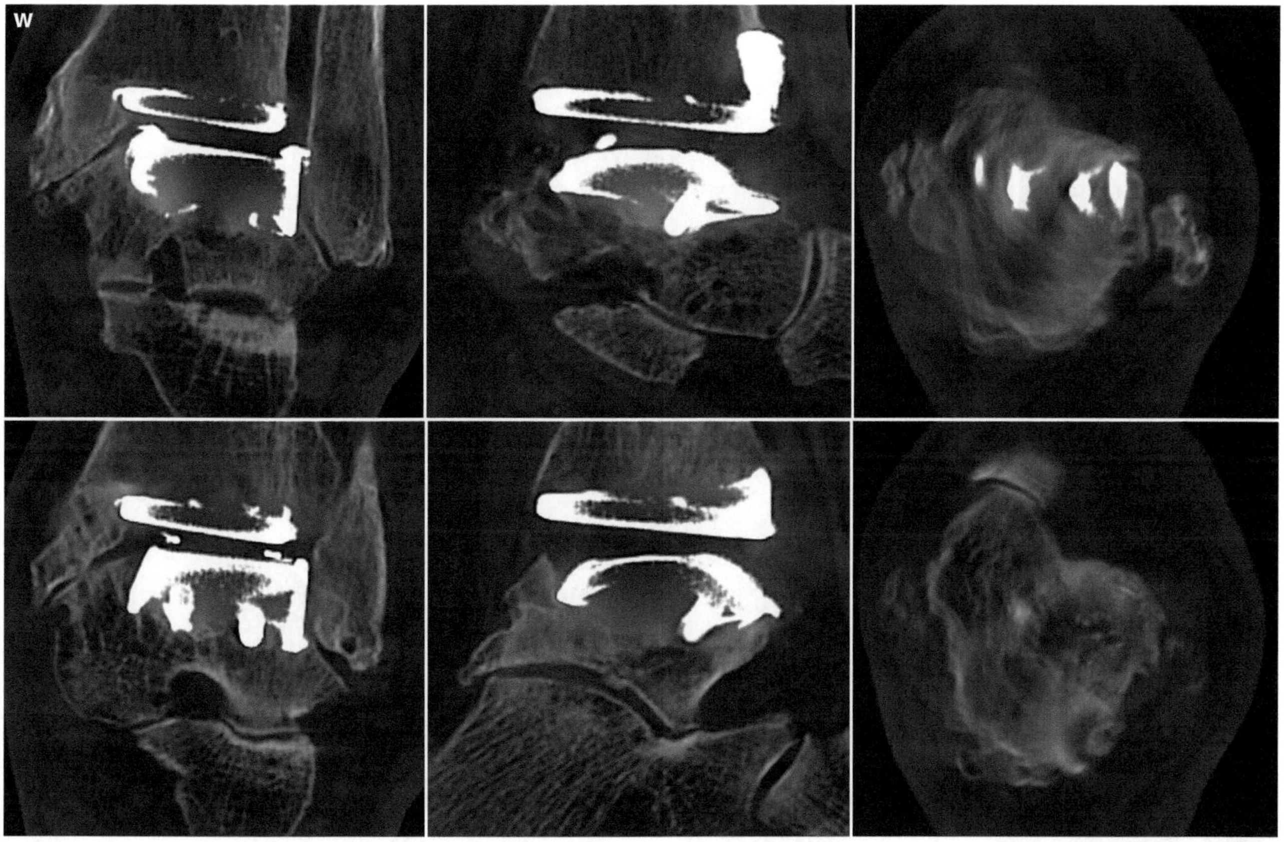

Fig. 15.12 (continued)

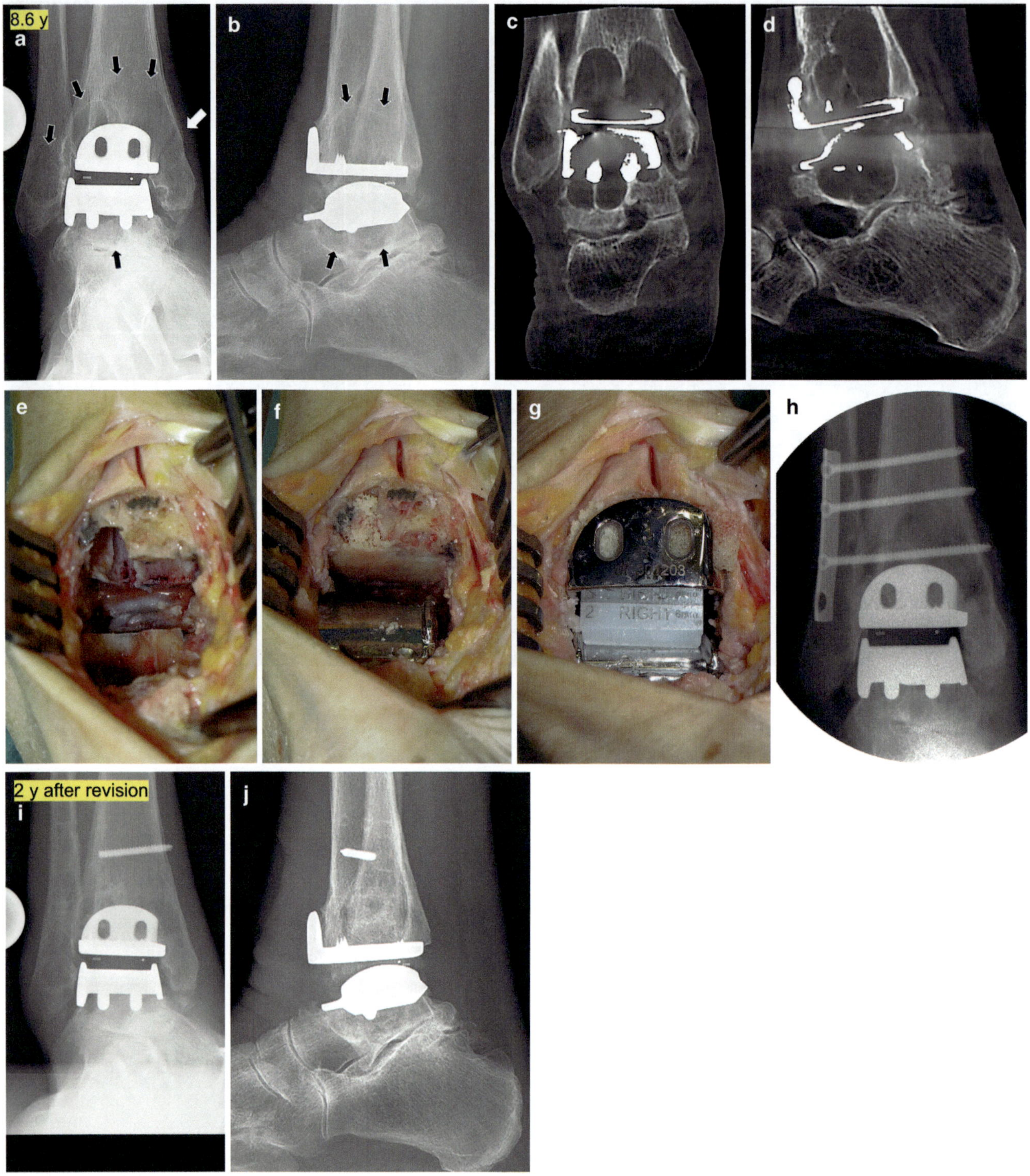

Fig. 15.13 Cyst debridement with grafting and tibial implant exchange. A 72-year-old female patient, 8.6 years after total ankle arthroplasty for post-traumatic osteoarthritis, complains of acute pain at the medial malleolus. (**a**) AP view shows a medial malleolus fracture (white arrow) and massive cyst formation at the tibial, talar, and fibular sites (black arrows), as also seen in the lateral view (**b**). (**c**, **d**) The extent of these lesions can be better seen with the CT scans. (**e**) Surgical view after carefully cleaning the cyst on the tibial and talar side. (**f**) After the talus revision and implant insertion using the technique shown in Fig. 15.12, the defects of the distal tibia were filled by allograft and bone matrix analogously to the talar side while leaving the genuine bone as it is (no additional cut). (**g**) After that, a standard tibial implant one size bigger than the previous one was inserted, followed by a polyethylene insert. (**h**) Finally, the distal tibiofibular joint was fused to enhance the stability of the ankle mortise. (**i**, **j**) The implants were stable 2 years after the revision surgery, and the allografts were well-osseointegrated. The fibular plate was removed 8 months after the surgery because of local discomfort

15.5 Conclusions

- Despite a slightly higher risk of failure and reoperation than primary replacement surgery, revision of primary total ankle arthroplasty can be an effective procedure with improved functional outcomes.
- Most challenging in revision arthroplasty of the ankle is the anchorage of the components in deficient bone stock.
- In contrast to the hip and the knee, stemmed and bulky implants might not work in the ankle; newer studies have shown that flat components can accommodate the force transmission at the bone-implant interface, although the contact area is often decreased.
- New perspectives may arise with custom-made implants using 3D-printing techniques.
- Revision arthroplasty of a failed total ankle arthroplasty is a viable alternative to extended ankle arthrodesis.

References

1. Bonnin M, Gaudot F, Laurent JR, Ellis S, Colombier JA, Judet T. The Salto total ankle arthroplasty: survivorship and analysis of failures at 7 to 11 years. Clin Orthop Relat Res. 2011;469(1):225–36.
2. Clough T, Bodo K, Majeed H, Davenport J, Karski M. Survivorship and long-term outcome of a consecutive series of 200 Scandinavian Total Ankle Replacement (STAR) implants. Bone Joint J. 2019;101-B(1):47–54.
3. Daniels TR, Mayich DJ, Penner MJ. Intermediate to long-term outcomes of total ankle replacement with the Scandinavian Total Ankle Replacement (STAR). J Bone Joint Surg Am. 2015;97(11):895–903.
4. Mann JA, Mann RA, Horton E. STAR ankle: long-term results. Foot Ankle Int. 2011;32(5):S473–84.
5. Barg A, Zwicky L, Knupp M, Henninger HB, Hintermann B. HINTEGRA total ankle replacement: survivorship analysis in 684 patients. J Bone Joint Surg Am. 2013;95(13):1175–83.
6. Kvarda P, Peterhans US, Susdorf R, Barg A, Ruiz R, Hintermann B. Long-term survival of HINTEGRA total ankle replacement in 683 patients: a concise 20-year follow-up of a previous report. J Bone Joint Surg Am. 2022;
7. Yoon YK, Park KH, Park JH, Lee W, Han SH, Lee JW. Long-term clinical outcomes and implant survivorship of 151 total ankle arthroplasties using the HINTEGRA prosthesis: a minimum 10-year follow-up. J Bone Joint Surg Am. 2022;104(16):1483–91.
8. Wood PL, Prem H, Sutton C. Total ankle replacement: medium-term results in 200 Scandinavian total ankle replacements. J Bone Joint Surg Br. 2008;90(5):605–9.
9. Yang HY, Wang SH, Lee KB. The HINTEGRA total ankle arthroplasty: functional outcomes and implant survivorship in 210 osteoarthritic ankles at a mean of 6.4 years. Bone Joint J. 2019;101-B(6):695–701.
10. Pedowitz DI, Kane JM, Smith GM, Saffel HL, Comer C, Raikin SM. Total ankle arthroplasty versus ankle arthrodesis: a comparative analysis of arc of movement and functional outcomes. Bone Joint J. 2016;98-B(5):634–40.
11. Valderrabano V, Hintermann B, Nigg BM, Stefanyshyn D, Stergiou P. Kinematic changes after fusion and total replacement of the ankle: part 2: Movement transfer. Foot Ankle Int. 2003;24(12):888–96.
12. Sokolowski M, Krahenbuhl N, Wang C, Zwicky L, Schweizer C, Horn Lang T, et al. Secondary subtalar joint osteoarthritis following total ankle replacement. Foot Ankle Int. 2019;40(10):1122–8.
13. Joo SD, Lee KB. Comparison of the outcome of total ankle arthroplasty for osteoarthritis with moderate and severe varus malalignment and that with neutral alignment. Bone Joint J. 2017;99-B(10):1335–42.
14. Lee GW, Wang SH, Lee KB. Comparison of intermediate to long-term outcomes of total ankle arthroplasty in ankles with preoperative varus, valgus, and neutral alignment. J Bone Joint Surg Am. 2018;100(10):835–42.
15. Queen RM, Adams SB Jr, Viens NA, Friend JK, Easley ME, Deorio JK, et al. Differences in outcomes following total ankle replacement in patients with neutral alignment compared with tibiotalar joint malalignment. J Bone Joint Surg Am. 2013;95(21):1927–34.
16. Sadoghi P, Liebensteiner M, Agreiter M, Leithner A, Bohler N, Labek G. Revision surgery after total joint arthroplasty: a complication-based analysis using worldwide arthroplasty registers. J Arthroplast. 2013;28(8):1329–32.
17. Trajkovski T, Pinsker E, Cadden A, Daniels T. Outcomes of ankle arthroplasty with preoperative coronal-plane varus deformity of 10 degrees or greater. J Bone Joint Surg Am. 2013;95(15):1382–8.
18. Henricson A, Skoog A, Carlsson A. The Swedish ankle arthroplasty register: an analysis of 531 arthroplasties between 1993 and 2005. Acta Orthop. 2007;78(5):569–74.
19. Carlsson A. Single- and double-coated star total ankle replacements: a clinical and radiographic follow-up study of 109 cases. Orthopade. 2006;35(5):527–32.
20. Kumar A, Dhar S. Total ankle replacement: early results during learning period. Foot Ankle Surg. 2007;13:19–23.
21. Haskell A, Mann RA. Perioperative complication rate of total ankle replacement is reduced by surgeon experience. Foot Ankle Int. 2004;25(5):283–9.
22. Doets HC, Brand R, Nelissen RG. Total ankle arthroplasty in inflammatory joint disease with use of two mobile-bearing designs. J Bone Joint Surg Am. 2006;88(6):1272–84.
23. Henricson A, Ågren PH. Secondary surgery after total ankle replacement. The influence of preoperative hindfoot alignment. Foot Ankle Surg. 2007;13:41–4.
24. Hintermann B. Total ankle arthroplasty—historical overview, current concepts and future perspectives. Wien-New York: Springer; 2004. 195 p
25. Richter D, Krahenbuhl N, Susdorf R, Barg A, Ruiz R, Hintermann B. What are the indications for implant revision in three-component total ankle arthroplasty? Clin Orthop Relat Res. 2021;479(3):601–9.
26. Anderson T, Montgomery F, Carlsson A. Uncemented STAR total ankle prostheses. Three to eight-year follow-up of fifty-one consecutive ankles. J Bone Joint Surg Am. 2003;85(7):1321–9.
27. Spirt AA, Assal M, Hansen ST Jr. Complications and failure after total ankle arthroplasty. J Bone Joint Surg Am. 2004;86(6):1172–8.
28. Hosman AH, Mason RB, Hobbs T, Rothwell AG. A New Zealand national joint registry review of 202 total ankle replacements followed for up to 6 years. Acta Orthop. 2007;78(5):584–91.
29. Henricson A, Carlsson A, Rydholm U. What is a revision of total ankle replacement? Foot Ankle Surg. 2011;17(3):99–102.
30. Daniels TR, Younger AS, Penner M, Wing K, Dryden PJ, Wong H, et al. Intermediate-term results of total ankle replacement and ankle arthrodesis: a COFAS multicenter study. J Bone Joint Surg Am. 2014;96(2):135–42.
31. Hintermann B, Zwicky L, Knupp M, Henninger HB, Barg A. HINTEGRA revision arthroplasty for failed total ankle prostheses. J Bone Joint Surg Am. 2013;95(13):1166–74.
32. Steck JK, Schuberth JM, Christensen JC, Luu CA. Revision total ankle arthroplasty. Clin Podiatr Med Surg. 2017;34(4):541–64.

33. Hintermann B, Peterhans US, Susdorf R, Horn Lang T, Ruiz R, Kvarda P. Survival and risk assessment in revision arthroplasty of the ankle. Bone Joint J. 2024;106-B(1):46–52.
34. Hintermann B, Zwicky L, Knupp M, Henninger HB, Barg A. HINTEGRA revision arthroplasty for failed total ankle prostheses: surgical technique. JBJS Essent Surg Tech. 2014;3(2):e12.
35. Meeker J, Wegner N, Francisco R. Revision techniques in total ankle arthroplasty utilizing a stemmed tibial arthroplasty system. Tech Foot Ankle Surg. 2013;12(2):99–108.
36. Schuberth JMS, Steck JK, Christensen JC. Ankle replacement arthroplasty. In: Southerland JTB, Boberg JS, Downey MS, editors. McGlarmy's comprehensive textbook of foot and ankle surgery. 4th ed. Philadelphia: Wolters/Kluwer//Lippincott Williams & Wilkins Health; 2012. p. 717–56.
37. Myerson MS, Won HY. Primary and revision total ankle replacement using custom-designed prostheses. Foot Ankle Clin. 2008;13(3):521–38.
38. Haddad SL, Coetzee JC, Estok R, Fahrbach K, Banel D, Nalysnyk L. Intermediate and long-term outcomes of total ankle arthroplasty and ankle arthrodesis. A systematic review of the literature. J Bone Joint Surg Am. 2007;89(9):1899–905.
39. Li SY, Myerson MS. Management of Talar component subsidence. Foot Ankle Clin. 2017;22(2):361–89.
40. Behrens SB, Irwin TA, Bemenderfer TB, Schipper ON, Odum SM, Anderson RB, et al. Clinical and radiographic outcomes of revision total ankle arthroplasty using an intramedullary-referencing implant. Foot Ankle Int. 2020;41(12):1510–8.
41. Wagener J, Gross CE, Schweizer C, Lang TH, Hintermann B. Custom-made total ankle arthroplasty for the salvage of major talar bone loss. Bone Joint J. 2017;99-B(2):231–6.
42. Morita S, Taniguchi A, Miyamoto T, Kurokawa H, Tanaka Y. Application of a customized total talar prosthesis for revision total ankle arthroplasty. JBJS Open Access. 2020;5(4)
43. Yamamoto T, Nagai K, Kanzaki N, Kataoka K, Nukuto K, Hoshino Y, et al. Comparison of clinical outcomes between ceramic-based total ankle arthroplasty with ceramic total talar prosthesis and ceramic-based total ankle arthroplasty. Foot Ankle Int. 2022;43(4):529–39.
44. Johnson LG, Anastasio AT, Fletcher AN, Hendren S, Adams SB. Outcomes following total talus replacement: a systematic review. Foot Ankle Surg. 2022;28(8):1194–201.
45. Hodel S, Calek AK, Cavalcanti N, Fucentese SF, Vlachopoulos L, Viehofer A, et al. A novel approach for joint line restoration in revision total ankle arthroplasty based on the three-dimensional registration of the contralateral tibia and fibula. J Exp Orthop. 2023;10(1):10.
46. Jonck JH, Myerson MS. Revision total ankle replacement. Foot Ankle Clin. 2012;17(4):687–706.
47. Rodriguez D, Bevernage BD, Maldague P, Deleu PA, Tribak K, Leemrijse T. Medium term follow-up of the AES ankle prosthesis: high rate of asymptomatic osteolysis. Foot Ankle Surg. 2010;16(2):54–60.
48. Cracchiolo A 3rd, Deorio JK. Design features of current total ankle replacements: implants and instrumentation. J Am Acad Orthop Surg. 2008;16(9):530–40.
49. Saltzman CL, Mann RA, Ahrens JE, Amendola A, Anderson RB, Berlet GC, et al. Prospective controlled trial of STAR total ankle replacement versus ankle fusion: initial results. Foot Ankle Int. 2009;30(7):579–96.
50. Kim BS, Knupp M, Zwicky L, Lee JW, Hintermann B. Total ankle replacement in association with hindfoot fusion: outcome and complications. J Bone Joint Surg Br. 2010;92(11):1540–7.
51. Kotnis R, Pasapula C, Anwar F, Cooke PH, Sharp RJ. The management of failed ankle replacement. J Bone Joint Surg Br. 2006;88(8):1039–47.
52. Castro MD. Insufficiency fractures after total ankle replacement. Tech Foot Ankle Surg. 2007;6:15–21.
53. Taniguchi A, Tanaka Y. An alumina ceramic total talar prosthesis for avascular necrosis of the talus. Foot Ankle Clin. 2019;24(1):163–71.
54. Tsukamoto S, Tanaka Y, Maegawa N, Shinohara Y, Taniguchi A, Kumai T, et al. Total talar replacement following collapse of the talar body as a complication of total ankle arthroplasty: a case report. J Bone Joint Surg Am. 2010;92(11):2115–20.
55. Currier BH, Currier JH, Collier JP, Mayor MB, Scott RD. Shelf life and in vivo duration. Impacts on performance of tibial bearings. Clin Orthop Relat Res. 1997;342:111–22.
56. Espinosa N, Walti M, Favre P, Snedeker JG. Misalignment of total ankle components can induce high joint contact pressures. J Bone Joint Surg Am. 2010;92(5):1179–87.
57. Hauer G, Hofer R, Kessler M, Lewis J, Leitner L, Radl R, et al. Revision rates after total ankle replacement: a comparison of clinical studies and arthroplasty registers. Foot Ankle Int. 2022;43(2):176–85.
58. Gougoulias N, Khanna A, Maffulli N. How successful are current ankle replacements? A systematic review of the literature. Clin Orthop Relat Res. 2010;468(1):199–208.
59. Gadd RJ, Barwick TW, Paling E, Davies MB, Blundell CM. Assessment of a three-grade classification of complications in total ankle replacement. Foot Ankle Int. 2014;35(5):434–7.
60. Glazebrook MA, Arsenault K, Dunbar M. Evidence-based classification of complications in total ankle arthroplasty. Foot Ankle Int. 2009;30(10):945–9.
61. Brunner S, Barg A, Knupp M, Zwicky L, Kapron AL, Valderrabano V, et al. The Scandinavian total ankle replacement: long-term, eleven to fifteen-year, survivorship analysis of the prosthesis in seventy-two consecutive patients. J Bone Joint Surg Am. 2013;95(8):711–8.
62. Wood PL, Karski MT, Watmough P. Total ankle replacement: the results of 100 mobility total ankle replacements. J Bone Joint Surg Br. 2010;92(7):958–62.
63. Labek G, Todorov S, Iovanescu L, Stoica CI, Bohler N. Outcome after total ankle arthroplasty-results and findings from worldwide arthroplasty registers. Int Orthop. 2013;37(9):1677–82.
64. Yoon HS, Lee J, Choi WJ, Lee JW. Periprosthetic osteolysis after total ankle arthroplasty. Foot Ankle Int. 2014;35(1):14–21.
65. Vaupel Z, Baker EA, Baker KC, Kurdziel MD, Fortin PT. Analysis of retrieved agility total ankle arthroplasty systems. Foot Ankle Int. 2009;30(9):815–23.
66. Kobayashi A, Minoda Y, Kadoya Y, Ohashi H, Takaoka K, Saltzman CL. Ankle arthroplasties generate wear particles similar to knee arthroplasties. Clin Orthop Relat Res. 2004;424:69–72.
67. Jiang H, Wu L, Randsborg PH, Houck J, Sun L, Marine M, et al. Analysis of polyethylene-related revisions after total ankle replacements reported in US Food and Drug Administration Medical Device Adverse Event Database. Foot Ankle Int. 2023;44(1):13–20.
68. Lee GW, Lee KB. Periprosthetic osteolysis as a risk factor for revision after total ankle arthroplasty: a single-center experience of 250 consecutive cases. J Bone Joint Surg Am. 2022;104(15):1334–40.
69. Arcangelo J, Guerra-Pinto F, Pinto A, Grenho A, Navarro A, Martin OX. Peri-prosthetic bone cysts after total ankle replacement. A systematic review and meta-analysis. Foot Ankle Surg. 2019;25(2):96–105.
70. Besse JL, Lienhart C, Fessy MH. Outcomes following cyst curettage and bone grafting for the management of periprosthetic cystic evolution after AES total ankle replacement. Clin Podiatr Med Surg. 2013;30(2):157–70.
71. Khademi M, Ferrao P, Saragas N. Medium-term results of the HINTEGRA total ankle arthroplasty. J Foot Ankle. 2020;14(3):121–8.

72. Mehta N, Serino J, Hur ES, Smith S, Hamid KS, Lee S, et al. Pathogenesis, evaluation, and management of osteolysis following total ankle arthroplasty. Foot Ankle Int. 2021;42(2):230–42.
73. Besse JL, Brito N, Lienhart C. Clinical evaluation and radiographic assessment of bone lysis of the AES total ankle replacement. Foot Ankle Int. 2009;30(10):964–75.
74. Deleu PA, Devos Bevernage B, Gombault V, Maldague P, Leemrijse T. Intermediate-term results of mobile-bearing total ankle replacement. Foot Ankle Int. 2015;36(5):518–30.
75. Hanna RS, Haddad SL, Lazarus ML. Evaluation of periprosthetic lucency after total ankle arthroplasty: helical CT versus conventional radiography. Foot Ankle Int. 2007;28(8):921–6.
76. Jensen J, Frokjaer J, Gerke O, Ludvigsen L, Torfing T. Evaluation of periprosthetic bone cysts in patients with a Scandinavian total ankle replacement: weight-bearing conventional digital radiographs versus weight-bearing multiplanar reconstructed fluoroscopic imaging. AJR Am J Roentgenol. 2014;203(4):863–8.
77. Kohonen I, Koivu H, Pudas T, Tiusanen H, Vahlberg T, Mattila K. Does computed tomography add information on radiographic analysis in detecting periprosthetic osteolysis after total ankle arthroplasty? Foot Ankle Int. 2013;34(2):180–8.
78. Koivu H, Kohonen I, Mattila K, Loyttyniemi E, Tiusanen H. Medium to long-term results of 130 ankle evolutive system total ankle replacements-inferior survival due to peri-implant osteolysis. Foot Ankle Surg. 2017;23(2):108–15.
79. Koivu H, Kohonen I, Sipola E, Alanen K, Vahlberg T, Tiusanen H. Severe periprosthetic osteolytic lesions after the Ankle Evolutive System total ankle replacement. J Bone Joint Surg Br. 2009;91(7):907–14.
80. Kokkonen A, Ikavalko M, Tiihonen R, Kautiainen H, Belt EA. High rate of osteolytic lesions in medium-term followup after the AES total ankle replacement. Foot Ankle Int. 2011;32(2):168–75.
81. Kopp FJ, Patel MM, Deland JT, O'Malley MJ. Total ankle arthroplasty with the agility prosthesis: clinical and radiographic evaluation. Foot Ankle Int. 2006;27(2):97–103.
82. Lintz F, Mast J, Bernasconi A, Mehdi N, de Cesar NC, Fernando C, et al. 3D, Weightbearing topographical study of periprosthetic cysts and alignment in total ankle replacement. Foot Ankle Int. 2020;41(1):1–9.
83. Schutte BG, Louwerens JW. Short-term results of our first 49 Scandanavian total ankle replacements (STAR). Foot Ankle Int. 2008;29(2):124–7.
84. Naude JJ, Saragas NP, Ferrao PNF. CT scan assessment and functional outcome of periprosthetic bone grafting after total ankle arthroplasty at medium-term follow-up. Foot Ankle Int. 2022;43(5):609–19.
85. Lundeen GA, Barousse PS, Moles LH, Whitlow SR, Cassinelli S. Technique tip: endoscopic-assisted curettage and bone grafting of periprosthetic total ankle arthroplasty bone cysts. Foot Ankle Int. 2021;42(2):224–9.
86. Gross CE, Huh J, Green C, Shah S, DeOrio JK, Easley M, et al. Outcomes of bone grafting of bone cysts after total ankle arthroplasty. Foot Ankle Int. 2016;37(2):157–64.
87. van Wijngaarden R, van der Plaat L, Nieuwe Weme RA, Doets HC, Westerga J, Haverkamp D. Etiopathogenesis of osteolytic cysts associated with total ankle arthroplasty, a histological study. Foot Ankle Surg. 2015;21(2):132–6.
88. Easley ME, Vertullo CJ, Urban WC, Nunley JA. Total ankle arthroplasty. J Am Acad Orthop Surg. 2002;10(3):157–67.
89. Viste A, Al Zahrani N, Brito N, Lienhart C, Fessy MH, Besse JL. Periprosthetic osteolysis after AES total ankle replacement: Conventional radiography versus CT-scan. Foot Ankle Surg. 2015;21(3):164–70.
90. Singh G, Reichard T, Hameister R, Awiszus F, Schenk K, Feuerstein B, et al. Ballooning osteolysis in 71 failed total ankle arthroplasties. Acta Orthop. 2016;87(4):401–5.
91. Hur ES, Mehta N, Lee S, Bohl DD. Management of periprosthetic bone cysts after total ankle arthroplasty. Orthop Clin North Am. 2023;54(1):109–19.

16 Salvage of the Failed Ankle

When a total ankle arthroplasty fails, revision arthroplasty is not always possible due to severe loss of tibia or talus bone stock, soft tissue problems, or infection. In such situations, the salvage options are tibiotalar (ankle) arthrodesis, a tibiotalocalcaneal arthrodesis, or an amputation. Many techniques for arthrodesis after total ankle arthroplasty failure have been described, including the use of plates and screws, retrograde intramedullary nails with or without structural bone graft, prefabricated metal implants, or custom three-dimensional printed implants. Circular external fixation has also been described in the setting of infection and proximal bone transport for acute shortening due to inadequate bone loss.

16.1 Preoperative Considerations and Decision-Making

Factors influencing the type of treatment include the quality of bone, the degree of bone loss, previous ipsilateral foot and ankle surgical procedures, patient comorbidities, and patient choice. A lack of available bone stock is the most important since it precludes any revision. Including the subtalar joint into the fusion has the advantage of performing a single definitive surgery but has downsides, including leg length discrepancy, nonunion, and ongoing symptoms [1, 2]. Conversion of a failed total ankle arthroplasty to fusion also has a high nonunion rate of 13% [3]. The decision on the fusion technique will depend on many factors. Unfortunately, many papers did not differentiate the results between techniques, and it is therefore impossible to conclude as to the relative outcomes.

The Authors' Preference
If a periprosthetic infection cannot be excluded, we consider first removing the prosthesis and inserting a gentamycin-Palacios spacer. The fusion procedure is initiated once the probe results clarify the situation, or the infection is treated appropriately. A tibiotalar arthrodesis is our favorable choice to preserve subtalar and hindfoot motion whenever possible. However, a tibiotalocalcaneal arthrodesis must be considered if there is a limited bone stock of talus for adequate fixation, a subtalar osteoarthritis, or damage to the subtalar joint by a subsided talar component. The treatment should also be tailored to the individual needs of each patient.

16.2 Tibiotalar (Ankle) Arthrodesis

Once the implant and nonviable bone are removed and the joint surfaces are prepared for fusion, the amount and configuration of the residual talar bone stock should be assessed regarding the potential implant fixation. If the remaining bone stock permits anchorage of implants for fixation, an isolated tibiotalar fusion can be considered. An in situ tibiotalar arthrodesis can be performed if there is a minor bone defect (<2 cm) and no significant expected limb length shortening. It is essential to take note of any malleolar impingement that occurs when compression between the joints is applied. Suppose the bone defect is larger than 2 cm, a structural allograft or autograft allows for a stable fusion construct, restores limb length, and keeps the muscles/tendons about the ankle working in a biomechanically advantageous position (Fig. 16.1) [4, 5]. Berkowitz et al. [6] recommended different bone grafting strategies for talar bone stock, including an in situ arthrodesis supplemented with local bone graft or a lengthening procedure with structural allograft. This fusion may be supplemented with allograft or autograft from the local bone or iliac crest (Fig. 16.2). Preferred fixation techniques include plate and screw fixation [4, 7–12].

B. Hintermann, R. Ruiz, *Total Ankle Replacement*, https://doi.org/10.1007/978-3-031-56810-7_16

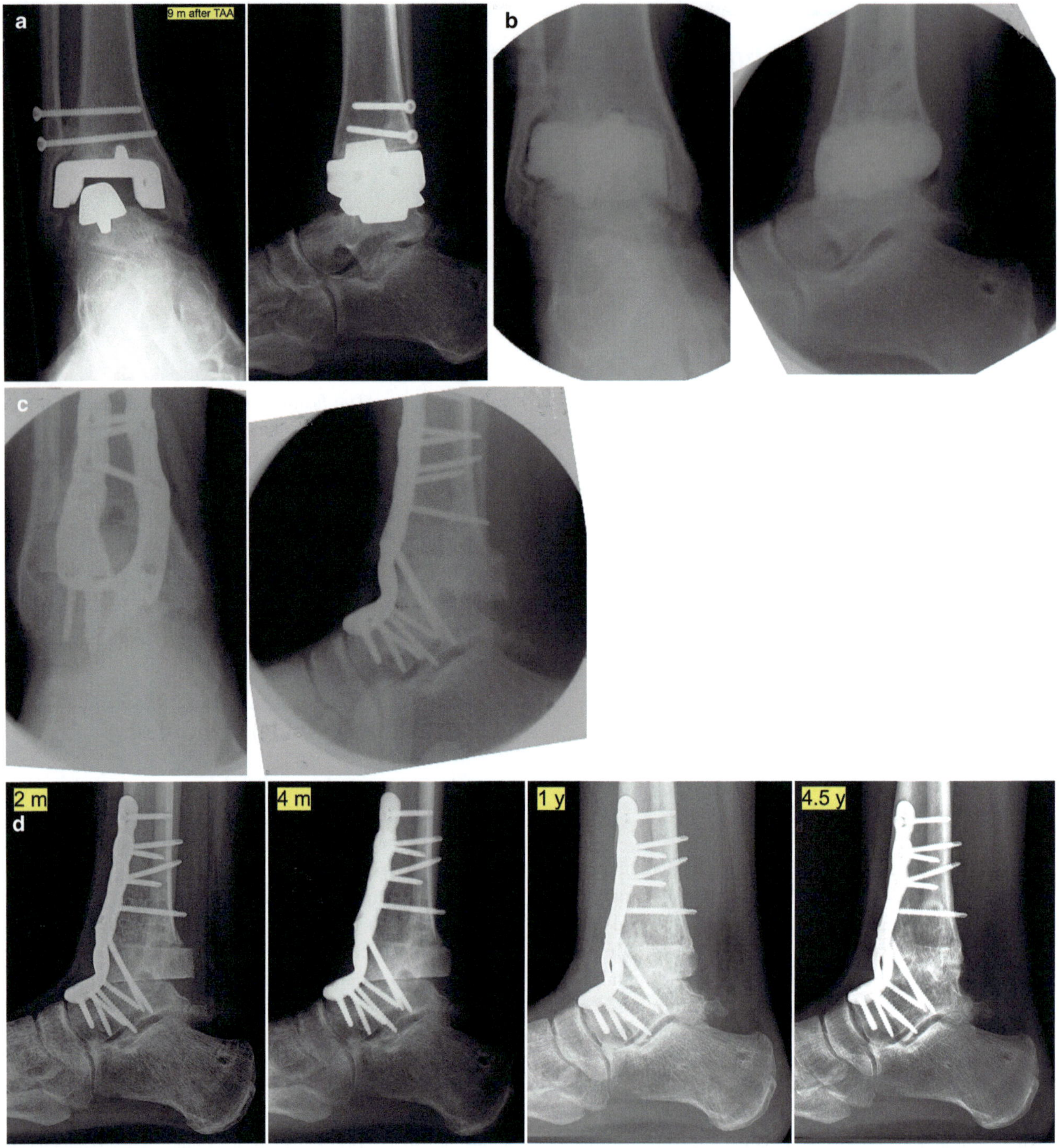

Fig. 16.1 Salvage with tibiotalar arthrodesis using an allograft. A 26-year-old female patient 9 m after total ankle arthroplasty with pain. (**a**) The standard radiographs evidence primary loosening of the tibial component and a subsided and tilted talar component. (**b**) The implants were removed, and a gentamycin-Palacios spacer was inserted as a spacer. (**c**) One week after excluding an infection, a tibiotalar arthrodesis was performed through the same anterior approach. A fresh-frozen femoral head allograft was shaped and inserted in the bone defect. A double plate anterior plate construct was used for fixation. (**d**) Series showing the healing process. The incorporation of the graft was typically seen earlier at the tibial side. The remodeling process started after 4 months and w1as completed after 4.5 years. Notably, full-weight-bearing was permitted after 2 months

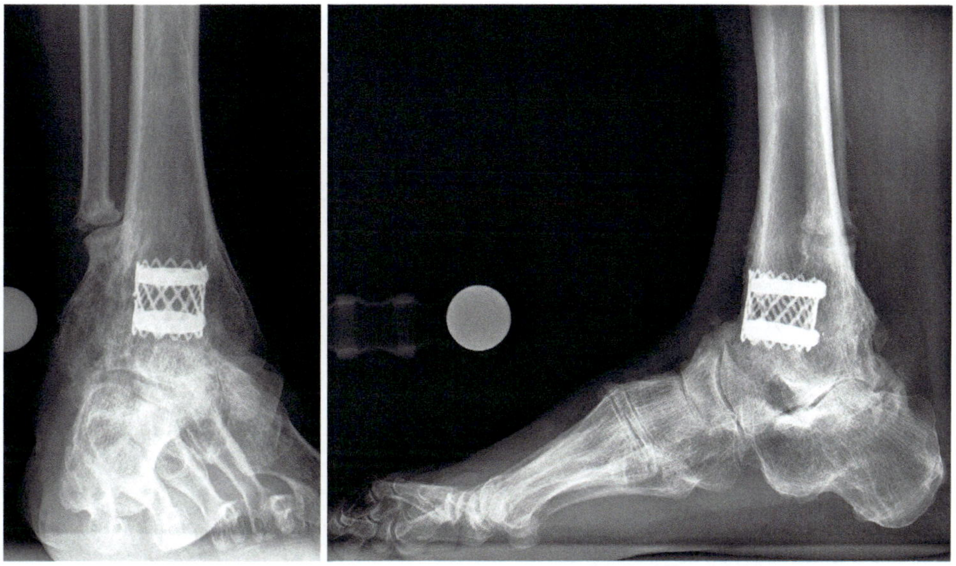

Fig. 16.2 Salvage with tibiotalar arthrodesis using autograft. In this case, autograft from the iliac crest was combined with a cage to enhance mechanical strength

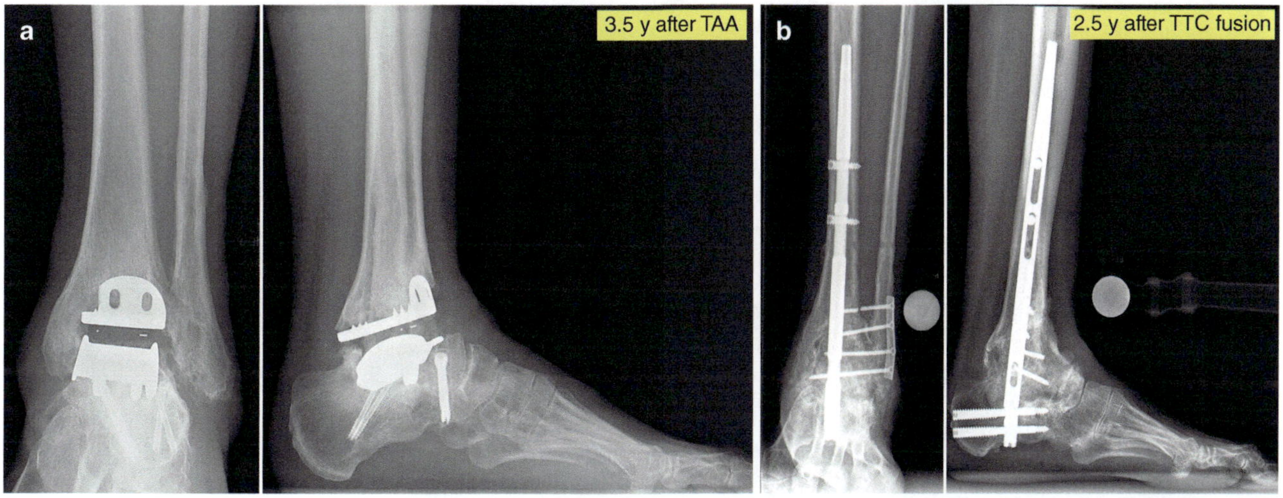

Fig. 16.3 Salvage tibiotalocalcaneal arthrodesis using intramedullary fixation. This 54-year-old patient underwent total ankle arthroplasty combined with a subtalar fusion for post-traumatic osteoarthritis after a talar fracture. (**a**) After 3.5 years, subsidence of the talar component was noticed due to avascular necrosis and subsequent collapse of the talar body. A fresh-frozen femoral head allograft and intramedullary fixation with a nail were used for tibiotalocalcaneal arthrodesis. Per our rule, the fibula was preserved and used as an additional stabilizer and vital bone to enhance the graft incorporation and the healing process of the arthrodesis. (**b**) 2.5 years postoperatively, the graft was fully incorporated. Notice the fusion achieved between the distal fibula and the talus

16.3 Tibiotalocalcaneal Arthrodesis

If there is symptomatic subtalar arthritis or if the talus has collapsed because of osteonecrosis, then a tibiotalocalcaneal fusion is indicated (Fig. 16.3). Management of the bone defect is similar to that described above for tibiotalar arthrodesis, but in most instances, the surgeon is faced with a larger bone defect. In general, the preferred fixation technique is using intramedullary nailing [2, 8, 9, 11–14]. However, if firm anchorage in the remaining calcaneal is impossible, plate and screw fixation must be considered (Fig. 16.4).

The Authors' Preference

Whenever possible, the fibula should be preserved. First, it is an essential lateral stabilizer of the ankle, and second, it serves as a vascularized bone graft in the case of a fusion, thus being beneficial for the healing process. In addition, it

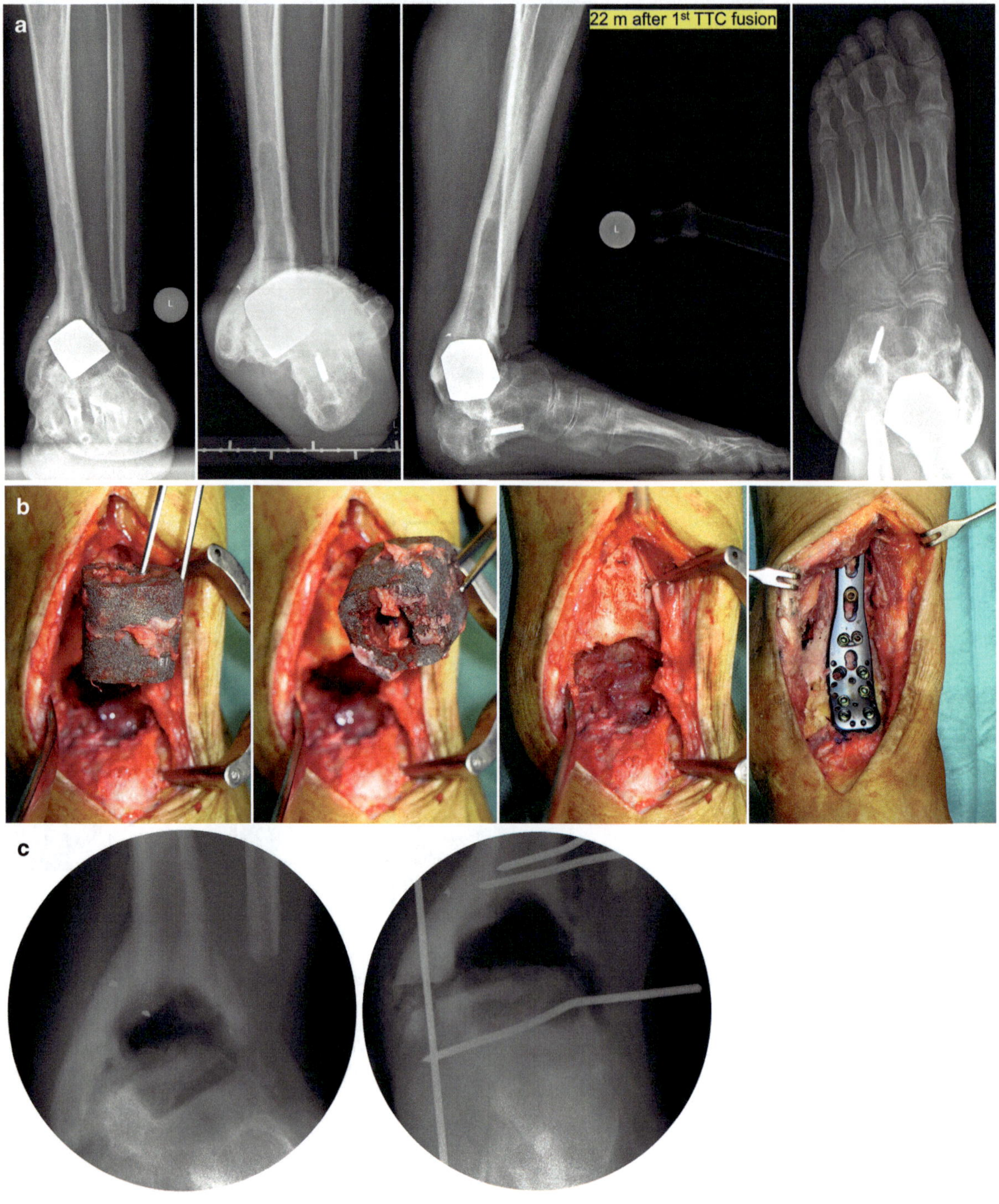

Fig. 16.4 Salvage tibiotalocalcaneal arthrodesis using plate fixation. This 48-year-old patient complained about progressive pain and shortening of his left leg after having undergone salvage tibiotalocalcaneal fusion for a failed total ankle arthroplasty through a lateral transfibular approach. A trabecular metal implant was used to accomplish the bone defect, and the remaining fibula was used as a morselized bone graft. Fixation was achieved with a retrograde nail. Because of a deep infection, the nail was removed after 9 months. (**a**) Standard radiographs show the metallic spacer tilted into the valgus and impacted into the tibia, associated with a hindfoot valgus deformity. The intramedullary bone loss from previous nail fixation was significant, especially on the calcaneus side, revising with a nail being thus critical. (**b**) The spacer was not incorporated. After having impacted an allograft into the defect in the calcaneus originating from the previous nail, a fresh-frozen femoral head added with allograft was used to fill the bone void. Finally, an anterior plate and screws were used for fixation. (**c**) Intraoperative fluoroscopies showing the extent of the bone defect. (**d**) Two months after the surgery, the fusion construct looked stable, with some valgus left. (**e**) Seven months after surgery, the patient felt a cracking in his foot when walking down the stairs. The radiographs evidenced a rupture of the fixation material associated with a recurrent valgus deformity. (**f**) After removing the implants, a retrograde nail was used for fixation; however, the hindfoot was not completely realigned because the defect in the calcaneus from the previous nail fixation did provoke a medial displacement of the nail. (**g**) As the valgus deformity progressed, the nail was revised to a longer nail with a more lateral fixation in the calcaneus, resulting in a well-aligned hindfoot. Nine months later, the arthrodesis seems stable, but the bone remodeling process has not yet been completed

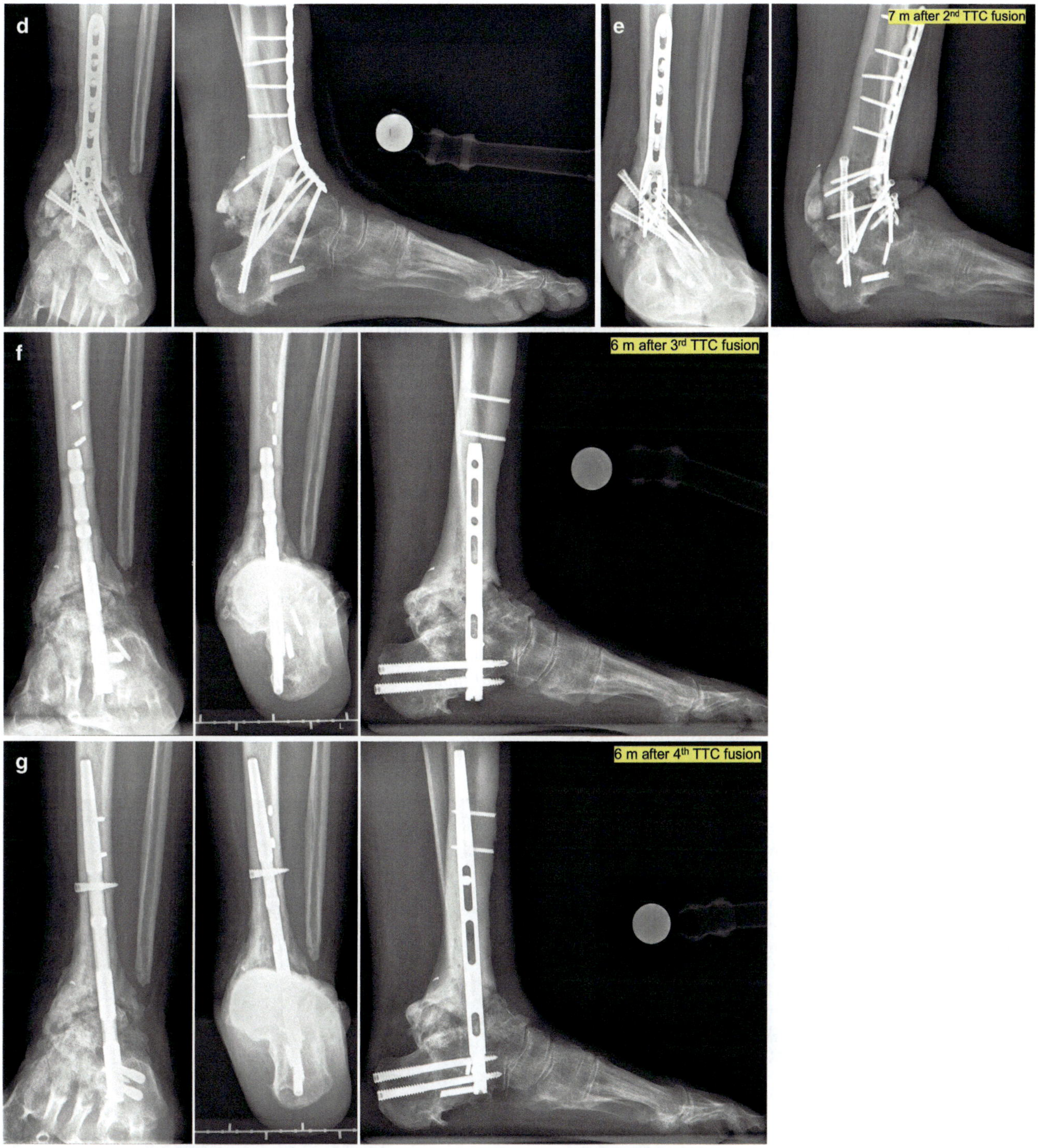

Fig. 16.4 (continued)

stabilizes the foot against rotational forces and serves as a reference for defining the rotational position during the arthrodesis surgery.

16.4 Outcome of Salvage Arthrodesis

In a systematic review on salvage arthrodeses after failed total ankle arthroplasties, Gross et al. [2] found an overall first-attempt fusion rate of 84% for tibiotalar and tibiotalocalcaneal arthrodeses. Tibiotalar arthrodesis had a higher first-attempt fusion rate of 94% compared with 65% for tibiotalocalcaneal cases. A blade plate provided the highest union rate of 100%, and a tibiotalocalcaneal fusion cage provided the lowest union rate of 50%. However, the tibiotalocalcaneal arthrodeses were undertaken in cases with more significant bone loss, thereby making the achievement of union more challenging. The most extensive study on failed total ankle arthroplasties reported 118 salvage arthrodeses [15]. The overall first-attempt successful fusion rate was 90%; however, they did not indicate the numbers of tibiotalar versus tibiotalocalcaneal arthrodeses. In another report on 17 patients, 13 (76%) achieved radiographic fusion on the first attempt [16]. While all five tibiotalar arthrodeses healed, four of the 12 tibiotalocalcaneal arthrodeses did not. Ali et al. [17] reported 23 tibiotalocalcaneal arthrodeses for aseptic loosening using a retrograde intramedullary nail without any interpositional spacer or graft. The union rate for the ankle was 95%, and for the subtalar joint, it was 91%.

Resection of the ankle components often leaves a large bone void. In a small series of 5 patients, Halverson et al. [18] reported using fresh frozen femoral heads for tibiotalocalcaneal salvage arthrodesis. Three of the five patients (60%) demonstrated complete healing of the graft after an average of 5 years. Alternatives to using femoral heads include acute shortening with proximal bone transport, so-called off-the-shelf metal implants, and custom 3D-printed implants. Recently, a trabecular metal implant was proposed, with a satisfactory outcome (Fig. 16.5) [19]. Aubret et al. [14], in contrast, reported continued pain and difficulty assessing arthrodesis in a series of 11 patients who received trabecular metal implants for failed total ankle arthroplasties. At a mean follow-up of 19.3 months, five patients achieved a fusion of the subtalar joint, and eight achieved a fusion of the tibiotalar joint. Three patients (27%) required surgical revision. Dekker et al. [13] reported on 15 patients who received a custom 3D cage for large bone defects in the ankle. There were two failures, one for nonunion and one for infection.

The Authors' Preference

*If a large bone void is left after implant removal, we consider using a vascularized bone graft to bridge the gap. An ipsilateral fibular graft is the most convenient because of its mechanical strength and high remodeling capability (*Fig. 16.6*).*

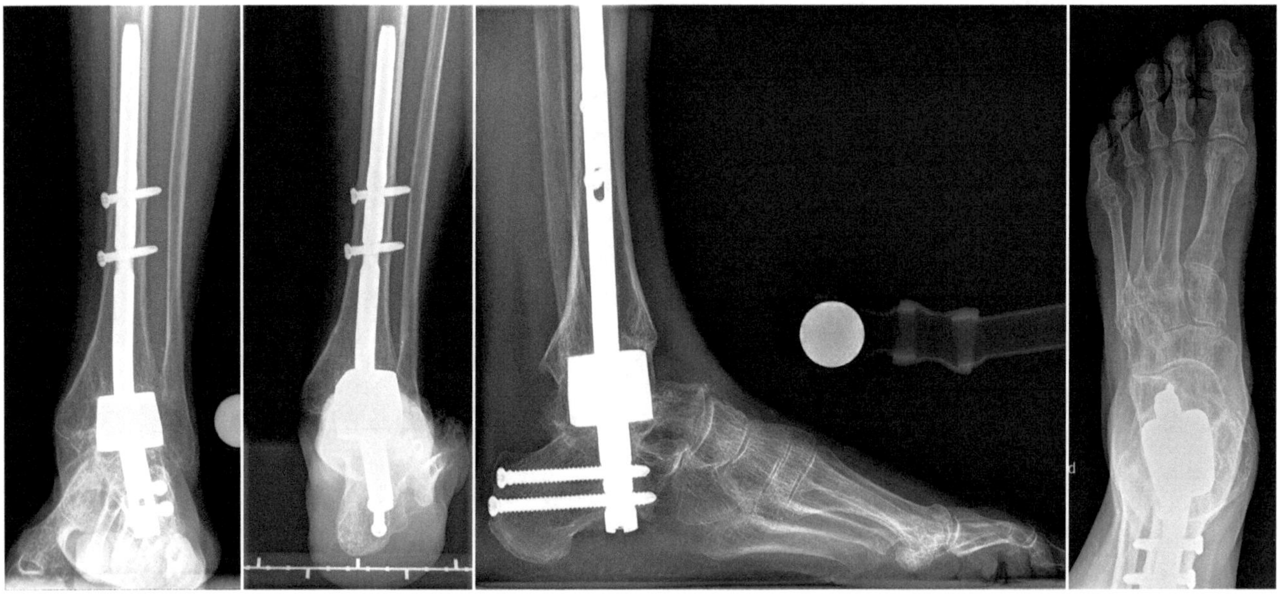

Fig. 16.5 Salvage tibiotalocalcaneal arthrodesis using a trabecular metal implant. Tibiotalocalcaneal arthrodesis was achieved in this patient using a trabecular metal implant and an intramedullary rod fixation. Notably, the preserved malleoli and bone formation on the posterior and anterior aspects might have been essential for achieving stable arthrodesis

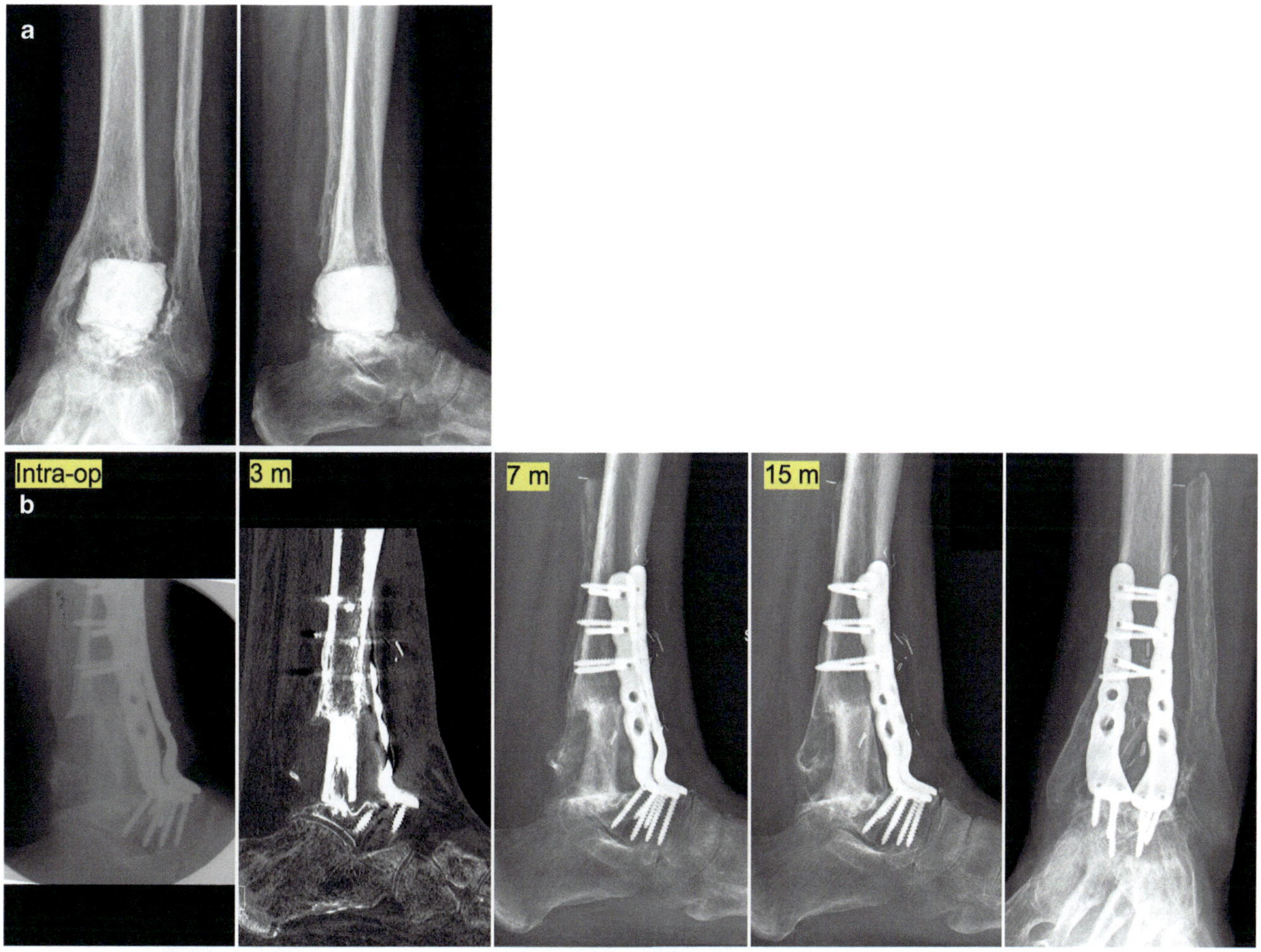

Fig. 16.6 Salvage tibiotalar arthrodesis using a vascularized fibular graft. After the removal of the loose components and nonviable bone, the bone defect was significant. The remaining bone stock of the talus was minimal. To preserve the subtalar joint in this 39-year-old patient, a vascularized fibular graft was used to bridge the defect. (**a**) Preoperative situation with the cement spacer in place. (**b**) Series of radiographs showing the incorporation of the graft. Notably, incorporation on the tibial and talar side is seen already after 3 months. Remodeling of the graft is seen to start after that

16.5 Below-the-Knee Amputation

Below-the-knee amputation should be considered an ultimate solution after other limb salvage procedures have failed (Fig. 16.7). Indications include extensive soft tissue deficit that cannot be addressed even with plastic surgery expertise, persistent infection with drainage even after hardware removal and antibiotic spacer insertion, and severe pain [15, 20, 21].

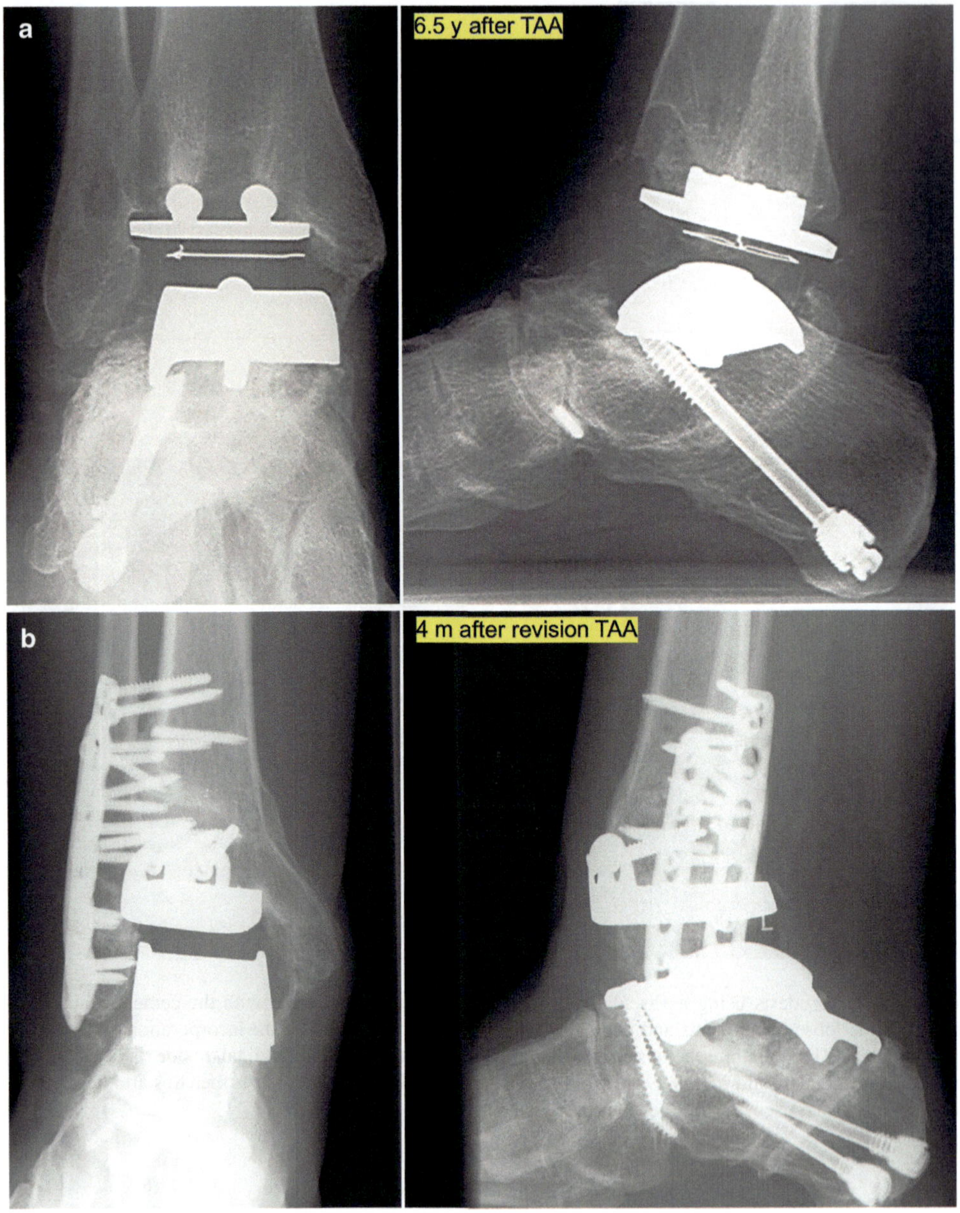

Fig. 16.7 Below-knee amputation for failed revision total ankle arthroplasty. This 56-year-old female with lupus disease treated with immunosuppression therapy underwent a total ankle arthroplasty for secondary arthritis due to circumscribed avascular necrosis of the talus 24 years ago. (**a**) 6.5 years after the replacement surgery, she presented with pain because of subsidence of the talar component. (**b**) Revision arthroplasty was performed using a custom-made talar component. (**c**) 17 years later, she experienced pain again due to the subsidence of the talar component. (**d**) Implant removal with the insertion of a gentamycin-Palacios spacer was performed. After extended discussions, the patient decided against the proposed tibiocalcaneal arthrodesis using a vascularized fibular graft instead of going for below-knee amputation. Her statement was: "24 years ago, I decided against a fusion, though I knew about the risk of replacement surgery. I had so many years of a beautiful time with my ankle prostheses, allowing me to pursue a professional career and visit many countries with my husband. It was my best decision. Why should I go now for a solution I rejected 24 years ago and assume the huge effort needed and its associated risks?"

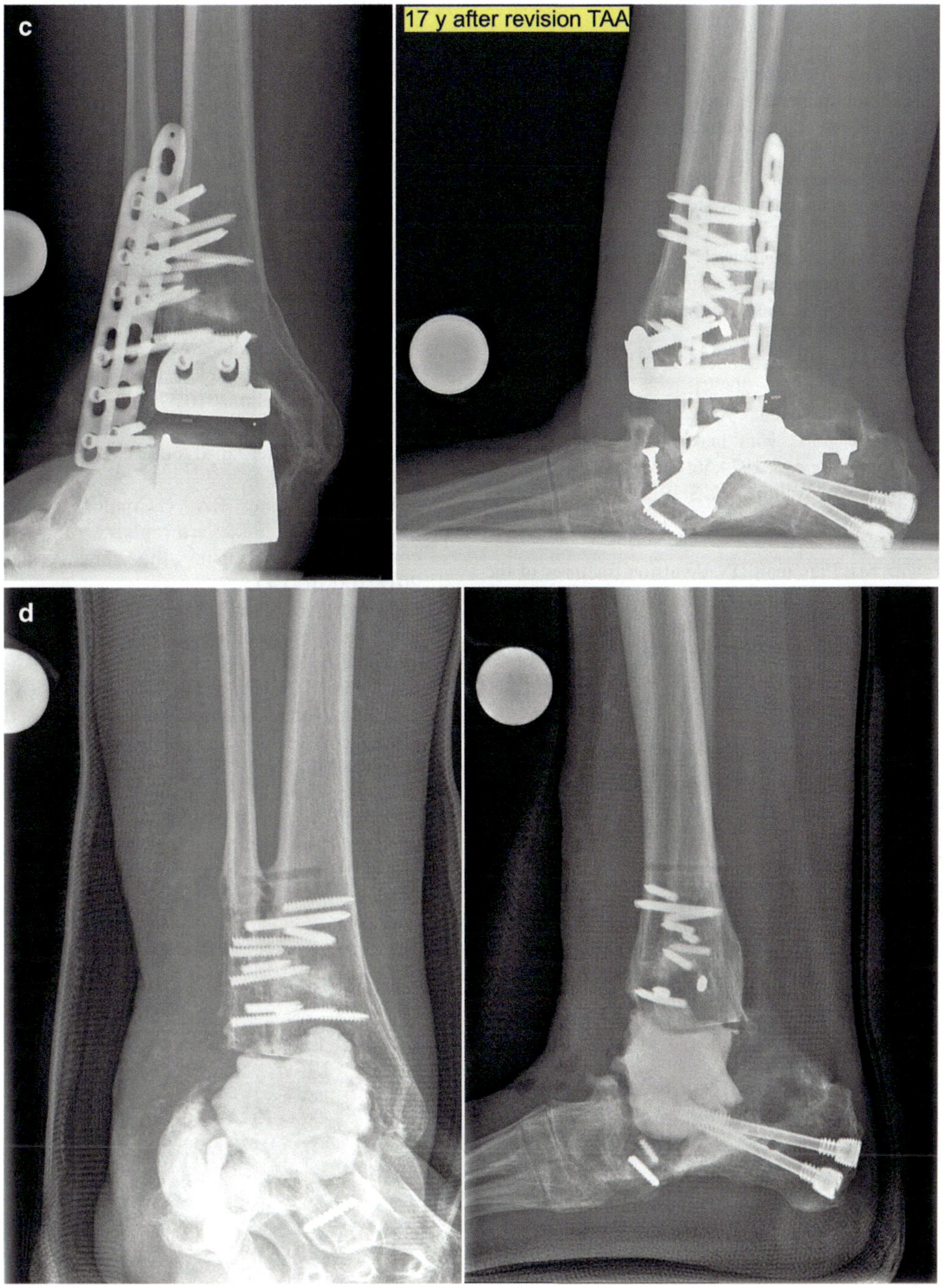

Fig. 16.7 (continued)

16.6 Conclusions

- Salvage arthrodesis is a reliable treatment option for failed total ankle arthroplasties, especially in severe loss of bone stock (tibia, talus, or both), inadequate soft tissue coverage, or the inability to eradicate infection.
- Tibiotalar arthrodesis is preferred over tibiotalocalcaneal arthrodesis to maintain function across the subtalar joint because the union rate is higher for tibiotalar arthrodesis.
- In cases of inadequate talus bone stock, tibiotalocalcaneal arthrodesis is necessary.
- Autograft or allograft bone can be used to maintain length.
- Metal implants have been proposed as an alternative, but they must prove their reliability in further studies.
- The fibula should be preserved whenever possible.
- Based on the literature data, the expected success rate is between 80% and 95%.

References

1. Donnenwerth MP, Roukis TS. Tibio-talo-calcaneal arthrodesis with retrograde compression intramedullary nail fixation for salvage of failed total ankle replacement: a systematic review. Clin Podiatr Med Surg. 2013;30(2):199–206.
2. Gross C, Erickson BJ, Adams SB, Parekh SG. Ankle arthrodesis after failed total ankle replacement: a systematic review of the literature. Foot Ankle Spec. 2015;8(2):143–51.
3. Jennison T, Spolton-Dean C, Rottenburg H, Ukoumunne O, Sharpe I, Goldberg A. The outcomes of revision surgery for a failed ankle arthroplasty : a systematic review and meta-analysis. Bone Jt Open. 2022;3(7):596–606.
4. Bruggerman NB, Kiataoka HB. Arthrodesis after failed total ankle arthroplasty. Tech Foot Ankle Surg. 2002:1.
5. Campbell CJ, Rinehart WT, Kalenak A. Arthrodesis of the ankle. Deep autogenous inlay grafts with maximum cancellous-bone apposition. J Bone Joint Surg Am. 1974;56(1):63–70.
6. Berkowitz MJ, Sanders RW, Walling AK. Salvage arthrodesis after failed ankle replacement: surgical decision making. Foot Ankle Clin. 2012;17(4):725–40.
7. Kim DH, Berkowitz MJ, Pressman DN. Avulsion fractures of the medial tubercle of the posterior process of the talus. Foot Ankle Int. 2003;24(2):172–5.
8. Kruidenier J, van der Plaat LW, Sierevelt IN, Hoornenborg D, Haverkamp D. Ankle fusion after failed ankle replacement in rheumatic and non-rheumatic patients. Foot Ankle Surg. 2019;25(5):589–93.
9. Gross CE, Lewis JS, Adams SB, Easley M, DeOrio JK, Nunley JA 2nd. Secondary arthrodesis after total ankle arthroplasty. Foot Ankle Int. 2016;37(7):709–14.
10. Rahm S, Klammer G, Benninger E, Gerber F, Farshad M, Espinosa N. Inferior results of salvage arthrodesis after failed ankle replacement compared to primary arthrodesis. Foot Ankle Int. 2015;36(4):349–59.
11. Pfahl K, Roser A, Eder J, Gottschalk O, Horterer H, Mehlhorn A, et al. Outcomes of salvage procedures for failed total ankle arthroplasty. Foot Ankle Int. 2023;44(4):262–9.
12. Adams SB. Salvage arthrodesis for failed total ankle replacement. Foot Ankle Clin. 2020;25(2):281–91.
13. Dekker TJ, Steele JR, Federer AE, Hamid KS, Adams SB Jr. Use of patient-specific 3D-printed titanium implants for complex foot and ankle limb salvage, deformity correction, and arthrodesis procedures. Foot Ankle Int. 2018;39(8):916–21.
14. Aubret S, Merlini L, Fessy M, Besse JL. Poor outcomes of fusion with trabecular metal implants after failed total ankle replacement: Early results in 11 patients. Orthop Traumatol Surg Res. 2018;104(2):231–7.
15. Kamrad I, Henricson A, Magnusson H, Carlsson A, Rosengren BE. Outcome after salvage arthrodesis for failed total ankle replacement. Foot Ankle Int. 2016;37(3):255–61.
16. Deleu PA, Devos Bevernage B, Maldague P, Gombault V, Leemrijse T. Arthrodesis after failed total ankle replacement. Foot Ankle Int. 2014;35(6):549–57.
17. Ali AA, Forrester RA, O'Connor P, Harris NJ. Revision of failed total ankle arthroplasty to a hindfoot fusion: 23 consecutive cases using the Phoenix nail. Bone Joint J. 2018;100-B(4):475–9.
18. Halverson AL, Goss DA Jr, Berlet GC. Ankle arthrodesis with structural grafts can work for the salvage of failed total ankle arthroplasty. Foot Ankle Spec. 2020;13(2):132–7.
19. Sagherian BH, Claridge RJ. Salvage of failed total ankle replacement using tantalum trabecular metal: case series. Foot Ankle Int. 2015;36(3):318–24.
20. Myerson MS, Shariff R, Zonno AJ. The management of infection following total ankle replacement: demographics and treatment. Foot Ankle Int. 2014;35(9):855–62.
21. Patton D, Kiewiet N, Brage M. Infected total ankle arthroplasty: risk factors and treatment options. Foot Ankle Int. 2015;36(6):626–34.

17 Conversion of Painful Ankle Arthrodesis to Total Ankle Arthroplasty

The debate about the best treatment for end-stage ankle osteoarthritis continues. Even though ankle replacements are becoming more reliable, many foot and ankle surgeons still treat their patients with fusions. The main arguments are that tibiotalar (ankle) range of motion is somewhat limited, and additional movement is generated from the adjacent foot joint [1]. Because of satisfactory success rates and low morbidity with an ankle fusion, it remained the gold standard for a long time [2–6].

Ankle fusions are not without complications. Several patients complain about persistent pain around the ankle because of nonunion, malunion, or malpositioning of the joint [7]. Initially, patients could gain motion through the talonavicular and subtalar joints after ankle fusions, but the incongruent movement could lead to progressive degenerative joint disease [8–12]. It is also known that younger patients submitted to ankle fusions more rapidly develop osteoarthritis of the adjacent joints caused by added stress because the ankle is not moving [10, 11]. Approximately 50% of patients have clinically significant hindfoot arthritis eight years after ankle arthrodesis [13], indicating that many patients predictably develop degenerative changes in surrounding joints as abnormal loads are shifted to neighboring joints [1, 10, 11, 13–15]. These patients cannot walk properly, have difficulties performing their daily duties, and cannot participate in most active sports activities [10]. The known long-term issues with ankle fusions could lead to further surgeries ranging from fusion revision, correcting alignment osteotomies, or fusions of adjacent joints [16]. The results of these complex operations are generally satisfactory but only sometimes as favorable as anticipated [10, 14]. Arthrodesis to relieve the pain in the subtalar or talonavicular joints increases morbidity and clinical limitations over time [17]. Recent articles have shown that converting an ankle fusion to an ankle replacement has promising results and could be the better option [7, 18–23].

17.1 Preoperative Considerations

17.1.1 Analysis of the Fusion and Feasibility for Conversion

Fusions, where no bone was removed, are the easiest to convert, particularly if the lateral and the medial gutters were not fused (Fig. 17.1). Transfibular and flat cut fusions are much more difficult (Fig. 17.2). A fusion where the fibula was removed is very critical for replacement and mostly considered contraindicated (Fig. 17.3). To the authors' experience, a fusion that was made through a medial approach with resection of the medial malleolus is contraindicated (Fig. 17.4). Malunited fusions are most challenging and may need first a correcting surgery before considering a conversion to a total ankle arthroplasty (Fig. 17.5).

17.1.2 Hardware

Often, hardware is in place. Removing complex hardware first is advised, especially if there is a posterior tibial plate (Fig. 17.6).

17.1.3 Imaging Evaluation

Evaluating the preoperative radiographs is crucial for a successful surgery to understand where the joint line should be created (Fig. 17.7a). Using radiographs of the non-affected

B. Hintermann, R. Ruiz, *Total Ankle Replacement*, https://doi.org/10.1007/978-3-031-56810-7_17

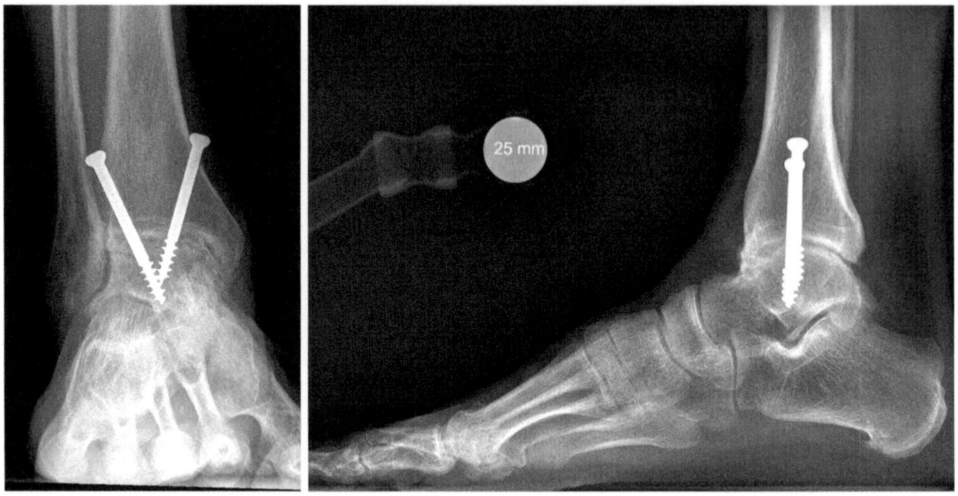

Fig. 17.1 Fusion without bone removal. In this arthroscopically fused ankle 6.5 years ago, the bone stock and the previous articular references are preserved, facilitating conversion to a total ankle arthroplasty

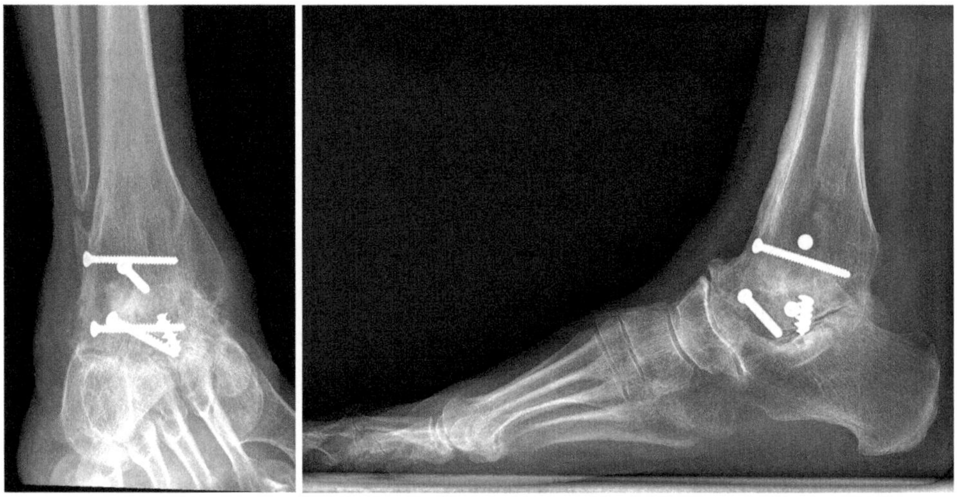

Fig. 17.2 Fusion with bone removal. This ankle was fused nine years ago through a transfibular approach, using one part of the fibula as a morselized bone graft and the other as a structural bone graft. A conversion of the ankle to a total ankle arthroplasty is critical because of the minimal bone left to create a sufficient lateral buttress. Of note is the equinus malunion with degenerative disease of the peritalar joints

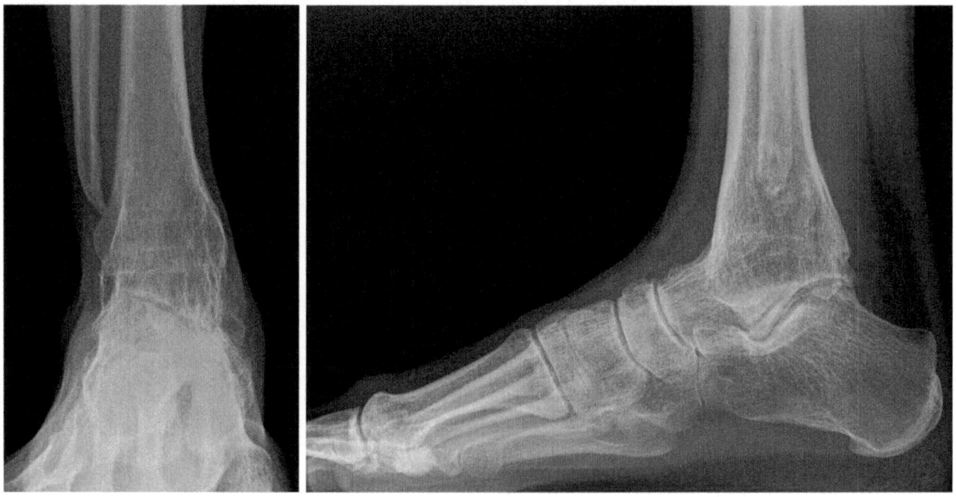

Fig. 17.3 Fusion with resection of distal fibula. This ankle was fused 11 years ago through a transfibular approach, using the fibula as a morselized bone graft. A conversion of the ankle to a total ankle arthroplasty would need reconstruction of the fibula with an increased risk of failure; a conversion to an ankle replacement is feasible but highly risky and thus considered contraindicated

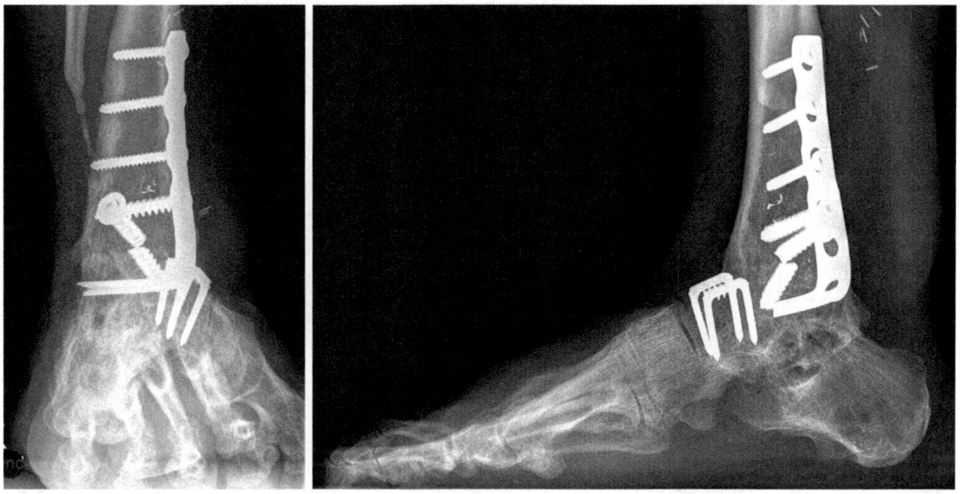

Fig. 17.4 Fusion with resection of both malleoli. This ankle was fused 13 years ago through a transfibular approach, using the fibula as a morselized bone graft and revised four times. Fusion was finally achieved by fixation with a blade plate through a medial approach, scarifying the medial malleolus. Notice that the extended fusion includes the subtalar and the talonavicular joint. A conversion to a total ankle arthroplasty is contraindicated

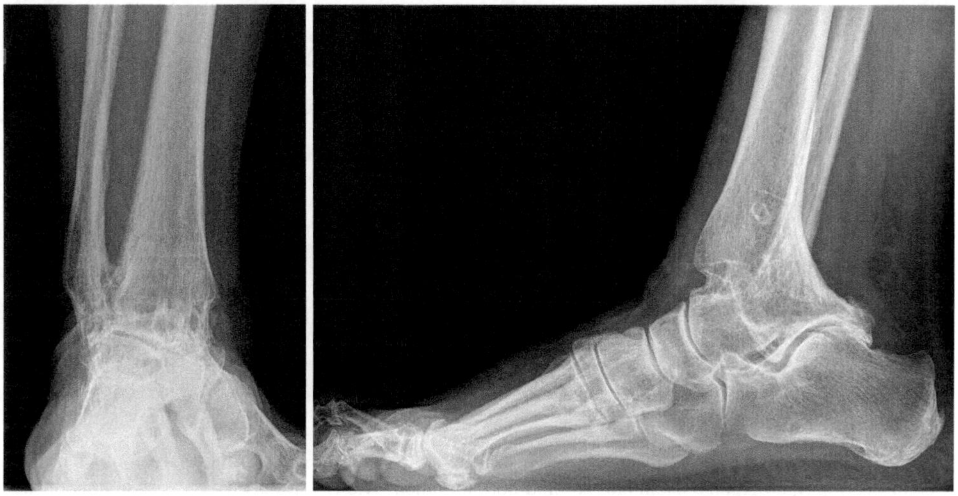

Fig. 17.5 Malunited fusion. This ankle was fused 7.8 years ago, secondary to a failed ankle fracture treatment with the development of septic arthritis. Because of this, healing was achieved by immobilization in plaster, which resulted in an equinus malunion. Conversion to total ankle arthroplasty is challenging for making resection cuts and is complicated by partial loss of both malleoli

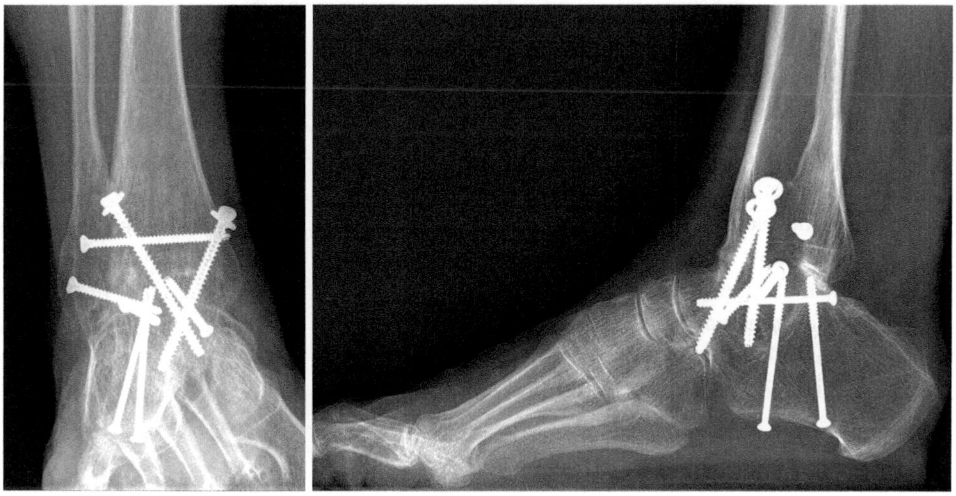

Fig. 17.6 Fusion with hardware in place. This ankle underwent six surgeries since the first attempt for fusion. Hardware removal first is advised since screw removal might be challenging and unpredictable about the time needed and the bad soft tissues

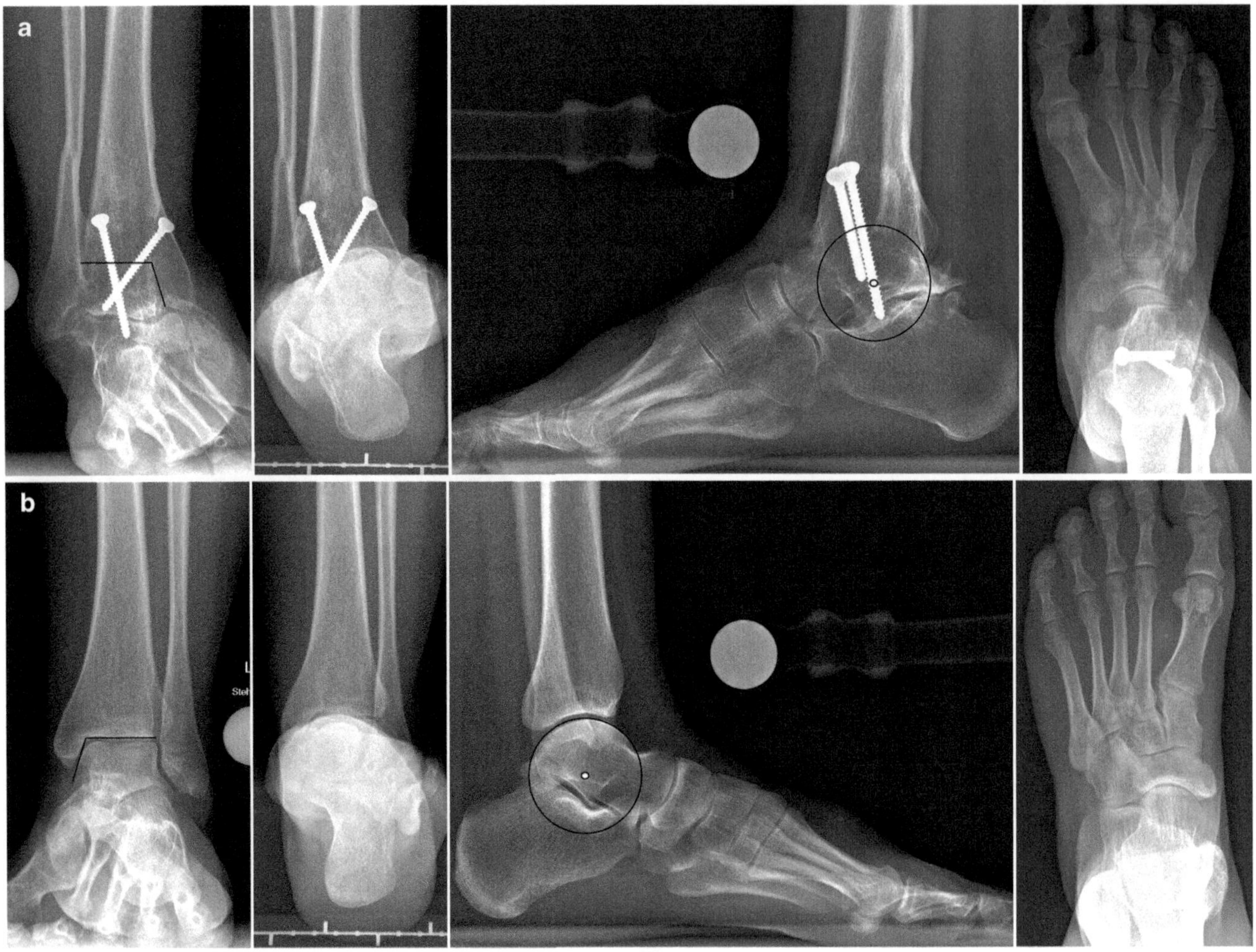

Fig. 17.7 Radiographic assessment of the fused ankle. Standard weight-bearing radiographs, including a hindfoot alignment view, assess the fused ankle. (**a**) In this 37-year-old female patient, the fusion was made at 17 years and 22 months after an ankle fracture that was treated conservatively. Arthroscopic fusion of the ankle without addressing the incompetent lateral soft tissue structures resulted in a progressive varus-supination deformity. (**b**) Standardized radiographs of the contralateral ankle are used to determine the references and the height of the resection cuts

contralateral ankle as the reference may be helpful (Fig. 17.7b).

Pain that develops after an initial successful, pain-free ankle fusion is most often due to adjacent joint osteoarthritis or mechanical changes from a fused joint. Pain in the ankle itself is only if there is a nonunion present. Therefore, further investigation of the peritalar joints by CT scan (Fig. 17.8) or Spect CT (Fig. 17.9) is generally recommended.

17.1.4 Preoperative Planning

The joint line should be established at, or as close as possible, to the original joint line. This is best done by using bilateral radiographs. In the AP view, the medial corner of the tibiotalar joint of the presumed ankle is determined as shown in Fig. 17.7. In the lateral view, the height of the talus is defined as shown in Fig 17.7.

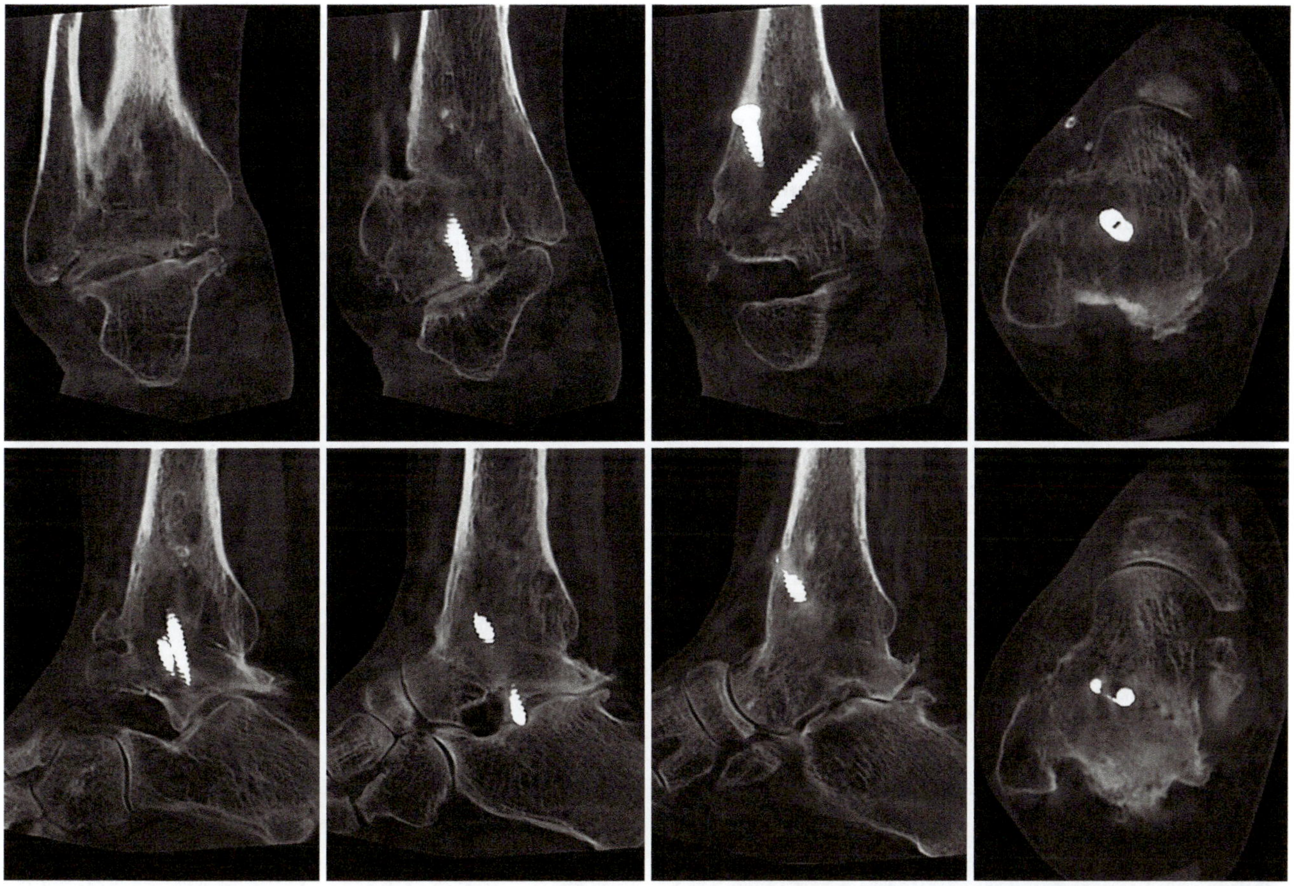

Fig. 17.8 Weight-bearing CT scan. A CT scan is used to understand the malposition of the peritalar joints, the extent of osteoarthritic changes at the subtalar joint, and overall deformity of the hind- and midfoot (same patient as Fig. 17.7)

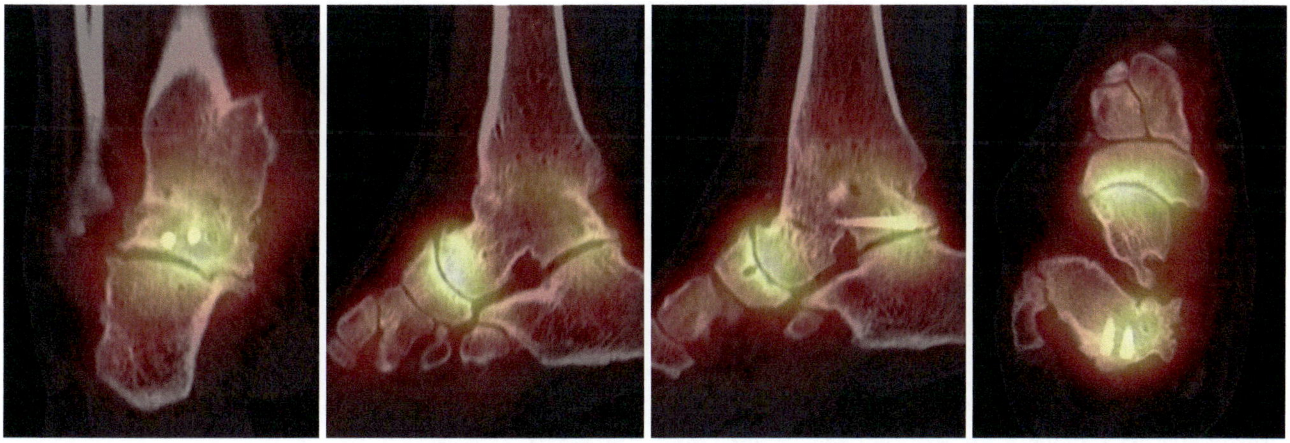

Fig. 17.9 Spect CT. A Spect CT was used in this patient 8.2 y after ankle fusion to assess the underlying cause of massive pain. It reveals an activity process in the posterior subtalar and the talonavicular joint, indicating that a fusion of the subtalar and talonavicular joints should be considered

17.2 Surgical Technique

Fusion of the adjacent joints (subtalar and talonavicular) should be done only in the case of an advanced stage of osteoarthritis in fear of devascularization of the talus with the dome, the lateral and medial gutter, and then either subtalar or talonavicular preparation. Restoring ankle motion may also reduce the stress and load in the adjacent joints and reduce pain. If in doubt, we preoperatively use a Spect CT (Fig. 17.9) to decide.

We have described our surgical technique previously in detail [24]. For didactic reasons, we present below our technique of converting the fusion to total ankle arthroplasty in combination with a subtalar fusion. However, we don't fuse the subtalar joint in most cases.

17.2.1 Conversion of the Fusion with a Subtalar Fusion

If a subtalar fusion is planned, the subtalar joint is exposed and debrided first (Fig. 17.10). After wound closure, a 12- to 14-cm longitudinal anterior approach is used to expose the arthrodesis site. The incision may be adapted for previous skin incisions from the fusion. The anterior aspect of the tibia and the talar neck is identified after subperiosteal dissection. The anteromedial corner of the original tibiotalar joint is identified and marked with a K-wire (Fig. 17.11). The jig with the tibial resection block is mounted proximally to the tibial tuberosity and distally to the K-wire as the reference. The width of the tibial resection is determined with a trial component, and a 2nd K-wire is inserted at its lateral

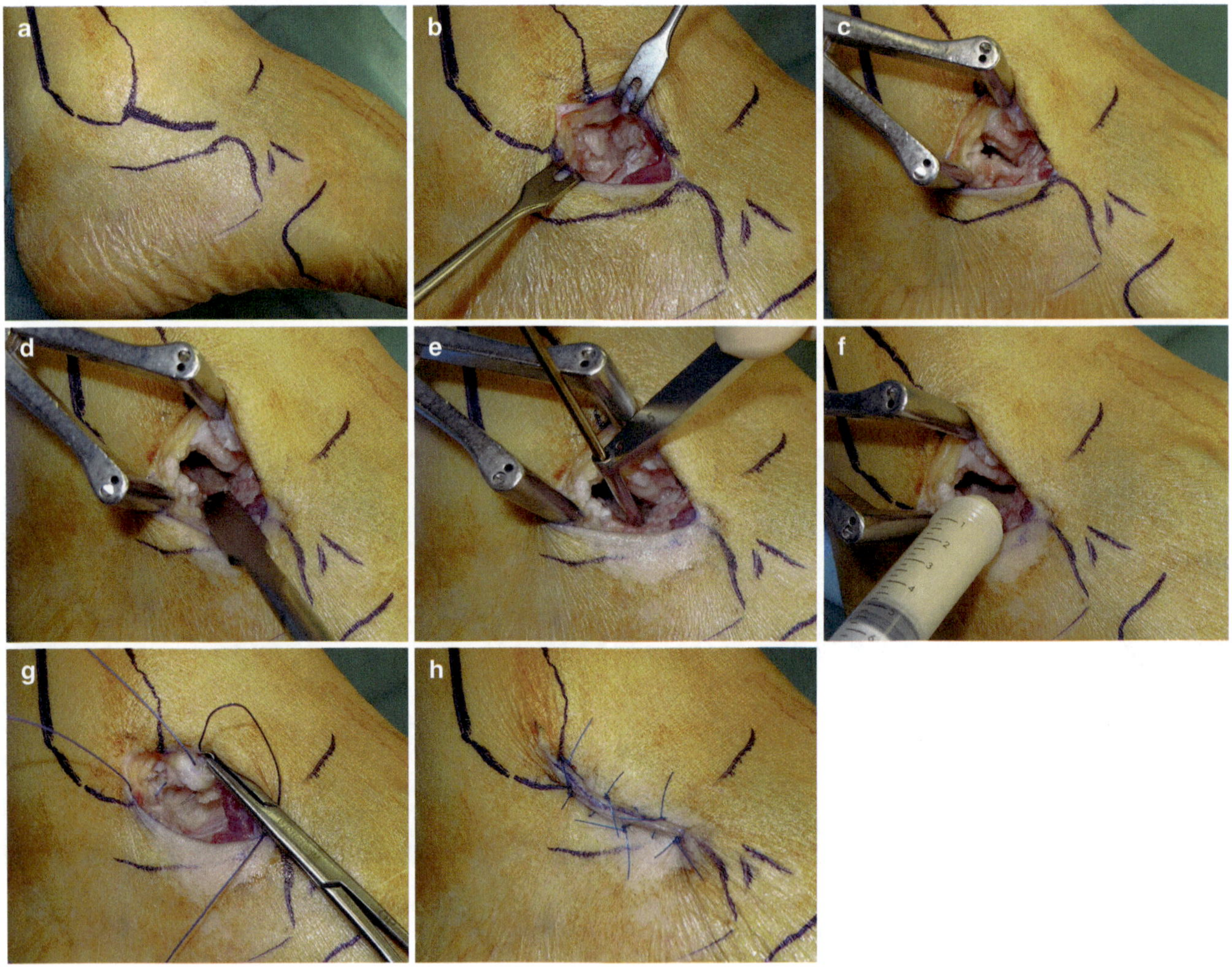

Fig. 17.10 Debridement of the subtalar joint for fusion. (**a**) A 3- to 4-cm-long incision is made over the sinus tarsi. (**b**) Arthrotomy of the subtalar joint by sharp dissection. The sinus tarsi is not cleaned not to compromise the vascularity of the talus. (**c**) The subtalar joint is distracted over 2 K-wires, allowing insight into the posterior aspect of the subtalar joint. (**d**) The posterior facet is debrided to the subchondral bone. (**e**) Drillings are made to perforate subchondral sclerosis. (**f**) Bone matrix or cancellous auto- or allograft may enhance bone healing. (**g**) The deep layers are adapted to get a firm closure to prevent postoperative bleeding. (**h**) The skin is finally closed by interrupted sutures (same patient as Fig. 17.7)

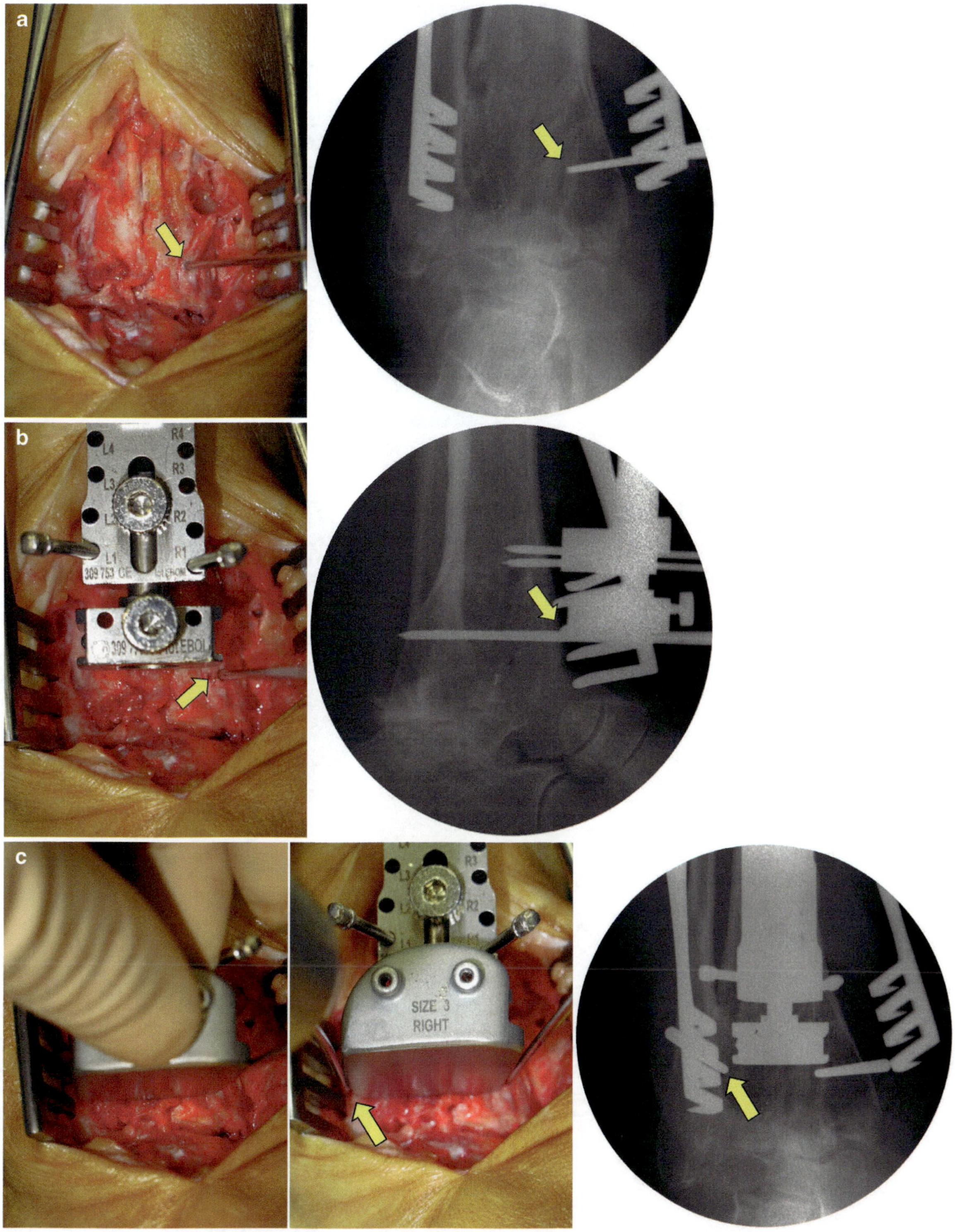

Fig. 17.11 Desarthrodesis of the ankle. (**a**) The arthrodesis site is exposed through a 12- to 14-cm longitudinal incision followed by sharp dissection of the extensor retinaculum along the lateral border of the anterior tibial tendon. Sharp dissection to the tibia and subperiosteal exposure of the arthrodesis site. The anteromedial corner of the tibiotalar joint is determined with fluoroscopy (arrow), and a K-wire is inserted 2–4 mm above, accounting for the thickness of the tibial implant. (**b**) The tibial resection block is mounted proximally to the tibial tuberosity and distally to the K-wire (arrow) as the reference and checked by fluoroscopy. (**c**) As planned on radiographs, a trial tibial component of the selected size is positioned to determine the width of the mortise to be created. A 2nd K-wire is inserted along the lateral border of the component (arrow). (**d**) An additional K-wire is inserted distally on the medial and lateral sides (arrows) to mark the gutters under fluoroscopic control. (**e**) The tibial resection cut is made along the resection block as controlled medially and laterally by the K-wires (arrows). (**f**) A smaller oscillating or reciprocal saw makes the medial and lateral gutter cuts (arrows), using the K-wires as a guide. (**g**) If the ankle is fused in a well-aligned position, the tibial resection block is moved 6–8 mm distally, and the talar cut is performed parallel to the tibial cut. In the case of a malalignment, the cut is made freehand with an angulation according to the needed correction. The bone block is removed, and the ankle is mobilized (same patient as Fig. 17.7)

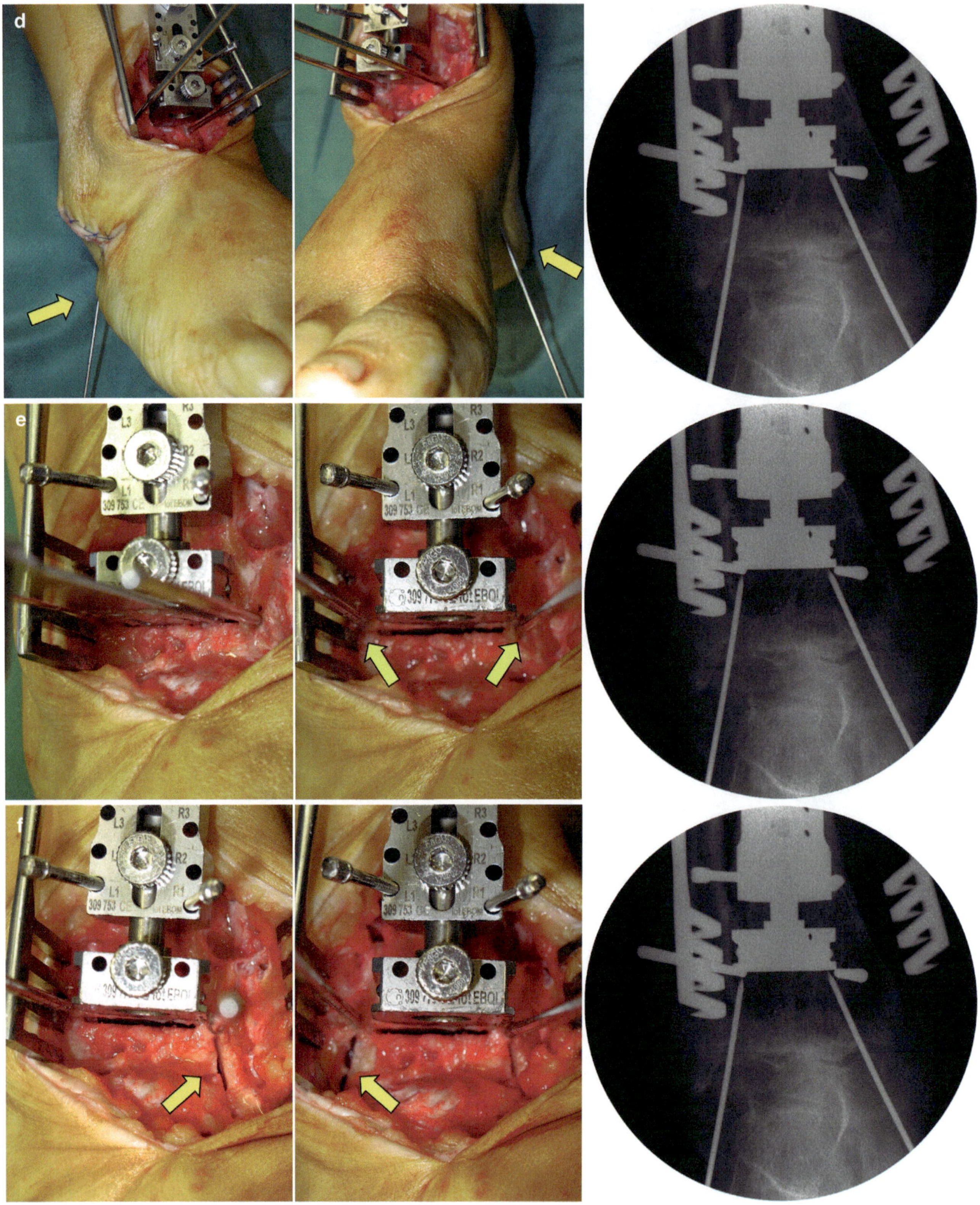

Fig. 17.11 (continued)

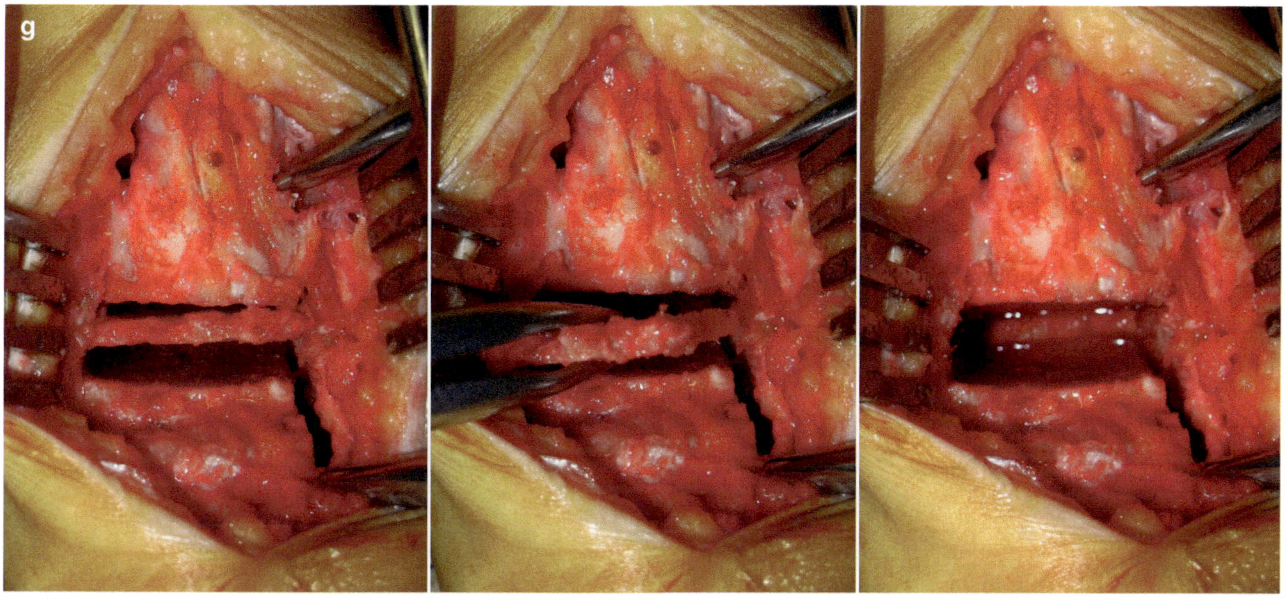

Fig. 17.11 (continued)

margin. A K-wire is inserted distally on the medial and lateral sides to mark the gutters under fluoroscopic control. At this point, additional K-wires can be inserted to protect the malleoli from a fracture. The tibial cut is performed with an oscillating saw through the guide, perpendicular to the long axis of the tibial shaft. The vertical medial and lateral cuts are made along the K-wires with an end-cutting reciprocating saw or an oscillating saw recreating the medial and lateral gutters. The tibial resection block is moved 6–8 mm distally, and the talar cut is performed parallel to the tibial cut. If any coronal or sagittal plane deformity correction needs to be done, the correction is done at this stage, holding the foot in the desired position and doing the talar cut on the proper angulation. The created ankle joint is distracted over 2 K-wires, and the bone block from the fusion is removed. To fix the subtalar fusion, the foot is held in the neutral position while the ankle joint is still distracted. A first K-wire is directed from the center of the talar body to the calcaneal tuberosity and forwarded until its end reaches the level of the resection surface (Fig. 17.12). A second K-wire is inserted from the talar neck into the anterior process of the calcaneus. One canulated screw is inserted retrograde in the talar body, and another screw anterograde in the calcaneus.

The length of the tibial resection surface in the anteroposterior direction is measured to determine the size of the tibial implant; as a rule, the same or slightly smaller component is used for the talus. The talus is further prepared according to the implant's needs (Fig. 17.13). After insertion of the implants and fluoroscopic control (Fig. 17.14), the ankle is aggressively mobilized into dorsiflexion to release the scared soft tissue structures (Fig. 17.15). The heel cord should be released if the achieved dorsiflexion is less than 5°. We consider lengthening the Achilles tendon even when the dorsiflexion does not reach 10°. The motion will not improve as time passes, so time zero should be more than needed. Lateral or medial ligament reconstructions or release, calcaneal osteotomies, or other associated procedures are completed. The wound is closed step-by-step over a drain left without suction for 24 h. After the dressing is made, the ankle is protected with a splint.

The postoperative rehabilitation protocol is the same as for primary total ankle arthroplasties. Usually, weight-bearing as tolerated is permitted from the 2nd day postoperatively.

17.2.2 Fibular Reconstruction

If the fibula was osteotomized during the fusion to be used partially as a morselized bone graft and the other as a structural bone graft, the remaining bone might be critical to providing enough lateral buttress for conversion to a total ankle arthroplasty. If a tiny bone shelf can be preserved, the procedure is feasible (Fig. 17.16) However, the ankle must be well

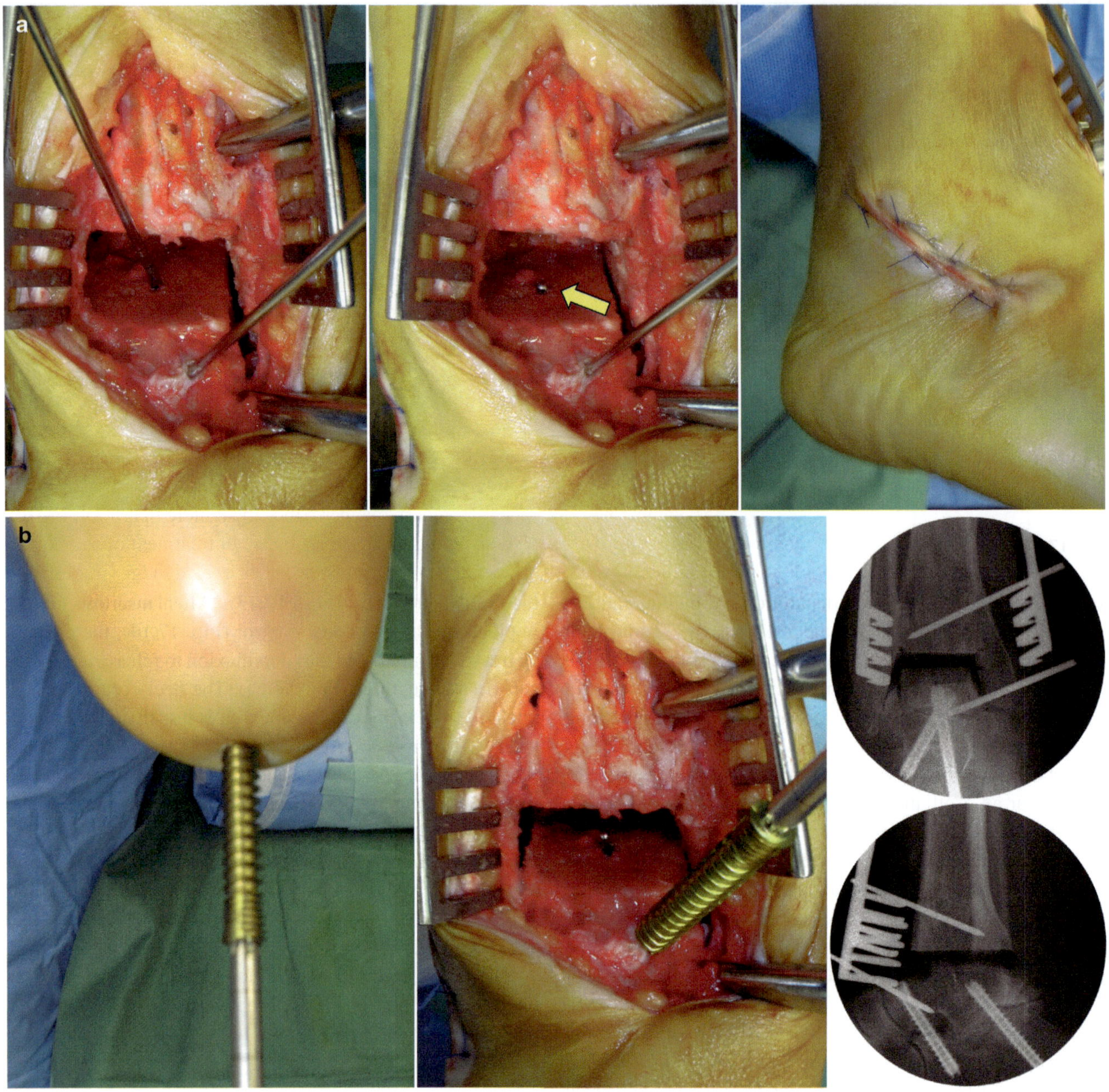

Fig. 17.12 Fixation of subtalar joint. (**a**) While the ankle joint is distracted and the foot is held in a neutral position, a K-wire is inserted into the center of the talar body and directed to the calcaneal tuberosity. After perforating the heel, the K-wire is pulled out until its proximal end reaches the resection surface (arrow). A 2nd K-wire is inserted into the talar head and directed into the anterior process of the calcaneus. (**b**) After determining the distance from the heel to the talar resection surface with the aid of another K-wire and deduced 6–10 mm (to preserve a distance to the implant), a canulated screw is inserted into the talar body. The 2nd canulated screw is inserted anterograde from the talar head into the anterior calcaneus. The screw position is checked by fluoroscopy (same patient as Fig. 17.7)

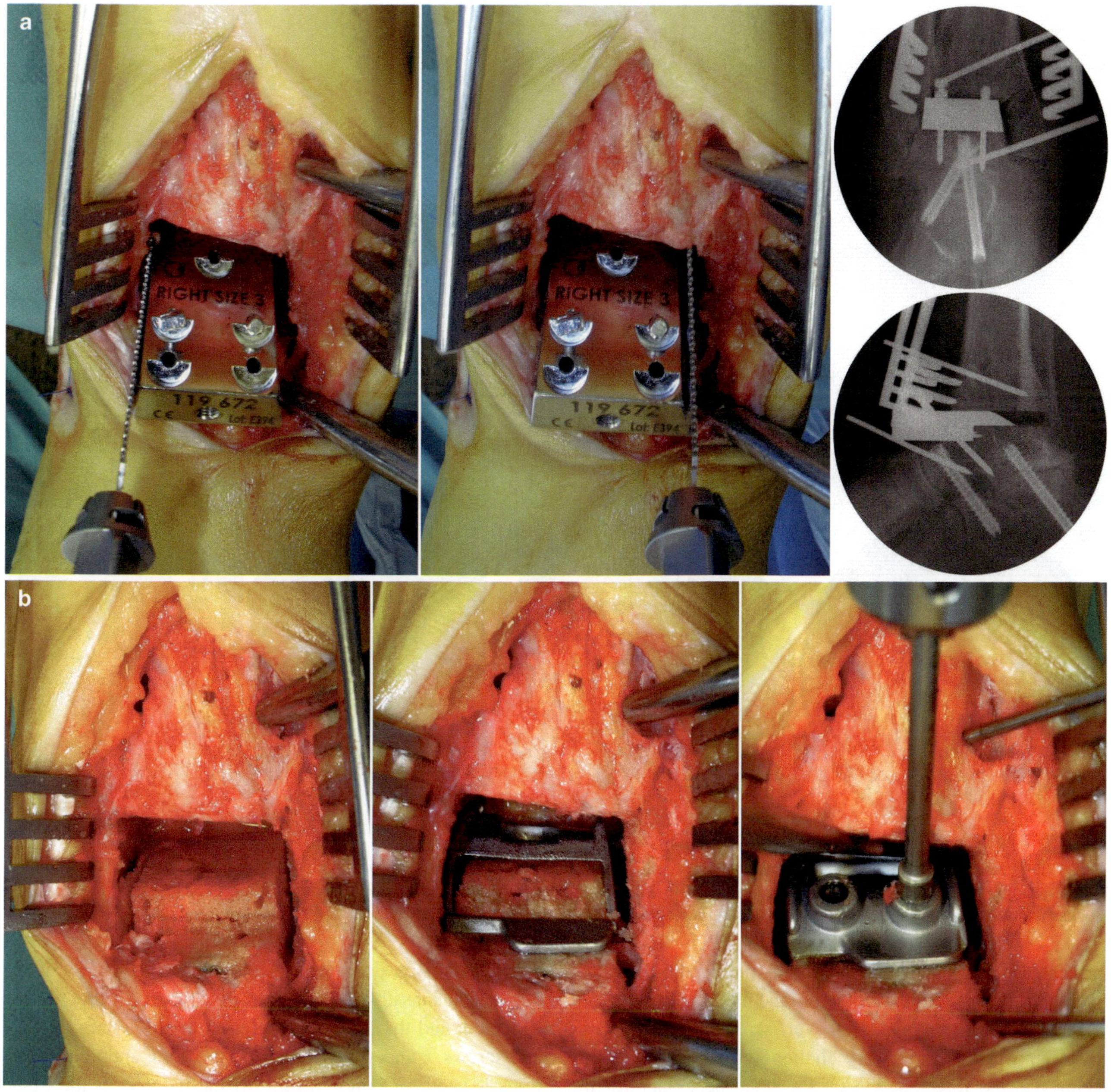

Fig. 17.13 Resection cuts of the talus. (**a**) The talus is further prepared according to the implant's needs. For this ankle design, the talar resection block is mounted on the talus and adjusted, taking the medial and posterior border of the talus as the reference. The aim is to resect approximately 2 mm of the medial and posterior surfaces. The talar resection block is fixed by 2–4 pins, and fluoroscopy can check the position. The resection cuts are made, and the resection block is removed. (**b**) After cleaning the medial and lateral gutters, the posterior aspect of the joint is meticulously cleaned. The posterior capsule is also resected, giving free sight to the flexor hallucis longus tendon. The flexor digitorum longus tendon should also be visible on the posteromedial corner, confirming that the posteromedial capsule is completely removed. The final resection block is mounted, and the anterior resection is made. Finally, with the next resection block in place, the holes for the pegs are reamed (same patient as Fig. 17.12)

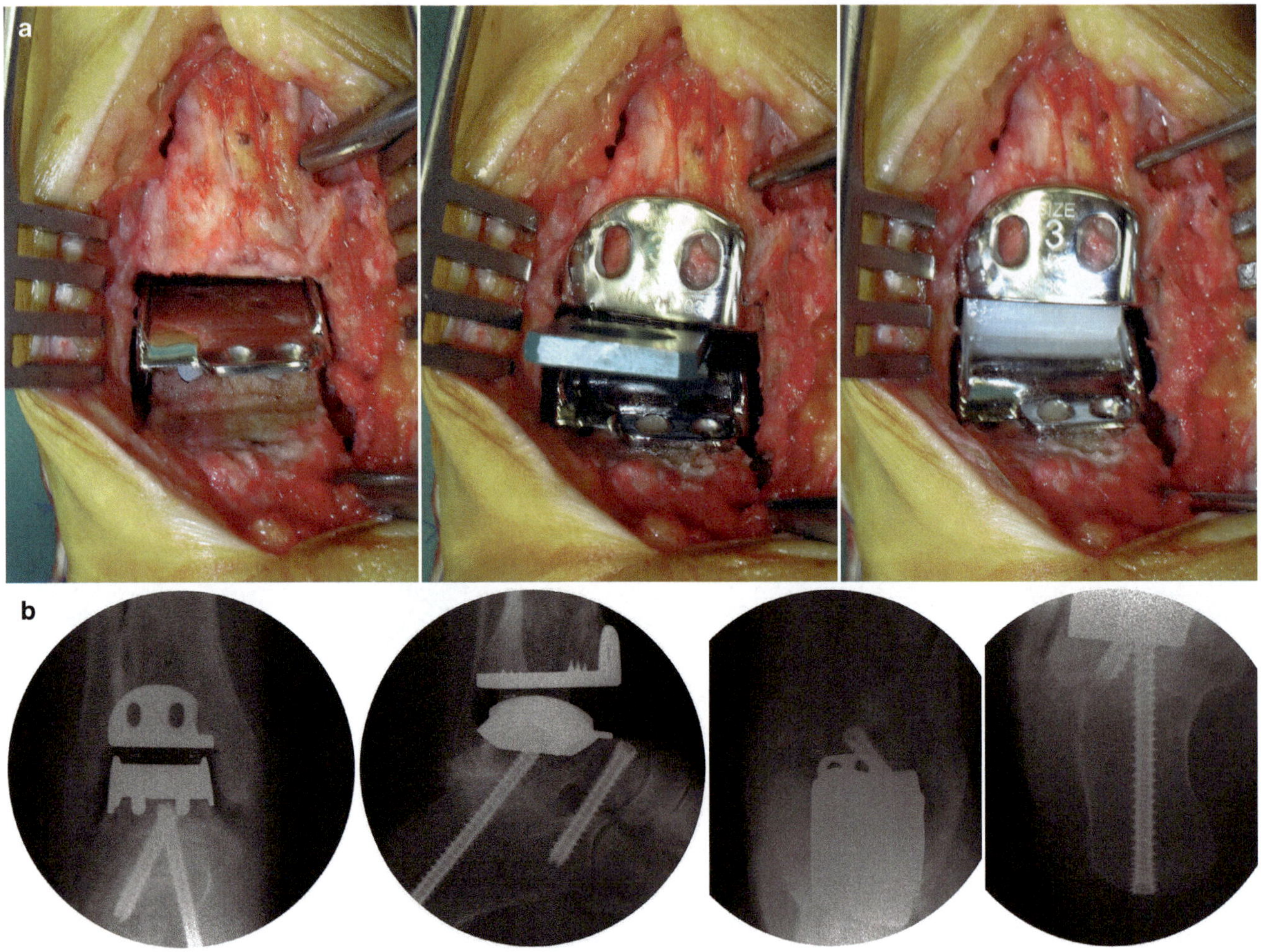

Fig. 17.14 Insertion of implants. (**a**) First, the talar component is inserted and impacted using the pegs as guidance. Then, the tibial component is inserted while the trial insert serves as a protection to avoid metal-to-metal contact. Finally, the polyethylene liner is inserted. (**b**) The position of the components is checked by fluoroscopy (same patient as Fig. 17.12)

protected during the first 3–4 months until remodeling has increased bone strength. Protecting the fibula with screws or a plate is an alternative. However, screw insertion in the remaining bone can be very challenging, and a plate may neutralize the forces acting on the bone necessary for the physiologic remodeling. Most importantly, the heel cannot be left in a valgus at the time of the surgery as it would create lateral translational forces that may exceed the strength of the remaining bone.

If the fibula is missing because of a prior resection at the time of the ankle fusion, a lateral longitudinal incision is made to approach the distal aspect of the residual fibula (Fig. 17.17). An osteotomy is performed 6–8 cm proximal to its distal end. Then, the fibula is mobilized and moved distally until its distal end meets the lateral aspect of the talus. The lateral aspect of the distal part of the tibia is debrided, and the fibula is secured to the tibia using a plate and screws. Cancellous bone from the tibial and talar resections is used for bone grafting. If the fixation of the fibula directly onto the tibia creates a too-narrow mortise, a resected bone from the tibia is used to be interposed between the tibia and the talus.

The peroneal tendons are used for ligament reconstruction because the residual lateral ligaments are usually too sparse for any reconstruction (Fig. 17.17d). After fibular resection at previous fusion surgery, they are generally nonfunctional following the longstanding dislocation. They are exposed at the level of the distal part of the fibula and

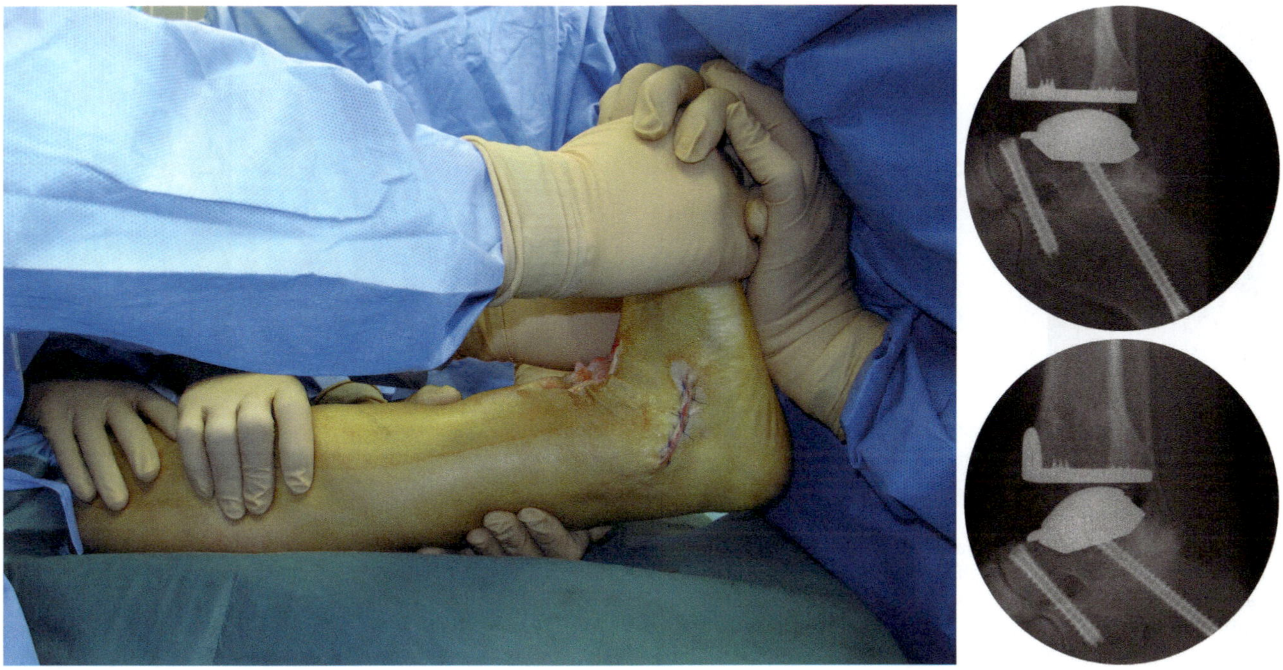

Fig. 17.15 Mobilization of the joint. The ankle is aggressively mobilized into dorsiflexion to release the scared soft tissue structures. The heel cord should be released if the achieved dorsiflexion is less than 5°. We consider lengthening the Achilles tendon even when the dorsiflexion does not reach 10° (same patient as Fig. 17.7)

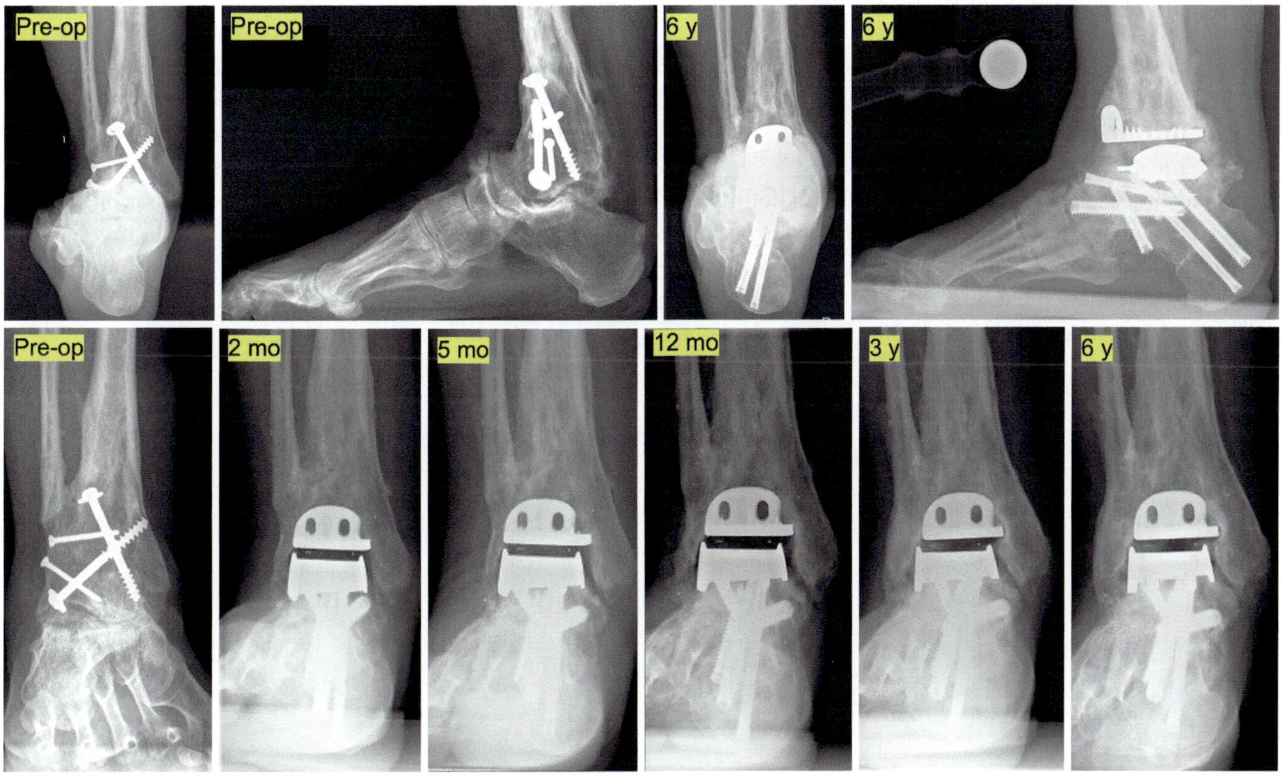

Fig. 17.16 Conversion with a minimized fibula. This ankle was fused 22 years ago through a transfibular approach, using one part of the fibula as a morselized bone graft and the other as a structural bone graft. Preoperatively, the peritalar joints were worn out with significant osteoarthritic changes associated with a valgus malalignment of the heel. A tiny shelf of bone was preserved, and a subtalar fusion and a medial sliding osteotomy were performed. The series of AP views shows the remodeling process of the fibula over the 6-year follow-up

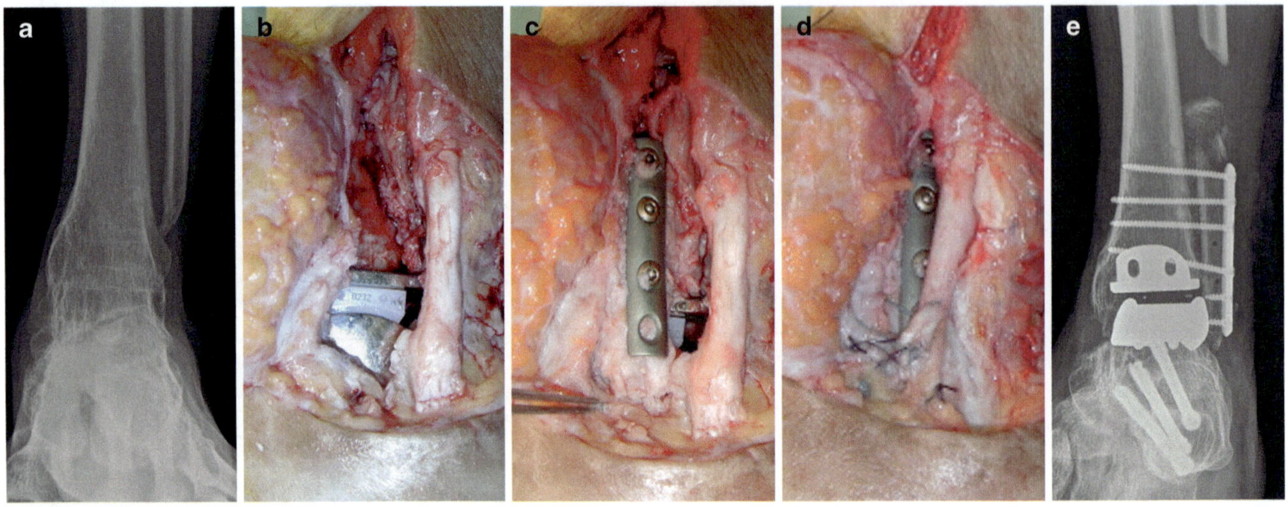

Fig. 17.17 Conversion with fibular reconstruction. This ankle was fused 13 years ago through a transfibular approach, using the fibula as a morselized bone graft. The ankle was four times revised because of deep infection with wound necrosis, and it finally healed after a free flap cover of the defect. (**a**) Preoperative status with the absence of the fibula. (**b**) The fusion was taken down, and the replacement surgery was made through an anterolateral approach, as the free flap gave. Notice the hypertrophic peroneal tendons that were dislocated since the fusion surgery. (**c**) After osteotomy of the fibula 5 cm above its distal end, it was transferred distally and fixed by a plate. (**d**) The peroneal tendons were fixed to the tip of the fibula (tenodesis). (**e**) Postoperative radiograph showing the fibular reconstruction

transposed behind the fibula. While the foot is held in a neutral position, transosseous sutures are used to obtain strong fixation to the posterior aspect of the distal part of the fibula [24].

17.2.3 Inframalleolar Correction

Understanding and addressing an inframalleolar deformity is often challenging because of the structural changes in the peritalar joints. A stable hindfoot in a neutral position is paramount for the replacement surgery. In some instances, using a distractor or compression clamp on the lateral side and the distraction clamp on the medial side is very helpful in correctly positioning the talus on top of the calcaneus (Fig. 17.18).

Residual valgus malalignment is detrimental to the success of this conversion to total ankle arthroplasty, especially when using the three-component ankle prosthesis [7, 19]. Eccentric pull of the Achilles tendon leads to a valgus thrust within the joint, shifting the talus against the medial malleolus at the interface between the tibial component and the polyethylene insert. This can result in painful overstress of the medial malleolus. Therefore, we do not tolerate hindfoot valgus, often present during the surgery. In these cases, a medial sliding osteotomy of the calcaneus is done.

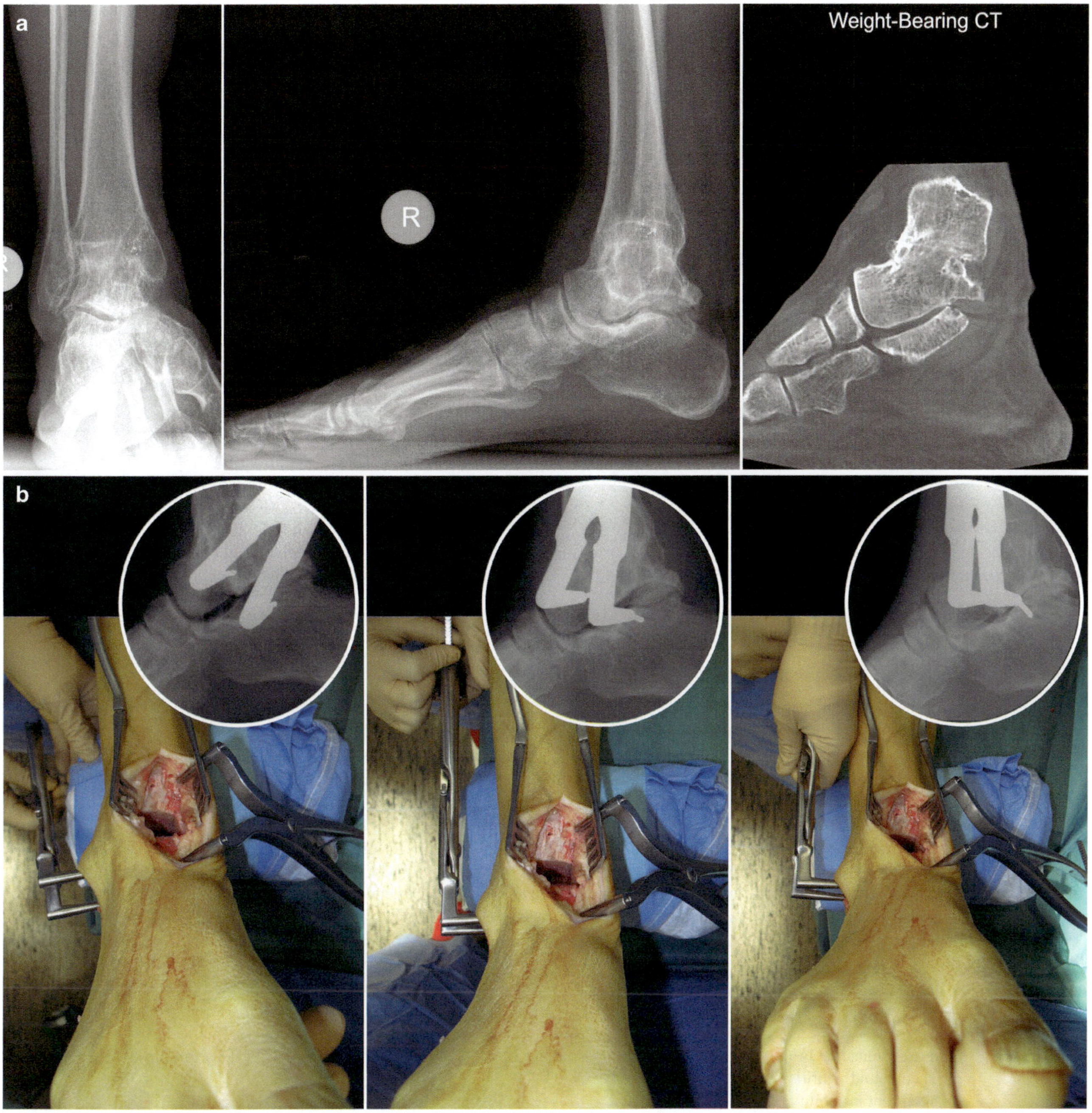

Fig. 17.18 Inframalleolar correction. (**a**) This ankle was fused 16.5 years ago in a slight equinus position, resulting in significant compensatory peritalar instability. (**b**) A correct talus position on top of the calcaneus was achieved with a distraction clamp on the medial side and a compression clamp on the lateral side. This first allowed repositioning maneuvers by rotating the clamp until the forefoot was in a neutral position and then applying compression at the subtalar site

17.3 Outcomes

Little data is available on the take-down of a painful fusion and conversion to a total ankle arthroplasty (Table 17.1). In most cases, the surgeon was faced with high multiple problems, as demonstrated by the number of adjunctive procedures necessary for the replacement surgery (Table 17.2). Though the functional outcome, including the achieved range of motion, is lower than after the primary total ankle arthroplasty, the overall result is satisfactory indicating that an ankle replacement is a valuable option for salvaging a painful ankle fusion (Table 17.3).

Table 17.1 Demographic data of reported studies

Author (year)	Patients (n)	Ankles (n)	Age (mean)	Time from fusion (months)	Implant type	Follow-up (months)
Geisberg (2004)	18	19	52.0	94.0	Agility	39 (7–69)
Hintermann (2009)	28	30	57.8	141.6	Hintegra	55.6
Pellegrini (2015)	23	23	59.0	84.5	STAR (7) Inbone (14) Salto Talaris (2)	33.1 (12–101)
Huntington (2016)	5	5	62.5	20.9	Inbone I or II	21.3
Preis (2017)	18	18	51.0	75.0	Hintegra	54
Schubert (2020)	77	77	58.9	103.2	Agility (23) Salto Talaris (14) STAR (26) Infinity (3) Inbone (11)	84.7 (25–191)
Coetzee (2021), Lundeen (2022)	51	52	62.2	Minimally 96.0	Salto Talaris	50.6 (24–138)

Table 17.2 Indications and adjunctive procedures

Author (year)	Indication for ankle arthrodesis	Indication for conversion to TAA	Adjunctive procedures
Geisberg (2004)	Post-traumatic OA (13), rheumatoid arthritis (3), recurrent sprains (2), idiopathic DJD (1)	STJ OA (5), non-union (2), misalignment (3), pain of uncertain etiology (9)	STJ fusion (4), medial column reconstruction/ calcaneal osteotomy (1), ATL (9), tendon transfers (2)
Hintermann (2009)	Post-traumatic OA (23), primary OA (4), secondary inflammatory joint disease (3)	Painful limitation of mobility (30), malunion (28), secondary OA of adjacent joints (18), non-union of ankle (5), non-union of STJ (2), stress fracture (1)	STJ fusion (14), TN fusion (7), TMT fusion (2), fibular reconstruction (2), calcaneal osteotomy (1), ligament reconstruction (3), ATL (6), other (4)
Pellegrini (2015)	NA	Secondary OA of adjacent joints (12), non-union of STJ or tibiotalar joint (11)	Prophylactic malleoli fixation (16), STJ fusion (6), gastrocnemius recession or ATL (6), ORIF of fibular non-union (2), periarticular (gutter) debridement (1), prophylactic radial forearm free flap (1), TN fusion (1)
Huntington (2016)	Post-traumatic OA (2), rheumatoid arthritis (2), recurrent instability (1)	Painful tibiotalar non-union (5)	ATL (1), 2nd and 3rd PIPJ arthroplasty (1)
Preis (2017)	Post-traumatic OA (13), rheumatoid arthritis (1), hemophilic (4)	Malunion (18), non-union (2)	Fibular reconstruction (2), medial malleolus reconstruction (1), TN fusion (1), calcaneal osteotomy (1), ATL (13), lateral ligament reconstruction (2)
Schubert (2020)	NA	Painful ankle arthrodesis (77)	Gastrocnemius recession (48), STJ fusion (29), ATL (2), lateral ligament reconstruction (1), syndesmotic fusion (2)
Coetzee (2021) Lundeen (2022)	NA	Symptomatic nonunion (5), malunion (16), severe STJ OA (5), severe TN OA (3)	NA

NA not applicable, *DJD* degenerative joint disease, *OA* osteoarthritis, *STJ* subtalar joint, *TN* talonavicular, *ATL* Achilles tendon lengthening, *TN* talonavicular, *TMT* tarsometatarsal, *ORIF* open reduction internal fixation, *PIPJ* proximal interphalangeal joint

Table 17.3 Outcome

Author (year)	VAS (mean)		AOFAS Score (mean)		ROM
	Pre-op	Post-op	Pre-op	Post-op	(degree)
Geisberg (2004)	NA	NA	42	68	26.0
Hintermann (2009)	7.5	1.8	34	71	24.3
Pellegrini (2015)	6.5	1.8	NA	NA	21.9
Huntington (2016)	NA	NA	NA	NA	35.5
Preis (2017)	9.0	2.0	23	68	23.5
Schubert (2020)	8.0	3.0	33	75	20.1
Coetzee (2021)	6.4	2.9	NA	NA	29.6
Lundeen (2022)					

NA not applicable, *VAS* Visual Analogue Scale, *AOFAS* American Orthopaedic Foot and Ankle Society, *ROM* range of motion

17.3.1 Determining Factors of Motion

A major problem in analyzing the reported results of the available literature is the variety of pathologies, ranging from simple arthroscopic fusions with minimal soft tissue compromises to complex posttraumatic ankles with extended soft tissue damages, deformities, and malunions. Most studies also include ankle arthrodeses and nonunions. Huntington et al. [25], for instance, reported on a series of five patients who underwent the conversion to a total ankle arthroplasty for a nonunited ankle fusion with a range of motion as high as 35.5°. In a series of 23 ankles, of which 11 (48%) were treated for a tibiotalar nonunion, Pellegrini et al. [22], in contrast, reported a significantly lower range of motion of 21.9°. In other series with <10% nonunited ankle fusions, gained motion ranged between 20.1 and 29.6° [7, 18, 19, 21, 26, 27] indicating that the functional recovery of soft tissues immobilized over a more extended period is limited. This corresponds with the findings of Hintermann et al. [19] that patients with more than four previous procedures on the ankle or having had surgery less than one year before the conversion to ankle replacement had poorer results with more pain and worse functional values. Preis et al. [28], in contrast, reported in a series of six patients who underwent a replacement surgery 9.1 years after tibiotalocalcaneal fusion gained 29.8° of motion, 6.6° more than reported earlier on 18 patients after conversion of a tibiotalar fusion [21]. It remains unclear whether patients with initial tibiotalocalcaneal arthrodesis have less favorable outcomes than patients who initially underwent tibiotalar arthrodesis. Pellegrini et al. [33] reported on outcomes of 23 conversion procedures, 11 performed on patients with tibiotalocalcaneal arthrodesis. However, no comparison between both subgroups was performed.

17.3.2 Motion and Patient Satisfaction

From all these studies, it is generally agreed that massive soft tissue injury at the original injury with significant soft tissue scarring will limit the ability to regain motion with a conversion to replacement and should be a relative contraindication. However, whether patient satisfaction is associated with gained motion still needs clarification. From our experience, the stress released within the surrounding joints by gaining some motion at the created tibiotalar joint is the main contribution to the patient's perception and satisfaction.

17.3.3 The Role of the Implant

An ongoing concern is the apparent higher rate of implant subsidence observed after ankle fusions converted to total ankle arthroplasty compared to primary replacement procedures. One reason could be that the bone is soft on the tibial and talar side once the bone block is removed, which differs from the usual dense subchondral bone of a normal ankle. Therefore, implant choice is essential. The tibial and talar components should cover as much of the bone surface as possible and have anterior and posterior cortical coverage. Flat resurfacing implants are suggested to be superior to implants using fixation features that might further weaken the bone when preparing the resection surface for receiving the implant. Out of the 54 patients with a mobile-bearing ankle design with flat surfaces, as reported in three studies [19, 21, 28], only one component loosening and no subsidence was observed.

17.3.4 Fixed-Bearing Versus Mobile-Bearing

A primary challenge in total ankle arthroplasty is to restore the center of rotation as close as possible to the individual anatomy (Fig. 17.19). Theoretically, a mobile-bearing ankle is superior to a fixed-bearing ankle because it permits the talus to take its position within the created ankle mortise given by the tension of the soft tissue structures (Fig. 17.20). However, consistency in available data would be necessary to compare the two ankle designs.

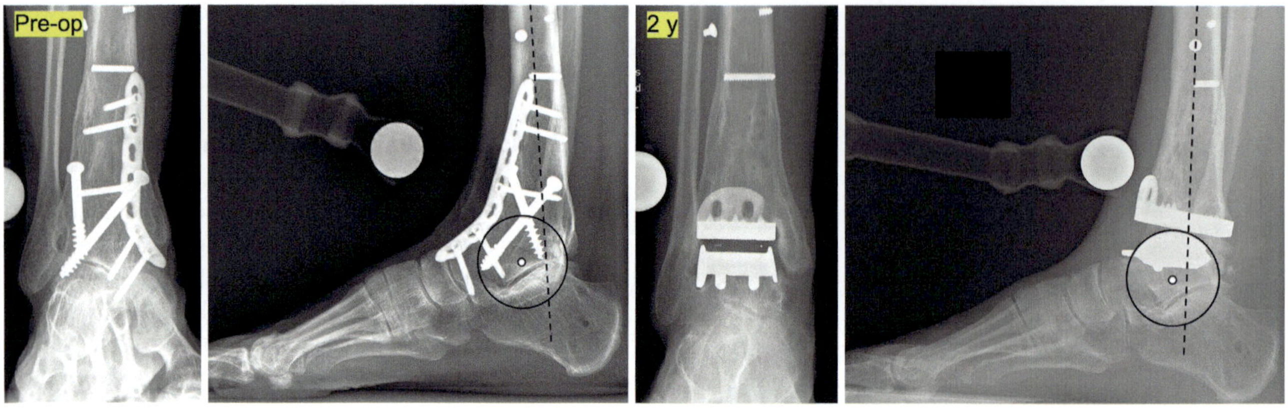

Fig. 17.19 The advantage of a fixed-bearing ankle. This ankle was fused 2.5 years ago using an anterior plate in a too-anterior talus position. A fixed-bearing ankle was selected to provide intrinsic stability in the sagittal plane while the alignment was restored

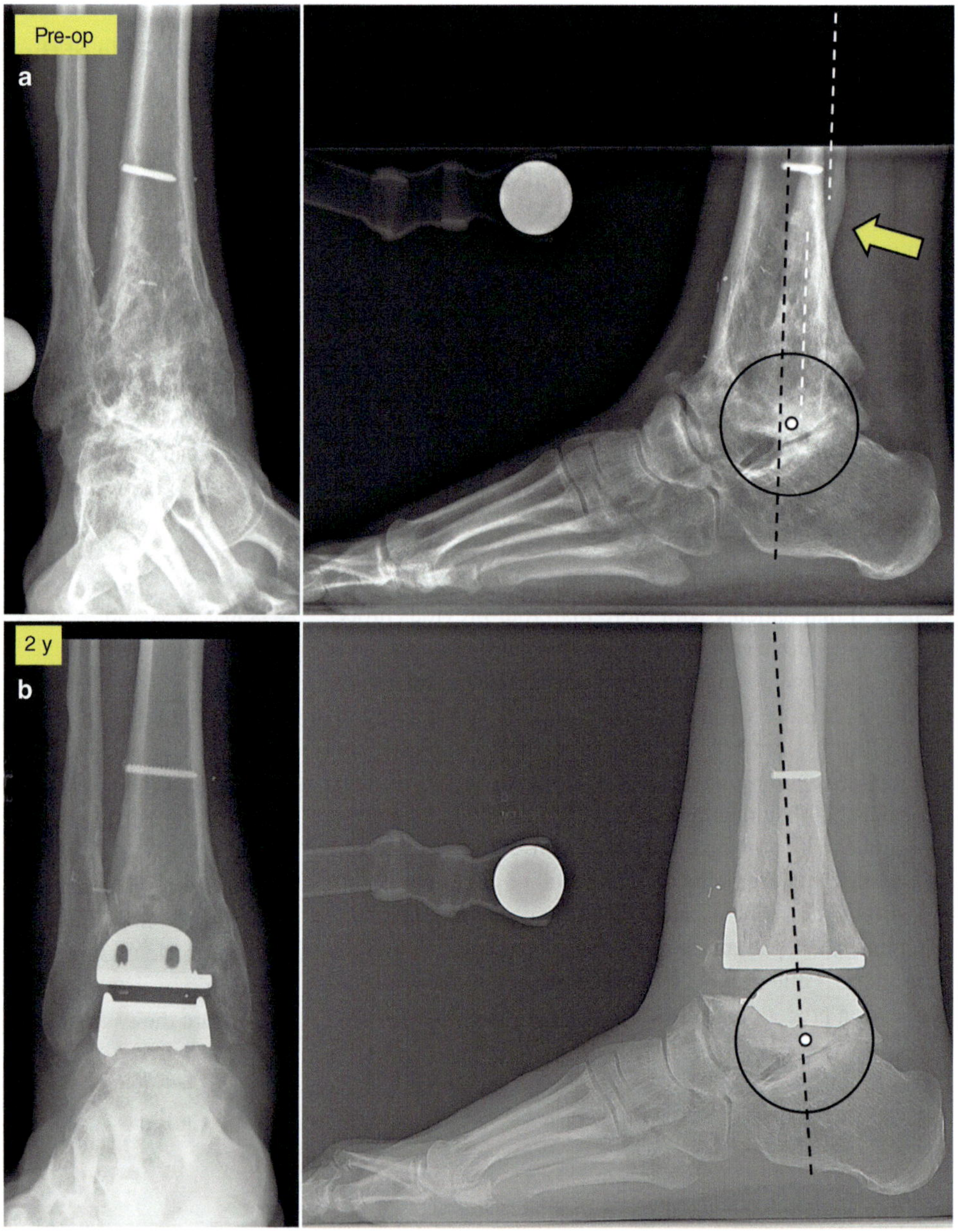

Fig. 17.20 The advantage of a mobile-bearing ankle. (**a**) This ankle was fused 12 years ago in an internally malrotated foot position of 20°, caused by the not-addressed fibular malunion (arrow). The conversion in a total ankle arthroplasty using a mobile-bearing ankle allowed free-positioning of the talus within the created ankle mortise. (**b**) After taking down the fusion and replacing the ankle, the internal rotation of the foot disappeared, thus making a fibular correcting osteotomy, as considered preoperatively, unnecessary

17.4 Risks and Complications

Conversion of a fusion to total ankle arthroplasty is a technically challenging procedure with a high potential complication rate (Table 17.4).

An intraoperative malleolar fracture rate of 18.5% to 43% has been reported in previous studies [18, 19, 21, 26]. Prophylactic malleolar fixation efficiently lowered the prevalence of intraoperative fractures [7, 22].

A significant concern is a high incidence of postoperative arthrofibrosis and periarticular ossifications that might progressively reduce motion and become a source of pain (Fig. 17.21). Though not proven, an essential factor may be the preexistent soft tissue damage with loss of elasticity and gliding properties after a previous long-standing ankle fusion. Specific studies need to be done to get more insight into the underlying causes and how they can be recognized, thus facilitating patient selection for this complex procedure.

Table 17.4 Complications, reoperations, and revisions

	Complications		Reoperations	Revisions			
Author (year)	Peri-op	Late		Exchange MC	Exchange PI	TTC fusions	Amputations
Geisberg (2004)	Lateral malleolar fracture (4), medial malleolar fracture (3), bimalleolar fracture (3)	Valgus malalignment (3), medial malleolar nonunion (1), deep infection (1)	5	5	0	0	3
Hintermann (2009)	Lateral malleolar fracture (1), medial malleolar fracture (3), bimalleolar fracture (1), FHL transection (1), wound complication (2)	Painful arthrofibrosis (4), impingement (3), medial instability (1), tarsometatarsal OA (1), valgus malalignment (3), lymphedema (1)	8	0	1	1	0
Pellegrini (2015)	Malleolar fracture (2), wound complication (5), transient nerve irritation (3)	STJ OA (1), varus malalignment (2), impingement (3)	5	3	1	1	0
Huntington (2016)	Wound complication (2)	None	0	0	0	0	0
Preis (2017)	Medial malleolar fracture (2), CRPS (1), wound complication (3), painful arthrofibrosis (2)	Painful arthrofibrosis (2)	0	2	0	1 planned TTC fusion	0
Schubert (2020)	Medial malleolar fracture (8)	Impingement (9), stress fracture (2), talar subsidence (5)	NA	8	0	2	1
Cotzee (2021) Lundeen (2022)	Medial malleolar fracture (1)	Painful arthrofibrosis (6), STJ OA (2), nonunion STJ fusion (1), periprosthetic joint infection (1) Achilles repair (1), pes cavus correction (1)	10	0	0	1	0

NA not applicable, *FHL* flexor hallucis longus, *CRPS* complex regional pain syndrome, *TTC* tibiotalocalcaneal, *MC* metallic component, *PI* polyethylene insert, *STJ* subtalar joint, *OA* osteoarthritis

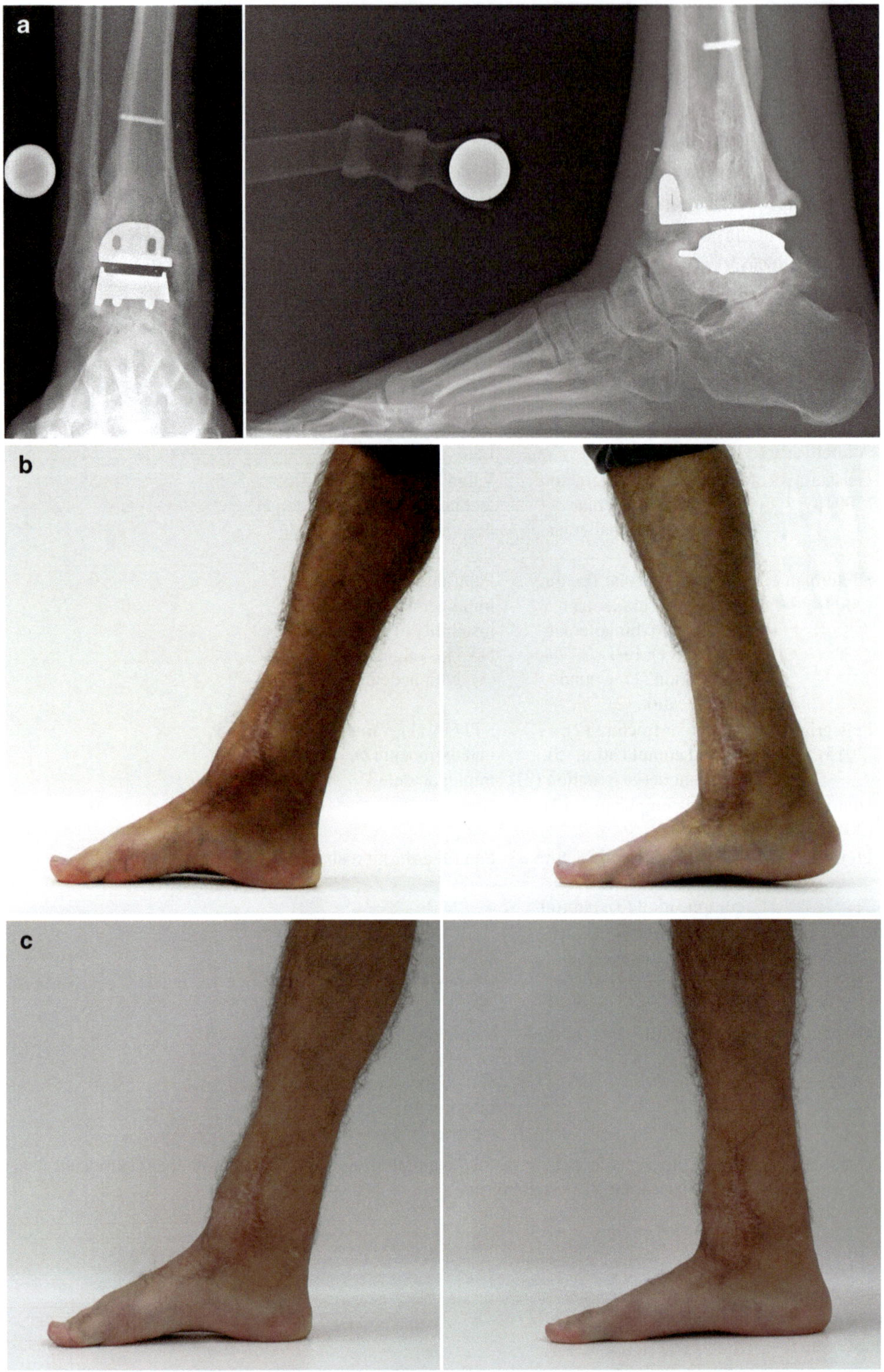

Fig. 17.21 Periarticular ossifications. (**a**) At the 5-year follow-up, the radiographs show significant periarticular ossifications (same patient as Fig. 17.20). (**b**) Range of motion at the 2-year follow-up. (**c**) It was significantly decreased at the 5-year follow-up. The patient was pain-free and satisfied with the regained motion; thus, he did not consider a debridement of the joint as we proposed

17.5 Conclusions

- There is increasing evidence that a conversion to an ankle replacement is a reasonable option for a painful ankle fusion.
- A significant soft tissue envelope compromise is a relative contraindication for a fusion takedown. It is unpredictable if a reasonable range of motion would be obtained.
- The fusion method also plays a role in predicting outcomes in total ankle arthroplasty. The less destructive fusions are easier to convert, with better long-term results.
- The absence of a distal fibula is critical and should thus be a contraindication for conversion to a total ankle arthroplasty.
- From a technical perspective, using a flat cut instead of a chamfer cut talus for conversions is easier.
- Most adjacent joint pain might resolve or become manageable once the ankle joint moves and acts as a stress reliever for the other joints. Fusions of the adjacent joints at the time of the fusion takedown to replacement should thus be carefully initiated.
- Heterotopic bone formation that will limit motion and cause pain is probably the most frequent complication; therefore, postoperative rehabilitation should be pretty aggressive to maintain the intraoperative range of motion.

References

1. Mazur JM, Schwartz E, Simon SR. Ankle arthrodesis. Long-term follow-up with gait analysis. J Bone Joint Surg Am. 1979;61(7):964–75.
2. Haddad SL, Coetzee JC, Estok R, Fahrbach K, Banel D, Nalysnyk L. Intermediate and long-term outcomes of total ankle arthroplasty and ankle arthrodesis. A systematic review of the literature. J Bone Joint Surg Am. 2007;89(9):1899–905.
3. Adukia V, Mangwani J, Issac R, Hussain S, Parker L. Current concepts in the management of ankle arthritis. J Clin Orthop Trauma. 2020;11(3):388–98.
4. Bloch B, Srinivasan S, Mangwani J. Current concepts in the management of ankle osteoarthritis: a systematic review. J Foot Ankle Surg. 2015;54(5):932–9.
5. Kim HJ, Suh DH, Yang JH, Lee JW, Kim HJ, Ahn HS, et al. Total ankle arthroplasty versus ankle arthrodesis for the treatment of end-stage ankle arthritis: a meta-analysis of comparative studies. Int Orthop. 2017;41(1):101–9.
6. Veljkovic AN, Daniels TR, Glazebrook MA, Dryden PJ, Penner MJ, Wing KJ, et al. Outcomes of total ankle replacement, arthroscopic ankle arthrodesis, and open ankle arthrodesis for isolated non-deformed end-stage ankle arthritis. J Bone Joint Surg Am. 2019;101(17):1523–9.
7. Coetzee JC, Raduan F, McGaver RS. Converting ankle arthrodesis to a total ankle Arthroplasty. Orthop Clin North Am. 2021;52(2):181–90.
8. Sealey RJ, Myerson MS, Molloy A, Gamba C, Jeng C, Kalesan B. Sagittal plane motion of the hindfoot following ankle arthrodesis: a prospective analysis. Foot Ankle Int. 2009;30(3):187–96.
9. Ahlberg A, Henricson AS. Late results of ankle fusion. Acta Orthop Scand. 1981;52(1):103–5.
10. Fuchs S, Sandmann C, Skwara A, Chylarecki C. Quality of life 20 years after arthrodesis of the ankle. A study of adjacent joints. J Bone Joint Surg Br. 2003;85(7):994–8.
11. Coester LM, Saltzman CL, Leupold J, Pontarelli W. Long-term results following ankle arthrodesis for post-traumatic arthritis. J Bone Joint Surg Am. 2001;83(2):219–28.
12. Aaron AD. Ankle fusion: a retrospective review. Orthopedics. 1990;13(11):1249–54.
13. Muir DC, Amendola A, Saltzman CL. Long-term outcome of ankle arthrodesis. Foot Ankle Clin. 2002;7(4):703–8.
14. Easley ME, Montijo HE, Wilson JB, Fitch RD, Nunley JA 2nd. Revision tibiotalar arthrodesis. J Bone Joint Surg Am. 2008;90(6):1212–23.
15. Ling JS, Smyth NA, Fraser EJ, Hogan MV, Seaworth CM, Ross KA, et al. Investigating the relationship between ankle arthrodesis and adjacent-joint arthritis in the hindfoot. A systematic review. J Bone Joint Surg Am. 2015;97(9):e43.
16. Lenz AL, Nichols JA, Roach KE, Foreman KB, Barg A, Saltzman CL, et al. Compensatory motion of the subtalar joint following tibiotalar arthrodesis: an in vivo dual-fluoroscopy imaging study. J Bone Joint Surg Am. 2020;102(7):600–8.
17. Papa JA, Myerson MS. Pantalar and tibiotalocalcaneal arthrodesis for post-traumatic osteoarthrosis of the ankle and hindfoot. J Bone Joint Surg Am. 1992;74(7):1042–9.
18. Greisberg J, Assal M, Flueckiger G, Hansen ST Jr. Takedown of ankle fusion and conversion to total ankle replacement. Clin Orthop Relat Res. 2004;424:80–8.
19. Hintermann B, Barg A, Knupp M, Valderrabano V. Conversion of painful ankle arthrodesis to total ankle arthroplasty. J Bone Joint Surg Am. 2009;91(4):850–8.
20. Preis M, Bailey T, Jacxsens M, Barg A. Total ankle replacement in patients with haemophilic arthropathy: primary arthroplasty and conversion of painful ankle arthrodesis to arthroplasty. Haemophilia. 2017;23(4):e301–e9.
21. Preis M, Bailey T, Marchand LS, Barg A. Can a three-component prosthesis be used for conversion of painful ankle arthrodesis to total ankle replacement? Clin Orthop Relat Res. 2017;475(9):2283–94.
22. Pellegrini MJ, Schiff AP, Adams SB Jr, Queen RM, DeOrio JK, Nunley JA 2nd, et al. Conversion of tibiotalar arthrodesis to total ankle arthroplasty. J Bone Joint Surg Am. 2015;97(24):2004–13.
23. Chu AK, Wilson MD, Houng B, Thompson J, So E. Outcomes of ankle arthrodesis conversion to total ankle arthroplasty: a systematic review. J Foot Ankle Surg. 2021;60(2):362–7.
24. Hintermann B, Barg A, Knupp M, Valderrabano V. Conversion of painful ankle arthrodesis to total ankle arthroplasty. Surgical technique. J Bone Joint Surg Am. 2010;92(Suppl. 1 Pt. 1):55–66.
25. Huntington WP, Davis WH, Anderson R. Total Ankle arthroplasty for the treatment of symptomatic nonunion following tibiotalar fusion. Foot Ankle Spec. 2016;9(4):330–5.
26. Schuberth JM, King CM, Jiang SF, Ross JS, Christensen JC, Steck JK. Takedown of painful ankle arthrodesis to total ankle arthroplasty: a case series of 77 patients. J Foot Ankle Surg. 2020;59(3):535–40.
27. Lundeen AL, Raduan FC, Stone McGaver R, Seiffert KJ, Fritz JE, Giveans MR, et al. Takedown of ankle fusions and conversion to total ankle replacements. Foot Ankle Int. 2022;43(11):1402–9.
28. Preis M, Bailey T, Marchand LS, Weinberg MW, Jacxsens M, Barg A. Conversion of painful tibiotalocalcaneal arthrodesis to total ankle replacement using a 3-component mobile bearing prosthesis. Foot Ankle Surg. 2019;25(3):286–93.

Future Prospectives in Total Ankle Arthroplasty

18

The ideal total ankle prosthesis has yet to be determined, but much has been learned from early experiences in total ankle arthroplasty. Modern implants typically respect anatomic concerns more and have found new approaches to decrease interface stress. Biologic fixation has improved upon cemented results. Surgical techniques and understanding of associated ligamentous deficiency, malalignment, and deformity have advanced. The current series still has varied results, and longer follow-up is needed. Despite this, some modern ankle replacements represent significant progress, with improved results and survival rates challenging those of arthrodesis. Further, preserved motion benefits and foot osteoarthritis avoidance outstrip the "gold standard."

18.1 Current Concerns to Be Addressed

With the increased experience from the past, most patients with painful ankle osteoarthritis can receive a total ankle arthroplasty as a viable alternative to ankle arthrodesis. The main concerns remain concerning its long-term success, however.

18.1.1 Prospective Studies

Despite the numerous prosthetic designs introduced on the market, a major concern is the need for well-documented prospective studies. By meticulously analyzing each case, learning from the successes and failures would help increase current knowledge and improve total ankle arthroplasty.

Another issue is the selection of patients, which differs markedly among surgeons. Consequently, obtained results can only be compared with caution.

There is, therefore, a need for extensive, well-documented prospective studies that use standardized protocols with comparable parameters.

18.1.2 Prosthetic Design

Each prosthetic design introduced on the market has been an attempt to address the specific demands of the ankle joint. However, the fact that each new prosthesis has included several new features and changes compared to previous designs has made it extremely difficult to evaluate new ideas and changes for their success. Nevertheless, the current concepts have supported the belief that anatomy should be respected as much as possible [1, 2].

As the mechanical demands on an ankle prosthesis change entirely in the hindfoot after extensive fusion [3], it probably needs special designs to address these cases.

Custom-made ankle prostheses based on CT scan data could also be advantageous for severely traumatized ankles, particularly for total ankle revisions [4].

18.1.3 Preoperative Planning and Implantation Technique

The techniques for implantation can still be improved by more accurate instrumentation and better pre- and intraoperative planning tools to help achieve optimal component positioning. Computer-assisted preoperative planning may be particularly sought to enhance surgical implantation and improve the clinical outcomes of total ankle replacement [5–7]. Such planning may be based on minimizing changes in ligament length and the amount of bone stock to be removed. The main output report might be a detailed picture of the replaced ankle, with indications for component loca-

B. Hintermann, R. Ruiz, *Total Ankle Replacement*, https://doi.org/10.1007/978-3-031-56810-7_18

tions and quantitative bone-cut measures. Likely, future design improvements may help to reduce ligament strain, restore normal axes of rotation, and maintain mobile bearing stability.

18.1.4 Stability of Bone-Implant Interface

Another issue to be addressed is the long-term stability of the bone-component interface. It still needs to be determined whether double-coated surfaces (with or without hydroxyapatite coating) can create stable bony ingrowth and long-term interface stability, as has been the case in total hip and knee replacements [8].

Although early results with semi- and nonconstrained ankle designs are encouraging, it still needs to be clarified to what extent the current designs can dissipate rotational forces while maintaining the joint's stability [9]. Careful assessment of long-term follow-up will determine how closely the present designs mimic the unique requirements of the arthritic foot and ankle. Further work in biomechanics is necessary to better understand the kinematic changes of the arthritic ankle joint and to estimate the forces acting on the implant-bone interface.

18.1.5 Periprosthetic Osteolysis

As experience with total ankle arthroplasty broadens, ankle component wear and related long-term durability will become the next primary concern. Like hip and knee arthroplasty, periprosthetic osteolysis has been seen as a risk factor for failure and revision surgery of total ankle arthroplasty [8]. Adverse responses in periprosthetic bone and soft tissues to implant-derived material components of wear debris have been recognized as relevant factors inducing aseptic implant failure [10]. Whether and to which extent polyethylene wear contributes to periprosthetic osteolysis and whether this is associated with failure in total ankle arthroplasties is not understood in detail. It was shown that wear rate depends on implant design and material properties [11, 12]. However, polyethylene particles were not necessarily found in the synovial fluid of ankles with osteolysis, indicating that mechanisms other than polyethylene wear alone may be responsible for or promote the development of osteolysis [13–16]. Micromotion at the bone-implant interface might promote the development of periprosthetic osteolysis [17]. The initial stability and alignment achieved during surgery are vital to reduce micromotion and avoid premature loosening. High fluid pressure has also been identified as a possible causative factor regarding the development of periprosthetic osteolysis [18–21]. To conclude, though a tremendous scientific effort has been made to explain the underlying mechanisms, periprosthetic loosening still needs to be better understood.

18.2 Further Success Will Increase Patient Demand

Successful total ankle arthroplasty may relieve pain and restore some motion, allowing patients to return to certain physical activities they could not perform before implantation. Consequently, the physical demands of patients may increase, and successful primary replacements may fail because the replaced ankle is subjected to too much stress. Analogously, increased success may lead to indications for total ankle arthroplasty being extended to pathologic conditions that are probably not suitable for replacement surgery.

18.3 Further Research

More accurate research is necessary to understand better the mechanics of the intact and replaced ankle joint complex. First, this should help to improve the implants further, and second, it should help to elaborate guidelines for better planning and more accurate implantation techniques, which would result in more reliable and effective total ankle replacement.

The surgeon's cognitive and psychomotor skills improve as experience is acquired, leading to better preoperative planning and technical execution of the replacement surgery. With the emergence of navigated-assisted total ankle replacement systems, the question is whether a computer-assisted strategy can improve surgical precision in achieving an individualized predefined target, especially whether the additional cost of both surgeon and engineering time and the cost of the advanced imaging are justified [22]. First reports on patient-specific instrumentation still needed to provide a meaningful initial advantage in the standard ankle replacement regarding the accuracy of coronal or sagittal plane positioning for both tibial and talar component. This is also the case for implant size estimation and operative time. Another concern is that patient-specific instrumentation requires extensile periosteum stripping to guarantee adequate bony contact with the customized guides, which may carry the risk of impaired bony ingrowth of the implants [23–25]. The potential advantages may be flattening the learning curve, enhanced accuracy, and reproducibility across various clinical challenges.

The 3D-printing technology has enlarged the possibilities in total ankle arthroplasty. First reports on partial or total talus replacement as a treatment option for talar AVN that allows for preservation of the tibiotalar articulation showed encouraging results in the short term, but still need to prove the long-term efficiency [26–32]. Concerns persist about the potential salvage procedure should the surgery fail.

Although first long-term results are available, future studies emphasizing the objective analysis of long-term clinical results are still necessary to define and delineate the role of total ankle arthroplasty.

18.4 Summary and Conclusions

As total ankle arthroplasty continues to evolve as a viable treatment option for end-stage ankle osteoarthritis, the adverse clinical and biomechanical consequences of ankle arthrodesis are far more apparent. Proper patient selection is a critical aspect of promoting successful results. Acceptable results have been reported in older, low-demand patients with osteoarthritis or rheumatoid arthritis. However, a significant percentage of patients with end-stage ankle osteoarthritis are younger patients with post-traumatic osteoarthritis. However, the use of ankle replacement in younger, more physically active patients and those with significant deformity in the ankle or hindfoot remains a debate. More studies must be completed, and further developments must be made to maximize the longevity and functional results of total ankle arthroplasty in future designs and applications.

Along with improved implants that are typically more respectful of anatomic concerns, proper positioning of the implants (particularly of the talar component about the center of rotation of the talus), accurate balancing of the soft tissues, and appropriate correction of malalignment are far more important for the success of total ankle arthroplasty than previously believed. Careful clinical investigation and reliable diagnostic tools should thus be used to identify all the associated problems so that they can be appropriately addressed during ankle replacement.

Further research is necessary to understand better potential risk factors and underlying causes of failures in total ankle arthroplasty, such as age, body weight, activity lesions, implant design, fixation method, material properties, immunologic responses, and biomechanical adaptations to total ankle arthroplasty. This may help to lower the failure rate further and to define more appropriate and reliable solutions for the revision of failed total ankle arthroplasties. There is also a need to identify the potential benefit of patient-specific instrumentation and navigation in ankle replacement surgery.

References

1. Valderrabano V, Hintermann B, Nigg BM, Stefanyshyn D, Stergiou P. Kinematic changes after fusion and total replacement of the ankle: Part 3: Talar movement. Foot Ankle Int. 2003;24(12):897–900.
2. Espinosa N, Walti M, Favre P, Snedeker JG. Misalignment of total ankle components can induce high joint contact pressures. J Bone Joint Surg Am. 2010;92(5):1179–87.
3. Hintermann B, Nigg BM. Influence of arthrodeses on kinematics of the axially loaded ankle complex during dorsiflexion/plantarflexion. Foot Ankle Int. 1995;16(10):633–6.
4. Wagener J, Gross CE, Schweizer C, Lang TH, Hintermann B. Custom-made total ankle arthroplasty for the salvage of major talar bone loss. Bone Joint J. 2017;99-B(2):231–6.
5. Leardini A, Rapagna L, Ensini A, Catani F, Cappello A. Computer-assisted preoperative planning of a novel design of total ankle replacement. Comput Methods Programs Biomed. 2002;67(3):231–43.
6. Berlet GC, Penner MJ, Lancianese S, Stemniski PM, Obert RM. Total ankle arthroplasty accuracy and reproducibility using preoperative CT scan-derived, patient-specific guides. Foot Ankle Int. 2014;35(7):665–76.
7. Hsu AR, Davis WH, Cohen BE, Jones CP, Ellington JK, Anderson RB. Radiographic outcomes of preoperative CT scan-derived patient-specific total ankle arthroplasty. Foot Ankle Int. 2015;36(10):1163–9.
8. Espinosa N, Klammer G, Wirth SH. Osteolysis in total ankle replacement: how does it work? Foot Ankle Clin. 2017;22(2):267–75.
9. Hintermann B, Susdorf R, Krahenbuhl N, Ruiz R. Axial rotational alignment in mobile-bearing total ankle arthroplasty. Foot Ankle Int. 2020;41(5):521–8.
10. Athanasou NA. The pathobiology and pathology of aseptic implant failure. Bone Joint Res. 2016;5(5):162–8.
11. Sundfeldt M, Carlsson LV, Johansson CB, Thomsen P, Gretzer C. Aseptic loosening, not only a question of wear: a review of different theories. Acta Orthop. 2006;77(2):177–97.
12. Sochart DH. Relationship of acetabular wear to osteolysis and loosening in total hip arthroplasty. Clin Orthop Relat Res. 1999;363:135–50.
13. Dalat F, Barnoud R, Fessy MH, Besse JL, French Association of Foot Surgery A. Histologic study of periprosthetic osteolytic lesions after AES total ankle replacement. A 22 case series. Orthop Traumatol Surg Res. 2013;99(Suppl. 6):S285–95.
14. Vaupel Z, Baker EA, Baker KC, Kurdziel MD, Fortin PT. Analysis of retrieved agility total ankle arthroplasty systems. Foot Ankle Int. 2009;30(9):815–23.
15. Kobayashi A, Minoda Y, Kadoya Y, Ohashi H, Takaoka K, Saltzman CL. Ankle arthroplasties generate wear particles similar to knee arthroplasties. Clin Orthop Relat Res. 2004;424:69–72.
16. van Wijngaarden R, van der Plaat L, Nieuwe Weme RA, Doets HC, Westerga J, Haverkamp D. Etiopathogenesis of osteolytic cysts associated with total ankle arthroplasty, a histological study. Foot Ankle Surg. 2015;21(2):132–6.
17. Goodman SB, Huie P, Song Y, Lee K, Doshi A, Rushdieh B, et al. Loosening and osteolysis of cemented joint arthroplasties. A biologic spectrum. Clin Orthop Relat Res. 1997;337:149–63.
18. Linder L. Implant stability, histology, RSA and wear--more critical questions are needed. A view point. Acta Orthop Scand 1994;65(6):654-658.
19. Alidousti H, Taylor M, Bressloff NW. Periprosthetic wear particle migration and distribution modelling and the implication for osteolysis in cementless total hip replacement. J Mech Behav Biomed Mater. 2014;32:225–44.
20. Catelas I, Jacobs JJ. Biologic activity of wear particles. Instr Course Lect. 2010;59:3–16.
21. Skripitz R, Aspenberg P. Pressure-induced periprosthetic osteolysis: a rat model. J Orthop Res. 2000;18(3):481–4.
22. Reb CW, Berlet GC. Experience with navigation in total ankle arthroplasty. Is it worth the cost? Foot Ankle Clin. 2017;22(2):455–63.
23. Escudero MI, Symes M, Bemenderfer TB, Barahona M, Anderson R, Davis H, et al. Does Patient-specific instrumentation have a

higher rate of early osteolysis than standard referencing techniques in total ankle arthroplasty? A radiographic analysis. Foot Ankle Spec. 2020;13(1):32–42.
24. Escudero MI, Le V, Barahona M, Symes M, Wing K, Younger A, et al. Total ankle arthroplasty survival and risk factors for failure. Foot Ankle Int. 2019;40(9):997–1006.
25. Heisler L, Vach W, Katz G, Egelhof T, Knupp M. Patient-specific instrumentation vs standard referencing in total ankle arthroplasty: a comparison of the radiologic outcome. Foot Ankle Int. 2022;43(6):741–9.
26. Kadakia RJ, Akoh CC, Chen J, Sharma A, Parekh SG. 3D Printed total talus replacement for avascular necrosis of the talus. Foot Ankle Int. 2020;41(12):1529–36.
27. Harnroongroj T, Harnroongroj T. The talar body prosthesis: results at ten to thirty-six years of follow-up. J Bone Joint Surg Am. 2014;96(14):1211–8.
28. Taniguchi A, Takakura Y, Sugimoto K, Hayashi K, Ouchi K, Kumai T, et al. The use of a ceramic talar body prosthesis in patients with aseptic necrosis of the talus. J Bone Joint Surg Br. 2012;94(11):1529–33.
29. Tsukamoto S, Tanaka Y, Maegawa N, Shinohara Y, Taniguchi A, Kumai T, et al. Total talar replacement following collapse of the talar body as a complication of total ankle arthroplasty: a case report. J Bone Joint Surg Am. 2010;92(11):2115–20.
30. Kurokawa H, Taniguchi A, Morita S, Takakura Y, Tanaka Y. Total ankle arthroplasty incorporating a total talar prosthesis: a comparative study against the standard total ankle arthroplasty. Bone Joint J. 2019;101-B(4):443–6.
31. Morita S, Taniguchi A, Miyamoto T, Kurokawa H, Tanaka Y. Application of a customized total talar prosthesis for revision total ankle arthroplasty. JBJS Open Access. 2020;5(4)
32. Ketz J, Myerson M, Sanders R. The salvage of complex hindfoot problems with use of a custom talar total ankle prosthesis. J Bone Joint Surg Am. 2012;94(13):1194–200.

GPSR Compliance

The European Union's (EU) General Product Safety Regulation (GPSR) is a set of rules that requires consumer products to be safe and our obligations to ensure this.

If you have any concerns about our products, you can contact us on ProductSafety@springernature.com

In case Publisher is established outside the EU, the EU authorized representative is:

Springer Nature Customer Service Center GmbH
Europaplatz 3
69115 Heidelberg, Germany

Batch number: 10731524

Printed by Printforce, the Netherlands